WOMEN IN SPORT

VOLUME VIII OF THE ENCYCLOPAEDIA OF SPORTS MEDICINE

AN IOC MEDICAL COMMITTEE PUBLICATION

IN COLLABORATION WITH THE

INTERNATIONAL FEDERATION OF SPORTS MEDICINE

EDITED BY

BARBARA L. DRINKWATER

b

**Blackwell
Science**

©2000 by
Blackwell Science Ltd
Editorial Offices:
Osney Mead, Oxford OX2 0EL
25 John Street, London WC1N 2BL
23 Ainslie Place, Edinburgh EH3 6AJ
350 Main Street, Malden
  MA 02148 5018, USA
54 University Street, Carlton
  Victoria 3053, Australia
10, rue Casimir Delavigne
  75006 Paris, France

Other Editorial Offices:
Blackwell Wissenschafts-Verlag GmbH
Kurfürstendamm 57
10707 Berlin, Germany

Blackwell Science KK
MG Kodenmacho Building
7–10 Kodenmacho Nihombashi
Chuo-ku, Tokyo 104, Japan

The right of the Authors to be
identified as the Authors of this Work
has been asserted in accordance
with the Copyright, Designs and
Patents Act 1988.

First published 2000

DISTRIBUTORS

Marston Book Services Ltd
PO Box 269
Abingdon, Oxon OX14 4YN
(*Orders*: Tel: 01235 465500
         Fax: 01235 465555)

USA
Blackwell Science, Inc.
Commerce Place
350 Main Street
Malden, MA 02148 5018
(*Orders*: Tel: 800 759 6102
           781 388 8250
      Fax: 781 388 8255)

Canada
Login Brothers Book Company
324 Saulteaux Crescent
Winnipeg, Manitoba R3J 3T2
(*Orders*: Tel: 204 837-2987)

Australia
Blackwell Science Pty Ltd
54 University Street
Carlton, Victoria 3053
(*Orders*: Tel: 3 9347 0300
       Fax: 3 9347 5001)

A catalogue record for this title
is available from the British Library

ISBN 0-632-05084-5

Library of Congress
Cataloging-in-publication Data

Women in sport / edited by Barbara L. Drinkwater; in collaboration with the International Federation of Sports Medicine.
        p.   cm. — (The encyclopaedia of sports medicine; v. 8)
    Includes index.
    ISBN 0-632-05084-5
    1. Woman athletes—Health and hygiene. I. Drink-
water, Barbara L., 1926–   II. International Federation of
Sports Medicine.   III. Series.

RC1218. W65   W664   2000
617.1′027′082—dc21
                                          99-057719

For further information on
Blackwell Science, visit our website:
www.blackwell-science.com

Contents

v

Part 6: The Female Athlete Triad

Part 7: Psychosocial Issues

**Part 8: Sport-specific Injuries:
Prevention and Treatment**

List of Contributors

R. AGOSTINI MD, *Virginia Mason Medical Center, 904 7th Avenue, Seattle, Washington 98104, USA*

J.B. ALLEN MS, *School of Physical Education, Sport and Leisure, De Montefort University, Bedford MK40 2BZ, UK*

A.J. AMOROSE PhD, *Memorial Gym, Curry School of Education, University of Virginia, Charlottesville, Virginia 22903, USA*

E. ARENDT MD, *Department of Orthopaedic Surgery, 350 Variety Club Research Center, 401 East River Road, Minneapolis, Minnesota 55455, USA*

M.M. BAKER MD, *Center for Bone and Joint Surgery, 832 Georgiana Street, Port Angeles, Washington 98362, USA*

C. BRACKENRIDGE MA, *Leisure and Sport Research Unit, Cheltenham and Gloucester College of Higher Education, Swindon Road, Cheltenhan GL50 4AZ, UK*

M. CALE'-BENZOOR PT MSc, *Ribstein Center for Sport Medicine Sciences and Research, Wingate Institute, Netanya 42902, Israel*

B.N. CAMPAIGNE PhD, *Eli Lilly and Co., Lilly Corporate Center, Drop Code 2044, Indianapolis, Indiana 46285, USA*

P.M. CLARKSON PhD, *Department of Exercise Science, Totman Building, University of Massachusetts, Amherst, Massachusetts 01003, USA*

N. CONSTANTINI MD, *Ribstein Center for Sport Medicine Sciences and Research, Wingate Institute, Netanya 42902, Israel*

M.E. CRESS PhD, *Gerontology Center and Department of Exercise Science, University of Georgia, Athens, Georgia 30602-6554, USA*

J.A. CRUSSEMEYER PhD, *Department of Kinesiology and Physical Education, California State University, 1250 Bellflower Boulevard, Long Beach, California 90840-4901, USA*

K.P. DePAUW PhD, *Graduate School, Washington State University, Pullman, Washington 99164-1030, USA*

B.L. DRINKWATER PhD, *Pacific Medical Center, 1200 12th Avenue South, Seattle, Washington 98144, USA*

J.L. DUDA PhD, *School of Sport and Exercise Sciences, University of Birmingham, Edgbaston, Birmingham B15 2TT, UK*

J.S. DUFEK PhD, *Human Performance and Wellness Inc., 3265 Chambers Street, Eugene, Oregon 97405, USA*

W.M. EY Med, *Executive Director, Womensport West, Perth, Western Australia, Australia (Dr W.M. Ey unfortunately passed away during publication of this volume)*

K. FASTING PhD, *Norwegian University of Sport and Physical Education, Sognsveien 220, PO Box 4014, Kringsja N-0806, Oslo, Norway*

P.S. FREEDSON PhD, *Department of Exercise Science, University of Massachusetts, 110 Totman Gymnasium, Box 37805, Amherst, Massachusetts 01003-7805, USA*

J. GIBSON MD, *Rheumatic Diseases Unit, Cameron Hospital, Windygates, Fife KY8 5RR, UK*

A.C. GRANDJEAN EdD, *International Center for Sports Nutrition, 502 South 44th Street, Room 3007, Omaha, Nebraska 68105-1065, USA*

L. GRIFFIN MD, *Suite 705, 2001 Peachtree Road NE, Atlanta, Georgia 30309, USA*

J.A. HANNAFIN MD, PhD, *Sports Medicine and Shoulder Service, Hospital for Special Surgery, 535 East 70th Street, New York, New York 10021, USA*

S.S. HARRIS MD, MPH, *Palo Alto Medical Clinic, Department of Sports Medicine, El Camino Real, Palo Alto, California 94301, USA*

E.M. HAYMES PhD, *Department of Nutrition, Food and Exercise Sciences, Florida State University, Tallahassee, Florida 32306-1493, USA*

A. HEINONEN PhD, *President Urho Kaleva Kekkonen, Institute for Health Promotion Research, PO Box 30, Fin-335000 Tampere, Finland*

M.D. JOHNSON MD, *Department of Pediatrics, University of Washington, Seattle, Washington 98195, USA*

K. KENAL MD, *University of Utah Health Network, Greenwood Medical Center, 7495 South State Street, Midvale, Utah 84047, USA*

W.M. KOHRT PhD, *Department of Medicine, Division of Geriatrics, University of Colorado Health Sciences Campus, 4200 East Ninth Avenue, Box B179, Denver, Colorado 80262, USA*

L. LAMOREAUX MD, *1990 Cook Road, Centralia, Washington 98531, USA*

C.M. LEBRUN MD, *Fowler–Kennedy Sport Medicine Clinic, 3M Center, University of Western Ontario, London, Ontario N6A 3K7, Canada*

A. LJUNGQVIST MD, PhD, *Swedish Sports Confederation RF, Idrottens Hus, S-12387 Farsta, Sweden*

M.M. MANORE PhD, *Department of Family Research and Human Development, Arizona State University, Tempe, Arizona 85287, USA*

L.A. MARSHALL MD, *Virginia Mason Clinic, 1100 9th Avenue, Seattle, Washington 98111, USA*

C.E. MATTHEWS PhD, *Division of Preventive and Behavioral Medicine, University of Massachusetts Medical Center, Worcester, Massachusetts 01655, USA*

K.D. MITTLEMAN PhD, *DesignWrite Inc., 189 Wall Street, Princeton, New Jersey 08540, USA*

J.M. MORAN MD, *Summit Injury Management Inc., 605 Discovery Street, Victoria, British Columbia V8T 5G4, Canada*

M.F. MOTTOLA PhD, *Department of Anatomy and Cell Biology, School of Kinesiology, University of Western Ontario, Thames Hall, London, Ontario N6A 3K7, Canada*

P.C. NASCA PhD, *Department of Biostatistics and Epidemiology, University of Massachusetts, 110 Totman Gymnasium, Box 37805, Amherst, Massachusetts 01003-7805, USA*

A. NATTIV MD, *UCLA Department of Family Medicine, Room 50-071, Center for the Health Sciences, 10833 Le Conte Avenue, Los Angeles, California 90095-1683, USA*

C.L. OTIS MD, *WTA Tour, 1247 Devon Avenue, Los Angeles, California 90024, USA*

M.L. O'TOOLE PhD, *Department of Obstetrics and Gynecology, St Louis University, 1031 Bellevue Avenue, St Louis, Missouri 63117, USA*

G. PFISTER PhD, *Institut für Sportwissenschaft, Freie Universität Berlin, Schwendener Strasse 8, D-14195 Berlin, Germany*

M. PUTUKIAN MD, *Center for Sports Medicine, Penn State University, 1850 East Park Avenue, Suite 112, University Park, Pennsylvania 16803, USA*

K.J. REIMERS MS RD, *International Center for Sports Nutrition, 502 South 44th Street, Room 3007, Omaha, Nebraska 68105-1065, USA*

J.S. RUUD MS RD, *International Center for Sports Nutrition, 502 South 44th Street, Room 3007, Omaha, Nebraska 68105-1065, USA*

S.W. RYAN MD, *Denver Center for Sports and Family Medicine, Suite 210, 210 University Boulevard, Denver, Colorado 80206, USA*

P. SANGENIS MD, *Institute for Sportsmedicine, 'Deporte y Salud' Buenos Aires, Santa Fe 782, Acassuso 1640, Buenos Aires, Argentina*

A. SCHNEIDER PhD, *International Centre for Olympic Studies, Faculty of Health Sciences, University of Western Ontario, London, Ontario N6A 5C1, Canada*

A.D. SMITH MD, *Department of Orthopedics and Pediatrics, Case Western Reserve University School of Medicine, 11100 Euclid Avenue, Cleveland, Ohio 44106, USA*

J. SUNDGOT-BORGEN PhD, *Department of Sports Medicine, Norwegian University of Sport and Physical Education, PO Box 40, Kringsja N-0807, Oslo, Norway*

P. TRELA PT, *University of Utah Sports Medicine Center, Physical Therapy Clinic, 546 Chipeta, Suite G-300, Salt Lake City, Utah 84108, USA*

I. VUORI MD, *President Urho Kaleva Kekkonen Institute for Health Promotion Research, PO Box 30, Fin-335000 Tampere, Finland*

M.R. WEISS PhD, *Memorial Gym, Curry School of Education, University of Virginia, Charlottesville, Virginia 22903, USA*

C.L. WELLS PhD, *President Emeritus of Exercise Science and Physical Education, Arizona State University, Tempe, Arizona 85287-0404, USA (current address: PO Box 730, Arroyo Seco, New Mexico 87514, USA)*

L.A. WOLFE PhD, *School of Physical Education and Health, Queen's University, Kingston, Ontario K7L 3N6, Canada*

C.M. ZACHER BSc, *Department of Exercise Science and Sport Studies, Rutgers University, PO Box 270, New Brunswick, New Jersey 08903, USA*

Forewords

On behalf of the International Olympic Committee, I should like to welcome Volume VIII of the Encyclopaedia of Sports Medicine series. This new volume is devoted to women in sport. The advancements made in women's sports during the last quarter century have been astounding. The end result has been a consistent increase in the quality of performance at all ages and levels of competition and an improvement in national, regional and Olympic records. This volume addresses both the basic science underlying the performance of the woman athlete and the special issues involved in sports training and sports participation.

I should like to thank all those involved in the preparation of this volume whose work is highly respected and appreciated by the whole Olympic Family.

JUAN ANTONIO SAMARANCH
Marqués de Samaranch

As opportunities for competitive participation and access to skilled coaching were presented, girls and women came in increasing numbers to experience sport competitions. Women clinicians and scientists identified special issues and needs for these athletes and diligent researchers have provided a strong foundation of science as related to conditioning, nutrition, competitive performance, injury prevention and treatment, and general health issues.

On behalf of the International Olympic Committee and its Medical Commission I should like to thank Professor Barbara Drinkwater and over 50 internationally recognized sports medicine clinicians and sports science researchers who cooperated to produce this important volume. *Women in Sport* will stand as the single best source of information on the topic for many years to come.

PRINCE ALEXANDRE DE MERODE
Chairman, IOC Medical Commission

Preface

The Sydney Olympics in the year 2000 will mark the 100th anniversary of women's participation in the Olympic Games. Although the modern Olympic Games actually began in 1896, women were not permitted to participate. If the father of the modern Olympics, Baron Pierre de Coubertin, had prevailed the Olympics would have remained the '. . . solemn and periodic exaltation of male athleticism, with internationalism as a base, loyalty as a means, art for its setting and female applause as reward'. Women's lack of enthusiasm for their assigned role led them to challenge the status quo and undertake the long and arduous task of achieving acceptance as athletes and equal participants in the Games. Year by year the number of events open to women and the number of female athletes has increased. In the Atlanta Games, two-thirds of the competitors were women competing in 58% of the events. Even better representation is expected in the Sydney 2000 Games.

Support for increasing women's representation on IOC committees and other decision-making positions has come from an unexpected source. IOC President Samaranch initiated and led an effort to achieve gender equality in these positions by establishing the goal of increasing women's representation in leadership roles within the IOC, National Olympic Committees and International Federations to 10% by the end of the year 2000 and to 20% by the end of 2005. The recommendation was approved by the General Session of the IOC in Atlanta. Now it will be up to each of these groups to implement these initial steps toward gender equity.

Along with the increase in the number of women athletes has come a parallel increase in the number of women sports medicine physicians and exercise physiologists. Many of these women had their initial experience with sport as athletes and later chose a career that combined a commitment to sport with their professional path. Twenty years ago it would have been difficult to find women scientists and physicians to write chapters for this volume, *Women in Sport*. For this publication it was a matter of selecting a few women from among many equally qualified to write about medical issues specific to women.

The volume is divided into eight sections. Part 1 surveys the history of women's participation in the Olympic Games. Today's young athletes would do well to read about how their opportunities today came about through the efforts of strong and determined women long before they were born. Part 2 examines the physiology of female athletes. Are there gender differences in the qualities that mark the skilled athlete? How does she respond to environmental challenges and how does the menstrual cycle affect her performance? In Part 3 the authors look at the basic factors involved in training an athlete, whether they differ between women and men, and if so how this affects training regimens. The growth of masters' competition has extended the competitive career of many women. Part 4 discusses how the physiological changes that occur with ageing may affect a woman's performance and how the hormonal changes following menopause may affect her success. There are a number of medical issues that are specific to the female athlete as well as areas of general concern which have unique factors relating to gender. These are covered in Part 5. The potentially serious consequences of a preventable problem, the female athlete triad, are covered in Part 6. In Part 7, three psychosocial areas are explored: the psychological effect of intense competition and parental involvement on the child athlete; ethical issues affecting women in sport and sports medicine; and the increasing presence and influence of women on sports governing bodies. Finally, in Part 8, physicians apply their experience treating women athletes in discussing injuries that are specific to or more common to women in 12 different sports. Although space limited the number of sports that could be included, an effort was made to select events from both team and individual events representing the Summer and Winter Games.

It has been a pleasure to work with so many outstanding authors from around the world to add this volume, *Women in Sport*, to the IOC series, The Encyclopaedia of Sports Medicine.

Dedication

Finally, I would like to dedicate this volume to Wendy Ey (1938–1997), who exemplified the passion and dedication of all the women who have furthered the cause of women's sport. Wendy was a Commonwealth Games silver medallist in 1958, a state sprint and hurdles champion in Australia from 1954 to 1960, and a masters world champion. An author, administrator and untiring advocate for women athletes of all ages, she was the first woman to manage an Australian track and field team at the Commonwealth and Olympic Games. For her services to sport, Wendy received an Award of Merit from the Confederation of Australian Sport and the British Empire Medal in 1977. Although very ill, Wendy travelled from Australia to the United States to speak at the 1996 Pre-Olympic Congress in Dallas to dispute what she considered an unfair application of the doping regulations to postmenopausal women on hormone therapy. Chapter 11, addressing that topic, was written during her final illness. Wendy was an outstanding athlete and an extraordinary woman. In his eulogy to Wendy, Dr John Daly included this appropriate quotation, '. . . don't grieve at the loss of a friend, rejoice at having been privileged to have know them . . . learn something from their courage, their commitment, their life . . .'.

PART 1

HISTORY

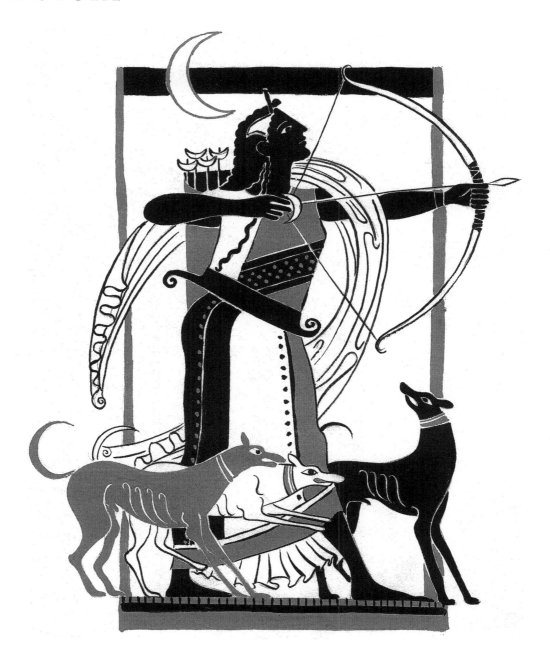

Chapter 1

Women and the Olympic Games

GERTRUD PFISTER

Introduction

For a long time women played no more than a marginal role in the Olympic movement. Even in 1992 women represented less than 30% of the competitors at the Summer Olympic Games. On their way to Olympia women were faced with a great number of obstacles. The opposition which they met was directed at not only women's participation in sport but also the masculinization that this was alleged to produce as well as the 'emancipation' of women and the perceived threat of change in the gender order itself. In an age when the ideals, duties and roles of the two sexes in everyday life were being radically transformed by processes of modernization, it was hoped that sport and the Olympic Games might contribute towards upholding the myth of the male as the 'stronger sex'.

The main parties in the controversy over the participation of women in the Olympic Games were groups with divergent interests, such as the International Olympic Committee (IOC), the international sports federations and the international women's sport federation. The demands, strategies and ideologies of these various groups are examined in this chapter. In the reconstruction of the controversy it becomes apparent that, even among the women who took part in the debate, the integration of women into the male-dominated world of the Olympic Games did not go unquestioned.

Onlookers at the Olympic Games: 1900–12

In the 19th century, women, like the ovens they cooked on, belonged in the home and not on the sportsground. This was true of both Europe and the USA. It lay 'in the nature of things' that girls should be excluded from the first initiatives and concepts of physical education which, like German *Turnen* or Swedish gymnastics, began to appear in the early 19th century. Girls and women, for example, were not allowed on the first German *Turnen* grounds opened in 1811 in a Berlin park known as Hasenheide; they could only admire the feats of the *Turner* from the perimeter (Pfister, 1996a). Modern sport of English origin was, in its early phase, also an exclusively male domain. Although physical exertion and competition were held to be contrary to a woman's nature, by the end of the 19th century a few women did take part in bicycle racing, swimming contests and even in parachuting or ski jumping, much to the horror of the public (Hargreaves, 1994; Hult, 1996; Pfister, 1996b).

It was no wonder then that the Olympic Games were considered to be a male preserve as they had been in ancient Greece. Throughout his life, de Coubertin, a typical man of his times, thought that women should not sully the Games with their sweat but should merely crown the victors (Leigh, 1974; Simri, 1977; Boutilier & San Giovanni, 1991; Welch & Costa, 1994; Wilson, 1996). However, he only succeeded in excluding

3

women once, in 1896. The bold intention of a Greek woman to compete in the first Olympic marathon was firmly rejected. However, she was not to be deterred from carrying out her plan and ran the full distance of 42 km 194 m alone some days before the Games began. She completed the course in 4.5 hours. Another woman, a 35-year-old mother of seven children, was so excited about the victory of Spyros Louis that after the games she tried to emulate him. She, too, was able to run the full distance without any difficulty in 5.5 hours (Odenkirchen, 1996).

Since the following Games in 1900 and 1904 were connected with World Fairs, the selection of events to be included in the Olympic programme was mainly in the hands of the Fairs' organizing committees and thus to a large extent beyond the control of the IOC. Therefore, in many respects, a move was made away from the 'Olympic spirit'. One of the developments that de Coubertin criticized as 'incompatible with the Olympic idea' was the participation of women in a festival which he described as 'l'exaltation solennelle et périodique de l'athlétisme mâle' (de Coubertin, 1912). As early as 1900, at the second Olympic Games in Paris, 12 women took part in the tennis and golf competitions, typical upper-class sports (Fig. 1.1). Seven of them were Americans and all seven came from rich families. They had all come to Europe more or less by chance and regarded golf and tennis mainly as social events (Welch & Costa, 1994). In 1900 women were also allowed to take part in sailing, a so-called 'mixed' event, and it was here that a woman first won a gold medal as a crew member of one of the winning yachts (Wilson, 1996).

However, women participated in the Games 'without the official consent of or comment from the IOC' (Mitchell, 1977; Simri, 1977). At the St Louis Games in 1904 only eight American women represented their country, this time in archery, although IOC members, who were strong opponents of competitive sport for women, declared the archery competition to be an exhibition only (Welch & Costa, 1994). It was not until 1908, when the Olympic Games were held in England, the birthplace of modern

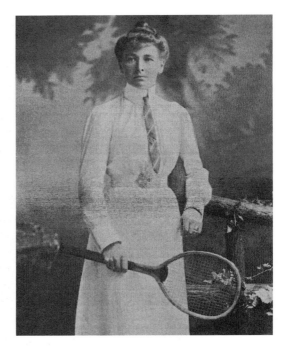

Fig. 1.1 Charlotte Cooper (1870–1966), Great Britain, won a gold in tennis singles and a gold in tennis mixed doubles outdoors at the 1900 Olympic Games in Paris.

sport, that women's sports achieved a modest upswing, with women competing in four disciplines – tennis, sailing, ice-skating and archery – all of them sports with high social prestige. The battle for metres and seconds was first opened to women in 1912 when, according to the minutes of the IOC assembly in 1911, the 'feminist' Swedes allowed women to compete in swimming events (Mitchell, 1977). The inclusion of such a popular sport as swimming in the women's programme contributed considerably to the participation of women athletes from many other countries, and 11 nations sent women athletes to Stockholm. As many as 55 women, representing 2.2% of all competitors, took part in these Olympic Games. Nevertheless, women's sports remained a marginal phenomenon and were still not officially recognized by the IOC. Furthermore, women were not allowed to compete in those sports that involved visible exertion, physical strength or bodily contact. The femininity of female athletes was to be safe-guarded as far as possible (Spears, 1976; Pfister, 1981; Simri, 1984).

The first women Olympic competitors came predominantly from the countries hosting the Games, but the only women athletes who took part in the Olympic Games with any regularity before the First World War were those from Great Britain, the country with the longest sporting tradition. British women were absent only at the 1904 Games in St Louis.

Women's Olympiads: the interwar years

In the 1920s, women who had learned to take over men's roles during the First World War fought increasingly for their rights. In many countries women acquired the right to vote in the 1920s and were also given access to university study and the academic professions. The fashion of short skirts and short hair freed women from many restrictions and granted them new freedom of movement. The fashionable ideal was now the 'new woman' with a slim body, no hips and long legs, gainfully employed and successful in love as well as in sport. But this ideal, which was transported via the mass media, especially popular movies, did not influence the lives of the great majority of women, who had no money for silk stockings or tennis club fees and had to work hard in order to maintain their families. Women remained disadvantaged in many areas of the labour market, discriminated against not only by law but also by social norms and values. Sport, especially competitive sport, was also a domain in which women had to fight for their rights. The opposition towards the participation of the 'weaker sex' in sporting competitions and in the Olympic Games had not yet been overcome (Hargreaves, 1994; Vertinski, 1994a,b).

Track and field events were particularly controversial since they had been the classic domain of male athletes from the very beginning. Karl Ritter von Halt, for example, a renowned German athlete and IOC member from 1929 to 1964, claimed in the 1920s that 'Men were born

to compete; competition is alien to a woman's nature. So let us do away with women's athletics championships' (Kühn, 1926). In spite of the stereotypes of women taking part in track and field events, women started to enter sports stadiums in a number of countries. In Germany, for instance, the Athletics Association, which had experienced a heavy loss of members during the First World War, encouraged sports clubs in 1920 to create womens' sections. In the same year the first women's athletics championships were organized.

The International Women's Sport Federation and the Women's Olympic Games

There were two possibilities open to women who wished to practise sport in general and competitive sports in particular: they could either try to integrate and become part of 'men's sports' or they could establish their own associations and organize their own competition. Among the first opportunities women had to take part in international athletics contests, and especially in 'unfeminine' track and field events, were the Women's Olympiads that took place in 1921, 1922 and 1923 in Monte Carlo (Bernett, 1988; Meyer, 1988). These first 'Olympic Games for Women' were organized by the International Sporting Club of Monaco in Monte Carlo in order to attract and entertain wealthy sports enthusiasts on their visits to the Principality of Monaco (Meyer, 1988).

Grounds below the casino normally used for clay-pigeon shooting served as a stadium. The first Women's Olympiad in 1921 lasted 5 days, with 300 sportswomen from France, England, Switzerland and Italy competing against each other in track and field events (including those held to be male domains like shot-putting and the 800 m) as well as in basketball and pushball. In addition, there were presentations of dancing that combined strong elements of gymnastics. It was this mixture of a sporting contest and artistic performance that made this sports festival so distinctive and contributed to the enthusiastic reception it had among the public and press alike. In 1922 the number of women who travelled to Monte Carlo to take part in either the sports contests or the gymnastic dance performances rose to as many as 700 from nine different countries. The third and last Women's Olympiad in Monte Carlo, which took place the following year and opened with a 3-day gymnastics festival, 'La fête fédérale de gymnastique', was also an outstanding success.

The success of the first Women's Olympiad made it much easier to organize further international sports meetings for athletic events and even for such 'unfeminine' competitions as soccer matches (Fischer, 1983; Pfister, 1999a). These included, on 30 October 1921, a two-nation championship contest between England and France in athletics and soccer, initiated by the French Women's Sport Federation (FSFSF). The federation's president, Alice Milliat, took advantage of this international event to invite representatives of women's sports from various countries, including England and the USA, to a conference. The 12 delegates attending, among them two women, founded the Fédération Sportive Féminine Internationale and appointed Alice Milliat as its president (FSFI, 1928; Webster, 1930; Pallett, 1955; Durry, 1992). The official reason for founding FSFI was the refusal of the International Amateur Athletic Federation (IAAF) to support and represent women's athletics (FSFI, 1936). The main tasks of the new international body were the drawing up of rules, the acknowledgement and supervision of records and, above all, the promotion of women's sports in general (FSFI, 1928).

This initiative to further women's sports at an international level was helped by a favourable constellation of circumstances then prevailing in French sports politics. For one thing, women's sports organizations, several of which had been founded and sponsored by influential figures (including men), thrived at club and association level. For another, a female sports culture had developed in France that had no inhibitions about practising types of sport which were considered to be 'male' sports like soccer or barette (a game similar to rugby) (Laget *et al.*, 1982; Durry,

1992). In women's sports clubs like Femina Sport or in the FSFSF it was usual for women to play both 'male' and 'female' sports. At the 'Fête du Printemps', for example, organized by the FSFSF and held in the Pershing Stadium in Paris, there were performances of formation gymnastics and ballet in addition to athletic contests and basketball matches. This combination of events as well as the moderate objectives of the FSFI helped to take the wind out of the sails of all those opposed to women's sports. The aim of sport, Milliat stressed, was to improve health and strength, and to foster the 'proper balance between the body and spirit' in order for women to be able to 'found a healthy and robust family, help the country in the fight against all social disease and contribute to the preservation of world peace' (Milliat, 1928). It can also be assumed that the rivalry between the various organizations involved in women's sports, and thus also between different definitions of femininity and different physical cultures in France, encouraged the striving for distinction and the international commitment of the FSFSF and its president.

The most important activities of the FSFI were the organization of the Olympic Women's Games, which took place in 1922 (Paris), in 1926 (Gothenburg), in 1930 (Prague) and in 1934 (London). Not only the name, which had later to be given up, but also the overall planning of the women's games, including individual elements of staging like the entrance of the athletes with their national flags, were borrowed from the men's Olympic Games (Bergmann, 1925). The first Games were opened by Alice Milliat with the words: 'I declare the world's first Olympic Games for Women open' (Eyquem, 1944).

As a whole, the Olympic Women's Games documented the capacity for high performance by female athletes and found a positive echo among the general public (Pfister, 1996b). They also proved to be a trump card in the struggle for women's Olympic sport. Not only did they provide women athletes with the chance of overcoming the marginalization of women's sports by competing in international contests, but they also served the FSFI as a way of exerting pressure on the IOC as well as influencing the development of women's sports as a whole (Leigh & Bonin, 1977).

Struggles and conflicts

The growing significance of women's sports and the increasing activities of the FSFI forced the IOC at regular intervals to turn its attention to the role of women in the 'Olympic family'. At the IOC assembly in 1920, for example, de Coubertin announced that women should be excluded from the Games. In 1923 there was renewed debate in the IOC about the 'abus et excès' of this new women's sports movement and it was recommended that women's sport should be placed under the supervision of the international sports federations. From then on the 'women's issue' was on the agenda of almost all IOC meetings, and the international federations started to play a major role in the debate on 'Olympic Women' (Pfister, 1999a). It was above all the intrusion of women into the very heart of the Olympic Movement, the stadium, that gave rise to the vigorous, obstinate, but ultimately fruitless opposition of de Coubertin and many IOC members. The dispute between the FSFI and its president, Alice Milliat, on the one side and the IOC and the IAAF on the other did not end until 1936 when the FSFI gradually lost power and was more or less forced to disband (Pfister, 1999a).

The 15-year history of the FSFI is marked by the shifting focus of its objectives. At first the FSFI fought for the right of women to compete in track and field, then for the expansion of the athletic programme at the Olympic Games, and later for the establishment of separate Olympic Games for women in a wide variety of disciplines. The separatist cause was especially taken up by the FSFI delegates from Great Britain, who argued that the integration of women into 'men's sport' would have to be paid for by giving up much of their power and influence. Although the delegates from the USA backed Alice Milliat and her efforts to be admitted into the 'men's Olympic club', they knew that they would meet with great opposition at home. In the USA a broad movement of resistance had developed in the 1920s that rejected competitive sports for women (Hult, 1989) and which was strongly supported by physical training teachers at colleges and universities. Their goal was the spread of sports for all, their motto being: 'A sport for every girl and every girl in a sport' (Guttmann, 1991).

In the committees of the IOC and the IAAF various strategies were developed. At first there was a general consensus that women should be prevented from competing in Olympic track and field disciplines, but later the men were forced to concede a minimum degree of integration in order not to lose their influence on women's sport completely. The main strategy used was that of limiting women's participation to only a small number of disciplines. However, the attitudes of IOC and IAAF members to the 'women's issue' varied, not least because they also followed the interests and directives of national sports federations. One result of this is to be seen in the run-up to the 1932 Olympics in Los Angeles, where the American members of the IOC supported the participation of women in track and field events since they were aware that there were good chances of their female athletes winning medals in these disciplines (Müller, 1983).

The Olympic woman: developments in the interwar years

After the First World War the women's Olympic programme was extended slightly. In 1924 women were allowed to compete in foil fencing and in 1928 they also took part in the team contests in gymnastics. However, the demands of the FSFI that women should be provided with an extensive track and field programme including at least 10 disciplines at the 1928 Olympics were only partly fulfilled, although it must be added that for the first time women were allowed to compete in an Olympic stadium. Of the disciplines included in the programme (high jump, discus, 100 m, 4×100 m relay and 800 m) it was the 800 m that caused by far the most controversy. That several of the women dropped to the ground exhausted at the end of the race seemed to confirm the worst fears of all those opposed to women's sports. Although the athletes quickly recovered and put their exhaustion down to insufficient training, their behaviour was deemed both scandalous and unaesthetic and generally regarded as proof that women were not made for sports which required stamina. The 800 m race provided the IOC with an opportunity to reconsider the question of women's track and field events. Although the resolution put forward in 1930 by IOC President Baillet-Latour to abolish all women's track and field events was not carried by the majority of members, the 800 m was excluded from the Olympic programme of the 1932 Games (Hargreaves, 1994; Welch & Costa, 1994; Pfister, 1999a). It is interesting to note that it was not only men who were against the participation of women at the Olympic Games. In the 1920s wide-ranging opposition to women's competitive sports had formed, especially in the USA (Hult, 1989). A major role in this opposition was played by the Committee on Women's Athletics of the American Physical Education Association and by the women's division of the National Amateur Athletic Federation (NAAF) (Gerber *et al.*, 1974; Lucas & Smith, 1982; Guttmann, 1991). These groups were of the opinion that female physical education and training had to take into account the purported natural physical and psychological differences between the sexes and had to prepare girls for their future roles as mothers and 'worthy citizens'. Enjoyment of sport and team spirit were considered more important than individual performance and achievement. Competitions ought to be kept to a minimum, if not entirely abolished. As an alternative some colleges began to organize 'play days' where fun and recreation, cooperation, and playing together were intended to take the place of contests and competing for first place (Guttmann, 1991).

In spite of the opposition described above, women's sport enjoyed further success at the 1928 Games in Amsterdam with regard to both the number of disciplines included in the pro-

gramme as well as the numbers of women competing: 11.5% of the events were contested by female athletes and 9.6% of all competitors were women, a ratio not attained again until 1952. German Olympic teams included a relatively large proportion of women. A large number of German women athletes were also selected for track and field events even though these were considered 'unfeminine' in Germany too. These athletes were successful in both the 1928 and 1936 Olympics. In 1928 Lina Radke-Batschauer won the first gold medal for Germany in a track and field event when she came first in the 800 m (Pfister & von der Lippe, 1994) (Fig. 1.2). By contrast, some other European countries, Norway for example, sent only a few women to the Olympic Games. Even in the years 1912 and

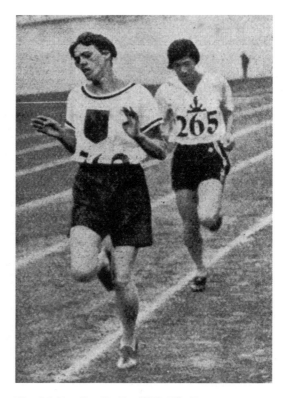

Fig. 1.2 Karoline Radke (1903–83), Germany, won a gold in the 800 m in the 1928 Olympics; Kinue Hitomi of Japan took the silver.

1920, when the Games took place virtually around the corner in Stockholm and Antwerp, thus theoretically allowing Norway to send large teams, the percentages of Norwegian women competitors were a mere 0.5% and 1% respectively. In 1928 and 1932 not a single Norwegian woman took part in the Games. Not one of the seven women who represented Norway at the Summer Games before the Second World War took part in events held to be 'unfeminine', such as track and field or fencing; four competed in swimming events, one in figure skating and two in tennis (Pfister & von der Lippe, 1994). Because of the opposition to women's athletics in the USA, American women also only played a minor role at the Olympic Games. However, at the 1932 Games in Los Angeles, women's sports in the USA received a new and positive impetus. The American athlete, Mildred 'Babe' Didrikson, became the first female idol of the sporting public (Fig. 1.3). An all-round athlete and winner of three medals, she seemed to personify America's capabilities. However, apart from the great controversy about her amateur status, she

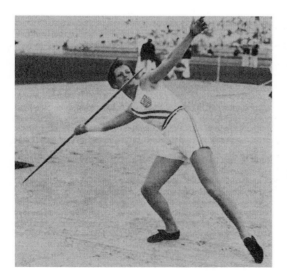

Fig. 1.3 Mildred 'Babe' Didrikson (1911–56) won a gold in both the javelin and the 80 m hurdles and a silver in the high jump at the 1932 Los Angeles Olympic Games.

was also faced with conflicting ideals of femininity (Borish, 1996).

A short interlude: the Workers' Olympiads

Besides the Women's Olympiads and the 'official' Olympic Games there were also workers' sports Olympiads, which took place in Frankfurt in 1925, Vienna in 1931 and Antwerp in 1937 (Krüger & Riordan, 1996). In Germany in 1893 a national federation of gymnasts had been founded with socialist objectives and, in the period that followed, it grew into the largest and most influential workers' sports organization in Europe. Workers' sports federations were formed in other European countries as well, and these amalgamated into the Socialist Workers' Sport International and the Red Sport International, both founded in 1921. In the 1920s roughly 15% of the members of the German Workers' Gymnastics and Sports Federation were women (Pfister, 1994). Female athletes of the workers' sports movement were able to compete in track and field events as early as 1925 at the games in Frankfurt, where the German women's team even set a world record in the 4×100 m relay. In Germany, the workers' sports movement was abolished by the National Socialist regime in 1933. In protest against, and in opposition to, the Olympic Games to be held in National Socialist Germany, the International Socialist Workers' Sports Movement organized alternative Olympic Games in Antwerp in 1937. The poster announcing the Workers' Olympiad in Antwerp depicted a muscular woman athlete throwing the discus, showing that women in the workers' sports movement were faced with less opposition than their fellow athletes in bourgeois sports clubs (Guttmann, 1991).

The Olympic Games in National Socialist Germany

At the 1936 Games in Berlin, organized and exploited for propaganda purposes by the National Socialists, Germany put together the strongest women's team, not only in track and field but also in the overall reckoning, winning 13 of the 45 medals. Although women's competitive sports ran counter to the principles of 'racial hygiene' and national socialist ideals of femininity, top women athletes like Christl Cranz and Gisela Mauermayer were given intensive backing since they were supposed to demonstrate the superiority of the Nazi system. On the other hand, there was no increase in the proportion of women competitors in 1936, neither was the programme of women's events extended.

The female image at the 1936 Olympics was not only shaped by female athletes. In the decorative sculptures adorning the Olympic stadium, in the mass outdoor exercises of Berlin schoolchildren and, particularly, in the festival performance created by Carl Diem, the prevailing gender hierarchy was 'staged' (Alkemeyer, 1994). The huge, solid, rigidly erect male statues in and around the stadium 'embodied' ideals of masculinity; they signalled firmness, strength and a combative spirit. The mass performance 'Olympic Youth' glorified the 'Combat of Youths' that ended with their 'sacred, sacrificial death' (Alkemeyer, 1994). The bodies of girls and women were used as decorative ornaments and as framework and backdrop to an event on which they had no influence.

In Leni Riefenstahl's film of the 1936 Games, especially in the sequence introducing the 'festival of nations', nude men with oiled, muscular bodies and powerful movements are glorified as ancient as well as contemporary heroes. Women, on the other hand, are presented in the first frames of the film as creatures of nature, their movements representing billowing grain and the opening of blossoms, their bodies girlish, graceful and flower-like. In his analysis of the 'Olympic film' Müller (1993) comments: 'Mysterious familiarity seems to envelop the women, who do not have the straightforward muscular character of men. Nor are muscular women considered desirable. . . . Thus, it is not surprising that the athletic victories of women are not emphasised as much as those of men'. It was a film that expressed the ambivalent attitude

of the National Socialists towards women's bodies and women's athletics.

Digression: women's sport as reflected in the medical discourse

The great controversy about allowing women to compete in sports events is closely connected with the stereotype views on the nature of women and the myth of the 'weaker sex'. In the 1920s the arguments put forward in this debate were wholly supported, like all the popular theories on the abilities and roles of the sexes both in sport and elsewhere, by mainstream medicine. The central issues of the medical discourse focused on the forms of physical activities suitable for women as well as the participation of female athletes in competitive sports. In the view of the medical profession, forms of women's physical culture were determined by their obligation to bear children. Women seemed to be both the products and the captives of the reproductive system. For most doctors, therefore, the only question raised by women's participation in sports was that of its possible effects on childbirth. It was the general belief that 'all sporting activities undertaken by adult women have to be judged from the point of view of reproduction' (Küstner, 1931). Although there was little knowledge about the effects of physical exertion and athletic activity on the number of children a woman might have or on the course of childbirth, most doctors discouraged women from participating in competitive and strenuous sports. With the authority of medical science they constructed a variety of theories on the negative effects of sports on the female body (Pfister, 1990; Vertinsky, 1990; Park 1991, 1994). The 'vitalistic' theory, popular in the 19th century, contended that the human body contained only a limited, unrenewable amount of energy. Applied to women's sports, this meant that women had to conserve their energy for their essential purpose in life, i.e. for bearing and looking after children: 'Its premature exhaustion [by sporting activities] violates the nature of girls and women' (Müller, 1927). In the 19th century it was a widespread belief that the uterus was the most vulnerable and fragile part of the female body. Even in the 1920s gynaecologists were still of the opinion that the uterus 'pulls at its sinews with every vigorous jump a woman makes, and may even tilt backwards' (Sellheim, 1931). In addition, excessive physical exercise was said to hinder the development of the pelvis and, as a result, cause difficulty during childbirth. A further, very influential theory put forward by a well-known gynaecologist claimed that women should have slack muscles capable of expansion: 'Each attempt to train the muscles of the female abdomen and pelvis leads to a tautening of the muscle fibres so that childbirth becomes much more difficult, if not impossible' (Sellheim, 1931).

The notion that women might lose their ability to bear children was closely linked with the fear that they could become physically and psychically more masculine and, as a result, turn away from heterosexuality. According to Sellheim (1931), 'femininity and masculine build are contradictions . . . Too frequent exercise, as practised by males, will lead to masculinisation. . . . The female abdominal organs wither and the artificially created virago is complete'. Furthermore, the perceived 'masculinization' of women represented a threat to the division of labour between men and women and hence to the structure of society as a whole. The polarity of the sexes, not their assimilation, was believed to guarantee the progress of civilization. Major importance was therefore attached to the physical differences between the sexes. In many standard works on medicine, anatomical and physiological differences between the sexes were generalized and often exaggerated. In medical literature man was the norm; women, accordingly, were described as deviant and deficient. For example, Sellheim (1931) characterized the female organs as 'incomplete', while Müller (1927) held women to be physically 'underprivileged'.

Although most doctors were against competitive sports for women, their recommendations were quite contradictory, rhythmical gymnastics being the only form of physical exercise that was universally accepted. Exercises that required strength, daring and endurance, or other traits men considered 'unfeminine', were especially discouraged by the medical profession and branded as potentially dangerous.

Scarcely any male doctors and only a handful of female doctors were convinced that women by nature were not as weak and needful of care and rest as was claimed in the medical textbooks. Many of the first doctors (in Germany, at least) to begin systematic research into the effects of physical activities on the female body were women. Female doctors, for example, interviewed and examined more than 1500 participants at a sports festival in 1928. They were, like many of their colleagues, unable to discover any negative effects of sporting activities on the women they examined (Pfister, 1990). The results of investigations into women's sports were summarized at an international congress of women doctors in 1934. By that year 120 scientific publications on women's sports had already appeared in Germany, and some 10 000 girls and women who practised sport had been examined. There were no results presented from any of the studies, carried out according to scientific standards, that might have justified the reservations about women's competitive sports. However, it must be taken into consideration that standards of performance and the corresponding training differed fundamentally from the world records and training practices of today.

The findings of scientific research into the effects of physical activity on the female body were scarcely acknowledged by the mainstream of medicine and failed to convince the opponents of women's sports, who continued to believe in the myth of the weaker sex. On the whole, the medical discourse, with its warnings and prescriptions, contributed quite considerably to the marginalization of women in competitive sport (Pfister, 1990).

Women athletes in the limelight

The debate on the participation of women in the Olympic Games went on after the Second World War. In 1952 it was IOC President Avery

Brundage who advocated the removal of women's contests from the Olympic programme (Mayer, 1960); as late as 1966 the IOC was still discussing whether or not to exclude the shot-put and discus from the women's Olympic programme (Hargreaves, 1994). This would further the IOC's objectives in two ways: for one thing, it was thought increasingly necessary to reduce the number of Olympic events; for another, IOC members still wished to prevent women from taking part in all too 'unfeminine' sporting activities. This time, the IOC's wishes were not fulfilled; on the contrary, there was a continual increase in the number of competitions open to women in the Olympic Games.

Important milestones in the history of women's Olympic sports have been the participation of strong teams of female athletes from the Soviet Union since 1952. In the wake of political and economic consolidation in Europe in the postwar period, sport began to flourish again in the 1950s. In the following decades it became also an increasingly important factor in the conflict between East and West; sport became a weapon in the cold war. The result was the same intense competition in the stadium as in the arms race, marked by a sharp rise in the performance and achievements of athletes from the socialist countries especially. A great deal was invested by these countries in the success of their athletes (partly at the expense of providing sports for all) in order to 'demonstrate' the superiority of their political and economic system. On the Olympic stage, upon which it was possible to achieve not only international recognition but also political success, the gender of medal-winners was of no great importance. Since women played only a minor role in sport in many western countries, investing in women's sport was especially worthwhile. Consequently, in the German Democratic Republic (GDR) and other countries of eastern Europe competitive sports for girls and women were given particularly intensive support. As a result, women became an increasingly important factor in sport, and the Western countries were forced to make a greater effort in the field of women's competitive sports.

It was above all the participation of strong teams of sportswomen from the Soviet Union from 1952 onwards that led to rapid integration of women in the Olympic movement. And it was above all the Soviet IOC members who, in order to increase their chances of winning more medals, demanded a wider Olympic programme for women. Even though the IOC rejected Constantin Andrianov's proposal, put forward in 1957, that all women's events should be included in which officially recognized world championships were held, new disciplines were successively added to the women's programme (Wilson, 1996).

It must be added, however, that the medical reservations about women taking part in competitive sports as well as in numerous other types of sport had by no means been given up. Especially difficult to shake off was the idea that prolonged exertion might be harmful to the health of girls and women. Physical contests and aggressive body contact were also claimed to have negative effects on the female body, with doctors continuing to provide arguments for excluding women from long-distance running and team sports; among the latter, soccer especially was considered too rough for women. The first team sport in which women were allowed to take part in the Olympic Games was volleyball in 1964. This was followed by basketball and handball in 1976 and hockey in 1980. Soccer, long considered a typical male preserve, was not open to women as an Olympic discipline until 1996.

How suitable endurance sports were for the purportedly weaker sex was a subject which proved particularly controversial. Women, it was said, should be spared from strenuous long-distance racing, especially such inhuman tortures as the marathon (Pfister, 1999b). Furthermore, the legendary Boston Marathon was not to be debased by the participation of the 'weaker sex'; thus, in 1966, Roberta Gibb had to run this traditional race without a start number. In 1967, giving her name simply as K.V. Switzer, Kathrine Switzer also tried to take part in the Boston Marathon. In the very first miles she was discovered and attacked by an official, who attempted to pull her out of the race by force. However, her coach and her boy friend came to her aid and she was able to continue and complete the marathon. It was not until 1972 that women were officially allowed to take part in this race without having to disguise themselves (Blue, 1988). Nevertheless, women marathon runners still had to wait more than 10 years before they were able to run in their event in the Olympic Games.

In the 1980s a break was made with persistent conventions and traditions when women were finally allowed to take part in the Olympic Games in both endurance sports and team sports with body contact (Pfister, 1981; Simri, 1984). In 1984, not only cycling and the marathon were made women's Olympic disciplines but also rhythmical gymnastics and synchronized swimming, events in which only women compete. It was not until 1988, however, that women were allowed to compete in the Olympic 10 000 m. Since then the women's programme has steadily been extended to include sports that were previously male domains, such as judo (1992) and soccer (1996). In 1980 only about 25% of the events were exclusively women's events, whereas in 1996 this figure increased to 36% in the Games in Atlanta. In addition to these, there were also 11 events open to both men and women, so that women were able to compete in 40% of the disciplines (Théberge, 1991; Wilson, 1996). Women continue to be excluded from three types of sport, boxing, wrestling and weight-lifting, although the International Weight-lifting Federation is currently trying to have the latter included in the women's Olympic programme.

As the number of women's Olympic disciplines has progressively risen, so too has the number of women competitors. In 1980, the percentage of women athletes competing in the Games amounted to just under 22%; by 1996 this figure had risen to 34.3% (Table 1.1). The gradual increase in the number of women competitors

Table 1.1 Women's participation in the Olympic Games

Year	No. of national Olympic committees	Nations with female athletes (%)	No. of sports	No. of events	Events with female athletes (%)	No. of participants	Female athletes (%)
1896	14	–	9	43	–	245	–
1900	19	26.3	17	86	3.5	1 078	1.1
1904	13	7.7	14	89	2.2	687	0.9
1908	22	18.2	20	107	2.8	2 035	1.8
1912	28	39.3	13	102	5.9	2 437	2.3
1920	29	44.8	19	152	3.9	2 607	2.5
1924	44	45.5	17	126	8.7	3 072	4.3
1928	46	54.3	14	109	12.8	2 884	9.5
1932	37	48.6	14	117	12.0	1 333	9.3
1936	49	53.1	19	129	11.6	3 936	8.4
1948	59	55.9	17	136	14.0	4 092	9.5
1952	69	59.4	17	149	16.8	5 429	9.3
1956	67	58.2	17	151	17.2	3 337	11.2
1960	83	54.2	17	150	19.3	5 313	11.2
1964	93	57.0	19	163	20.2	5 133	13.3
1968	112	48.2	18	172	22.7	5 498	14.1
1972	121	53.7	21	195	22.1	7 121	14.9
1976	92	71.7	21	198	24.7	6 043	20.8
1980	80	67.5	21	203	24.6	5 283	21.5
1984	140	67.1	21	221	28.1	6 802	23.1
1988	159	73.6	23	237	36.3	8 473	26.1
1992	169	80.5	25	257	38.1	9 368	28.9
1996	197	85.8	26	271	39.9	10 744	34.3

obscures the fact that a woman's chance of competing at the Olympic Games depends to a large extent on her nationality. Even among European nations there are considerable differences. At the Seoul Olympics, for example, the proportion of women in the Great Britain team was 35%, while that of the Spanish delegation was only 18%. In the 1972 Games at Munich only 12% of all women competitors came from Africa, Latin America and Asia; in Barcelona these women accounted for 34% of the total women athletes (Wilson, 1996). Since the Tokyo Olympics in 1964 the number of female athletes from Asian countries has increased especially (Welch & Costa, 1994). Furthermore, in 1996, approximately 86% of the participating countries sent a women's team to the Games.

It is still generally true that the greater a country's economic resources, the greater the proportion of women athletes in the country's Olympic team. However, this rule does not hold true for Cuba and China. As soon as China reappeared on the Olympic stage in 1984, it presented a remarkably strong women's delegation and in 1988 the proportion of women in the Chinese team (46%) was higher than that of any other country competing in the Games. In comparison, the proportion of women athletes in the US team was 37%; the overall proportion was only 26% when all countries are taken into account. The success of the Chinese women was not only in numbers and percentages but also in performance and achievement. Within a few years they had shaken off their image as 'nobodies' to become world champions and gold-medal winners. Contributing to this success, besides the favourable conditions prevailing in China for high-level sports and the intensive support given to women's sports, was an image of sport that was not traditionally associated with masculinity. On the other hand, Chinese sporting success is also attributable to stringent training methods and the use of pharmaceuticals (Riordan & Jinxia, 1996). The example of Chinese women athletes illustrates the two sides of the Olympic medal: the opportunities sport can open up and the price that must often be paid.

Although women were represented on 160 teams in 1988, only 28 countries (18%) won any women's medals (Boutilier & San Giovanni, 1991); 79% of these medals were won by seven countries (five eastern bloc countries, the USA and West Germany), 23% being won by women of the GDR. The efficient system of selecting talent, the excellent training conditions and the concentration of sport sciences on high-level sports, in fact the whole material and human resources that the eastern countries and especially the GDR invested in women's sports, yielded an excellent return. It must be added, however, that the price for this sporting success was high, both from a socioeconomic and from an individual point of view. The funds chanelled into sport were taken from areas in which they were urgently needed, and the women athletes not infrequently put their health at risk for the sake of success in sport.

Also conspicuous in recent decades has been the great increase in, as well as success of, black women athletes at the Olympics. In 1932 and 1936, on the orders of the trainers, these women were not allowed to compete even in events in which they had qualified. It was not until 1948 that black women, all of them students at black colleges, took part in Olympic competitions (Welch & Costa, 1994). In 1952, Alice Coachman was the first black female to win a gold medal, taking first place in the high jump. At the 1960 Olympics, Wilma Rudolph was made a star after winning three gold medals and thus became the most successful woman athlete of the Games. In the 1970s and 1980s, black athletes like Valerie Briskoe-Hooks, Evelyn Ashford, Florence Griffith-Joyner and Jackie Joyner-Kersee were outstanding Olympic champions. 'Black women have led the way for America's pursuit of Olympic gold medals in track and field' (Davis, 1992).

During the 1990s, women's sport has increasingly found its way into the limelight. In the 1930s and 1940s, athletes like Babe Didrikson, Sonja Henie and Fanny Blankers-Koen, 'the flying Dutch housewife' and mother of two children who won four gold medals in 1948, became

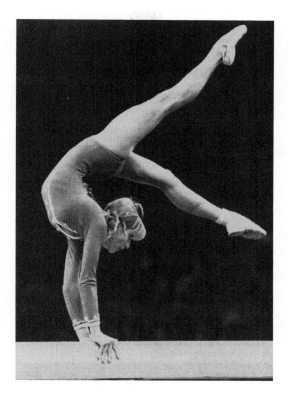

Fig. 1.4 Olga Korbut (born 1955), the Soviet Union, won three golds in the 1972 games in Munich: the balance beam, floor exercises and all-round team. She also won a silver in the uneven parallel bars.

celebrities. In the television age and the age of the media, Wilma Rudolph and Olga Korbut and later Nadia Comaneci and Katharina Witt have been turned into idols representing contemporary ideals of the female, slim, graceful, not too muscular and, above all, 'feminine' (Fig. 1.4). The star of the Seoul Games, Florence Griffith-Joyner, made up for her androgynous figure by wearing extremely feminine clothes. Highly marketable in recent years have been young-looking women ('women in girls' bodies'), who combine excellent athletic performance with the looks of a model and signal female eroticism in the way they move and dress. Today, representations of female Olympic athletes play a decisive role in popular culture and, with their help, fashion, beauty and other products can be marketed. In

this process gender images and stereotypes are seized upon by the advertising industry, which exploits the athletes' sporting achievements and successes, thus creating roots for new meanings and cultural indicators of femininity and masculinity in the material world.

Equal opportunities for women and then what?

The development of women's participation at the Olympic Games reflects both the increasing integration of women in sport and the continuing male dominance of sport. Even today approximately 65% of all Olympic athletes are men. Of the 160 countries that took part in the Seoul Olympics, 42 (including 21 Islamic countries) sent only male athletes (Hargreaves, 1994); in Barcelona 33 countries and in Atlanta 28 countries did not include women on their teams. In many developing nations, and above all in Islamic countries, women's sport is confronted with numerous difficulties, ranging from the lack of physical education for girls at school and the limited opportunities women have of practising sports to the prohibition of joint training sessions for men and women. Religious precepts in particular (having to cover the body in public, not being able to take part in sporting activities with men) are barriers that prevent or at least hinder the spread of sporting practices that are customary in Western countries. Furthermore, in many countries, sport is incompatible with the prevailing somatic culture of girls and women and/or cannot be integrated into the context of their lives (Hargreaves, 1994). Current debate on these issues centres on two antithetical strategies and perspectives. On one side, the initiative Atlanta+, founded by French women politicians and today a worldwide organization, has formulated the demand that nations which do not send women to the Games should be excluded from membership of the Olympic family. On the other side, Islamic Women's World Games have taken place (Teheran in 1993) from which men are barred, even as spectators. The IOC has rejected the demands of Atlanta+, calling them 'anti-Islamic' and referring to them as interfering in the internal affairs of sovereign countries. However, this does not solve the problems raised by Atlanta+. As Wilson (1996) has pointed out, 'Nevertheless, the issue raised by Atlanta+ is a legitimate one that will not go away'.

According to Hargreaves, a further problem plaguing the international sports movement is that of the distribution of resources. In many countries poverty is linked with gender, women being affected by it to a much greater extent than men. Moreover, the opportunities available to women for taking part in any kind of sporting activity are extremely limited. Hargreaves therefore asks, in view of the daily struggle for survival of many women in the world, whether it is right to spend resources on high-level sport, from which men chiefly benefit.

In recent years women have been admitted to a wider range of Olympic contests, including disciplines that require endurance and which were long considered harmful to women's health. In the 1996 Games in Atlanta, women's teams competed for medals in soccer for the first time, and thus a sport that until recently was regarded as a male preserve has now become a women's Olympic discipline. Nevertheless, women continue to be barred from a great number of disciplines, including boxing and wrestling (i.e. especially combative sports and those involving body contact), which are also considered to have an adverse effect on women's health. Hargreaves disputes the reasons given for excluding these sports from the women's Olympic programme, pointing out that the medical arguments only serve to legitimize and preserve the differences between the sexes: 'The ethics of arguments to ban dangerous sports such as boxing are as appropriate to men as they are to women; the reason they are applied only to women is cultural, not biological' (Hargreaves, 1994). Not only the exclusion of women from certain types of sport but also the inclusion of disciplines open to women alone (synchronized swimming and rhythmical gymnastics since 1984) help to strengthen the view that men and women are born with different attributes, women, for example, being the more graceful of the two

sexes. As Borish (1996) has noted: 'In fact, gender lines remained in force, and the status quo held sway in the history of the modern Olympic Games, delineating the control of women's participation. The female body existed [and still exists] as a zone of conflict in the social discourse'. It must also be pointed out that in the typically feminine disciplines like rhythmic gymnastics and gymnastics on apparatus girls are most successful when their bodies are not 'feminine'. This means that girl gymnasts must start training at an ever earlier age and that they must be extremely careful to keep their weight low and thus expose themselves to the risk of anorexia. The growing problems linked with gymnastics on apparatus have prompted Blue (1988) to speak of 'killer gymnastics'.

Responsibility for the Olympic programme lies with international sports federations and the IOC. However, the decision-makers in the IOC, the national Olympic committees and the international sports federations have almost always been exclusively male; in 1995 only five of the 196 national Olympic committees were chaired by a woman. A survey carried out by the Amateur Athletic Foundation in Los Angeles revealed that only 5% of the approximately 13000 positions in executive bodies of sport around the world are occupied by women (DeFrantz, 1991). Today, the issue of power and responsibility can no longer be swept aside. As noted above in the dispute between the IOC and the FSFI, the role of women in the Olympic family was a result of a struggle for power and influence. It was not until 1981 that the first two women (Pirjo Haggmann from Finland and Flor Isava-Fonseca from Venezuela) were appointed members of the IOC; by 1995 only seven of the 107 members were female, women thus making up a tiny minority (Davenport, 1996; Wilson, 1996). Although medical questions have always played a key role in the various discussions of women and sport, the Medical Commission of the IOC includes not a single woman. Without any influence in decision-making bodies and without any say in the destiny of the Olympic movement, women will remain outsiders, dependent upon the attitudes and interests of male functionaries. It must be recognized that in the practice of sport, women have different needs and pursue different objectives.

In recent years there has been a growing awareness of the problems that women face in the Olympic movement. One result of this was the addition in 1991 of a clause to the Olympic Charter ruling out sexual discrimination. In 1995, at the Centennial Olympic Congress, the small number of women in leading positions was discussed and recommendations made. In addition, a working group was set up 'to advise the IOC Executive Board and its President on the measures which should be taken to enhance women's participation in sport and in its administrative structures' (International Olympic Committee, 1996). Four concrete proposals, addressed to each and every organization of the Olympic movement, were drafted and later adopted at the 105th IOC Session in Atlanta. In 1996 a World Conference on Women and Sport was held in Lausanne, Switzerland, at which the participants could exchange views and draw up perspectives for the future.

Equality in the Olympic movement: what might this signify? Interpreting equal participation with equality is problematical, not least because the sporting activities, performance and achievements of men and women have different meanings and can convey different messages. Sport, with its seemingly impartial hierarchy of achievement, contributes in no small way to the construction of the gender order, and above all to the naturalization of gender and gender differences (Théberge, 1991).

Today, the Olympic movement, like competitive sports generally, is subject to all kinds of influence and developments, many of which lie beyond the control of the IOC and the sports federations. These include factors such as commercialization, the drastic increase in hours and resources spent on training, and the constant raising of standards and performance. Many of the problems arising from these factors affect women and men differently, if only because in a great number of sports women athletes are considerably younger than their male counterparts.

Observable progress has been made in the struggle for equal opportunities among men and women in the Olympic movement, but is this enough? When women have achieved integration and are thus potentially able to exert influence, are they not called upon at the same time to play a more active role than they have done up to the present in seeking solutions for the problems connected with high-level sports? Furthermore, in many countries women have scarcely any opportunity of taking up a sport in their leisure time. In a time of economic austerity and limited resources, the question here is how and where priorities are to be set. Whatever conclusions are reached, it must always be borne in mind that women's Olympic successes are good publicity for women's sport in general and that this publicity must at the same time be used to help dismantle the barriers which prevent or hinder the active participation of women in sport.

References

Alkemeyer, T. (1994) *Vom Wettstreit der Nationen zum Kampf der Völker. Aneignung und Umdeutung der 'Olympischen Idee' in deutschen Faschismus.* Unpublished PhD thesis, Berlin.

Bergmann, W. (1925) *Die Frau und der Sport.* Stalling, Oldenburg.

Bernett, H. (1988) Die ersten 'olympischen' Wettbewerbe im internationalen Frauensport. *Sozial und Zeitgeschichte des Sports* **2**, 66–87.

Blue, A. (1988) *Faster, Higher, Further. Women's Triumphs and Disasters at the Olympics.* Virago Press, London.

Borish, L.J. (1996) Women at the modern Olympic Games: an interdisciplinary look at American culture. *Quest* **48**, 43–56.

Boutilier, M.A. & San Giovanni, L.F. (1991) Ideology, public policy and female Olympic achievement: a cross-national analysis of the Seoul Olympic Games. In F. Landry, M. Landry & M. Yerlès (eds) *Sport: The Third Millennium*, pp. 397–409. Les Presses de l'Université Laval, Sainte-Foy.

Davenport, J. (1996) Breaking into the rings: women on the IOC. *Journal of Physical Education, Recreation, and Dance* **67**, 26–30.

Davis, M. (1992) *Black American Women in Olympic Track and Field.* McFarland & Company, Jefferson/London.

De Coubertin, P. (1912) Les femmes aux Jeux Olympique. *Revue Olympique* July, 109–110.

DeFrantz, A.L. (1991) Progress made, pitfalls and conditions for further advancement of women in the Olympic movement. In F. Landry, M. Landry & M. Yerlès (eds) *Sport: The Third Millenium*, pp. 413–417. Les Presses de l'Université Laval, Sainte-Foy.

Durry, J. (1992) Le combat des femmes et l'évolution des structures. In R. Hubscher (ed.) *L'Histoire en Mouvements*, pp. 287–313. Arman Colin, Paris.

Eyquem, M.-T. (1944) *La Femme et le Sport*. J. Susse, Paris.

Fédération Sportive Feminine Internationale (1928) *Fédération Sportive Feminine Internationale*. FSFI, Paris.

Fédération Sportive **Feminine Internationale** (1936) *Fédération Sportive Feminine Internationale*. FSFI, Paris.

Fischer, H. (1983) *Der Weltverband für Frauensport und seine besonderen Aufgaben*. Unpublished Master thesis, Köln.

Gerber, E.R., Felshin, J., Berlin, P. & Wyrick, W. (1974) *The American Woman in Sport*. Addison Wesley, New York.

Guttmann, A. (1991) *Women's Sports: A History*. Columbia University Press, New York.

Hargreaves, J. (1994) *Sporting Females*. Routledge, London.

Hult, J. (1989) Women's struggles for governance in U.S. amateur athletics. *International Review for the Sociology of Sport* **24**, 249–261.

Hult, J. (1996) Women's sports, North America. In D. Levinson & K. Christensen (eds) *Encyclopedia of World Sport: From Ancient Times to the Present*, Vol. III, pp. 1170–1182. ABC-CLIO, Santa Barbara.

International Olympic Committee (1996) *Women in the Olympic Movement*. IOC, Lausanne.

Krüger, A. & Riordan, J. (eds) (1996) *The Story of the Worker Sport*. Human Kinetics Publishers, Champaign, Illinois.

Kühn, W. (1926) Wohin führt der Weg? Eine kritische Betrachtung zur Frauensportbewegung. *Leibesübungen* **8**, 193–196.

Küstner, H. (1931) Frau und sport. *Medizinische Welt*, 757–758; 791–793.

Laget, F., Laget, S. & Mazot, J.-P. (1982) *Le Grand Livre du Sport Féminin*. SIGEFA, Belle Ville.

Leigh, M. (1974) Pierre de Coubertin: a man of his time. *Quest* **22**, 19–24.

Leigh, M. & Bonin, T. (1977) The pioneering role of Madame Allice Milliat and the FSFI in establishing international track and field competition for women. *Journal of Sport History* **4**, 72–83.

Lucas, J. & Smith, R. (1982) Women's sport: a trial of equality. In R. Howell (ed.) *Her Story in Sport*, pp. 239–265. Leisure Press, Westpoint.

Mayer, O. (1960) *A Travers les Anneaux Olympiques*. Cailler, Genf.

Meyer, H.P. (1988) *Die ersten 'Olympischen Spiele' der Frauen 1921 in Monte Carlo*. Unpublished Master thesis, Köln.

Milliat, A. (1928) FSFI. *Der Leichtathlet* **5**, 19.

Mitchell, S. (1977) Women's participation in the Olympic Games 1926. *Journal of Sport History* **4**, 208–228.

Müller, J. (1927) *Eignung der Frauen und Mädchen für Leibesübungen*. Naumann, Leipzig.

Müller, N. (1983) *Von Paris bis Baden-Baden. Die Olympischen Kongresse 1894–1981*. Schors, Niedernhausen.

Müller, U. (1993) Ausgrenzende Vor-Bilder. In Sportmuseum Berlin (ed.) *Sportstadt Berlin in Geschichte und Gegenwart*, pp. 199–207. Sportmuseum Berlin, Berlin.

Odenkirchen, E. (1996) Auch Frauen beteiligt. In K. Lennartz (ed.) *Die Olympischen Spiele 1896 in Athen. Erläuterungen zum Neudruck des Offiziellen Berichts*, pp. 133–135. Agon, Kassel.

Pallet, G. (1955) *Women's Athletics*. Normal Press, Dulwich.

Park, R. (1991) Physiology and anatomy are destiny!? Brains, bodies and exercise in nineteenth century American thought. *Journal of Sport History* **18**, 31–64.

Park, R. (1994) A decade of the body: researching and writing about health, fitness, exercise and sport, 1983–1993. *Journal of Sport History* **21**, 59–82.

Pfister, G. (1981) Les femmes et les Jeux Olympiques. In B. Errais (ed.) *La Femme d'Aujourd'hui et le Sport*, pp. 39–51. Amphora, Paris.

Pfister, G. (1990) The medical discourse on female physical culture in Germany in the 19th and early 20th centuries. *Journal of Sport History* **17**, 183–199.

Pfister, G. (1994) Demands, realities and ambivalences: women in the proletarian sports movement in Germany (1893–1933). *Women in Sport and Physical Activity Journal* **3**, 39–69.

Pfister, G. (1996a) Physical activity in the name of the fatherland: Turnen and the National Movement (1810–1820). *Sporting Heritage* **1**, 14–36.

Pfister, G. (1996b) Women's Sports, Europe. In D. Levinson & K. Christensen (eds) *Encyclopedia of World Sport: From Ancient Times to the Present*, Vol. III, pp. 1159–1169. ABC-CLIO, Santa Barbara.

Pfister, G. (1999a) Die Frauenweltspiele. In Sportmuseum Berlin (ed.) *Jahrbuch 1999*. Sportmuseum Berlin, Berlin.

Pfister, G. (1999b) Vom schwachen zum starken Geschlecht? Frauensport im medizinischen Diskurs in denersten 30 Jahren der Bundesrepublik Deutschland. In T. Terret (ed.) *Sport and Health in History*. Proceedings of the 4th ISHPES Congress, Lyon, 1997, pp. 202–214. Academia, St Augustin.

Pfister, G. & Reese, D. (1995) Gender, body culture, and body politics in National Socialism. *Sport Science Review* **4**, 91–122.

Pfister, G. & von der Lippe, G. (1994) Women's participation in sports and the Olympic Games in Germany and Norway: a sociohistorical analysis. *Journal of Comparative Physical Education and Sport* **16**, 30–41.

Riordan, J. & Jinxia, D. (1996) Chinese women and sport: success, sexuality and suspicion. *China Quarterly* **145**, 130–152.

Sellheim, H. (1931) Auswertung der Gymnastik der Frau für die ärztliche Praxis. *Medizinische Klinik* **27**, 1439–1442.

Simri, U. (1977) *Women at the Olympic Games*. Wingate Institute, Natanya, Israel.

Simri, U. (1984) Frauen und Olympia: Sport und Emanzipation. In M. Blödorn (ed.) *Sport und Olympische Spiele*, pp. 89–104. Rororo, Reinbek bei Hamburg.

Théberge, N. (1991) Women and the Olympic Games: a consideration of gender, sport and social change. In F. Landry, M. Landry & M. Yerlès (eds) *Sport:*

The Third Millennium, pp. 385–395. Les Presses de l'Université Laval, Sainte-Foy.

Vertinsky, P. (1990) *The Eternally Wounded Woman. Woman, Exercise and Doctors in the Late Nineteenth Century*. Manchester University Press, Manchester.

Vertinsky, P. (1994a) Gender relations, women's history and sport history: a decade of changing enquiry, 1983–1993. *Journal of Sport History* **21**, 1–24.

Vertinsky, P. (1994b) Sport history and gender relations. *Journal of Sport History* **21**, 25–58.

Webster, S.A.M. (1930) *Athletics of To-Day for Women*. Frederick Waren, London/New York.

Welch, P. & Costa, D.M. (1994) A century of Olympic competition. In D.M. Costa & S.R. Guthrie (eds) *Women and Sport: Interdisciplinary Perspectives*, pp. 123–138. Human Kinetics Publishers, Champaign, Illinois.

Wilson, W. (1996) The IOC and the status of women in the Olympic Movement: 1972–1996. *Research Quarterly for Exercise and Sport* **67**, 183–192.

PART 2

PHYSIOLOGY OF
THE FEMALE ATHLETE

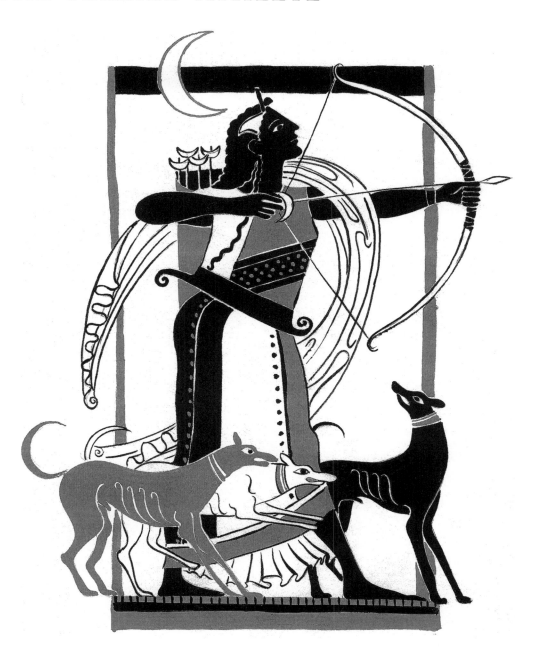

Chapter 2

Factors Influencing Endurance Performance, Strength, Flexibility and Coordination

KAREN D. MITTLEMAN AND CRISTINE M. ZACHER

Introduction

When Joan Benoit Samuelson crossed the finish line of the inaugural women's Olympic marathon in the 1984 Los Angeles Games the long-standing myth perpetuated in the 1920s that 'women were considered to be physiologically incapable of prolonged physical activity' (Lucas & Smith, 1982) was officially laid to rest. However, for most individuals involved in sport, the notion of the 'weaker sex' had previously been demystified in scientific reviews (Drinkwater, B.L., 1973; Drinkwater, B.A., 1984) and textbooks (Wells, 1991) devoted to the physiological aspects of sport and exercise in women.

In the years since women have competed in officially sanctioned endurance events, the dramatic improvements in their performance times, especially in running events, led to the speculation that in the near future women's and men's running times would coincide (Whipp & Ward, 1992). Although this speculation has been questioned (Joyner, 1993; Sparling et al., 1993), recent studies in ultra-endurance athletes have confirmed this hypothesis. As shown in Fig. 2.1, Bam and colleagues (1997) studied equally trained men and women and reported that at distances greater than 42.2 km sex differences in running speeds are negligible, with women potentially outperforming men at distances greater than 70 km. Research in male and female ultra-endurance athletes matched for marathon (42.2 km) performances has indicated that women

had better performances at 90 km (Speechly et al., 1996). However, certain biological differences discussed below will probably preclude élite women athletes from surpassing their male counterparts, especially in events in which strength and power predominate.

The gains in performance that women athletes have achieved over the last 20 years are not limited to endurance events. This chapter summarizes the research literature since 1985 and investigates the factors that may influence endurance performance, strength, flexibility and coordination in women athletes.

Endurance performance

Endurance performance is determined by the complex integration of a number of physiological indices, including maximal oxygen uptake ($\dot{V}_{O_{2max}}$), economy of movement and lactate threshold (see Joyner, 1993 and Coyle, 1995 for detailed discussion). These major components are influenced by morphological and functional characteristics (e.g. stroke volume, muscle fibre type, aerobic enzyme activity, haemoglobin concentration, muscle capillaries) that are, to some extent, genetically determined (Bouchard et al., 1992). In addition, the ability to sustain relatively high exercise intensities (65–75% $\dot{V}_{O_{2max}}$) over long periods is also dependent on the utilization and availability of energy substrates (Gollnick, 1988). Although there are few investigations of the interaction of these factors in determining endurance performance in women, Joyner (1993)

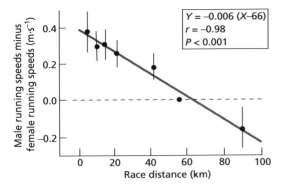

$$Y = -0.006\ (X\text{–}66)$$
$$r = -0.98$$
$$P < 0.001$$

Fig. 2.1 Differences in running speeds of matched men and women racing at increasing distances. Results are means ± SEM. The 95% confidence intervals of the differences between the men's and women's running speeds were significantly greater than zero over distances of 5–42.2 km. (From Bam *et al.*, 1997 with permission of Williams & Wilkins.)

suggests that they are probably similar in men and women.

Determinants of $\dot{V}O_{2max}$

In a previous review of the literature on women in sport, Drinkwater (1984) reported average values for aerobic power around 55 ml·kg^{-1}·min^{-1} for women distance runners. Since that time $\dot{V}O_{2max}$ values of 67–68 ml·kg^{-1}·min^{-1} have been measured in élite women distance runners (Pate *et al.*, 1987; Daniels & Daniels, 1992; Bunc & Heller, 1993). This dramatic improvement probably reflects improvements in training methodology. Despite these gains, the $\dot{V}O_{2max}$ values of women athletes are typically reported to be 10–15% lower than comparably trained men (Joyner, 1993). Exceptions to these gender differences have been noted in studies with competitive triathletes, where running $\dot{V}O_{2max}$ values, ranging from 58 to 68 ml·kg^{-1}·min^{-1}, were similar in men and women (O'Toole *et al.*, 1987; Kohrt *et al.*, 1989). Although a higher body fat has often been implicated in the lower aerobic power measured in endurance-trained women (Drinkwater, 1984; Pate *et al.*, 1987; Ogawa *et al.*, 1992), relative

$\dot{V}O_{2max}$, corrected for lean body mass, does not always negate these differences. Additional factors related to oxygen delivery may also play a role: the importance of alterations in haemoglobin concentration and blood volume, both of which are lower in women, in determining $\dot{V}O_{2max}$ have been demonstrated (Warren & Cureton, 1989).

Telford and Cunningham (1991) investigated haematological variables in nationally ranked male and female athletes from a variety of sports and reported haemogloblin values for women (144 g·l^{-1}, average for eight sports, 190 athletes) that were 10% lower than men (159 g·l^{-1}, average for eight sports, 249 athletes) who were matched by sport. Durstine *et al.* (1987) noted similar differences in haemoglobin values between male and female distance runners, while others have reported sex differences that range from 2.5 to 15% in runners and cross-country skiers (Berglund *et al.*, 1988; Weight *et al.*, 1992). Whether the linear relationship between haemoglobin concentration and body size (body mass index) observed by Telford and Cunningham (1991) may account, in part, for the variability in sex differences between studies is not known.

However, the influence of lower haemoglobin values on $\dot{V}O_{2max}$ and ultimately endurance performance in women athletes may not be as important as previously proposed (Joyner, 1993). In a study of 34 male and 16 female distance runners, Weight and colleagues (1992) found higher concentrations of 2,3-diphosphoglycerate (a phosphate compound that enhances release of oxygen to the tissues) in the women, which the authors suggest compensates for the lower haemoglobin values. Similar findings were reported by Pate *et al.* (1985) in their study of male and female distance runners, matched for performance time over 24.2 km. Sex differences have not been found in serum erythropoietin, a regulatory hormone for red blood cell formation (Berglund *et al.*, 1988; Weight *et al.*, 1992), or in the rightward shift of the oxygen dissociation curve following exercise (Weight *et al.* 1992) in endurance athletes.

Total blood volumes are approximately 30% lower in women than men (see Sanborn & Jankowski, 1994 for review). However, when expressed relative to body weight, Weight and colleagues (1991) reported similar blood and plasma volumes in female (blood volume 78 ± 8 ml·kg^{-1}, plasma volume 52 ± 6 ml·kg^{-1}) and male (blood volume 86 ± 10 ml·kg^{-1}, plasma volume 53 ± 8 ml·kg^{-1}) endurance-trained athletes. This expansion in blood volume with endurance training, measured using radiolabelling techniques, resulted in values that were 36% and 16% higher than those in non-exercising men and women respectively. This training-induced increase in blood volume has been linked to the lower haemoglobin values (i.e. dilutional effect) observed in endurance athletes of both sexes (Weight et al., 1991; Eichner, 1992), although its role in enhancing $\dot{V}_{O_{2max}}$ is questionable (Rowell, 1993).

As reviewed by Saltin and Strange (1992) the importance of the pumping capacity of the heart on $\dot{V}_{O_{2max}}$ has been studied for over 100 years. The smaller heart volume in women results in lower maximal values for both cardiac output and stroke volume compared with men (see Wells, 1991 for review). Meanwhile, exercise training results in an increased maximal cardiac output that can be explained to a large extent by the increase in stroke volume (Saltin & Strange, 1992). Although it is generally accepted that cardiovascular adaptations to exercise training (i.e. increased stroke volume) are similar in men and women (Drinkwater, 1984; Mitchell et al., 1992), Ogawa and colleagues (1992) noted subtle sex differences in the contribution of the cardiovascular alterations to $\dot{V}_{O_{2max}}$. These authors reported that training had a larger effect on maximal cardiac output and stroke volume but a smaller effect on maximal arteriovenous oxygen difference in men compared with women. These sex differences were more prevalent in older than younger individuals, leading to the speculation that sex hormones may modulate the cardiovascular adaptations with exercise training. However, it should be noted that the subjects in the previous study were not competitive athletes. In a study of similarly trained male and female endurance athletes, Hutchinson et al. (1991) determined that the reduced left ventricular mass of the women accounted for 68% of the difference in $\dot{V}_{O_{2max}}$. This effect of cardiac size, in combination with the higher fat mass in the women athletes, accounted for almost 99% of the $\dot{V}_{O_{2max}}$ differential they observed.

The proposal by Dempsey (1985) that the pulmonary system may limit $\dot{V}_{O_{2max}}$ in highly trained athletes has led to the speculation that this may influence female athletes to a greater extent due to their smaller pulmonary capillary volumes (Mitchell et al., 1992). To date, this hypothesis has not been addressed.

Lactate threshold

Although $\dot{V}_{O_{2max}}$ is an important determinant of endurance performance, Coyle and colleagues (1988) demonstrated, in trained male cyclists with similarly high $\dot{V}_{O_{2max}}$ values, a strong relationship between the lactate threshold (defined as the percentage $\dot{V}_{O_{2max}}$ corresponding to an increase in blood lactate of 1 mmol·l^{-1}) and endurance performance. Lactate threshold values are reported to be similar in male and female endurance athletes (Iwaoka et al., 1988; Kohrt et al., 1989; Weyand et al., 1994). Because the lactate threshold has been closely linked to aerobic enzyme activity (see Coyle, 1995 for discussion), the findings of similar enzyme adaptations in women matched to men trained for the same distances (Costill et al., 1987) further supports this concept.

The trainability of the lactate threshold in women athletes is evident from a unique study of an élite marathon runner whose exercise training was studied for 16 weeks following childbirth (Potteiger et al., 1993). Although minimal changes were observed in $\dot{V}_{O_{2max}}$, her postpartum lactate threshold increased from 68% $\dot{V}_{O_{2max}}$ at 4 weeks to 82% $\dot{V}_{O_{2max}}$ at 8 weeks and remained stable for the duration of training. This final value is similar to that reported in female collegiate distance runners (Weyand et al., 1994).

Economy/efficiency of movement

Economy of movement, generally defined as the oxygen uptake ($\dot{V}_{O_2}$) needed to maintain a given velocity of movement, interacts with $\dot{V}_{O_2max}$ and lactate threshold to affect endurance performance (Joyner, 1993; Coyle, 1995). In an earlier review, Wells (1991) reported equivocal results from previous studies citing sex differences in running economy, although the studies in highly trained men and women indicated that running economies were similar. Data from more recent studies continue to provide inconsistent results. A number of studies in equally trained men and women have shown no sex differences in running economy (Pate et al., 1985, 1987; Billat et al., 1996; Speechly et al., 1996), while others have reported advantages for men (Helgerud et al., 1990; Daniels & Daniels, 1992) or women (Helgerud, 1994; Weyand et al., 1994). Although it has been postulated that gender effects on the biomechanics of running (e.g. stride length, vertical displacement, pelvic width) may affect running economy (Wells, 1991), Williams and colleagues (1987) reported minimal correlations between running economy and biomechanical variables in élite female distance runners.

Studies addressing the importance of the contribution of running economy to endurance performance in women have also produced equivocal results. Evans et al. (1995) investigated 10-km performance correlates in endurance-trained women. Lactate threshold and $\dot{V}_{O_2max}$, but not running economy, were significantly related to performance. Helgerud and colleagues (1990) studied sex differences in performance-matched marathon runners. While $\dot{V}_{O_2max}$ was similar between the groups, running economy was poorer in the women. In contrast, others have reported a high correlation between running economy and endurance performance in trained women (Pate et al., 1987; Daniels & Daniels, 1992).

Coyle (1995) has suggested that during endurance cycling mechanical efficiency, defined as the ratio of work performed to energy expended, may influence economy. Although the majority of work on cycling efficiency has been performed in male cyclists, Berry et al. (1993) reported that cycling efficiency in women was related to body mass, work rate and pedal frequency, correlates previously demonstrated in men. Also, since the percentage of type I muscle fibres has been linked to cycling efficiency (Coyle et al., 1992), similarities in mechanical efficiency between trained men and women are not surprising as muscle fibre type distribution is also similar in sport-matched élite male and female athletes (see review by Drinkwater, 1984).

Substrate utilization

The importance of the availability of muscle glycogen and blood glucose on endurance performance is well established and has been previously reviewed (Gollnick, 1988). Because of the potential lipolytic action of female sex hormones (Bunt, 1990), a number of studies have focused on the effect of menstrual cycle phase on substrate utilization during endurance exercise; these are discussed in Chapter 3.

Whether sex differences in substrate utilization contribute to differences in endurance performance is also of interest. Based on the data shown in Fig. 2.1, Bam et al. (1997) suggest that their findings of better performances in women running distances greater than 42.2 km may be partially explained by greater glycogen sparing due to increased fat oxidation. Since 1985, several studies in comparably trained men and women (Tarnopolsky et al., 1990, 1995) support this conclusion, although others do not (Friedmann & Kindermann, 1989). During prolonged (90–100 min) treadmill exercise at 65% $\dot{V}_{O_2max}$, Tarnopolsky and colleagues (1990) observed greater lipid utilization (calculated from non-protein respiratory exchange ratio) in the female runners, which the authors suggest accounted for the smaller reduction in muscle glycogen compared with the male runners. In a follow-up study, Tarnopolsky et al. (1995) confirmed their previous findings of greater lipid utilization in women compared with men during prolonged exercise at 75% $\dot{V}_{O_2max}$. In contrast, Friedmann and Kindermann (1989) found no gender differences in lipid metabolism or in the regulatory hormones (e.g. growth hormone, insulin, adrenaline, noradrenaline, cortisol) in endurance-trained women and men who ran at 80% $\dot{V}_{O_{2max}}$ for 14 and 17 km respectively. Although Tarnopolsky *et al.* (1990) observed sex differences in growth hormone, insulin and adrenaline responses during prolonged exercise, these alterations could not account for the observed differences in substrate metabolism. These equivocal findings for the influence of gender on lipid metabolism during endurance exercise may be related to the different exercise intensities and durations among the protocols.

The potential impact of gender differences in glycogen sparing on substrate metabolism during endurance exercise, with and without carbohydrate (CHO) loading, was investigated by Tarnopolsky and colleagues (1995). Somewhat surprisingly, the women athletes failed to respond to a 75% CHO diet with increased muscle glycogen, although muscle glycogen increased by 41% in similarly trained men. The authors speculated that potential differences in glucose transporters may be responsible for the gender differences; however, this hypothesis has not been investigated in endurance-trained men and women. Gulve and Spira (1995) reported that short-term endurance training (7–10 days) increased the glucose transport protein, GLUT-4, in muscle of previously untrained men and women; no sex differences were reported by these authors.

In contrast to their previous study (Tarnopolsky *et al.*, 1990) demonstrating glycogen sparing in endurance-trained women following 1.5 hours of exercise at 65% $\dot{V}_{O_{2max}}$, Tarnopolsky *et al.* (1995) failed to find gender differences in muscle glycogen use during exercise at 75% $\dot{V}_{O_{2max}}$ for 1 hour on a 55–60% CHO diet. When a high CHO diet (75% over 4 days) was consumed, glycogen use was greater in the men. In terms of performance, the women's time to fatigue at 85% $\dot{V}_{O_{2max}}$ was similar for both dietary regimens, while the men improved their performance by approximately 6% on the 75%

CHO diet. Of interest is that performance times were similar between men and women when 55–60% CHO was consumed. Since the relative intensities sustained by endurance-trained women during long-term exercise (i.e. distances >21 km) are reported to be below 80% $\dot{V}_{O_{2max}}$ (Speechly *et al.*, 1996), the relevance of these findings to endurance performance is questionable. In a study recently completed in our laboratory (Fig. 2.2; S.P. Bailey *et al.*, unpublished data), supplementation with a 6% CHO drink every 30 min prolonged exercise time to fatigue by 14% in trained women ($\dot{V}_{O_{2max}}$ ~50 ml·kg^{-1}·min^{-1}) who cycled at 70% $\dot{V}_{O_{2max}}$ (Fig. 2.3).

In addition to the potential gender effects on lipid and carbohydrate utilization during prolonged exercise, data from Tarnopolsky *et al.* (1990, 1995) and Phillips *et al.* (1993) indicate that endurance-trained women oxidize less protein than similarly trained men. Although the contribution of protein to energy metabolism during prolonged exercise is relatively small (Gollnick, 1988), the relationship between protein, fat and carbohydrate availability has been proposed to influence fatigue during prolonged exercise via the central nervous system (see Davis &

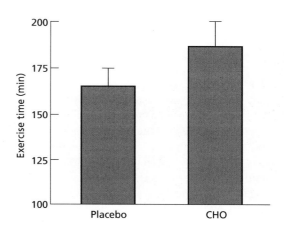

Fig. 2.2 Exercise time to exhaustion (mean ± SEM) for nine subjects who cycled at 70% $\dot{V}_{O_{2max}}$. Subjects ingested a drink containing flavoured water (placebo) or a 6% carbohydrate solution (CHO) every 30 min. Exercise time was significantly greater ($P < 0.05$) during the CHO trial.

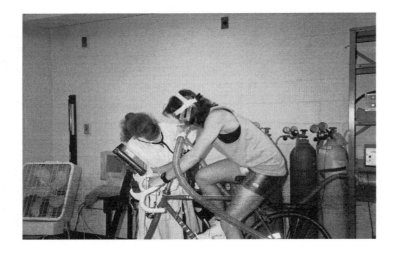

Fig. 2.3 Subject and researcher during blood sampling.

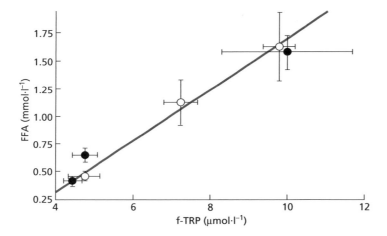

Fig. 2.4 Relationship between plasma free tryptophan (f-TRP) and plasma free fatty acids (FFA) during cycling at 70% $\dot{V}_{O_{2max}}$ to exhaustion. Subjects either ingested a placebo drink (○) or a 6% carbohydrate drink (●) every 30 min. Blood samples were taken at the end of each hour and at fatigue. Each symbol represents the means ± SEM for eight subjects.

Bailey, 1997 for review). These authors discuss the mechanisms by which the ratio of free-tryptophan (f-TRP) to branched chain amino acid (BCAA) concentrations may influence central nervous system fatigue by modulating the production of serotonin. In trained male cyclists, dietary supplementation with a CHO drink (6% or 12% CHO) suppressed mobilization of plasma free fatty acids (FFA), resulting in a reduction in f-TRP:BCAA and prolonged exercise time to exhaustion (Davis *et al.*, 1992). Although we similarly observed a linear relationship between FFA and f-TRP (Fig. 2.4; S.P. Bailey *et al.*, unpublished data) as well as a reduction in FFA with

CHO supplementation in trained women, f-TRP:BCAA was not reduced during the CHO trial even with a greater exercise time to fatigue. Whether these disparate results are due to gender differences in protein catabolism during exercise requires further study.

Summary and future directions

The complex integration of physiological factors that influence endurance performance presents a challenge to our understanding of the women athletes who compete in these events. Although the last 25 years have resulted in an exponential increase in studies of endurance-trained women, a great deal of our knowledge of endurance performance and its correlates are based on research primarily performed on male athletes. The impact of cardiac size on the delivery of oxygen is a factor that will probably preclude most élite women from achieving the same $\dot{V}_{O_{2max}}$ values as sport-matched élite men. However, the evidence that ultra-endurance events favour women's performances over similarly trained men reveals physiological advantages for female athletes that override the importance of $\dot{V}_{O_{2max}}$ in endurance performance. Although lactate threshold and economy of movement have been shown to interact with $\dot{V}_{O_{2max}}$ in determining endurance performance in men, it is not clear how these factors are integrated to affect women's performances. Further studies of the regulatory enzymes and hormones that control energy metabolism in women athletes during prolonged endurance events are also necessary. It is important that future studies in this area take into consideration factors that may influence exercise responses. These include, but are not limited to, sex hormones, training status and history, dietary status, circadian effects, body size and composition, and intensity and duration of the exercise stimulus. The smaller differential in performance times between men and women over the last 20 years indicates that the adaptability of the human body to exercise training is not as sexually dimorphic as previously proposed by those who opposed women's participation in endurance events.

Strength

Muscular strength, defined as the maximum force or tension generated by a muscle, is a requirement for all athletic events. Physiological factors that contribute to the development of muscular strength include neurological adaptations (e.g. recruitment of motor units, disinhibition), muscle hypertrophy, alterations in muscle fibre composition, and hormonal responses. These have been recently reviewed by Kraemer *et al.* (1996). Although the majority of human

studies that have investigated training influences on muscular strength have focused on men, research on women has dramatically increased over the last two decades.

Neural adaptation

It is well accepted that the gains in muscular strength observed in the initial phases (2–8 weeks) of a resistance training programme are a result of neural alterations with little change in muscle cross-sectional area (CSA) (see Sale, 1988 and Kraemer *et al.*, 1996 for reviews). Moritani and deVries (1979) investigated the role of neural factors and hypertrophy in the time course of gains in muscle strength in seven men and eight women who performed progressive resistance exercise training for 8 weeks. These authors reported identical time-course responses for strength gains between the men and women, noting that neural factors were predominant in the initial (<4 weeks) gains in strength. Staron and colleagues (1994) confirmed the influence of neural factors in maximal dynamic strength gains in both men and women following an 8-week heavy resistance training programme. Although muscle fibre size was not increased in this short-term training programme, these authors noted alterations in muscle fibre type composition and phenotypic expression of contractile proteins (myosin heavy chain content) concomitant with the early strength gains in both sexes.

Whole muscle hypertrophy

Prior to the 1980s, strength gains following resistance training in women were reported to be accompanied by minimal muscle hypertrophy (Brown & Wilmore, 1974; Wilmore, 1974) or hypertrophy that was approximately 50% of that observed in men (Moritani & deVries, 1979). However, more recent studies using computerized tomography or muscle biopsies for measurement of muscle CSA and muscle fibre area have demonstrated that women respond with similar hypertrophic adaptations as those seen in men following heavy resistance training (Cureton *et al.*, 1988; Hickson *et al.*, 1994; Staron *et al.*, 1994). Cureton *et al.* (1988) reported significant increases in strength in both men and women following a 16-week progressive resistance training protocol. Although the men exhibited a greater absolute change in arm strength, the relative change in arm strength did not differ between men and women. Absolute increases in muscle CSA of the upper arm were the same for women and men. Cureton *et al.* attributed the greater gains in absolute arm strength to the larger pretraining muscle fibre size and number in men compared with women that had previously been reported by Sale *et al.* (1987).

Muscle fibre type and cross-sectional area

Although previous research elucidated the importance of muscle fibre type on sport performance in women athletes (Drinkwater, 1984), few of these studies investigated the influence of resistance training on alterations in muscle fibre types in women. Staron *et al.* (1990) studied 24 women who participated in a heavy resistance training programme (6–8 repetition maximum (RM), three sets) designed to elicit an increase in thigh muscle strength. In addition to significant improvements in maximal dynamic strength (1 RM), histochemical and photomontage analyses of muscle biopsies of the vastus lateralis before and after training showed significant increases in CSA of type I (slow-twitch), type IIA (fast-twitch oxidative–glycolytic) and type IIAB + IIB [combination of fast-twitch glycolytic (IIB) and intermediate between types IIA and IIB], with the greatest gains observed in the fast-twitch fibres. The distribution of fibre types was also altered following the training programme: the percentage of type IIB fibres decreased with a reciprocal increase in percentage of type IIA fibres, suggesting conversion of type IIB to IIA. The muscle hypertrophy detected by histochemical techniques was not confirmed by anthropometric measurement of thigh girth, which the authors attributed to a decrease in thigh subcutaneous skinfold thickness.

As part of a follow-up study, Staron *et al.* (1991) investigated the effects of detraining and retraining on muscle strength, hypertrophy and fibre type conversions. Of the women that participated in the heavy resistance training programme in the previous study (Staron *et al.*, 1990) six underwent long-term (30–32 weeks) detraining. During this time the women were not involved in any type of endurance or resistance training. Following detraining the subjects were retested and resumed the training protocol for 6 weeks (neural adaptation phase) followed by an additional 7 weeks of training (muscle hypertrophy phase, *n* = 4). Detraining resulted in a decrease in strength, although values remained greater than those measured prior to the initial training protocol. Similar changes were noted in the CSA of type IIAB + IIB fibres and, to a lesser extent, of type IIA and type I muscle fibres. In contrast, the detraining period resulted in a return of the composition of type II fibres to pretraining levels (i.e. increase in percentage of type IIB and decrease in percentage of type IIA). Following the 6-week retraining period, 1-RM values were comparable to those obtained at the conclusion of the initial 20-week training programme and the percentage of type IIB fibres significantly decreased. Muscle fibre CSA increased in type IIA and type IIAB + IIB fibres from their detrained values. The additional hypertrophic training period resulted in significant increases in percentage of type IIA fibres, with no further alterations in the CSA of any muscle fibre type. These data suggest that in women maximal dynamic strength and muscle fibre CSA may be retained over long periods of detraining and that a rapid return to the trained state is possible with short-term (6 weeks) heavy resistance training.

More recently, Staron and colleagues (1994) investigated the time course of alterations in muscle strength and morphology in women and men who performed an 8-week progressive resistance training protocol. Both men and women exhibited similar increases in absolute and relative dynamic strength of the lower extremity as well as decreases in the percentage of type IIB fibres. However, the hormonal mechanisms for these alterations were gender specific.

Hormonal factors

The hypertrophy that accompanies heavy resistance training is modulated by endocrine responses, which are both gender and protocol specific (Kraemer *et al.*, 1996). In men this response to training is believed to be mediated by an increase in several anabolic hormones, including testosterone and growth hormone (GH) (Kraemer *et al.*, 1990). Recently Staron *et al.* (1994) observed a correlation between the early changes in muscle fibre types with heavy resistance training and increased testosterone and decreased cortisol levels in men. However, these endocrine responses were not evident in the women who demonstrated similar muscular adaptations.

Previous studies investigating the hormonal factors that modify muscular strength and hypertrophy in women have produced equivocal results. While Cumming *et al.* (1987) found a significant increase in serum testosterone and cortisol values in women who performed resistance exercise, other researchers have found no increase in serum testosterone in women during resistance training (Krahenbuhl *et al.*, 1978; Westerlind *et al.*, 1987; Kraemer *et al.*, 1991, 1993, 1995). Heavy resistance exercise did result in significant increases in GH in women (Kraemer *et al.*, 1991, 1993); however, this was only observed if the exercise protocol was designed to induce hypertrophy rather than strength (i.e. lower resistance, more repetitions, shorter rest period). This protocol resulted in a greater elevation in lactic acid, which the authors suggest may have stimulated the release of GH. Cumming *et al.* (1987) also suggested that lactic acid concentrations were related to the hormonal responses to resistance training in the women they studied.

Muscle endurance

One of the potential reasons noted for the enhanced performance of women over men during running events greater than 42.2 km is a fatigue resistance of their musculature (Bam *et al.*, 1997). Two studies using physically active men and women provide evidence to support this suggestion. Clarke (1986) measured a hand-gripping exercise and reported a slower fatigue rate in the women compared with the men. Misner and colleagues (1990) observed similar results for both finger-flexion and leg-extension exercises. Although mechanisms for these differences have not been elucidated, Coetzer *et al.* (1993) have reported an inverse relationship between peak isometric torque and time to fatigue in élite black male distance runners. Whether the lower absolute strength reported in women compared with men (Heyward *et al.*, 1986; Sale *et al.*, 1987; Cureton *et al.*, 1988; Misner *et al.*, 1990) contributes to this fatigue resistance is unknown.

Summary and future directions

Since 1985 a large body of research has established that women respond to resistance training with similar hypertrophic adaptations as previously observed in men, although hormonal mechanisms responsible for these changes are sex specific. The smaller fibre CSA and total muscle CSA of women result in a sport-specific gender difference in absolute strength, although relative strength (per body mass or lean body mass) may be similar. It is interesting to note that the studies detailed above have not included women athletes in sports that depend on absolute strength for success (e.g. athletic field events). Further studies of the interrelationship between fatigue resistance, muscular strength and endurance performance are also warranted.

Flexibility

Flexibility, which may be defined as the athlete's ability to move a joint through a normal range of motion without undue musculotendinous stress (Chandler *et al.*, 1990), has been advocated for enhanced performance as well as reduced injury rates (Smith, 1994; Plowman & Smith,

1997), although conclusive evidence is lacking (Plowman, 1992; Plowman & Smith, 1997). The commonly stated assumption that women have greater flexibility than men has also been challenged by Plowman and Smith (1997), who suggest that evidence is based on tests of hip flexion, which has been shown to be greater in women than men (Shephard *et al.*, 1990; McHugh *et al.*, 1992) and does not necessarily reflect general flexibility. However, Kibler and colleagues (1989) studied total-body flexibility (11 measurements) in 629 female and 1478 male athletes participating in a variety of sports and found that the women were more flexible than the men on all measurements. In addition, these authors noted that lower-body female athletes had reduced flexibility compared with upper-body female athletes; this finding was not apparent in the male athletes. It was suggested that the discrepancy between the sexes was due to the initially reduced flexibility of the male athlete (i.e. less to lose). Caution is advised in interpreting these data as the athletes were recruited from junior high school through collegiate programmes but age was not factored into the analyses.

McHugh *et al.* (1992) compared the mechanical component of flexibility, assessed by viscoelastic stress relaxation, in men and women. Although the women had greater hip flexibility, the stretch-induced electromyographic response and viscoelastic stress relaxation were similar between the sexes. Differences in muscle mass, joint geometry or sex-specific collagenous muscle structure were suggested as factors potentiating the greater muscle extensibility in the women; however, these were not evaluated.

Support for the importance of flexibility and muscular strength in determining injury rates in women athletes is provided by the study of Knapik and colleagues (1991). These authors evaluated lower-body isokinetic knee torque and flexibility in 138 female collegiate athletes participating in eight weight-bearing varsity sports. Tests were conducted during the preseason and were related to occurrences of lower extremity injuries. Results indicated that imbalances in strength (flexion/extension ratio <0.75; right vs.

left knee flexor >15% at $180°·s^{-1}$) and flexibility (right hip vs. left hip >15%) were associated with the first incidence of lower extremity injury in these athletes. Over the course of the 3-year study, 40% of the women suffered one or more injuries.

Although laxity of joints is considered a primary factor in risk of injury in a number of sports in which women participate (Agostini, 1994), this is more likely a sport-specific rather than sex-specific issue.

Coordination

In their review of neurophysiology of motor skills in sport, Henatsch and Langer (1985) suggest that the development of precision in sport is the culmination of the motor learning process, which involves hierarchical levels of coordination (i.e. crude < fine < super-fine).

It has been postulated that the greater incidence of injury in female athletes compared with male athletes in the same sport may be due to inadequate skill development, which Beck and Wildermuth (1985) suggest is a result of poor training experience in the developmental years. In other words, the discrepancy in skill development is due to sociological rather than biological factors. Whether women athletes who have participated in organized youth sport programmes since their formative years are less prone to injury has not been studied, although more current information on athletes indicates that injury rates are more sport specific than sex specific, with minor exceptions (e.g. anterior cruciate ligament) (Arendt, 1994).

In contrast to this sociological argument, research studies have demonstrated sex differences in performance on motor tasks (Watson & Kimura, 1989; Hall & Kimura, 1995; Nicholson & Kimura, 1996), which Kimura (1992) attributes to the effect of sex hormones on brain organization during development. In general, women have been shown to be superior to men on tasks involving fine motor coordination (Kimura, 1992; Hall & Kimura, 1995) and speed of motor programming (Nicholson & Kimura, 1996), whereas men outperform women on target-directed motor skills (Watson & Kimura, 1989; Kimura, 1992). Watson and Kimura (1989) reported that the differential patterns of motor programming they observed in men and women performing target-throwing and interception tasks were not related to differences in physique or athleticism. However, the 'athleticism' of their subjects was determined by a self-rated questionnaire of experience in athletics and organized baseball. Whether similar results would be found in equally trained male and female athletes whose sport-specific training matched the motor skills evaluated is yet to be determined. The finding of improved manual coordination in women during the luteal phase of their menstrual cycle (Hampson & Kimura, 1988) further supports the hypothesis that sex hormones may influence motor skills.

Although the research on sex differences in motor learning is intriguing, there is no evidence to suggest that the final outcome of sport precision is different in men and women. Whether female athletes utilize a different motor programme strategy to achieve these skills may have implications for coaching practices. In addition, studies on coordination in women athletes and its potential role on injury rates and performance are warranted.

Conclusion

Over the last 25 years research has shown that the training response of the female athlete is similar to the male athlete, with minor exceptions. As young girls participate in sports from their formative years, many of the sex differences observed in the past will be reduced to the basic biological differences (e.g. cardiac size, muscle CSA) and women will achieve their true potential.

References

Agostini, R. (ed.) (1994) *Medical and Orthopedic Issues of Active and Athletic Women.* Hanley and Belfus, Philadelphia.

Arendt, E.A. (1994) Orthopaedic issues for active and athletic women. *Clinics in Sports Medicine* **13**, 483–503.

Bam, J., Noakes, T.D., Juritz, J. & Dennis, S.C. (1997) Could women outrun men in ultramarathon races? *Medicine and Science in Sports and Exercise* **29**, 244–247.

Beck, J.L. & Wildermuth, B.P. (1985) The female athlete's knee. *Clinics in Sports Medicine* **4**, 345–366.

Berglund, B., Birgegård, G. & Hemmingsson, P. (1988) Serum erythropoietin in cross-country skiers. *Medicine and Science in Sports and Exercise* **20**, 208–209.

Berry, M.J., Storsteen, J.A. & Woodard, C.M. (1993) Effects of body mass on exercise efficiency and V_{O_2} during steady-state cycling. *Medicine and Science in Sports and Exercise* **25**, 1031–1037.

Billat, V., Beillot, J., Jan, J., Rochcongar, P. & Carre, F. (1996) Gender effect on the relationship of time limit at 100% $V_{O_{2max}}$ with other bioenergetic characteristics. *Medicine and Science in Sports and Exercise* **28**, 1049–1055.

Bouchard, C., Dionne, F.T., Simoneau, J.-A. & Boulay, M.R. (1992) Genetics of aerobic and anaerobic performances. *Exercise and Sport Sciences Reviews* **20**, 27–58.

Brown, C.H. & Wilmore, J.H. (1974) The effects of maximal resistance training on the strength and body composition of women athletes. *Medicine and Science in Sports and Exercise* **6**, 174–177.

Bunc, V. & Heller, J. (1993) Ventilatory threshold in young and adult female athletes. *Journal of Sports Medicine and Physical Fitness* **33**, 233–238.

Bunt, J.C. (1990) Metabolic actions of estradiol: significance for acute and chronic exercise responses. *Medicine and Science in Sports and Exercise* **22**, 286–290.

Chandler, T.J., Kibler, W.B., Uhl, T.L., Wooten, B., Kiser, A. & Stone, E. (1990) Flexibility comparisons of junior elite tennis players to other athletes. *American Journal of Sports Medicine* **18**, 134–136.

Clarke, D.H. (1986) Sex differences in strength and fatigability. *Research Quarterly for Exercise and Sport* **57**, 144–149.

Coetzer, P., Noakes, T.D., Sanders, B. *et al.* (1993) Superior fatigue resistance of elite black South African distance runners. *Journal of Applied Physiology* **75**, 1822–1827.

Costill, D.L., Fink, W.J., Flynn, M. & Kirwin, J. (1987) Muscle fibre composition and enzyme activities in elite female distance runners. *International Journal of Sports Medicine* **8** (Suppl.), 103–106.

Coyle, E.F. (1995) Integration of the physiological factors determining endurance performance ability. *Exercise and Sport Sciences Reviews* **23**, 25–63.

Coyle, E.F., Coggan, A.R., Hopper, M.K. & Walters, T.J. (1988) Determinants of endurance in well trained cyclists. *Journal of Applied Physiology* **64**, 2622–2630.

Coyle, E.F., Sidossis, L.S., Horowitz, J.F. & Beltz, J.D. (1992) Cycling efficiency is related to the percentage of type I muscle fibres. *Medicine and Science in Sports and Exercise* **24**, 782–788.

Cumming, D.C., Wall, S.R., Galbraith, M.A. & Belcastro, A.N. (1987) Reproductive hormone responses to resistance exercise. *Medicine and Science in Sports and Exercise* **19**, 234–238.

Cureton, K.J., Collins, M.A., Hill, D.W. & McElhannon Jr, F.M. (1988) Muscle hypertrophy in men and women. *Medicine and Science in Sports and Exercise* **20**, 338–344.

Daniels, J. & Daniels, N. (1992) Running economy of elite male and elite female runners. *Medicine and Science in Sports and Exercise* **24**, 483–489.

Davis, J.M. & Bailey, S.P. (1997) Possible mechanisms of central nervous system fatigue during exercise. *Medicine and Science in Sports and Exercise* **29**, 45–57.

Davis, J.M., Bailey, S.P., Woods, J.A., Galiano, F.J., Hamilton, M.T. & Bartoli, W.P. (1992) Effects of carbohydrate feedings on plasma free tryptophan and branched-chain amino acids during prolonged cycling. *European Journal of Applied Physiology* **65**, 513–519.

Dempsey, J.A. (1985) Is the lung built for exercise? *Medicine and Science in Sports and Exercise* **18**, 143–155.

Drinkwater, B.A. (1984) Women and exercise: physiological aspects. *Exercise and Sport Sciences Reviews* **12**, 339–372.

Drinkwater, B.L. (1973) Physiological responses of women to exercise. *Exercise and Sport Sciences Reviews* **1**, 125–153.

Durstine, J.L., Pate, R.R., Sparling, P.B., Wilson, G.E., Senn, M.D. & Bartoli, W.P. (1987) Lipid, lipoprotein, and iron status of elite women distance runners. *International Journal of Sports Medicine* **8**, 119–123.

Eichner, E.R. (1992) Sports anemia, iron supplements, and blood doping. *Medicine and Science in Sports and Exercise* **24** (Suppl.), S315–S318.

Evans, S.L., Davy, K.P., Stevenson, E.T. & Seals, D.R. (1995) Physiological determinants of 10-km performance in highly trained female runners of different ages. *Journal of Applied Physiology* **78**, 1931–1941.

Friedmann, B. & Kindermann, W. (1989) Energy metabolism and regulatory hormones in women and men during endurance exercise. *European Journal of Applied Physiology* **59**, 1–9.

Gollnick, P.D. (1988) Energy metabolism and prolonged exercise. In D.R. Lamb and R. Murray (eds) *Perspectives in Exercise Science and Sports Medicine*, pp. 1–42. Benchmark Press, Indianapolis.

Gulve, E.A. & Spina, R.J. (1995) Effect of 7–10 days of cycle ergometer exercise on skeletal muscle Glut-4 protein content. *Journal of Applied Physiology* **79**, 1562–1566.

Hall, J.A. & Kimura, D. (1995) Sexual orientation and performance on sexually dimorphic motor tasks. *Archives of Sexual Behavior* **24**, 395–407.

Hampson, E. & Kimura, D. (1988) Reciprocal effects of hormonal fluctuations on human motor and perceptual–spatial skills. *Behavioral Neuroscience* **102**, 456–459.

Helgerud, J. (1994) Maximal oxygen uptake, anaerobic threshold and running economy in women and men with similar performance level in marathons. *European Journal of Applied Physiology* **68**, 155–161.

Helgerud, J., Ingjer, F. & Stromme, S.B. (1990) Sex differences in performance-matched marathon runners. *European Journal of Applied Physiology* **61**, 433–439.

Henatsch, H.-D. & Langer, H.H. (1985) Basic neurophysiology of motor skills in sport: a review. *International Journal of Sports Medicine* **6**, 2–14.

Heyward, V.H., Johannes-Ellis, S.M. & Romer, J.F. (1986) Gender difference in strength. *Research Quarterly for Exercise and Sport* **57**, 154–159.

Hickson, R.C., Hidaka, K. & Foster, C. (1994) Skeletal muscle fibre type, resistance training, and strength-related performance. *Medicine and Science in Sports and Exercise* **26**, 593–598.

Hutchinson, P.L., Cureton, K.J., Outz, H. & Wilson, G. (1991) Relationship of cardiac size to maximal oxygen uptake and body size in men and women. *International Journal of Sports Medicine* **12**, 369–373.

Iwaoka, K., Hatta, H., Atomi, Y. & Miyashita, M. (1988) Lactate, respiratory compensation thresholds, and distance running performance in runners of both sexes. *International Journal of Sports Medicine* **9**, 306–309.

Joyner, M.J. (1993) Physiological limiting factors and distance running: influence of gender and age on record performances. *Exercise and Sport Sciences Reviews* **21**, 103–133.

Kibler, W.B., Chandler, T.J., Uhl, T. & Maddus, R.E. (1989) A musculoskeletal approach to the preparticipation physical examination. *American Journal of Sports Medicine* **17**, 525–531.

Kimura, D. (1992) Sex differences in the brain. *Scientific American* **267**, 118–125.

Knapik, J.J., Bauman, C.L., Jones, B.H., Harris, J.M. & Vaughan, L. (1991) Preseason strength and flexibility imbalances associated with athletic injuries in female collegiate athletes. *American Journal of Sports Medicine* **19**, 76–81.

Kohrt, W.M., O'Connor, J.S. & Skinner, J.S. (1989) Longitudinal assessment of responses by triathletes to swimming, cycling, and running. *Medicine and Science in Sports and Exercise* **21**, 569–575.

Kraemer, R.R., Heleniak, R.J., Tryniecki, J.L., Kraemer, G.R., Okazaki, N.J. & Castracane, V.D. (1995) Follicular and luteal phase hormonal responses to low-volume resistive exercise. *Medicine and Science in Sports and Exercise* **27**, 809–817.

Kraemer, W.J., Marchitelli, L., Gordon, S.E. *et al.* (1990) Hormonal and growth factor responses to heavy resistance exercise protocols. *Journal of Applied Physiology* **69**, 1442–1450.

Kraemer, W.J., Gordon, S.E., Fleck, S.J. *et al.* (1991) Endogenous anabolic hormonal and growth factor responses to heavy resistance exercise in males and females. *International Journal of Sports Medicine* **12**, 228–235.

Kraemer, W.J., Fleck, S.J., Dziados, J.E. *et al.* (1993) Changes in hormonal concentrations after different heavy-resistance exercise protocols in women. *Journal of Applied Physiology* **75**, 594–604.

Kraemer, W.J., Fleck, S.J. & Evans, W.J. (1996) Strength and power training: physiological mechanisms of adaptation. *Exercise and Sport Sciences Reviews* **24**, 363–397.

Krahenbuhl, G.S., Archer, P.A. & Pettit, L.L. (1978) Serum testosterone and female trainability. *Ergonomics* **18**, 359–364.

Lucas, J.A. & Smith, R.A. (1982) Women's sport: a trial of equality. In R. Howell (ed.) *Her Story in Sport: A Historical Anthology of Women in Sports*, pp. 239–265. Leisure Press, West Point, New York.

McHugh, M.P., Magnusson, S.P., Gleim, G.W. & Nicholas, J.A. (1992) Viscoelastic stress relaxation in human skeletal muscle. *Medicine and Science in Sports and Exercise* **24**, 1375–1382.

Misner, J.E., Massey, B.H., Going, S.B., Bemben, M.G. & Ball, T.E. (1990) Sex differences in static strength and fatigability in three different muscle groups. *Research Quarterly for Exercise and Sport* **61**, 238–242.

Mitchell, J.H., Tate, C., Raven, P. *et al.* (1992) Acute responses and chronic adaptation to exercise in women. *Medicine and Science in Sports and Exercise* **24** (Suppl.), 258–265.

Moritani, T. & deVries, H.A. (1979) Neural factors vs. hypertrophy in the time course of muscle strength gain. *American Journal of Physical Medicine* **58**, 115–130.

Nicholson, K.G. & Kimura, D. (1996) Sex differences in speech and manual skill. *Perceptual and Motor Skills* **82**, 3–13.

Ogawa, T., Spina, R.J., Martin III, W.H. *et al.* (1992) Effects of aging, sex, and physical training on cardiovascular responses to exercise. *Circulation* **86**, 494–503.

O'Toole, M.L., Hiller, W.D.B., Crosby, L.O. & Douglas, P.S. (1987) The ultraendurance triathlete: a physiological profile. *Medicine and Science in Sports and Exercise* **19**, 45–50.

Pate, R.R., Barnes, C. & Miller, W. (1985) A physiological comparison of performance-matched female and male distance runners. *Research Quarterly for Exercise and Sport* **56**, 245–250.

Pate, R.R., Sparling, P.B., Wilson, G.E., Cureton, K.J. & Miller, B.J. (1987) Cardiorespiratory and metabolic responses to submaximal and maximal exercise in elite women distance runners. *International Journal of Sports Medicine* **8**, 91–95.

Phillips, S.M., Atkinson, S.A., Tarnopolsky, M.A. & MacDougall, J.D. (1993) Gender differences in leucine kinetics and nitrogen balance in endurance athletes. *Journal of Applied Physiology* **75**, 2134–2141.

Plowman, S.A. (1992) Physical activity, physical fitness, and low back pain. *Exercise and Sport Sciences Reviews* **20**, 221–242.

Plowman, S.A. & Smith, D.L. (1997) *Exercise Physiology for Health, Fitness, and Performance.* Allyn and Bacon, Boston.

Potteiger, J.A., Welch, J.C. & Byrne, J.C. (1993) From parturition to marathon: a 16-weeks study of an elite runner. *Medicine and Science in Sports and Exercise* **25**, 673–677.

Rowell, L.B. (1993) *Human Cardiovascular Control.* Oxford University Press, New York.

Sale, D.G. (1988) Neural adaptation to resistance training. *Medicine and Science in Sports and Exercise* **20** (Suppl.), S135–S145.

Sale, D.G., MacDougall, J.D., Alway, S.E. & Sutton, J.R. (1987) Voluntary strength and muscle characteristics in untrained men and women and male body-builders. *Journal of Applied Physiology* **62**, 1786–1793.

Saltin, B. & Strange, S. (1992) Maximal oxygen uptake: 'old' and 'new' arguments for a cardiovascular limitation. *Medicine and Science in Sports and Exercise* **24**, 30–37.

Sanborn, C.F. & Jankowski, C.M. (1994) Physiologic considerations for women in sport. *Clinics in Sports Medicine* **13**, 315–327.

Shephard, R.J., Berridge, M. & Montelpare, W. (1990) On the generality of the 'sit and reach' test: an analysis of flexibility data for an aging population. *Research Quarterly for Exercise and Sport* **61**, 326–330.

Smith, C.A. (1994) The warm-up procedure: to stretch or not to stretch. A brief review. *Journal of Orthopaedics and Sports Physical Therapy* **19**, 12–17.

Sparling, P.B., Nieman, D.C. & O'Connor, P.J. (1993) Selected scientific aspects of marathon racing. An update on fluid replacement, immune function, psychological factors and the gender difference. *Sports Medicine* **15**, 116–132.

Speechly, D.P., Taylor, S.R. & Rogers, G.G. (1996) Differences in ultra-endurance exercise in performance-matched male and female runners. *Medicine and Science in Sports and Exercise* **28**, 359–365.

Staron, R.S., Malicky, E.S., Leonardi, M.J., Falkel, J.E., Hagerman, F.C. & Dudley, G.A. (1990) Muscle hypertrophy and fast fibre type conversions in heavy resistance-trained women. *European Journal of Applied Physiology* **60**, 71–79.

Staron, R.S., Leonardi, M.J., Karapondo, D.L. *et al.* (1991) Strength and skeletal muscle adaptations in heavy-resistance-trained women after detraining and retraining. *Journal of Applied Physiology* **70**, 631–640.

Staron, R.S., Karapondo, D.L., Kraemer, W.J. *et al.* (1994) Skeletal muscle adaptations during early phase of heavy-resistance training in men and women. *Journal of Applied Physiology* **76**, 1247–1255.

Tarnopolsky, L.J., MacDougall, J.D., Atkinson, S.A., Tarnopolsky, M.A. & Sutton, J.R. (1990) Gender differences in substrate for endurance exercise. *Journal of Applied Physiology* **68**, 302–308.

Tarnopolsky, M.A., Atkinson, S.A., Phillips, S.M. & MacDougall, J.D. (1995) Carbohydrate loading and metabolism during exercise in men and women. *Journal of Applied Physiology* **78**, 1360–1368.

Telford, R.D. & Cunningham, R.B. (1991) Sex, sport, and body-size dependency of hematology of trained athletes. *Medicine and Science in Sports and Exercise* **23**, 788–794.

Warren, G.L. & Cureton, K.J. (1989) Modeling the effect of alterations in hemoglobin concentration on Vo_{2max}. *Medicine and Science in Sports and Exercise* **21**, 526–531.

Watson, N.V. & Kimura, D. (1989) Right-hand superiority for throwing but not for intercepting. *Neuropsychologia* **27**, 1399–1414.

Weight, L.M., Darge, B.L. & Jacobs, P. (1991) Athletes' pseudoanaemia. *European Journal of Applied Physiology* **62**, 358–362.

Weight, L.M., Alexander, D., Elliot, T. & Jacobs, P. (1992) Erythropoietic adaptations to endurance training. *European Journal of Applied Physiology* **64**, 444–448.

Wells, C.L. (1991) *Women, Sport and Performance.* Human Kinetics Publishers, Champaign, Illinois.

Westerlind, K.C., Byrnes, W.C., Freedson, P.S. & Katch, F.I. (1987) Exercise and serum androgens in women. *Physician and Sportsmedicine* **15**, 87–94.

Weyand, P.G., Cureton, K.J., Conley, D.S., Sloniger, M.A. & Liu, Y.L. (1994) Peak oxygen deficit predicts sprint and middle-distance track performance. *Medicine and Science in Sports and Exercise* **26**, 1174–1180.

Whipp, B.J. & Ward, S.A. (1992) Will women soon outrun men? *Nature* **355**, 25.

Williams, K.R., Cavanagh, P.R. & Ziff, J.L. (1987) Biomechanical studies of elite female distance runners. *International Journal of Sports Medicine* **8** (Suppl.), 107–118.

Wilmore, J.H. (1974) Alterations in strength, body composition and anthropometric measurements consequent to 10-week weight training program. *Medicine and Science in Sports and Exercise* **6**, 133–138.

Chapter 3

Effects of the Menstrual Cycle and Oral Contraceptives on Sports Performance

CONSTANCE M. LEBRUN

Introduction

Sports performance is a multifaceted entity, determined by a multitude of diverse cardio-pulmonary, musculoskeletal, biomechanical, cellular and enzymatic adaptations. In addition, there is intraindividual variability in body temperature, heart rate, ventilation and ventilatory responses, as well as in muscle fibre type. Psychological state (affect, perception, cognition) can also affect performance dramatically. Despite the typical selection bias of many investigations towards male subjects, it is currently accepted that women respond to physical training as do men, with decreased blood pressure and heart rate, reduced percentage body fat and increased maximal aerobic capacity.

Although aerobic capacity is the 'gold standard' by which fitness is evaluated, other parameters such as running economy and mechanical efficiency are equally important. Many of the measurable physiological differences between male and female athletes can be minimized if corrected for percentage lean body mass, as discussed in Chapter 2. Nevertheless there remain significant gender differences that are largely attributable to the influence of the male and female sex steroids, particularly after puberty. Women must also deal with fluctuating levels of endogenous hormones in the course of an ovulatory menstrual cycle, as well as during pregnancy, parturition and menopause. Combinations of exogenous hormones are frequently used in oral contraceptives (OCs) and for hor-

monal replacement therapy in postmenopausal women. There has been much debate about the effect of these variations on sports performance but relatively few valid scientific studies.

For the practitioner caring for the female athlete, it is important to have an understanding of the rhythmic alterations in female sex steroids that occur during the biological life cycle and their physiological implications. Knowledge in this area has advanced somewhat over the past few decades because of the substantial increase in women who are physically active and the larger population of well-trained female athletes for researchers to study. There are still many unanswered questions. This chapter reviews what is currently known about the impact of puberty, phases of the menstrual cycle and OCs on sports performance. Weaknesses of the evidence in the literature to date as well as areas for future research are also addressed.

Performance parameters

There are many components of sports performance (Table 3.1). Physical fitness is frequently defined by five physiological measures: aerobic fitness, local muscle endurance (anaerobic fitness), muscle strength and power, flexibility and body fat percentage. The relative importance of each depends upon the nature of the given sport. For example, success in long-distance endurance events is determined by a high-performance velocity maintained for a given distance. Other sports rely upon performance

Table 3.1 Components of sports performance. (From Winget *et al.*, 1985)

Sensory–motor: simple reaction time
Psychomotor: hand–eye coordination
Sensory perceptual: pain threshold
Cognitive: information processing
Neuromuscular: strength
Psychological
    Affective: mood
    Psychophysiological: arousal
Cardiovascular
    Heart rate
    Stroke volume
Metabolic
    Core body temperature
    Resting oxygen consumption
Aerobic capacity: $\dot{V}o_{2max}$

power or power output maintained for a given time. Still others require coordination and a steady hand and/or eye for athletic success.

Functionally, the onset of fatigue is linked to lactate concentration. Lactate concentration represents the balance between lactate production by muscle, diffusion into blood and its removal. The degree of muscle and blood lactate accumulation during exercise is also influenced by the amount of muscle mass sharing in the distribution of power output. Energy consumption depends upon oxygen consumption by the working muscles. Morphological components essential to oxygen delivery include heart rate, stroke volume, haemoglobin concentration, muscle capillary density and aerobic enzyme activity.

Power and strength, and aerobic and anaerobic capacity can all be documented quantitatively, but psychological conditions such as mood state, arousal level, etc. are not as easy to measure. Some factors are modifiable through sport-specific training or improvements in equipment. However, there are still a significant number of relevant physiological processes that can be altered by changes in the hormonal milieu, with subsequent implications for female sports performance.

Puberty and sports performance

Prior to puberty there is little difference between male and female athletes in terms of aerobic capacity (Turley & Wilmore, 1997), anaerobic capacity or muscle strength. In young females, menarche signals the monthly variation of the female sex steroids, oestrogen and progesterone. Oestrogen is either directly secreted from the ovary or formed from aromatization of testosterone in peripheral adipose tissues. Oestrogen is responsible for the development of primary and secondary sex characteristics but also plays an important role in fat accumulation and protein anabolism.

There is extensive debate regarding the potential delay in sexual development in female athletes who have been involved in very physical sports from an early age. It has previously been postulated that each year of hard training before puberty delays menarche by 5 months. More recently, these interpretations of the demographic data have been questioned. Stager *et al.* (1990) suggested that it would be more appropriate to state that age of menarche is 'later' rather than 'delayed'. This issue remains controversial, in part due to differences in research design. For example, Plowman *et al.* (1991) examined a cross-sectional group of 73 premenarcheal athletes and 53 non-athletes. Despite a lower percentage body fat in the athletes, the authors concluded that sexual maturation of the athletes was not impaired. In contrast, a recent prospective study from Sweden followed 22 female gymnasts and 22 inactive girls for 5 years, and demonstrated a delay in menarche and a reduction in peak height in the gymnasts (Lindholm *et al.*, 1994).

Menstrual phases

Review of normal menstrual physiology and changes with training

During the course of a normal ovulatory menstrual cycle, many hormonal changes occur in a well-defined predictable pattern. Gonadotrophin-releasing hormone (GnRH) from the hypothalamus initiate secretion of luteinizing hormone (LH) and follicle-stimulating hormone (FSH) at the pituitary level. Subsequent changes in the female sex steroids throughout the menstrual cycle modulate the endocrine events, leading to ovulation and preparation of the uterine endometrium for implantation of a fertilized ovum. During the follicular phase, levels of both oestrogen and progesterone are low. Immediately preceding ovulation, there is a peak in oestrogen levels and a change in the negative feedback to the hypothalamus. During the luteal phase of the cycle, secretion from the corpus luteum results in high concentrations of both hormones. If conception and implantation do not occur, falling levels of hormones cause the lining of the uterus to be shed as menstrual blood flow and the entire process begins anew (Fig. 3.1).

It is well accepted that strenuous physical training in conjunction with other factors such as an inadequate diet can lead to menstrual dysfunction, including short luteal phase, anovulatory cycles and amenorrhoea. It is less well understood whether the endogenous variations in female hormones during an ovulatory menstrual cycle or the administration of exogenous female hormones, such as in OCs or hormonal replacement therapy, have any impact on sports performance. In general, vigorous regular exercise is thought to decrease the physical perturbations related to phases of the menstrual cycle, such as pelvic and low back pain, headache, anxiety, depression and fatigue, and decrease the use of analgesics (Prior et al., 1987). However, there are myriad and complex physiological fluctuations throughout an ovulatory menstrual cycle with potential to alter performance, particularly at the élite level.

Physiological effects of the female sex steroids

The interrelationship of the various sex steroids is detailed in Fig. 3.2. Changing patterns of either endogenous or exogenous hormones may have multiple consequences for the cardiovascular, respiratory and metabolic systems. Depending upon the relative proportion of each hormone, there can be alterations in blood pressure and blood volume, heart rate and vascular tone. Body temperature, electrolyte and water exchange, respiration/ventilation and energy metabolism may also be affected to varying degrees.

ACTIONS OF OESTROGEN

The physiological actions of oestrogens in the body extend well beyond those related to development of secondary sexual characteristics (Bunt, 1990). Oestrogens promote deposition of fat in the typical female areas of the breasts, buttocks and thighs; more importantly, they have a number of significant actions on the cardiovascular system. The decrease in total and low-density lipoprotein cholesterol levels and increase in high-density lipoproteins confer protection against atherosclerosis, while alterations in plasma fibrinolytic activity and platelet aggregation can lead to a detrimental increase in thrombosis. Sodium and chloride retention can cause oedema, weight gain and increase in blood pressure. The latter actions are of particular concern when oestrogens are used in OCs.

Metabolic effects

Metabolic actions of oestrogen include facilitation of glycogen storage and uptake in both liver and muscle. This has been demonstrated in animals and humans. There is also a glycogen-sparing effect at rest and during exercise, with increased lipid synthesis, enhanced lipolysis in muscle and a shift in metabolism towards more utilization of free fatty acids (FFA) for fuel (Bunt, 1990). Compared with their male counterparts, female athletes have been shown to have a greater reliance on fat stores for energy at a specific exercise intensity, as reflected by lower blood lactate and respiratory exchange ratio (RER) values (Tarnolpolsky et al., 1990). Elevated levels of oestrogen promote lipolytic activity. This has been postulated to be due to an alteration of the sensitivity to lipoprotein lipase and by an increase in the levels of human growth

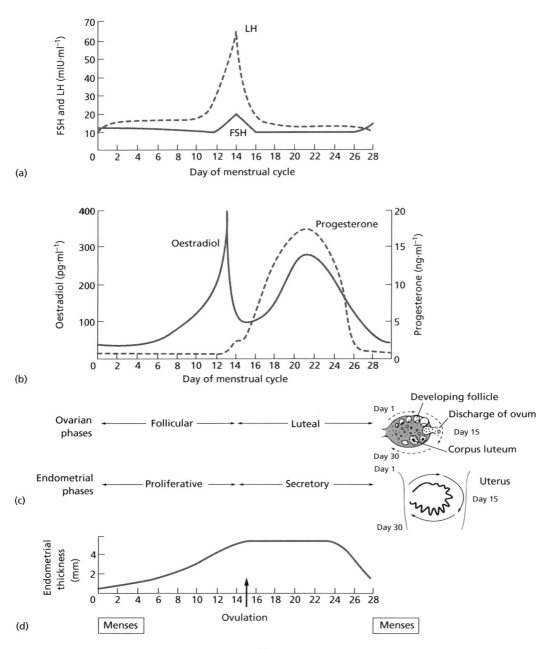

Fig. 3.1 Hormonal events of the menstrual cycle: (a) follicle-stimulating hormone (FSH) and luteinizing hormone (LH), (b) oestradiol and progesterone. (c) Phases of the ovarian and endometrial cycles. (d) Endometrial thickness throughout the menstrual cycle. (Adapted from Shangold & Mirkin, 1994.)

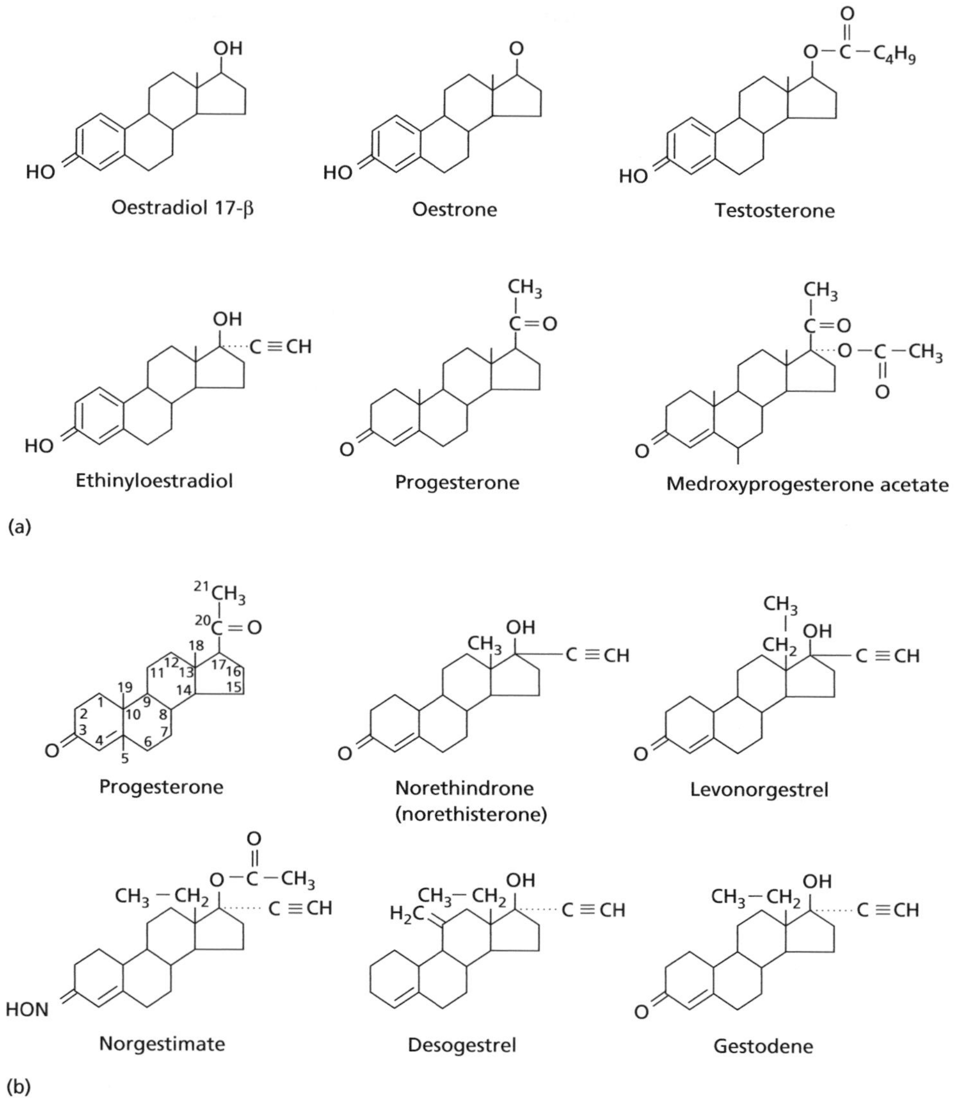

Fig. 3.2 Structural formulae of (a) the major sex steroids, and (b) progesterone and synthetic progestins used in oral contraceptives and contraceptive progestins.

hormone (GH), an activator of lipolysis (Ruby & Robergs, 1994). Recently, transdermal oestradiol has also been shown to modify glucose metabolism at rest and during moderate exercise as a result of decreased gluconeogenesis, adrenaline secretion and changes in glucose transport (Ruby

et al., 1997). These actions of oestrogens on substrate metabolism could potentially enhance sports performance, particularly for endurance and ultra-endurance events.

Effects on blood glucose and lactate production are less well characterized. However, it is known that oestradiol can precipitate glucose intolerance as a result of insulin insensitivity (Diamond *et al.*, 1988). With increasing doses of oestrogen or administration of synthetic oestrogens in OCs, the secondary effects of oestrogens (primarily an increase in corticosteroid activity) predominate, leading to deterioration in glucose tolerance and insulin resistance (Godsland, 1996). In addition, the metabolism of energy substrates probably varies with the subnormal levels of gonadotrophic hormones that occur secondary to menstrual dysfunction in female athletes.

Another essential action of oestrogen is the facilitation of calcium uptake into bone. Women with oligomenorrhoea or amenorrhoea may have a chronic oestrogen deficiency state similar to that of postmenopausal women and are susceptible to premature osteoporosis. Current clinical guidelines suggest the therapeutic use of replacement hormones such as OCs or various combinations of oestrogen and progesterone for protection of bone density in these populations. In this group of athletic women, the potential for hormonal effects on substrates for sports performance is a critical issue.

ACTIONS OF PROGESTERONE

In many ways, the progestin group of hormones have 'anti-oestrogenic' effects that seem to be proportional to their androgenicity. They can significantly modify body composition, thermoregulation, cardiorespiratory function and haemodynamics. Core body temperature is elevated by 0.3–0.5°C during the luteal phase of a normal menstrual cycle, giving the classic 'biphasic' curve characteristic of ovulation.

Respiratory effects

Minute ventilation and the hypercapneic and hypoxic respiratory drives are increased during the luteal phase (England & Fahri, 1976; Schoene *et al.*, 1981). In untrained subjects, this subjective sense of dyspnoea has been demonstrated to impair sports performance (Schoene *et al.*, 1981),

although it is likely that in more fit individuals the effects of training mitigate this to some degree.

Effects on fluid balance

Fluid dynamics are also altered under the simultaneous influence of progesterone and/or oestrogen, depending upon the ratio of the two hormones. Progesterone antagonizes the effects of aldosterone, which then leads to increased excretion of water and sodium from the kidney. This natriuresis in turn stimulates the renin–angiotensin system, which paradoxically increases aldosterone secretion and promotes an increase in antidiuretic hormone, thought to contribute to postovulatory fluid retention. Although it would seem that premenstrual symptoms might somehow be associated with these changes in fluid dynamics, a recent study was not able to correlate subjective breast tenderness and bloating with sodium retention in the luteal phase of the cycle (Olson *et al.*, 1996).

Metabolic effects

In terms of substrate metabolism, progestins cause a shift towards a greater dependence on fat. This is evidenced by lower RER values, lower blood lactate levels during submaximal exercise (Dombovy *et al.*, 1987) and higher circulating FFA (Reinke *et al.*, 1972). With special relevance for the population of female athletes, medroxyprogesterone acetate (Depo-Provera), administered intramuscularly (150 mg every 3 months) for contraception, has been found to cause deterioration of glucose tolerance or hyperinsulinaemia or both, possibly because of its glucocorticoid-like actions (Godsland, 1996).

Godsland (1996) has also summarized the research findings on the metabolic actions of the synthetic progestogens. The synthetic gonane progestogen levonorgestrel has been shown to induce deterioration in glucose tolerance and increased insulin levels when taken at a dose of 75 μg daily as a progestogen-only OC. The oestrane progestogens, ethynodiol diacetate and norethisterone (or norethindrone), appear to have little effect on glucose and insulin levels. There is insufficient information on the newer progestogens, desogestrel, gestodene and norgestimate, regarding their impact on glucose tolerance and insulin responses.

Hormones and cognitive functions

During the course of an ovulatory menstrual cycle, the luteal phase increase in both oestrogen and progesterone can cause a variety of symptoms collectively termed molimina. These include fluid retention, lateral breast tenderness, and appetite and mood changes. In moderation, this is a normal phenomenon and serves as a clinical indicator that the neuroendocrine axis is functioning adequately and that ovulation is occurring (Magyar et al., 1979). In most healthy young women these hormone-induced somatic changes are not accompanied by marked affective aberrations (Laessle et al., 1990). In some women, however, these symptoms are more troublesome and are termed premenstrual syndrome (PMS) (Mortola, 1996). Menstruation itself generally leads to relief from these symptoms but can be accompanied by dysmenorrhoea or significant menstrual cramps in association with prostaglandin-mediated uterine contractions. Both PMS and dysmenorrhoea can be disruptive to optimal sports performance on a cyclical basis. Fortunately, there is evidence that these symptoms can be somewhat ameliorated by regular physical exercise (Prior et al., 1987; Cowart, 1989). Antiprostaglandin medications are commonly prescribed for treatment of the discomfort of dysmenorrhoea.

There are other cognitive impacts of the female hormones, oestrogen in particular, that may also theoretically impair or enhance performance but which have not been systematically researched in athletes. In premenopausal women, changes in oestrogen levels are positively correlated with serotonin levels, serotonin being involved in the pathway for neurovascular headache. In low-oestrogen states (such as during menses, the placebo week of OCs or the postpartum period),

peripheral serotonin levels decrease causing an increase in migraines (Marcus, 1995). In postmenopausal women, oestrogen has been noted in a number of studies to have a beneficial effect on cognitive function and verbal memory, which may be modulated through alterations in the concentration and availability of neurotransmitters, including serotonin, in the brain. Oestrogen is also thought possibly to be protective against early onset of Alzheimer's dementia (Sherwin, 1996). It is interesting to speculate on potential future psychiatric implications of a prolonged hypooestrogenic state during the reproductive years in amenorrhoeic athletes.

Early studies of menstrual cycle and performance

Early anecdotal and retrospective studies on the effects of cycle phase on performance are inconsistent, although athletes generally reported their performances to be 'best' in the intermenstrual or immediate postmenstrual phase and 'worst' during the premenstrual phase (Erdelyi, 1962; Zaharieva, 1965; Bale & Davies, 1983; Lebrun, 1993, 1994). Some postulated mediators of these effects of the menstrual cycle include self-expectancies, a negative attitude towards menstruation, cultural restrictions and myths, and the coexistence of disturbing menstrual or premenstrual symptoms (Wells, 1991). Nevertheless, world records have been set and gold medals won by women in any phase of the cycle.

The major underlying fault of these early surveys, in addition to the known shortcomings of retrospective studies, was a failure adequately to identify the phase of the cycle. Basal body temperature (BBT) curves have been shown to be inaccurate in establishing cycle phase (Bauman, 1981). Quantitative analysis of BBT curves is slightly more efficacious in predicting the timing of ovulation and length of the luteal phase (Prior et al., 1990). More recently, urine testing to detect the mid-cycle LH surge has proved useful for estimation of the time of ovulation (Miller & Soules, 1996); however, adequate characterization of follicular, ovulatory and luteal phases of the cycle demands accurate documentation by serum hormonal measurements (Abraham *et al.*, 1974). These measurements must be made before exercise, as levels of both oestrogen and progesterone are thought to rise with exercise via alterations in hormone secretion or metabolic clearance (Jurkowski *et al.*, 1978; Bonen *et al.*, 1979). In contrast, Montagnani *et al.* (1992) found an increase in metabolic clearance rate with a 2-hour continuous treadmill test, leading to a decrease in hormone concentrations with exercise. It is probable that the wide circadian variation in hormonal secretion in normal women contributes to the incongruity of these results.

The first attempts to quantify scientifically these perceived differences in athletic performance were also flawed by numerous problems. Discrepancies in the timing of testing, inaccurate documentation of cycle phase, the use of small numbers of untrained subjects and a variety of physiological tests make accurate interpretation of the results difficult if not impossible. Testing protocols have generally used either a treadmill or cycle ergometer and have measured $\dot{V}_{O_{2max}}$ or submaximal oxygen uptake. Field studies examining the performance of adolescent swimmers found it best in the postmenstrual or menstrual phase and worst in the premenstrual phase or at the beginning of menses (Bale & Nelson, 1985; Brooks-Gunn *et al.*, 1986), while similar testing in older swimmers did not reveal any performance changes (Quadagno *et al.*, 1991). A study of cross-country skiers, using BBT and cervical mucus to pinpoint cycle phase, showed performance to be best in the postovulatory and postmenstrual phases (Fomin *et al.*, 1989). Others have observed a higher incidence of injuries in female soccer players during the premenstrual and menstrual phases, especially in those women with significant premenstrual symptoms (Möller-Nielson & Hammar, 1989). Dalton (1960) hypothesized lowered judgement and slower reaction time as causative factors for an increased accident rate during these phases. The results of these early studies are summarized in further detail elsewhere (Lebrun, 1993, 1994). There appears to be great interindividual variability in responses of female athletes to these cyclical hormonal changes.

Menstrual cycle and cardiovascular variables

As previously discussed, both oestrogen and progesterone can influence the cardiovascular system with different effects predominating at different phases of the cycle. Decreasing levels of oestrogen, such as seen in amenorrhoeic athletes, may increase peripheral resistance and decrease exercising muscle blood flow. During the menstrual cycle, changes in both oestrogen and progesterone levels have been shown to alter forearm skin blood flow and vascular reactivity (Bungum *et al.*, 1996), although the exact mechanisms remain speculative. Sita and Miller (1996) noted that higher oestradiol levels at different phases of the menstrual cycle contribute to a lowering of the cardiovascular responses to stress, most likely through an effect on arterial wall tone as well as a decrease in β-receptor sensitivity to catecholamines.

On the other hand, progesterone may increase cardiac excitability by its opposing effects on oestrogen. Rosano *et al.* (1996) documented an increase in the number and duration of episodes of paroxysmal supraventricular tachycardia during the late luteal phase that was positively correlated with plasma progesterone levels and inversely correlated with plasma oestradiol levels. Birch and Reilly (1997) examined cyclic variations in physiological responses to repeated lifting. They found that the heart rate response was elevated by approximately 10 beats min^{-1} during the postovulatory phase of cycle. Other investigators have also demonstrated a higher heart rate during this phase and have suggested that greater cardiovascular strain occurs at this time (Schoene *et al.*, 1981; Hessemer & Bruck, 1985b; Pivarnik *et al.*, 1992). These fluctuations in functional capacity are also associated temporally with body temperature and body mass increases, so it is difficult to pinpoint the cause with any certainty.

Oestrogen-related vasodilation, increased capillary membrane permeability/reactivity and possible shifts in plasma volume in the luteal phase may require cardiovascular compensation. The only study that has examined this in any detail did not use serum progesterone measurements (Gaebelein & Senay, 1982). A more recent study, utilizing menstrual diaries and BBT changes only, noted transient increases in plasma volume during the menstrual cycle that reached an initial peak within 2 days of the estimated day of ovulation and progressively increased during the luteal phase, peaking 2–3 days prior to menstruation (Fortney et al., 1994). Van Beek et al. (1996) studied peripheral haemodynamics and renal function during the follicular and luteal phases of the cycle in nine ovulatory subjects. Arterial blood pressure, vascular tone and blood flow to forearm and kidneys were similar, but the blood flow to the skin was consistently lower and the glomerular filtration rate higher during the luteal phase of the cycle. Any changes in haemoglobin concentration that have been documented over the menstrual cycle are small and probably due to shifts in plasma volume. Given the overriding adaptations of the cardiovascular system to exercise, it is doubtful that these cycle-phase alterations in haemodynamics significantly affect exercise performance.

Menstrual cycle and respiratory function

Under the influence of higher progesterone levels, minute ventilation and maximal exercise response are increased during the luteal phase, as is respiratory drive (Schoene et al., 1981; Dombovy et al., 1987; Dutton et al., 1989). Respiratory muscle endurance is also affected by cycle phase, being greatest in the luteal phase (Chen & Tang, 1989). It has been suggested that the pulmonary diffusing capacity of carbon monoxide (DL_{CO}) is lowest on the third day of menstrual flow (9% decrease) when progesterone and oestrogen levels are low and highest just prior to menses, with no associated changes in haemoglobin or carboxyhaemoglobin (Sansores et al., 1995). However, this particular study did not use serum progesterone levels to measure cycle phase. Endogenous carbon monoxide produc-

tion varies with menstrual phase, being twice as great in the progesterone phase as in the oestrogen phase (Coburn, 1970).

Endurance-trained athletes exhibit decreased hypoxic and hypercapneic respiratory drives both at rest and during exercise and this is thought to be a factor in their success. Therefore, any menstrual-cycle changes that affect respiratory drives have the potential to interfere with performance. The increase in hypercapneic ventilatory response is believed to be due to the ability of progesterone to lower the threshold of the medullary respiratory centre and increase its excitability. The higher ventilatory rate during the luteal phase of the cycle is associated with a greater oxygen demand as well as subjective dyspnoea. However, Schoene et al. (1981) reported no significant cycle-phase differences in exercise performance in eumenorrhoeic athletes in contrast to non-athletes, who had a greater perceived exertion during the luteal phase.

A recent phenomenon that has been identified is hormonal interaction and airway dysfunction in a subgroup of female asthmatic patients. The effect appears to be greater in severe compared with mild asthma (Gibbs et al., 1984). Premenstrual aggravation of asthma can be seen in 15–20% of female patients with asthma, although on many occasions the women themselves are unaware of this variation. Pauli et al. (1989) monitored the effect of cycle phase documented by hormonal measurements on daily records of asthma symptoms and measurements of peak expiratory flow rate in 11 asthmatic and 29 control subjects. The authors found an increase in asthma symptoms from the follicular to the luteal phases and a decrease in morning peak flows. Nevertheless, there were no correlations between changes in spirometry, airway reactivity as measured by a methacholine challenge test and absolute levels of either circulating progesterone or oestrogen. In another study, only 5 of 14 women reported premenstrual worsening of asthma symptoms at the time of enrolment, but all 14 had >20% decrease in peak expiratory flow rate and/or increase in symptoms premenstrually during the study itself (Chandler et al., 1997).

Administration of exogenous oestradiol resulted in a significant improvement in asthma symptoms and dyspnoea index scores, an effect that did not appear to be related to β_2 receptors.

The relevance of these findings remains speculative. In addition, it is thought that ventilation at rest is controlled by central and peripheral chemoreceptors, while during exercise neurogenic factors predominate. The changing hormonal patterns during the menstrual cycle may affect ventilatory control mechanisms differentially. It would be interesting to focus on the population of female athletes with asthma and more specifically those women with exercise-induced asthma.

Menstrual cycle and thermoregulation

The most obvious parameter to change throughout an ovulatory menstrual cycle is core body temperature, due to the central thermogenic action of progesterone. Carpenter and Nunneley (1988), among others, have documented the luteal-phase increase in core body temperature along with a slight fall in temperature around the time of ovulation. The exact dynamics of these shifts have been the basis of many studies; however, it is extremely difficult to separate thermoregulation from fluid volume or cardiovascular regulation. Frascarolo et al. (1990) measured metabolic heat production by indirect calorimetry and total heat loss by direct calorimetry and did not observe any significant changes between follicular and luteal phases (as documented by progesterone levels). They postulated that a decrease in thermal conductance allowed for maintenance of a higher internal temperature. Grucza et al. (1993) reported a greater temperature threshold and larger gains for sweating during the luteal phase compared with the follicular phase. Hirata et al. (1986) did not find any menstrual-phase differences in finger blood flow during exercise, and proposed that the thermoregulatory vasodilator response was attenuated by increasing exercise-induced vasoconstrictor tone in proportion to exercise intensity. During the luteal phase, the shift to a higher core or mean body temperature for the onset of a sudomotor, vasomotor and shivering response appears to be moderated by changes in either the central thermoreceptor cycle with no changes in either the thermosensitivity or the slope of the response (Kolka & Stephenson, 1989; Stephenson & Kolka, 1993).

In terms of sports performance, there are some hypothetical disadvantages for women performing prolonged exercise in the heat during the luteal phase of their cycle. Some investigators have demonstrated the variation in core temperature but no differences in response to short-term exercise or heat exposure (Wells & Horvath, 1973, 1974; Stephenson et al., 1982; Hessemer & Bruck, 1985a,b). Others have found an increase in heart rate and rating of perceived exertion (RPE) at the same intensity of exercise during the luteal phase (Schoene et al., 1981; Hessemer & Bruck, 1985b; Pivarnik et al., 1992; Birch & Reilly, 1997) and theorized a greater degree of cardiovascular strain. Differences in the thresholds for shivering and sweating have also been corroborated without any measurable impact on performance (Hessemer & Bruck, 1985a).

Menstrual cycle and metabolic rate

Energy and macronutrient intakes vary across the course of an ovulatory menstrual cycle as does energy expenditure. Basal and sleeping metabolic rates are elevated during the postovulatory or luteal phase and are lowest just before ovulation (Solomon et al., 1982; Bisdee et al., 1989). The putative cause is thought to be the increase in progesterone levels, but the associated temperature changes may also be a factor. Greater 24-hour energy expenditure has also been noted during the luteal phase (Webb, 1986). In a study by Dalvit (1981), energy intakes were approximately $2.1\,kJ\cdot day^{-1}$ ($0.5\,kcal\cdot day^{-1}$) higher during the 10 days before the onset of menses than after, but there were no hormonal measurements to substantiate cycle phase or examine correlations. Barr et al. (1995) also found that spontaneous energy intakes varied according to the phase of the cycle, being greater during the luteal phase. Interestingly, anovulatory women did not show any differences.

Menstrual cycle and substrate metabolism

As both oestrogen and progesterone promote glycogen uptake and storage and modify glycogen utilization, theoretically energy metabolism should be more efficient during the luteal phase when both oestrogen and progesterone levels are high. Muscle biopsy data have revealed an increase in muscle glycogen storage during this time (Nicklas *et al.*, 1989) that was associated with a non-significant trend towards improved endurance times on a cycle ergometer at 70% $\dot{V}O_{2max}$. Another study found that resting muscle glycogen was highest during the time of ovulation (Hackney, 1990). There is also thought to be greater protein catabolism during exercise in the luteal phase as measured by increased urea nitrogen excretion (Lamont *et al.*, 1987).

Blood lactate levels during different phases of the menstrual cycle are contradictory. Eston and Burke (1984) studied exercise responses in 21 physical education students and did not find any difference in lactate or RPE values or any other physiological parameters. However, the luteal phase was only documented by an increase in BBT of 0.4°C. Of the studies utilizing hormonal measurements, several have suggested a luteal-phase decrease in lactate production associated with an increase in endurance time (Jurkowski *et al.*, 1978, 1981; Dombovy *et al.*, 1987; Lavoie *et al.*, 1987). Others have not replicated this enhanced luteal-phase performance (Lebrun, 1995). Many other authors have been unable to demonstrate any significant differences in lactate during the menstrual cycle (Bonen *et al.*, 1983; Lamont, 1986; De Souza *et al.*, 1990; Kanaley *et al.*, 1992; Bemben *et al.*, 1995). This may be due to discrepancies in testing protocol, exercise intensity or pre-exercise nutritional status.

Some investigators have documented a lower RER during the luteal phase, suggesting an increased reliance on FFA for fuel, while others have not. One author documented greater fat utilization and oxidation at ovulation under the influence of higher oestrogen levels (Hackney, 1990). In another study, Hackney *et al.* (1994) further examined the responses of substrate metabolism to progressively increasing intensi-

ties of submaximal treadmill exercise (10 min at 35%, 10 min at 60% and 10 min at 75% $\dot{V}O_{2max}$) in nine eumenorrhoeic women. Cycle phases were determined by measurements of BBT but substantiated by urinary total oestrogen and pregnanediol (progesterone metabolite). At the low and moderate exercise intensities, carbohydrate utilization and oxidation rates were lower during the mid-luteal phase in association with greater lipid utilization and oxidation. At the highest exercise intensity, no differences in substrate metabolism were discernible between testing phases. However, a more recent study (also using BBT in association with urinary hormone levels) did find a difference in lactate levels at 3 and 30 min into recovery following an incremental treadmill run to exhaustion (McCracken *et al.*, 1994). There were no differences between mid-follicular and mid-luteal phases in either resting blood lactate levels or running time to exhaustion in the nine athletes in this study. Recovery lactate levels, however, were significantly lower during the luteal phase, again suggesting a preferential metabolism of lipid and a reduction in the degree of carbohydrate metabolized.

Investigations in this area are greatly influenced by the level of training and relative fitness of the individual. Subjects should also be carbohydrate replete in order to minimize any bias due to compromised nutrition. There appears to be a deterioration in carbohydrate metabolism during the luteal phase of the menstrual cycle. The complex metabolic effects of the female sex steroids lead to elevated glucose levels, increased area under the curve of a glucose tolerance test and glycosuria, although again nutritional status is a confounding variable. Other investigators have not shown a substantial change in blood glucose during the cycle (Nicklas *et al.*, 1989; Bonen *et al.*, 1991; Kanaley *et al.*, 1992).

Menstrual cycle and strength

Investigators have looked at various indices such as handgrip strength, strength and endurance of knee flexion and extension, leg press and bench press throughout the menstrual cycle. The majority of these studies have not noted any significant effects of menstrual phase, although they have been carried out without hormonal documentation (Higgs & Robertson, 1981; Dibrezzo *et al.*, 1991; Quadagno *et al.*, 1991). The only prospective study of this nature using hormonal measurements (Lebrun, 1995) did not find any variation in isokinetic strength of knee flexion and extension between follicular and luteal phases.

Several of the earliest studies have shown slight but contradictory variations. For example, the best achievement in hip strength (flexion and extension) and standing broad jump in a group of collegiate volleyball and basketball players was found during the premenstrual phase (Wearing *et al.*, 1972). One study (using BBT only) demonstrated a decrease in isometric handgrip endurance of forearm contraction during the luteal phase (Petrofsky *et al.*, 1976), with the highest value in the ovulatory phase and the lowest midway through the luteal phase. There was no difference over the menstrual cycle in the isometric strength of the forearm muscles. Wirth and Lohman (1982) found that maximal voluntary contraction of handgrip was significantly greater during the follicular phase. Davies *et al.* (1991) investigated changes in handgrip strength and standing long jump during the menstrual, ovulatory and luteal phases. They found a significantly stronger handgrip during the menstrual phase and attributed this to lower oestrogen and progesterone levels, despite the fact that they did not have any supportive evidence from blood measurements.

Testosterone has the potential to play a role in the variation in strength during the menstrual cycle because testosterone receptors are present in muscle, and blood levels of this hormone are increased at the time of ovulation. However, there is also a suggestion that strength peaks during the follicular phase just before ovulation (Phillips *et al.*, 1996) or at mid-cycle (Sarwar *et al.*, 1996) due to the stimulatory effect of oestrogen. There was no direct correlation with oestradiol levels in the study by Phillips *et al.* (1996), but if the mechanism is through the classic steroid

receptors it is possible that oestrogen has a delayed onset of action. The magnitude of the change is about 10–11%, and in one study was accompanied by a significant slowing of relaxation and increase in fatiguability at mid-cycle (Sarwar *et al.*, 1996). Progesterone does not appear to have any substantial effects on muscle strength or function.

Other investigators have demonstrated oestrogen and progesterone receptors localized to synoviocytes in the synovial lining of the knee, fibroblasts in the stroma of the anterior cruciate ligament and cells in the blood vessel walls of the ligaments in both males and females (Liu *et al.*, 1996). There are potential implications for increased laxity of the anterior cruciate ligament during the luteal phase. This may be one mechanism explaining the increased incidence of anterior cruciate ligament injuries in female soccer and basketball players compared with males at the same competitive level (Arendt & Dick, 1995), although other neuromuscular performance characteristics, such as gender differences in muscle strength, recruitment order and peak torque production, are probably of more importance (Huston & Wojtys, 1996).

Menstrual cycle and aerobic performance

In general, maximal oxygen capacity and submaximal exercise responses do not appear to be altered during a regular ovulatory menstrual cycle (De Souza *et al.*, 1990; Bemben *et al.*, 1995). The results of research using hormonal documentation of cycle phase are summarized in Table 3.2. One study of 16 élite athletes did find a slight decrement in $\dot{V}_{O_{2max}}$ of borderline statistical significance during the luteal phase (Lebrun, 1995). Some investigators have found a luteal-phase increase in oxygen consumption that was abolished by subsequent exercise (Wells & Horvath, 1974). Others have measured a 5.2% increase in $\dot{V}_{O_2}$ during exercise associated with a 5.6% increase in metabolic rate and a 5.3% decrease in net efficiency during the luteal phase (Hessemer & Bruck, 1985b).

Running economy, defined as the rate of

Table 3.2 Effects of menstrual-cycle phase on sports performance: studies with hormonal documentation of cycle phase. (Adapted from Lebrun, 1993)

Reference	No. of subjects	$\dot{V}O_{2max}$	Performance tests	Results
Bemben et al. (1995)	5	~ 3.0 l·min⁻¹	$\dot{V}O_{2max}$ (treadmill), incremental to exhaustion	No significant differences between early/late follicular and mid-luteal phases in $\dot{V}O_{2max}$, maximum ventilation, post-exercise lactate and time to exhaustion. However relative ventilatory threshold at higher percentage of $\dot{V}O_{2max}$ in early-follicular compared with mid-luteal and late-follicular phases
De Souza et al. (1990)	8 (N, T) 8 (A, T)	53.4 ml·kg⁻¹·min⁻¹ 55.4 ml·kg⁻¹·min⁻¹	$\dot{V}O_{2max}$ (treadmill) Submaximal test: 40 min at 80% $\dot{V}O_{2max}$	No significant differences in $\dot{V}O_{2max}$ or in any submaximal tests in either group or between phases
Dombovy et al. (1987)	8 (U)	34.4 ml·kg⁻¹·min⁻¹	$\dot{V}O_{2max}$ (bicycle ergometer); then constant load for 4 min above and below anaerobic threshold	No significant differences in $\dot{V}O_{2max}$, maximum exercise duration, work efficiency or maximum workload
Hackney et al. (1994)	9 (T)	46.0 ± 2.6 ml·kg⁻¹·min⁻¹	30-min graded treadmill run: 1–10 min, ~ 35% $\dot{V}O_{2max}$ 11–20 min, ~ 60 $\dot{V}O_{2max}$ 21–30 min, ~ 75% $\dot{V}O_{2max}$	No significant differences in $\dot{V}E$, $\dot{V}O_2$ or $\dot{V}CO_2$ between phases; mean RER at 35% and 60% intensities is lower in mid-luteal compared with mid-follicular phase
Hessemer & Bruck (1985b)	4 (U) 6 (T)	2.81 l·min⁻¹	Bicycle ergometer: 15 min at 18°C between 03.00 and 04.00	5.2% increase in mean $\dot{V}O_2$, 5.6% increase in metabolic rate and 5.3% decrease in net efficiency during luteal phase
Horvath & Drinkwater (1982)	4 (T)	39.0 ml·kg⁻¹·min⁻¹	Treadmill walk at 30% $\dot{V}O_{2max}$ at 28, 35 and 48°C	Highest resting $\dot{V}O_{2max}$ during luteal phase. Greater relative decrease in plasma volume during luteal phase following exercise at 48°C
Jurkowski et al. (1981)	9 (T)	41.8 ml·kg⁻¹·min⁻¹	Bicycle ergometer: 20 min at 30–35% $\dot{V}O_{2max}$ 20 min at 60–66% $\dot{V}O_{2max}$ 85–90% $\dot{V}O_{2max}$ to exhaustion	Time to exhaustion longer in luteal phase (1.57 ± 0.32 vs. 2.97 ± 0.63 min)

Continued p. 50

Table 3.2 (*Continued*)

Reference	No. of subjects	$\dot{V}O_{2max}$	Performance tests	Results
Lebrun (1995)	16 (T)	$53.7\,ml\cdot kg^{-1}\cdot min^{-1}$ $3.19\,l\cdot min^{-1}$	$\dot{V}O_{2max}$ (treadmill); time to exhaustion at 90% $\dot{V}O_{2max}$; anaerobic endurance	Slight decrease in $\dot{V}O_{2max}$ in luteal phase ($P = 0.04$), no other significant differences
McCracken *et al.* (1994)	9 (T)	$46.0 \pm 2.6\,ml\cdot kg^{-1}\cdot min^{-1}$	Treadmill run: 1–10 min at 35% $\dot{V}O_{2max}$ 11–20 min at 60% $\dot{V}O_{2max}$ 21–30 min at 75% $\dot{V}O_{2max}$ then at ~ 90% $\dot{V}O_{2max}$ to exhaustion	No differences in running time to exhaustion or in resting lactate levels; but recovery lactates at ~ 3 and 30 min after exercise lower in luteal phase
Nicklas *et al.* (1989)	6 (T)	$44.9\,ml\cdot kg^{-1}\cdot min^{-1}$	Bicycle ergometer: exercise to exhaustion, 90 min at 60% $\dot{V}O_{2max}$ followed by four 1-min sprints at 100% $\dot{V}O_{2max}$ 3 days rest, 60% carbohydrate diet, exercise time to fatigue at 70% $\dot{V}O_{2max}$, muscle biopsies for glycogen	Borderline increase in endurance time during luteal phase ($P < 0.07$), associated with increased muscle glycogen
Pivarnik *et al.* (1992)	9 (T)	$43.2\,ml\cdot kg^{-1}\cdot min^{-1}$	Bicycle ergometer: 60 min at 65% $\dot{V}O_{2max}$	No significant differences in performance, but an increase in cardiovascular strain and RPE during luteal phase
Robertson & Higgs (1983)	14		12-min submaximal run at 90% $\dot{V}O_{2max}$; all-out run at 100% $\dot{V}O_{2max}$	Endurance performance decreased in early menses compared with mid-follicular phase and increased in mid-luteal phase
Schoene *et al.* (1981)	6 (U) 6 (N, T) 6 (A, T)	$35.2\,ml\cdot kg^{-1}\cdot min^{-1}$ $49.6\,ml\cdot kg^{-1}\cdot min^{-1}$	$\dot{V}O_{2max}$ (bicycle ergometer): exercise time to exhaustion	Maximal exercise response better in follicular phase in non-athletes only
Williams and Krahenbuhl (1997)	8 (T)	$50.7 \pm 2.8\,ml\cdot kg^{-1}\cdot min^{-1}$	At rest and running on treadmill at speeds of 55 and 80% of $\dot{V}O_{2max}$; five cycle phases	Resting $\dot{V}O_{2}$ and ventilation higher in mid-luteal compared with mid-follicular phase; running economy at 55% $\dot{V}O_{2max}$ not different, but at 80% $\dot{V}O_{2max}$, economy significantly less in mid-luteal phase

A, amenorrhoeic; N, eumenorrhoeic; T, trained; U, untrained.
RER, respiratory exchange ratio; RPE, rating of perceived exertion.

oxygen consumption ($\dot{V}O_2$) during a given submaximal steady-state running speed, is probably a more accurate indicator of performance than maximal oxygen capacity. Williams and Krahenbuhl (1997) studied eight eumenorrhoeic runners at rest and at speeds corresponding to 55% and 80% of their maximal oxygen consumption. Measurements of $\dot{V}O_2$, progesterone and mood scores were taken at five different phases of the cycle: early follicular, late follicular, early luteal, mid-luteal and late luteal. At 80%, but not at 55%, of maximal speed, running economy was significantly less during the mid-luteal compared with the early-follicular phase. There were associated changes in ventilatory drives and fluctuations in mood state (Williams & Krahenbuhl, 1997).

Oral contraceptives

Contraceptive options for the female athlete

Athletic women during their reproductive years frequently require contraception. 'Natural' family planning is not usually a viable option because of the high prevalence of menstrual-cycle alterations in this physically active population. Spermicides and barrier methods, such as the condom, diaphragm or cervical cap, are popular due to lack of side-effects, including any perceived impact on performance. In addition, they provide protection from sexually transmitted diseases; however, they are less reliable than other methods and demand responsibility and consistency of use. The intrauterine device is more effective in preventing pregnancy but has the disadvantage of increasing menstrual cramping and monthly blood loss, both of which may adversely affect the competitive female athlete.

Previous estimates have suggested that 12–42% of female athletes preferentially use OCs (Shangold & Levine, 1982; Jarrett & Spellacy, 1983). This proportion is somewhat lower than in the general population but has probably increased in recent years. OCs are prescribed not only for contraception but also for cycle control,

management of dysmenorrhoea and PMS as well as for protection of bone density (Haberland *et al.*, 1995). In the absence of medical contraindications (Table 3.3), they can now be safely administered to women from either the age of 16 or 3 years past menarche (Committee on Sports Medicine, American Academy of Pediatrics, 1989) until the perimenopausal years. Despite the known health benefits of OCs (Table 3.4), many athletes still fear alterations in their sports performance. Given that a wide age range of physically active females may be taking these medications, it is somewhat surprising that relatively little is known in this area.

Table 3.3 Contraindications to oral contraceptives

Absolute contraindications
Thromboembolic disorders
Cerebrovascular accident
Coronary occlusion
Impaired liver function
Oestrogen-dependent neoplasia
Undiagnosed vaginal bleeding
Carcinoma of the breast

Relative contraindications
Hypertension [diastolic blood pressure > 90 mmHg (> 12 kPa)]
Hyperlipidaemia
Abnormal glucose tolerance
Renal, hepatic or gallbladder disease
Migraine headaches
Depression
Recent major elective surgery

Table 3.4 Health benefits of oral contraceptives

Elimination or reduction in dysmenorrhoea
Reduction in menstrually induced iron-deficiency anaemia
Reduced risk of endometrial and ovarian cancer
Reduced incidence of benign breast lesions, pelvic inflammatory disease, ovarian cysts, ectopic pregnancy, rheumatoid arthritis
Reduced risk of endometrial hyperplasia
Prevention of premature osteoporosis in amenorrhoeic athletes

Side-effects of oral contraceptives

Early contraceptive preparations consisted of much higher dosages than those in current use: contemporary OCs have a threefold to fourfold decrease in oestrogen content and a 10-fold decrease in progestin. In addition, the development of the second- and third-generation progestins has further attenuated adverse androgenic effects such as weight gain and fluid retention. As a result, it is likely that any significant changes in athletic performance are also lessened.

For both the younger and more mature athlete, beneficial side-effects include a reduction in dysmenorrhoea, PMS, menorrhagia and iron-deficiency anaemia secondary to excessive monthly blood loss. The frequency of dysfunctional uterine bleeding, common in both adolescents and perimenopausal women, is diminished (Burkman, 1994). A decrease in functional ovarian cysts and benign breast disease may also contribute to improved quality of active daily life for training and competition (Grimes, 1992).

Reports of significant adverse effects, such as mood and libido changes, headache, melanoma, gallbladder disease, liver tumours, exacerbation of sickle-cell disease, teratogenesis and 'postpill' amenorrhoea or infertility, have largely been disproved by better analysis of the existing data (Goldzieher & Zamah, 1995). Of more concern are potential cardiovascular and thrombotic complications, including myocardial infarction, embolic stroke and venous thrombosis (Carr & Ory, 1997). Healthy non-smoking women who are current or past users of OCs do not appear to have an increased risk of either myocardial infarction or stroke. In fact, the oestrogen in OCs may have direct cardioprotective effects on the walls of the coronary vessels. The oestrogen component of OCs also exerts a favourable action on lipoproteins, which may be opposed by the non-beneficial effect of the progestin component.

Oral contraceptives and the cardiovascular system

As previously discussed, the steroid hormones can precipitate certain alterations in the haematological and cardiovascular systems, although there is not universal agreement on any corresponding impact on performance. Research in this area is complicated by multiple factors, including the wide range of OCs on the market, the fitness level of the subjects, testing protocols and exercise-induced shifts in plasma volume. Antithrombin III, which accounts for at least 50% of the anticoagulant activity of the blood, is primarily affected in a dose-dependent fashion by the oestrogen component of the pill. Oestrogen also causes enhanced platelet aggregation and an increase in various coagulation factors. Formulations containing 35 µg or less of ethinyloestradiol theoretically have a lower thrombogenic potential, and there is evidence that administration of such an OC containing norethindrone did not have any adverse effects on haemostatic mechanisms in moderately active women (Notelovitz et al., 1987).

Regular physical activity has many health benefits in terms of prevention of coronary artery disease and atherosclerosis. Are female athletes who take OCs introducing a significant cardiovascular risk factor that may negate the advantages of their improved fitness levels? Exercise itself has an anticoagulatory effect and has been observed to act synergistically with some OCs to increase fibrinolytic activity (Huisveld et al., 1982, 1983). A more recent paper reported that the changes in the fibrinolytic system induced by physical exercise are not affected by OCs (De Paz et al., 1995). Detrimental changes in serum triglycerides, cholesterol and blood pressure are minimized by OCs containing the newer progestins, but are still detectable. In addition, regular conditioning exercise appears to attenuate any observed impact on plasma lipids (Gray et al., 1983; Merians et al., 1985).

Increases in blood pressure are usually manifest during the first few months of use, may diminish over time and are generally reversible on discontinuation of the pill. The postulated mechanism is related to increased liver synthesis of angiotensinogen, a precursor of angiotensin, and decreased renin secretion from the kidney. Exercise itself also causes physiological stimulation of the renin–angiotensin system, an effect that has been shown in at least one study to be suppressed in women taking OCs (Huisveld *et al.*, 1985). Recent data suggest that administration of combination OCs may be associated with an increase in systolic blood pressure of between 2 and 7 mmHg (0.26–0.93 kPa) and in diastolic pressure of between 1 and 3 mmHg (0.13–0.4 kPa). For the majority of women on OCs, these small changes do not have any clinical implications.

Theoretical cardiovascular advantages, such as increases in preload and stroke volume of the heart due to fluid retention, may augment the effective cardiac output and enhance performance. Seaton (1972) documented a higher pulmonary capillary blood volume in women on a variety of OCs, comparable to values in the second half of the cycle in a control group. A higher cardiac output has been demonstrated with several higher dosage combination pills, both at rest and during exercise, either with or without concomitant alterations in blood pressure and vascular volume (Walters & Lim, 1969; Littler *et al.*, 1974; Lehtovirta *et al.*, 1977). Low-oestrogen monophasic OCs containing levonorgestrel have also been reported to increase blood pressure depending on the dose of levonorgestrel, although triphasic preparations and OCs with the newer progestins appear to have little effect. For the most part, heart rate at rest and during exercise has not been shown to change significantly with administration of OCs.

Oral contraceptives and the respiratory system

Ventilatory changes have been documented in users of two different monophasic OCs. Montes *et al.* (1983) studied 12 women taking two different OCs and found no changes in $\dot{V}O_2$, either at rest or during exercise. There were increases in tidal volume, total minute ventilation and $\dot{V}CO_2$ that were greater at 3 months than at 6 months, suggesting some degree of accommodation to this effect. A different study with another monophasic OC measured an increase in oxygen consumption for standardized workloads on a cycle ergometer (McNeill & Mozingo, 1981). If ventilation increases, then there may be a concomitant increase in the work of breathing and hence oxygen consumption. However, two recent studies that demonstrated a slight decrement in aerobic capacity with administration of a low-dose OC did not document any associated ventilatory changes (Notelovitz *et al.*, 1987; C.M. Lebrun *et al.*, unpublished observation). An alternative explanation for increased oxygen consumption in women using OCs may be differences in the metabolic cost of releasing energy from various substrates, such as FFA and glycogen.

Oral contraceptives and energy metabolism

The interaction of OCs with systems regulating energy metabolism are somewhat more complex (Table 3.5). The oestrogen dose, as well as the type and dose of the progestin, modulate the overall metabolic impact of a given OC combination. Glucose production, both at rest and during exercise, is primarily determined by insulin, although other hormones such as thyroxine, the catecholamines, cortisol and GH can have a counter-regulatory effect. GH levels can be increased by high doses of oestrogen and decreased by progestins. Progesterone causes reduced insulin binding secondary to a decrease in insulin receptor concentration, both in the luteal phase of the cycle and when administered in a combination OC. The more androgenic progestins have the greatest detrimental impact on glucose transport and insulin secretion. Norgestrel and levonorgestrel are the most potent in this regard (Sondheimer, 1991). Depot medroxyprogesterone acetate also increases the insulin response, but norethindrone alone does not appear to have any significant effects.

Oestrogens and progesterone in combination

Table 3.5 Factors influencing substrate metabolism during endurance exercise

Endurance training and cardiorespiratory fitness
Exercise intensity and duration
Muscle morphology and histology
  Fibre distribution type and enzyme activity
  Succinate dehydrogenase
  Malate dehydrogenase
Hormones
  Stress hormones
    Catecholamines
    Cortisol
    Growth hormone
    Insulin
    Somatotrophin
    Thyroid hormones
  Gonadotrophic hormones
    Testosterone
    Oestrogen
    Progesterone
Cellular mechanisms
  Insulin receptors
  Glucose transporters (GLUT-4)
Diet and nutrition
  Glycogen status
    Before event
    During exercise
  Blood glucose homeostasis

OCs lead to a relatively consistent impairment of glucose tolerance and varying degrees of hyper-insulinaemia. Fasting glucose concentrations are also reduced in OC users. Postulated causative factors include reduced insulin receptor concentrations, increased FFA levels, increased GH concentrations, changes in alimentary absorption of glucose, increased glucocorticoid activity and disturbances in tryptophan metabolism (Godsland, 1996). The latter action is mainly mediated through increased activity of the enzyme tryptophan pyrrolase (increased by oestrogens), leading to a deficiency in vitamin B_6. By inference, there may be potential for improvement in glucose tolerance in OC users by administration of pyridoxine. The progestogen component may modify these oestrogen-induced changes by decreasing oestrogen elimination, via alterations in lipolytic rate or insulin half-life, or by direct opposition, as with megestrol.

There are no conclusive detrimental or beneficial effects on energy metabolism and sports performance. Some studies have shown an increase in FFA levels during mild exercise and lower blood glucose levels at rest and during exercise in OC users (Bonen *et al.*, 1991). Women on OCs have an elevated GH response to exercise as well as lower glucose and carbohydrate use, with a shift more towards FFA metabolism (Bemben *et al.*, 1992). There is an overall glycogen-sparing effect of the OCs and, theoretically, therapy with the 'right' OC might potentially provide a competitive advantage during prolonged intense exercise. Bemben (1993) has proposed a theoretical model for the potential impact of OCs on hormonal responses and substrate utilization during prolonged exercise (Fig. 3.3).

Results are complicated by many other variables, including pre-exercise nutritional status and the interaction of endogenous opioids released during exercise, which can also be independently affected by the steroid components in OCs. Greater ability to spare carbohydrate may be advantageous for prolonged exercise, but lower blood glucose levels may reflect decreased hepatic output (Bemben *et al.*, 1992). Alternatively, stimulation of lipolysis by GH might be a compensatory response to low blood glucose levels. To investigate these metabolic effects further, substrate turnover studies, controlling for all other variables, would be ideal.

Oral contraceptives and sports performance

Investigations reported in the literature are not in complete agreement about the potential physiological impacts of these synthetic sex steroids on athletic performance. Anecdotally, Bale and Davies (1983) noted a performance enhancement in 8% of women on OCs. Some studies have documented fewer musculoskeletal injuries in women taking OCs, probably secondary to an amelioration of symptoms of PMS and dysmenorrhoea (Möller-Nielson & Hammar, 1989, 1991). In élite athletes, the menstrual cycle can be

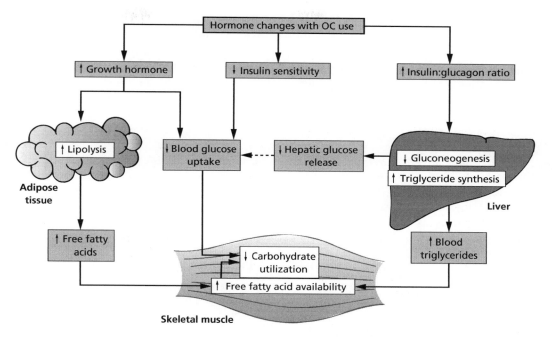

Fig. 3.3 Theoretical model for the potential impact of oral contraceptive (OC) use on hormonal responses and substrate utilization during prolonged exercise. (From Bemben, 1993 with permission.)

manipulated around the time of important competitions by extending the duration of active pills or the highest dose in a triphasic preparation. This can usually stave off menstruation successfully for at least 7–10 days, although Sulak *et al.* (1997) were able prospectively to stabilize 37 of 50 patients (74%) on an extended regimen of 6–12 weeks of consecutive days with active OCs. Therapeutically, this may decrease the frequency and alter the timing of menstrual-related problems, including dysmenorrhoea, menorrhagia, premenstrual-type symptoms and menstrual migraines. For the athlete concerned with performance, a better option might be to shorten the cycle progressively over a few months by decreasing the number of pills, so that the competition will occur after menstruation has finished, i.e. in the pill-free interval, in order to diminish any potential hormonal side-effects. The OC can also be stopped 10 days in advance of the anticipated competition. Of course, alternative methods of birth control must be used to protect against unwanted pregnancy.

It is less clear if there are any significant physiological performance-altering effects of steroid contraceptives. An early study by Daggett *et al.* (1983) demonstrated a detrimental impact on $\dot{V}_{O_{2max}}$ with administration of a higher-dose OC for 2 months that was reversible on discontinuation of the drug. There was an associated decrease in mitochondrial citrate, suggesting a possible cellular mechanism. Notelovitz *et al.* (1987) studied women on a lower-dose monophasic OC, containing 0.4 mg norethindrone, for 6 months. They also found a slight but significant change, with a 7% decrease in $\dot{V}_{O_{2max}}$ and an 8% deterioration in exercise performance as measured by oxygen pulse. C.M. Lebrun *et al.* (unpublished observations) studied seven women taking a lower-dose triphasic OC for 2 months compared with a similar group on placebo and found a decrement in $\dot{V}_{O_{2max}}$ that was not evident in the placebo group. Neither anaerobic capacity nor aerobic endurance were altered in this study. Recently, Bryner *et al.* (1996) prospectively randomized 10 moderately trained women to either placebo ($n = 3$) or an OC containing 1 mg norethindrone and 35 µg ethinyloestradiol ($n = 7$) for 21 days. Subjects were tested twice during a control menstrual cycle, performing a $\dot{V}_{O_{2max}}$ test and then 48 hours later a treadmill run to exhaustion at 80% of maximal heart rate. Testing was repeated during the first and third weeks of the treatment month. Serial transabdominal ultrasonography of the ovary was used to identify cycle phases in the placebo group. Neither the cycle phase nor the low-dose OC had any significant adverse effects on ventilatory frequency or athletic performance during the maximal treadmill test or endurance run.

Oral contraceptives and strength

Previously it was thought that the androgenic component of the pill might have an ergogenic action. In fact, in 1987 the International Olympic Committee seriously considered placing compounds containing norethindrone on the list of banned drugs, on the premise that they might potentially give an unfair advantage in terms of muscle strength and/or because of the possibility of masking other anabolic agents. Fortunately this ruling was successfully overturned by a group of determined physicians and scientists. More recently, women in the 1994 World Master's Games in Australia tested positive for steroids secondary to hormonal replacement therapy containing small amounts of testosterone in addition to the oestrogen. This has also been challenged and eliminated as a problem.

The thermogenic effect of progesterone seen during the luteal phase of the cycle is minimized by OCs (Grucza *et al.*, 1993), although with some of the biphasic or triphasic pills there may be a slight variation throughout the cycle. This may be the basis for the detrimental impact in forearm isometric endurance and muscle force output seen by Wirth and Lohman (1982); however, the

population group for this study consisted of 16 women on eight different OCs and testing in the 10 normal control subjects was determined by the calendar method. In another study of only seven women (three of whom were on different OCs), isometric endurance varied sinusoidally during the cycle (determined by BBT), with a peak value midway through the ovulatory phase and the lowest value midway through the luteal phase; the women on OCs did not show any variation in their test results across the cycle (Petrofsky *et al.*, 1976). In another study, isokinetic strength and endurance of knee flexors and extensors did not seem to be affected by administration of a low-dose triphasic OC (C.M. Lebrun *et al.*, unpublished observation). Although Sarwar *et al.* (1996) found menstrual-cycle variation of muscle strength, relaxation rate and fatiguability in 10 ovulatory women, they did not find any significant changes in a matched group taking a combined monophasic OC. Phillips *et al.* (1996) also found significant changes in menstruating subjects with no change in women on OCs.

Conclusion and recommendations for future research

This is a complex and fascinating field for clinicians, scientists, coaches and athletes alike. Although significant progress has been made in the understanding of the unique physiology of the female athlete during her reproductive years, there are still many unanswered questions. Are there inherent biological factors that limit the ability of women to transport and utilize oxygen or does the difference represent some factor amenable to training and sport experience? What are the most appropriate and accurate methods of matching male and female subjects on the fitness factor for comparative studies of oxygen delivery and utilization systems?

The evidence points to some influence of endogenous female sex steroids on various cardiovascular, respiratory and metabolic factors. These changes probably have minimal impact on the ability of most recreational athletes to participate in and enjoy their sport, but may have more significant impact at the élite level. Is it possible to clarify further the relationship between peripheral concentrations of the steroid hormones and their biological actions? What are the actions at the end-organ level and how can they be quantified? What additional effects can be accounted for by plasma volume shifts or changes in production or clearance of the hormones? Are the physiological responses linked to exercise intensity and/or duration with a certain 'threshold'?

For female athletes who choose OCs as a method of birth control or who may need to take them for therapeutic reasons, it is likely that any potential repercussions are lessened by use of the lower-dose triphasic pills and the newer progestins. However, it is necessary to acknowledge that there may be marked individual effects in some women. Although these may not achieve statistical significance, they may be of critical importance to the affected athlete. More large-scale, prospective, randomized clinical trials are required to delineate any advantage of one preparation over another. These must be carried out in trained individuals, using accurate hormonal measurements, particularly in the control groups not on OCs, in order to estimate the phase of the menstrual cycle precisely. The biggest benefit of OCs in the athletic population may be maintenance of a predictable hormonal milieu for training and competition.

As funding for research in women's issues hopefully continues to increase, there should be many more valid scientific studies addressing these and other critical problems. The next few decades should bring a plethora of interesting perspectives to the participation of women in sport and physical activity.

References

Abraham, G.E., Maroulis, G.B. & Marshall, J.R. (1974) Evaluation of ovulation and corpus luteum functioning using measurements of plasma progesterone. *Obstetrics and Gynecology* **44**, 522–525.

Arendt, E. & Dick, R. (1995) Knee injury patterns among men and women in collegiate basketball and soccer: NCAA data and review of literature. *American Journal of Sports Medicine* **23**, 694–701.

Bale, P. & Davies, J. (1983) Effect of menstruation and contraceptive pill on the performance of physical education students. *British Journal of Sports Medicine* **17**, 46–50.

Bale, P. & Nelson, G. (1985) The effects of menstruation on performance of swimmers. *Australian Journal of Science and Medicine in Sport* **17**, 19–22.

Barr, S.I., Janelle, K.C. & Prior, J.C. (1995) Energy intakes are higher during the luteal phase of ovulatory menstrual cycles. *American Journal of Clinical Nutrition* **61**, 39–43.

Bauman, J.E. (1981) Basal body temperature: unreliable method of ovulation detection. *Fertility and Sterility* **36**, 429–433.

Bemben, D.A. (1993) Metabolic effects of oral contraceptives. Implications for exercise responses of premenopausal women. *Sports Medicine* **16**, 295–304.

Bemben, D.A., Boileau, R.A., Bahr, J.M., Nelson, R.A. & Misner, J.E. (1992) Effects of oral contraceptives on hormonal and metabolic responses during exercise. *Medicine and Science in Sports and Exercise* **24**, 434–441.

Bemben, D.A., Salm, P.C. & Salm, A.J. (1995) Ventilatory and blood lactate responses to maximal treadmill exercise during the menstrual cycle. *Journal of Sports Medicine and Physical Fitness* **35**, 257–262.

Birch, K.M. & Reilly, T. (1997) The effect of eumenorrheic menstrual cycle phase on physiological responses to a repeated lifting task. *Canadian Journal of Applied Physiology* **22**, 148–160.

Bisdee, J.T., James, W.P. & Shaw, M.A. (1989) Changes in energy expenditure during the menstrual cycle. *British Journal of Nutrition* **61**, 187–199.

Bonen, A., Ling, W.Y., MacIntyre, K.P., Neil, R., McGrail, J.C. & Belcastro, A.N. (1979) Effects of exercise on serum concentrations of FSH, LH, progesterone, and estradiol. *European Journal of Applied Physiology* **42**, 15–23.

Bonen, A., Haynes, F.W., Watson-Wright, W. *et al.* (1983) Effect of menstrual cycle on metabolic responses to exercise. *Journal of Applied Physiology* **55**, 1506–1513.

Bonen, A., Haynes, F.W. & Graham, T.E. (1991) Substrate and hormonal responses to exercise in women using oral contraceptives. *Journal of Applied Physiology* **70**, 1917–1927.

Brooks-Gunn, J., Gargiulo, J.M. & Warren, M.P. (1986) The effect of cycle phase on the performance of adolescent swimmers. *Physician and Sportsmedicine* **14**, 182–192.

Bryner, R.W., Toffle, R.C., Ullrich, I.H. & Yeater, R.A. (1996) Effect of low dose oral contraceptives on exercise performance. *British Journal of Sports Medicine* **30**, 36–40.

Bungum, L., Kvernebo, K., Øian, P. & Maltau, J.M.

(1996) Laser Doppler-recorded reactive hyperemia in the forearm skin during the menstrual cycle. *British Journal of Obstetrics and Gynaecology* **103**, 70–75.

Bunt, J.C. (1990) Metabolic actions of estradiol: significance for acute and chronic exercise responses. *Medicine and Science in Sports and Exercise* **22**, 286–290.

Burkman, R.T. Jr (1994) Noncontraceptive effects of hormonal contraceptives: bone mass, sexually transmitted disease and pelvic inflammatory disease, cardiovascular disease, menstrual function and future fertility. *American Journal of Obstetrics and Gynecology* **170**, 1569–1575.

Carpenter, A.J. & Nunneley, S.A. (1988) Endogenous hormones subtly alter women's response to heat stress. *Journal of Applied Physiology* **65**, 2313–2317.

Carr, B.R. & Ory, H. (1997) Estrogen and progestin components of oral contraceptives: relationship to vascular disease. *Contraception* **55**, 267–272.

Chandler, M.H., Schuldheisz, S., Phillips, B.A. & Muse, K.N. (1997) Premenstrual asthma: the effect of estrogen on symptoms, pulmonary function, and beta2-receptors. *Pharmacotherapy* **17**, 224–234.

Chen, H.-I. & Tang, Y.-R. (1989) Effects of the menstrual cycle on respiratory muscle function. *American Review of Respiratory Disease* **140**, 1359–1362.

Coburn, R.F. (1970) Endogenous carbon monoxide production. *New England Journal of Medicine* **282**, 207–209.

Committee on Sports Medicine, American Academy of Pediatrics (1989) Amenorrhea in adolescent athletes. *Pediatrics* **84**, 394–395.

Cowart, V.S. (1989) Can exercise help women with PMS? *Physician and Sportsmedicine* **17**, 169–178.

Daggett, A., Davies, B. & Boobis, L. (1983) Physiological and biochemical responses to exercise following oral contraceptive use (abstract). *Medicine and Science in Sports and Exercise* **15**, 174.

Dalton, K. (1960) Menstruation and accidents. *British Medical Journal* **2**, 1425–1426.

Dalvit, S.P. (1981) The effect of the menstrual cycle on patterns of food intake. *American Journal of Clinical Nutrition* **34**, 1811–1815.

Davies, B.N., Elford, J.C.C. & Jamieson, K.F. (1991) Variations in performance of simple muscle tests at different phases of the menstrual cycle. *Journal of Sports Medicine and Physical Fitness* **31**, 532–537.

De Paz, J.A., Villa, J.G., Vilades, E., Martin-Nuño, M.A., Lasierra, J. & Gonzalez-Gallego, J. (1995) Effects of oral contraceptives on fibrinolytic response to exercise. *Medicine and Science in Sports and Exercise* **27**(7), 961–966.

De Souza, M.J., Maguire, M.S., Rubin, K. & Maresh, C.M. (1990) Effects of menstrual cycle phase and amenorrhea on exercise responses in runners. *Medicine and Science in Sports and Exercise* **22**, 575–580.

Diamond, M.P., Wentz, A.C. & Cherrington, A.D. (1988) Alterations in carbohydrate metabolism as they apply to reproductive endocrinology. *Fertility and Sterility* **50**, 387–397.

Dibrezzo, R., Fort, I.L. & Brown, B. (1991) Relationships among strength, endurance, weight and body fat during three phases of the menstrual cycle. *Journal of Sports Medicine and Physical Fitness* **31**, 89–94.

Dombovy, M.L., Bonekat, H.W., Williams, T.J. & Staats, B.A. (1987) Exercise performance and ventilatory response in the menstrual cycle. *Medicine and Science in Sports and Exercise* **19**, 111–117.

Dutton, K., Blankskby, B.A. & Morton, A.R. (1989) CO_2 sensitivity changes during the menstrual cycle. *Journal of Applied Physiology* **67**, 517–522.

England, S.J. & Farhi, L.E. (1976) Fluctuations in alveolar CO_2 and in base excess during the menstrual cycle. *Respiratory Physiology* **26**, 157–161.

Erdelyi, G.J. (1962) Gynecological survey of female athletes. *Journal of Sports Medicine and Physical Fitness* **2**, 174–179.

Eston, R.G. & Burke, E.J. (1984) Effects of the menstrual cycle on selected responses to short constant-load exercise. *Journal of Sports Sciences* **2**, 145–153.

Fomin, S.K., Pivovarova, V.I. & Voronova, V.I. (1989) Changes in the special working capacity and mental stability of well-trained women skiers at various phases of the biological cycle. *Sports Training Medicine and Rehabilitation* **1**, 89–92.

Fortney, S.M., Turner, C., Steinmann, L., Driscoll, T. & Alfrey, C. (1994) Blood volume responses of men and women to bed rest. *Journal of Clinical Pharmacology* **34**, 434–439.

Frascarolo, P., Schutz, Y. & Jéquier, E. (1990) Decreased thermal conductance during the luteal phase of the menstrual cycle in women. *Journal of Applied Physiology* **69**, 2029–2033.

Gaebelein, C.J. & Senay, L.C. Jr (1982) Vascular volume dynamics during ergometer exercise at different menstrual phases. *European Journal of Applied Physiology* **50**, 1–11.

Gibbs, C.J., Coutts, I.I., Lock, R., Finnegan, O.C. & White, R.J. (1984) Premenstrual exacerbation of asthma. *Thorax* **39**, 833–836.

Godsland, I.F. (1996) The influence of female sex steroids on glucose metabolism and insulin action. *Journal of Internal Medicine* **240** (Suppl. 738), 1–60.

Goldzieher, J.W. & Zamah, N.M. (1995) Oral contraceptive side effects: where's the beef? *Contraception* **52**, 327–335.

Gray, D.P., Harding, E. & Dale, E. (1983) Effects of oral contraceptives on serum lipid profiles of women runners. *Fertility and Sterility* **39**, 510–514.

Grimes, D.A. (1992) The safety of oral contraceptives:

epidemiologic insights from the first 30 years. *American Journal of Obstetrics and Gynecology* **166**, 1950–1954.

Grucza, R., Pekkarinen, H., Titov, E., Kononoff, A. & Hänninen, O. (1993) Influence of the menstrual cycle and oral contraceptives on thermoregulatory responses to exercise in young women. *European Journal of Applied Physiology* **67**, 279–285.

Haberland, C.A., Seddick, D., Marcus, R. & Bachrach, L.K. (1995) A physician survey of therapy for exercise-associated amenorrhea: a brief report. *Clinical Journal of Sport Medicine* **5**, 246–250.

Hackney, A.C. (1990) Effects of the menstrual cycle on resting muscle glycogen content. *Hormone and Metabolic Research* **22**, 647.

Hackney, A.C., McCracken-Compton, M.A. & Ainsworth, B. (1994) Substrate responses to submaximal exercise in the midfollicular and midluteal phases of the menstrual cycle. *International Journal of Sport Nutrition* **4**, 299–308.

Hessemer, V. & Bruck, K. (1985a) Influence of menstrual cycle on shivering, skin blood flow and sweating responses measured at night. *Journal of Applied Physiology* **59**, 1902–1910.

Hessemer, V. & Bruck, K. (1985b) Influence of menstrual cycle on thermoregulatory, metabolic and heart rate responses to exercise at night. *Journal of Applied Physiology* **59**, 1911–1917.

Higgs, S.L. & Robertson, L.A. (1981) Cyclic variations in perceived exertion and physical work capacity in females. *Canadian Journal of Applied Sport Sciences* **6**, 191–196.

Hirata, K., Nagasaka, T., Hirai, A., Hirashita, M., Takahata, T. & Nunomura, T. (1986) Effects of human menstrual cycle on thermoregulatory vasodilation during exercise. *European Journal of Applied Physiology* **54**, 559–565.

Horvath, S.M. & Drinkwater, B.L. (1982) Thermoregulation and the menstrual cycle. *Aviation Space and Environmental Medicine* **53**, 790–794.

Huisveld, I.A., Hospers, A.J.H., Bernink, M.J.E., Biersteker, M.W.A., Erich, W.B.M. & Bouma, B.N. (1982) Oral contraceptives and fibrinolysis among female cyclists before and after exercise. *Journal of Applied Physiology* **53**, 330–334.

Huisveld, I.A., Hospers, J.E.H., Bernink, M.J.E., Erich, W.B.M. & Bouma, B.N. (1983) The effect of oral contraceptives and exercise on hemostatic and fibrinolytic mechanisms in trained women. *International Journal of Sports Medicine* **4**, 97–103.

Huisveld, I.A., Derkx, F.M.H., Bouma, B.N., Erich, W.B.M. & Schalekap, M.A.D.H. (1985) Renin–angiotensin system: oral contraception and exercise in healthy female subjects. *Journal of Applied Physiology* **59**, 1690–1697.

Huston, L.J. & Wojtys, E.M. (1996) Neuromuscular

performance characteristics in elite female athletes. *American Journal of Sports Medicine* **24**, 427–436.

Jarrett, J.C. & Spellacy, W.N. (1983) Contraceptive practices of female runners. *Fertility and Sterility* **37**, 374–375.

Jurkowski, J.E.H., Jones, N.L., Walker, W.E., Younglai, E.V. & Sutton, J.R. (1978) Ovarian hormonal responses to exercise. *Journal of Applied Physiology* **44**, 109–114.

Jurkowski, J.E.H., Jones, N.L., Toews, C.J. & Sutton, J.R. (1981) Effects of menstrual cycle on blood lactate, O_2 delivery and performance during exercise. *Journal of Applied Physiology* **51**, 1493–1499.

Kanaley, J.A., Boileau, R.A., Bahr, J.A., Misner, J.E. & Nelson, R.A. (1992) Substrate oxidation and GH responses to exercise are independent of menstrual phase and status. *Medicine and Science in Sports and Exercise* **24**, 873–880.

Kolka, M.A. & Stephenson, L.A. (1989) Control of sweating during the human menstrual cycle. *European Journal of Applied Physiology* **58**, 890–895.

Laessle, R.G., Tuschl, R.J., Schweiger, U. & Pirke, K.M. (1990) Mood changes and physical complaints during the normal menstrual cycle in healthy young women. *Psychoneuroendocrinology* **15**, 131–138.

Lamont, L.S. (1986) Lack of influence of the menstrual cycle on blood lactate. *Physician and Sportsmedicine* **14**, 159–163.

Lamont, L.S., Lemon, P.W.R. & Brust, B.C. (1987) Menstrual cycle and exercise effects on protein catabolism. *Medicine and Science in Sports and Exercise* **192**, 106–110.

Lavoie, J.M., Dionne, N., Helie, R. & Brisson, G.R. (1987) Menstrual cycle phase dissociation of blood glucose homeostasis during exercise. *Journal of Applied Physiology* **62**, 1084–1089.

Lebrun, C.M. (1993) Effect of the different phases of the menstrual cycle and oral contraceptives on athletic performance. *Sports Medicine* **16**, 400–430.

Lebrun, C.M. (1994) The effect of the phase of the menstrual cycle and the birth control pill on athletic performance. *Clinics in Sports Medicine* **13**, 419–441.

Lebrun, C.M. (1995) Effects of menstrual cycle phase on athletic performance. *Medicine and Science in Sports and Exercise* **27**, 437–444.

Lehtovirta, P., Kuikka, J. & Pyorala, T. (1977) Hemodynamic effects of oral contraceptives during exercise. *International Journal of Gynaecology and Obstetrics* **15**, 35–37.

Lindholm, C., Hagenfeldt, K. & Ringertz, B.-M. (1994) Pubertal development in elite juvenile gymnasts. Effects of physical training. *Acta Obstetricia et Gynecologica Scandinavica* **73**, 269–273.

Littler, W.A., Bojorges-Bueno, R. & Banks, J. (1974) Cardiovascular dynamics in women during the menstrual cycle and oral contraceptive therapy. *Thorax* **29**, 567–570.

Liu, S.H., Al-Shaikh, R., Panossian, V. *et al.* (1996) Primary immunolocalization of estrogen and progesterone target cells in the human anterior cruciate ligament. *Journal of Orthopaedic Research* **14**, 526–533.

McCracken, M., Ainsworth, B. & Hackney, A.C. (1994) Effects of menstrual cycle phase on the blood lactate responses to exercise. *European Journal of Applied Physiology and Occupational Physiology* **69**, 174–175.

McNeill, A.W. & Mozingo, E. (1981) Changes in the metabolic cost of standardized work associated with the use of an oral contraceptive. *Journal of Sports Medicine* **21**, 238–244.

Magyar, D.M., Boyers, S.P., Marshall, J.R. & Abraham, G.E. (1979) Regular menstrual cycles and premenstrual molimina as indicators of ovulation. *Obstetrics and Gynecology* **53**, 411–414.

Marcus, D.A. (1995) Interrelationships of neurochemicals, estrogen and recurring headache. *Pain* **62**, 129–139.

Merians, D.R., Haskell, W.L., Vranizan, K.M., Phelps, J., Woods, P.D. & Superko, R. (1985) Relationship of exercise, oral contraceptive use and body fat to concentrations of plasma lipids and lipoprotein cholesterol in young women. *American Journal of Medicine* **78**, 913–919.

Miller, P.B. & Soules, M.R. (1996) The usefulness of a urinary LH kit for ovulation prediction during menstrual cycles of normal women. *Obstetrics and Gynecology* **87**, 13–17.

Möller-Nielson, J. & Hammar, M. (1989) Women's soccer injuries in relation to the menstrual cycle and oral contraceptive use. *Medicine and Science in Sports and Exercise* **21**, 126–129.

Möller-Nielson, J. & Hammar, M. (1991) Sports injuries and oral contraceptive use. Is there a relationship? *Sports Medicine* **12**, 152–160.

Montagnani, C.F., Arena, B. & Maffuli, N. (1992) Estradiol and progesterone during exercise in healthy untrained women. *Medicine and Science in Sports and Exercise* **24**, 764–768.

Montes, A., Lally, D. & Hale, R.W. (1983) The effects of oral contraceptives on respiration. *Fertility and Sterility* **39**, 515–519.

Mortola, J.F. (1996) Premenstrual syndrome. *Trends in Endocrinology and Metabolism* **7**, 184–189.

Nicklas, B.J., Hackney, A.C. & Sharp, R.L. (1989) The menstrual cycle and exercise: performance, muscle glycogen and substrate responses. *International Journal of Sports Medicine* **10**, 264–269.

Notelovitz, M., Zauner, C., McKenzie, L., Suggs, Y., Fields, C. & Kitchens, C. (1987) The effect of low-dose contraceptives on cardiorespiratory function, coagulation, and lipids in exercising young women: a pre-

liminary report. *American Journal of Obstetrics and Gynecology* **156**, 591–598.

Olson, B.R., Forman, M.R., Lanza, E. *et al.* (1996) Relation between sodium balance and menstrual cycle symptoms in normal women. *Annals of Internal Medicine* **125**, 564–567.

Pauli, B.D., Reid, R.L., Munt, P.W., Wigle, R.D. & Forkert, L. (1989) Influence of the menstrual cycle on airway function in asthmatic and normal subjects. *American Review of Respiratory Disease* **140**, 358–362.

Petrofsky, J.S., LeDonne, D.M., Rinehart, J.S. & Lind, A.R. (1976) Isometric strength and endurance during the menstrual cycle. *European Journal of Applied Physiology* **35**, 1–10.

Phillips, S.K., Sanderson, A.G., Birch, K., Bruce, S.A. & Woledge, R.C. (1996) Changes in maximal voluntary force of human adductor pollicis muscle during the menstrual cycle. *Journal of Physiology* **496**, 551–557.

Pivarnik, J.M., Marichal, C.J., Spillman, T. & Morrow, J.R. Jr (1992) Menstrual cycle phase affects temperature regulation during endurance exercise. *Journal of Applied Physiology* **72**, 543–548.

Plowman, S.A., Liu, N.Y. & Wells, C.L. (1991) Body composition and sexual maturation in premenarcheal athletes and nonathletes. *Medicine and Science in Sports and Exercise* **23**, 23–29.

Prior, J.C., Vigna, Y.M., Sciarretta, D., Alojado, N. & Schultzer, M. (1987) Conditioning exercise decreases premenstrual symptoms: a prospective, controlled 6-month trial. *Fertility and Sterility* **47**, 402–408.

Prior, J.C., Vigna, Y.M., Schultzer, M., Hall, J.E. & Bonen, A. (1990) Determination of luteal phase length by quantitative basal temperature methods: validation against the midcycle LH peak. *Clinical and Investigative Medicine* **13**, 123–131.

Quadagno, D., Faquin, L., Lim, G.-N., Kuminka, W. & Moffatt, R. (1991) The menstrual cycle: does it affect athletic performance? *Physician and Sportsmedicine* **19**, 121–124.

Reinke, U., Ansah, B. & Voigt, K.D. (1972) Effect of the menstrual cycle on carbohydrate and lipid metabolism in normal females. *Acta Endocrinologica* **69**, 762–768.

Robertson, L.A. & Higgs, L.S. (1983) Menstrual cycle variations in physical work capacity, post-exercise lactate, and perceived exertion (abstract). *Canadian Journal of Applied Sports Sciences* **8**, 220.

Rosano, G.M.C., Leonardo, F., Sarrel, P.M., Beale, C.M., De Luca, F. & Collins, P. (1996) Cyclical variation in paroxysmal supraventricular tachycardia in women. *Lancet* **347**, 786–788.

Ruby, B.C. & Robergs, R.A. (1994) Gender differences in substrate utilisation during exercise. *Sports Medicine* **17**, 393–410.

Ruby, B.C., Robergs, R.A., Waters, D.L., Burge, M., Mermier, C. & Stolarczyk, L. (1997) Effects of estradiol on substrate turnover during exercise in amenorrheic females. *Medicine and Science in Sports and Exercise* **29**, 1160–1169.

Sansores, R.H., Abboud, R.T., Kennell, C. & Haynes, N. (1995) The effect of menstruation on the pulmonary carbon monoxide diffusing capacity. *American Journal of Respiration and Critical Care Medicine* **152**, 381–384.

Sarwar, R., Niclos, B.B. & Rutherford, O.M. (1996) Changes in muscle strength, relaxation rate and fatiguability during the human menstrual cycle. *Journal of Physiology* **493**, 267–272.

Schoene, R.B., Robertson, H.T., Pierson, D.J. & Peterson, A.P. (1981) Respiratory drives and exercise in menstrual cycles of athletic and nonathletic women. *Journal of Applied Physiology* **50**, 1300–1305.

Seaton, A. (1972) Pulmonary capillary blood volume in women: normal values and the effect of oral contraceptives. *Thorax* **27**, 75–79.

Shangold, M.M. & Levine, H.S. (1982) The effect of marathon training upon menstrual function. *American Journal of Obstetrics and Gynecology* **143**, 862–869.

Shangold, M.M. & Mirkin, G. (eds) (1994) *Women and Exercise: Physiology and Sports Medicine*, 2nd edn. F.A. Davis, Philadelphia.

Sherwin, B.B. (1996) Hormones, mood, and cognitive functioning in postmenopausal women. *Obstetrics and Gynecology* **87**, 20S–26S.

Sita, A. & Miller, S.B. (1996) Estradiol, progesterone and cardiovascular response to stress. *Psychoneuroendocrinology* **21**, 339–346.

Solomon, S.J., Kurzer, M.S. & Calloway, D.H. (1982) Menstrual cycle and basal metabolic rate in women. *American Journal of Clinical Nutrition* **36**, 611–616.

Sondheimer, S.J. (1991) Update on the metabolic effects of steroidal contraceptives. *Endocrinology and Metabolism Clinics of North America* **20**, 911–923.

Stager, J.M., Wigglesworth, J.K. & Hatler, L.K. (1990) Interpreting the relationship between age of menarche and prepubertal training. *Medicine and Science in Sports and Exercise* **22**, 54–58.

Stephenson, L.A. & Kolka, M.A. (1993) Thermoregulation in women. *Exercise and Sport Sciences Reviews* **21**, 231–262.

Stephenson, L.A., Kolka, M.A. & Wilkerson, J.E. (1982) Metabolic and thermoregulatory responses to exercise during the human menstrual cycle. *Medicine and Science in Sports and Exercise* **14**, 270–275.

Sulak, P.J., Cressman, B.E., Waldrop, E., Holleman, S. &

Kuehl, T.J. (1997) Extending the duration of active oral contraceptive pills to manage hormone withdrawal symptoms. *Obstetrics and Gynecology* **89**, 179–183.

Tarnopolsky, L.J., MacDougall, J.D., Atkinson, S.A., Tarnopolsky, M.A. & Sutton, J.R. (1990) Gender differences in substrate for endurance exercise. *Journal of Applied Physiology* **68**, 302–308.

Turley, K.R. & Wilmore, J.H. (1997) Cardiovascular responses to submaximal exercise in 7- to 9-yr-old boys and girls. *Medicine and Science in Sports and Exercise* **29**(6), 824–832.

Van Beek, E., Houben, A.J.H.M., Van Es, P.N. *et al.* (1996) Peripheral haemodynamics and renal function in relation to the menstrual cycle. *Clinical Science* **91**, 163–168.

Walters, W.A.W. & Lim, Y.L. (1969) Cardiovascular dynamics in women receiving oral contraceptive therapy. *Lancet* **ii**, 879–881.

Wearing, M.P., Yuhasz, M., Campbell, R. & Love, E. (1972) The effect of the menstrual cycle on tests of physical fitness. *Journal of Sports Medicine and Physical Fitness* **12**, 38–41.

Webb, P. (1986) Twenty-four hour energy expenditure and the menstrual cycle. *American Journal of Clinical Nutrition* **44**, 614–619.

Wells, C.L. (1991) Effects of the menstrual cycle on physical performance. In C.L. Wells (ed.) *Women, Sport and Performance: A Physiological Perspective*, pp. 75–84. Human Kinetics Publishers, Champaign, Illinois.

Wells, C.L. & Horvath, S.M. (1973) Heat stress responses related to the menstrual cycle. *Journal of Applied Physiology* **35**, 1–5.

Wells, C.L. & Horvath, S.M. (1974) Responses to exercise in a hot environment as related to the menstrual cycle. *Journal of Applied Physiology* **36**, 299–302.

Williams, T.J. & Krahenbuhl, G.S. (1997) Menstrual cycle phase and running economy. *Medicine and Science in Sports and Exercise* **29**, 1609–1618.

Winget, C.M., DeRoshia, C.W. & Holley, D.C. (1985) Circadian rhythms and athletic performance. *Medicine and Science in Sports and Exercise* **17**, 498–516.

Wirth, J.C. & Lohman, T.G. (1982) The relationship of static muscle function to use of oral contraceptives. *Medicine and Science in Sports and Exercise* **14**, 16–20.

Zaharieva, E. (1965) Survey of sportswomen at the Tokyo Olympics. *Journal of Sports Medicine and Physical Fitness* **5**, 215–219.

Chapter 4

Environmental Challenges

EMILY M. HAYMES

Introduction

Many female athletes participate in competitive events that are held under various environmental conditions. Examples include the heat of the 1992 and 1996 Summer Olympics in Barcelona and Atlanta, the cold of the 1994 Winter Olympics in Lillehammer and the hypoxia due to an altitude of 2300 m at the 1968 Summer Olympics in Mexico City. Each of these environments can provide challenges not only to the physiological responses of the individual athlete but also may affect the athlete's performance. An example is the reduction in barometric pressure at altitude that reduces both oxygen transport in the blood and performance in endurance events.

Much of the research that has been conducted on the effects of different environments on the physiological responses to exercise used male subjects. Because the average female is smaller and has a higher proportion of body fat, some of the physiological responses to environmental challenges may be different in female athletes. Furthermore, female reproductive hormones influence thermoregulatory responses to warm and cold environments. The purpose of the present chapter is to examine the physiological responses of females to the environmental challenges most commonly experienced by competitive and recreational athletes.

Physiological responses to environmental challenges

This section focuses on the physiological responses to exercise in three types of environments: warm (both humid and dry), cold and altitude (hypobaric). The section begins with a brief description of the physiological responses to each environment. Observed differences in the responses of females and males to specific environmental challenges are then discussed.

Warm environments

Exercise in warm environments presents a challenge to the body's thermoregulatory system: to dissipate the metabolic heat produced when energy is released by the contracting muscles. The amount of heat produced is directly proportional to the intensity of the exercise. This heat must be transported by the blood to the body's surface where heat dissipation will occur. As the blood temperature increases and circulates through the anterior hypothalamus of the brain, neurones in the thermoregulatory centre stimulate blood vessels in the skin to dilate and the sweat glands to secrete sweat. In thermoneutral environments, a large thermal gradient exists between the temperatures of the skin and air that facilitates the loss of dry heat. Heat is also lost from the skin by evaporation of sweat. As air temperature rises in warm environments the gradient between skin and air diminishes, which reduces the amount of dry heat loss from the skin. Evaporation of sweat must increase in order to maintain thermal balance in warm environments. This is accomplished by increasing the sweat rate and is assisted by increasing blood flow to the skin. In warm humid environments, evaporation of sweat is limited because the air is saturated with water vapour. When the air temperature exceeds skin temperature (approximately 35°C), the body gains heat from the environment. The only avenue of heat loss at higher air temperatures is through the evaporation of sweat. Hot humid environments are particularly stressful because evaporative heat loss is limited. At air temperatures of 35°C or higher and relative humidity of 60% or above, runners are not able to achieve thermal balance because not enough sweat can evaporate (Nielsen, 1996). Failure to achieve thermal balance results in rising body core temperatures and increased risk of heat exhaustion.

Repeated exposure to warm environments increases an athlete's heat tolerance. Adaptations occur in several physiological responses that allow heat loss to begin earlier in the exercise bout and that reduce body temperatures and cardiovascular strain. This process, known as heat acclimatization, includes lower core temperatures for the onset of both sweating and vasodilation, increased plasma volume, lower core and skin temperatures, and a lower heart rate during exercise in the heat.

DESERT ENVIRONMENTS

The physiological responses of well-trained males and females to exercise in warm temperatures with low relative humidity are very similar. Although some early studies reported males were more tolerant of exercise in the heat than females, it appears that trained males were compared with sedentary females in some of these studies (Shapiro et al., 1980a, b). When heat-acclimatized male and female subjects were matched for fitness status, there were no differences in rectal temperature, heart rate or sweat rate during exercise at low and moderate intensi-

ties in hot (39–48°C) dry environments (Wells, 1980; Frye & Kamon, 1981).

It has been suggested that females may be at a disadvantage in hot dry environments because the average woman has a smaller plasma volume and a lower percentage of body water than the average man. The ratio of total body water to body weight is 50–55% in women and 55–60% in men (Van Loan & Boileau, 1996), while plasma volume is 13% less in women (Fortney, 1996). If male and female athletes lose sweat at the same rate, the rate of dehydration would be greater in the females because they are losing a higher proportion of their body water and plasma volume. It is recommended that female athletes consume fluids as frequently as males in order to replace the disproportionate loss of body fluids (Fortney, 1996).

TROPICAL ENVIRONMENTS

In the warm humid environments typical of the tropics, females appear to tolerate exercise better than males. Several studies have reported that unacclimatized females had lower rectal temperatures, heart rates and sweat rates (Paolone et al., 1978; Avellini et al., 1980; Shapiro et al., 1980a) and were able to exercise longer than unacclimatized males (Avellini et al., 1980). Following 10 days' acclimatization to a hot humid environment, both rectal temperature and heart rate were still significantly lower in females compared with males (Avellini et al., 1980). On the other hand, males have significantly higher sweat rates than females after acclimatization to a hot humid environment (Avellini et al., 1980). Acclimatization to humid heat also increases the sweat rate of females, but the increase (15%) is less than that observed in males (35%). Much of the males' additional sweat may have been wasted because high humidity limits evaporation. Lower sweat rates in humid environments would appear to be advantageous because body fluid and plasma volume losses would be reduced.

Several recent studies comparing male and female athletes competing in warm humid environments have reported that males lose significantly more sweat than females (Bergeron *et al.*, 1995; Millard-Stafford *et al.*, 1995). Female distance runners had lower sweat rates and smaller changes in plasma volume than male runners during a 40-km run (Millard-Stafford *et al.*, 1995). Over the last 10 km of the run the female runners also had lower rectal temperatures. A study of tennis players reported that females had significantly lower sweat rates than males during midday singles matches (Bergeron *et al.*, 1995). There were no significant differences in fluid replacement between males and females in either the 40-km run or tennis match. In both the runners and tennis players fluid intake did not replace fluid losses. Similar results have been reported for soccer and basketball players during training and competition in warm humid environments (Broad *et al.*, 1996). Failure to replace fluid losses during competition and training results in dehydration. The rate of fluid loss replacement among the female athletes ranged from 47% for the distance runners to 76% for the tennis players (Fig. 4.1). In some sports, like soccer and field hockey, fluid intake during competition is limited. Athletes in these sports should consume 500 ml of fluid prior to the match and at least 400 ml at half-time (Broad *et al.*, 1996). During tennis matches, fluid replacement should occur at each change-over at a rate of 120–240 ml (Bergeron *et al.*, 1995). Female runners should consume up to 1 litre of fluid in the hour prior to distance runs in warm environments and 150–300 ml every 15 min during the run (American College of Sports Medicine, 1996). Even female athletes competing and training in indoor environments (e.g. basketball, volleyball) need to replace fluids at the rate of 600–1000 ml·h^{-1} (Broad *et al.*, 1996).

EFFECTS OF TRAINING

Female athletes are able to tolerate exercise in hot dry environments better than untrained females (Fein *et al.*, 1975; Drinkwater *et al.*, 1976, 1977). There are several possible reasons why training improves heat tolerance. Athletes with higher

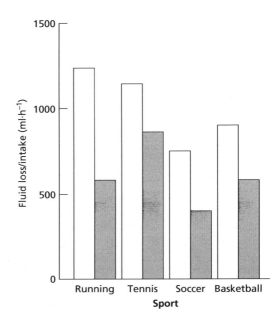

Fig. 4.1 Fluid loss (sweat rate, □) and fluid intake (■) of female athletes during competitive events in warm weather. (Data from Bergeron *et al.*, 1995; Millard-Stafford *et al.*, 1995; Broad *et al.*, 1996.)

aerobic fitness levels maintain lower heart rates and higher stroke volumes during prolonged exercise in the heat compared with non-athletes (Drinkwater *et al.*, 1976, 1977). Although there are no differences in sweat rate, female athletes are better able to maintain their plasma volumes during exercise due to a greater influx of proteins into the plasma (Drinkwater *et al.*, 1977). Increases in plasma volume and total plasma protein have been observed in females after an aerobic training programme (Fortney & Senay, 1979). An expanded plasma volume is an advantage because central blood volume, and therefore stroke volume, can be better maintained during exercise in warm environments.

It has also been observed that female athletes appear to be partially acclimatized on their first day of exposure to the heat (Fein *et al.*, 1975). Following an interval training programme, trained females were observed to acclimatize to the heat at a faster rate than untrained females (Cohen &

Gisolfi, 1982). The onset of sweating has been observed to occur earlier during an exercise bout in trained females (Araki *et al.*, 1981). Threshold core temperature for the onset of sweating decreases in females after training (Roberts *et al.*, 1977). Because sweating begins earlier in exercise, less heat will be stored and body temperatures will be lower. In warm humid environments, trained women's sweat rates were also found to decline (hidromeiosis) during prolonged exercise (Araki *et al.*, 1981). It has been suggested that training improves the efficiency of sweating in females by reducing wasteful sweating.

INFLUENCE OF THE MENSTRUAL CYCLE

The normal menstrual (ovarian) cycle is divided into two phases: the follicular phase, which begins on the first day of the menses and lasts until ovulation; and the luteal phase, which begins immediately following ovulation and lasts until the next menses. During the follicular phase, oestrogens are produced by the ovary in increasing amounts until shortly before ovulation. In the luteal phase, both oestrogens and progesterone are produced by the corpus luteum. After ovulation, the rising levels of progesterone are associated with a significant rise (0.3–0.6°C) in core and skin temperatures (Hessemer & Bruck, 1985a; Stephenson & Kolka, 1985). Thresholds for the onset of both sweating and cutaneous vasodilation are increased during the luteal phase of the menstrual cycle (Hessemer & Bruck, 1985b; Stephenson & Kolka, 1985). The effect of these shifts to higher thresholds on thermoregulatory responses during exercise has been the subject of several studies.

Higher core and skin temperatures were observed during the luteal phase throughout prolonged low-intensity exercise in a hot dry environment, but there was no impairment of heat tolerance and all subjects were able to complete the exercise bout (Carpenter & Nunneley, 1988). During moderate-intensity exercise in a thermoneutral environment (22°C), both core temperature and heart rate were significantly

higher in the luteal phase and perceived exertion was significantly greater near the end of exercise (Pivarnik *et al.*, 1992). Although core temperatures were higher during the luteal phase in both studies, no adverse effects on exercise performance were observed.

Plasma volume shifts during heat exposure and exercise have been observed to change during the menstrual cycle. Passsive heating produced a greater decrease in plasma volume (haemoconcentration) during the luteal phase, while high-intensity exercise produced a greater decrease in plasma volume during the follicular phase (Stephenson & Kolka, 1988). Greater decreases in plasma volume in the follicular phase have been observed during low-intensity exercise as well (Gaebelein & Senay, 1982). However, no adverse effect on endurance was observed in either study. The effect of menstrual-cycle phase on fluid replacement following exercise has been examined in a recent study (Maughan *et al.*, 1996). After exercising in a warm environment to reduce body weight by 1.8%, female subjects ingested enough carbohydrate–electrolyte drink to replace 150% of the weight lost over a 60-min period. The investigators found that there were no significant differences in fluid balance or urine volume in the different phases of the menstrual cycle (Maughan *et al.*, 1996). It should be noted, however, there have been no studies examining voluntary fluid replacement during the different phases of the menstrual cycle.

HEAT ILLNESS PREVENTION

Dehydration is fairly common in many sports events during the warm months of the year. As a result of dehydration, the athlete's body core temperature is elevated and may reach the hyperthermic range ($\geq 39°C$). Heat exhaustion and heat stroke are the two illnesses most likely to occur among athletes. Female athletes may experience heat illness in many sports, including running, soccer, field hockey, softball and tennis. Previous reports of the incidence of heat illness among athletes suggest that the rates for females and males are approximately the same (England *et al.*, 1982; Elias *et al.*, 1991).

The risk of heat illness can be reduced in athletes through the use of several strategies. One of the most important ways of preventing heat illness is to acclimatize athletes to the heat prior to competition. Allowing adequate time for full acclimatization (about 2 weeks) reduces the risk of heat illness and leads to improved performance in endurance events. During the first few days of acclimatization, athletes should reduce the intensity of training and the amount of time spent in the heat. Partial acclimatization to the heat occurs over the first 4–5 days, during which time heart rate and core and skin temperatures decrease and tolerance for exercise increases.

Another important strategy for reducing the risk of heat illness is to ensure adequate hydration. This should include consumption of fluids before exercise, at regular intervals during exercise and adequate amounts of fluids after exercise to replace sweat losses. Weighing athletes before and after practice each day is often used to identify individual athletes who are not replacing fluid losses.

Especially during the summer, scheduling training and competitive events during the cooler parts of the day (e.g. early in the morning or later in the evening) reduces the risk of heat illness (Fig. 4.2). The American College of Sports Medicine (1996) recommends that distance running events be rescheduled when the wet bulb globe temperature (WBGT) reaches 28°C. The combination of air temperature and relative humidity equivalent to a WBGT of 28°C is shown in Fig. 4.2 by the line separating the high and very high risks of heat illness. Athletes in many endurance events (e.g. soccer, field hockey) would reduce their risk of heat illness by following these same environmental stress guidelines recommended for runners.

Cold environments

In cold environments, exercise presents much less of a challenge to the thermoregulatory system because the large thermal gradient

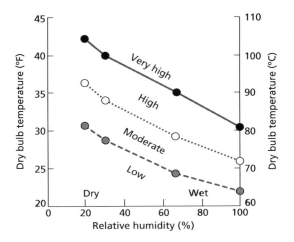

Fig. 4.2 Risk of heat exhaustion or heat stroke while racing in hot environments. (From American College of Sports Medicine, 1996 with permission.)

between the skin and air facilitates the loss of heat produced by the contracting muscles. If the rate of heat loss exceeds metabolic heat production, the decrease in core and skin temperatures stimulates vasoconstriction of the superficial blood vessels, which shunts more blood into the core and into deeper blood vessels in the extremities. The bloodless skin and subcutaneous fat serve as insulation against heat loss, helping to conserve body heat. Shivering, stimulated by a further drop in core temperature, increases metabolic heat production (thermogenesis).

Most studies of the physiological responses to cold environments have been conducted with male subjects. There is some evidence, however, that females may be able to work and even survive in cold environments better than males (Pugh, 1966; Hong *et al.*, 1986). It has been suggested that only females dive in the cold waters of Korea because they are better insulated against the cold than males (Hong *et al.*, 1986). After examining incidents of hypothermia in walkers, climbers and campers, Pugh (1966) concluded that females were more likely to survive cold exposure leading to hypothermia compared with males. Theoretically, females might be better insulated against the cold because the average female has a greater subcutaneous fat thickness than the average male. Fat is an excellent insulator against the cold: thickness of the subcutaneous fat layer is significantly related to maximal tissue insulation during cold exposure (Hong et al., 1986). It has been observed that females have greater tissue insulation during cold exposure than males (Rennie et al., 1962).

Body size is also an important factor determining heat loss. More heat is stored in a large body mass than a small body mass; however, the ratio of surface area to body mass (SA/M) determines the rate of heat loss from the body. Individuals with large SA/M lose heat more rapidly than individuals with small SA/M. Prepubertal swimmers have larger SA/M than adolescents and cool more rapidly in cold water (Sloan & Keatinge, 1973). The average female has a larger SA/M than the average male and should, based on geometrical considerations, lose heat more rapidly than males. The female's larger SA/M may negate part of the advantage provided by thicker subcutaneous fat layers in cold environments.

EXERCISE IN COLD ENVIRONMENTS

Gender differences in response to exercise in cold environments are complicated to study. When a person exercises, the metabolic rate is elevated in proportion to the exercise intensity and heat production rises. If males and females exercise at the same absolute intensity, the rate of heat production is equivalent. In exercise bouts at the same absolute intensity, the amount of heat produced is the same in both sexes and body temperatures will rise more rapidly in the females. If the women have a lower $\dot{V}_{O_{2max}}$ and are exercising at the same relative intensity (e.g. 70% $\dot{V}_{O_{2max}}$) as the men, the rate of heat production will be lower for the women. This latter situation exists in winter sports like cross-country skiing, where females ski at the same relative intensity but at slower speeds than males.

When males and females exercise at the same absolute intensity, females have been observed to have higher rectal temperatures in environments

at −5 and +5°C (Graham & Lougheed, 1985; Stevens et al., 1987). During the latter stages of prolonged intermittent periods of exercise and rest, the metabolic rate increased significantly in the males (Graham & Lougheed, 1985). In a subsequent study, no significant difference in rectal temperatures was observed between males and females exercising at the same absolute intensity in cold environments ranging from −10 to +10°C (Walsh & Graham, 1986). However, the females had lower metabolic rates during the latter part of the exercise compared with the males. Elevation of the metabolic rate suggests that thermogenesis was stimulated in the males but not the females.

Prolonged endurance events in cold environments may present more of a challenge to female athletes. In a study comparing males and females exercising at the same relative intensity (e.g. same percentage of $\dot{V}_{O_{2max}}$) in a −5°C environment, the females' rectal temperatures decreased significantly during the third hour of exercise (Graham, 1983). Heat production was significantly lower for the females who were exercising at a lower absolute intensity than the males. During the third hour of exercise net heat loss was significantly greater for the females. In a cold environment, a higher metabolic rate is advantageous in offsetting heat loss. Exercising in the wind further increases heat loss. Males and females wearing cross-country skiing uniforms were unable to maintain core temperatures when exercising at the same relative intensity in a 15 km·h⁻¹ wind at −20°C (Haymes et al., 1982).

Exercise in cold water presents even more of a challenge to the athlete. Because water is an excellent conductor of heat, heat loss occurs more rapidly in water than air at the same temperature. During exercise in cold water (20°C), both lean (9% body fat) and average (17% body fat) males increased their metabolic rates, while lean (18.5% body fat) females maintained relatively constant metabolic rates (McArdle et al., 1984). Decline in rectal temperature was greatest in the lean males after 1 hour of exercise, followed by the average males, lean females and average (25% body fat) females (Fig. 4.3). Similar results

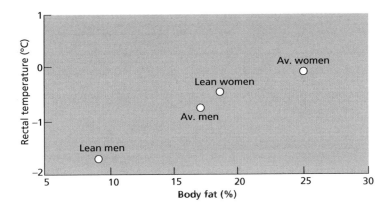

Fig. 4.3 Change in rectal temperature of lean men (9% fat), average men (17% fat), lean women (18.5% fat) and average women (25% fat) after exercise in water at 20°C for 1 hour. (Data from McArdle *et al.*, 1984.)

have been observed in younger males and females swimming in cold water (Sloan & Keatinge, 1973). The rate of body cooling while swimming was greater in males with less subcutaneous fat than in females with more subcutaneous fat.

INFLUENCE OF THE MENSTRUAL CYCLE

Thermoregulatory responses to the cold are influenced by the phase of the menstrual cycle. Not only were resting core temperatures significantly higher during the luteal phase but skin temperatures decreased at a faster rate (Hessemer & Bruck, 1985a). The threshold for shivering thermogenesis occurred at higher core temperatures in the luteal phase when the female subjects were exposed to cold. However, the metabolic rate increased during shivering at the same rate in both phases.

Because many female athletes are amenorrhoeic, the inclusion of female subjects who are amenorrhoeic may influence the responses to cold in comparison with males and eumenorrhoeic females. Amenorrhoeic females (less than one menstrual cycle per year) had significantly lower resting core temperatures than eumenorrhoeic females; however, the menstrual-cycle phase was not controlled in the eumenorrhoeic females (Graham *et al.*, 1989). During resting exposure to 5°C, amenorrhoeic females had lower metabolic rates than males and eumenor-

rhoeic females. The investigators concluded from their results that amenorrhoeic females are less sensitive to cold than males or eumenorrhoeic females (Graham *et al.*, 1989). Many of the earlier studies comparing females and males did not report any information concerning the menstrual status of their subjects. Onset of shivering thermogenesis in females who are amenorrhoeic may be delayed. Menstrual status and cycle phase should be controlled in future studies comparing females and males.

INFLUENCE OF IRON DEFICIENCY

Iron depletion without anaemia is relatively common among female athletes, with the reported incidence ranging from 20% to 47% (Clarkson & Haymes, 1995). Iron-deficiency anaemia is less common among athletes but is more prevalent in female than male athletes. Anaemia reduces the oxygen-carrying capacity of the blood and results in a greater cardiac output in order to supply oxygen to the tissues. Iron deficiency may deplete the tissues of iron-containing cellular enzymes (e.g. cytochromes) and impair cellular metabolism (e.g. thermogenesis). When anaemic males and females were compared with subjects who were iron deficient or had normal iron status, the decline in body temperature during exposure to cold water was 0.9°C in the anaemic subjects, 0.5°C in the iron-deficient subjects and 0.2°C in the normal subjects (Martinez-Torres *et al.*, 1984). During exposure to cold, metabolic rate was significantly higher in the anaemic and iron-deficient subjects compared with the normal subjects. Iron-deficient and anaemic subjects also had higher plasma noradrenaline levels than the normal subjects, which was the probably stimulus of the elevated metabolic rates.

The effects of iron depletion and iron repletion on responses to cold exposure were examined in a group of females. The females began shivering earlier during cold exposure following an 80-day period of iron depletion compared with 100 days of iron repletion (Lukaski *et al.*, 1990). Iron deficiency resulted in lower core and skin temperatures and metabolic rates were depressed even though noradrenaline levels were elevated. Thyroid hormones were slightly, but not significantly, lower in response to cold stimulus when the females were iron deficient. It appears that females who are iron deficient cannot produce as much heat during cold exposure due to a depressed thermogenic response. These results could have significant implications for female endurance athletes who compete in cold environments (e.g. cross-country skiers).

ACCLIMATIZATION TO THE COLD

The most comprehensive studies of cold acclimatization were conducted on female divers in Korea. Acclimatization to cold water reduced the core temperature at which these women began to shiver and increased their maximal tissue insulation (Hong *et al.*, 1986). The female divers allowed their core temperatures to drop to 35°C before terminating a diving session. These observations were made when the females wore only cotton suits during diving. Similar responses are likely to occur in female swimmers who train in cold water. After the Korean female divers switched to wet suits in 1977, cold acclimatization was gradually lost over the next 5 years (Hong *et al.*, 1986).

Most of the studies of acclimatization to cold air environments have been conducted with male subjects. Females who were repeatedly exposed to 10°C for 2 weeks had a delayed onset of shivering and a reduced thermogenic response following acclimatization (Silami-Garcia & Haymes, 1989). There were no significant changes in rectal or skin temperature reponses to cold following acclimatization. Reductions in the shivering response have also been reported in males acclimatized to 10°C for 3 weeks (Mathew *et al.*, 1981). Body temperature in the males did not drop as much during cold exposure after 3 weeks of acclimatization. The males' resting metabolism was elevated following acclimatization, a response similar to the elevated basal metabolic rates of the acclimatized diving females in Korea (Hong *et al.*, 1986). Due to insufficient data on cold acclimatization it is not possible to say whether females and males acclimatize to cold at the same rate. However, it appears that a delay in the onset of shivering and a reduction in shivering thermogenesis are the earliest responses seen in both sexes.

PREVENTING COLD ILLNESSES

Hypothermia and frostbite are the cold illnesses that athletes training and competing in cold environments are most likely to experience. The cause of hypothermia (core temperature <36°C) is failure of the metabolic rate to generate enough heat to counterbalance heat losses. Symptoms that suggest the onset of hypothermia include fatigue, weakness, inability to maintain pace, stumbling and falling (Pugh, 1966). Factors that contribute to the development of hypothermia in athletes are wet clothing, inadequate clothing, extreme cold, wind and low exercise intensities.

The insulation provided by clothing is greatly reduced when it is wet. Athletes training and competing in the rain and snow can reduce the risk of hypothermia by wearing an outer layer of clothing made of water-repellant material (Haymes & Wells, 1986). Although inadequate clothing is a factor in very cold environments, too much clothing may stimulate sweating during exercise and the inner layers of clothing become wet. It is recommended that athletes wear multiple layers of lightweight clothing when training in the cold, as it is the air trapped between the layers of clothing that is the best insulator. Because heat loss increases as wind speed increases, the risk of hypothermia also increases. Wearing outer garments made of wind-resistant materials (e.g. nylon) reduces heat loss from the skin.

The risk of hypothermia is greater when environmental temperatures are below 0°C; however, hypothermia can occur at temperatures below 10°C, especially in athletes wearing inadequate clothing (American College of Sports Medicine, 1996). Athletes at greatest risk of developing hypothermia are the slower runners and skiers in endurance events (e.g. marathon, 50-km ski race) because their exercise intensity is too low to generate enough heat to offset heat loss.

Frostbite occurs when the skin temperature falls below 0°C and fluids in the skin freeze. The risk of frostbite increases when the windchill index, a combination of air temperature and wind speed, exceeds −31°C. Coaches and athletes should monitor the windchill index when training in cold environments, especially when the ambient temperature is −10°C or below. At higher racing speeds in cross country skiing, the windchill is greater and races are postponed if the temperature is below −20°C (American College of Sports Medicine, 1996). Frostbite occurs most frequently on the exposed areas of the face, fingers and toes. In fact, some athletes may not realize that frostbite has occurred until they remove their gloves and boots. The skin is numb because sensory neurones are blocked by the cold. When the risk of frostbite is increased, companions should check for signs of frostbite on exposed areas of the face. The wearing of hats that cover the ears and bandanas or ski masks reduces the risk of frostbite to the face.

Altitude

Many athletes find exercise at altitude to be particularly challenging because of the earlier onset of fatigue. As altitude increases, barometric pressure decreases. Although the percentage of oxygen in the air remains constant (20.93%), the oxygen pressure (P_{O_2}) decreases. The higher the altitude, the greater the decrease in P_{O_2}. Reduction in P_{O_2} of the air leads to a lower P_{O_2} in the lungs and blood, which results in less oxygen being transported to the muscles. Thus, the performance of endurance athletes is more likely to be negatively affected at altitude.

On the other hand, some athletes may actually perform better at altitude. For example, at the 1968 Summer Olympics in Mexico City (altitude 2300 m), new world records were set in most of the sprinting events. The decline in air density as altitude increases results in a reduction in air resistance. Reductions in air resistance are particularly beneficial to athletes in sprinting, cycling, skiing and speed skating.

PHYSIOLOGICAL RESPONSES

Exercise at altitude at the same absolute intensity as at sea level (e.g. running at 16 km·h⁻¹) can put great strain on the cardiovascular system because the oxygen content of the blood will be reduced. This is especially true at altitudes of 2200 m and above. Although the P_{O_2} of the blood decreases linearly with altitude, the amount of oxygen bound to haemoglobin declines very little at low altitudes. At higher altitudes, cardiac output increases to compensate for the decrease in the blood oxygen content. The increase in cardiac output is due to increased heart rate. When males and females exercise at the same relative intensity (50% $\dot{V}_{O_{2max}}$), similar increases in heart rate have been observed as altitude increases (Elliott & Atterbom, 1978).

When females exercised at the same intensity relative to their $\dot{V}_{O_{2max}}$ at each altitude, heart rate, stroke volume and cardiac output were the same at altitudes ranging from sea level to 4270 m (Wagner et al., 1980). However, the respiratory exchange ratio (RER) was higher at altitude, indicating greater reliance on carbohydrates for energy, and blood lactate levels were elevated at 3050 and 4270 m. $\dot{V}_{O_{2max}}$ was reduced in females by 10% and 13% at 2130 and 3050 m respectively (Miles et al., 1980). During maximal exercise at 4100 m, females had significantly lower $\dot{V}_{O_{2max}}$,

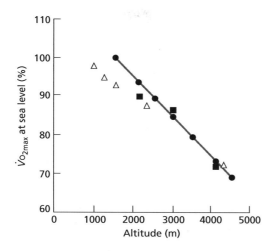

Fig. 4.4 Decline in $\dot{V}_{O_{2max}}$ at altitude in females (■) and males (△) compared with the predicted decline (●) of 1% per 100 m for altitudes above 1500 m. (Data from Drinkwater *et al.*, 1979; Miles *et al.*, 1980; Squires & Buskirk, 1982; Young *et al.*, 1982.)

maximal heart rate, RER and time to exhaustion but higher blood lactate compared with values at sea level (Drinkwater *et al.*, 1979). The decrease in $\dot{V}_{O_{2max}}$ for the females (26.7%) at this altitude was similar to that reported for males (27%) (Young *et al.*, 1982). The reduction in $\dot{V}_{O_{2max}}$ at altitude in females is very similar to the predicted decline of 1% for every 100 m above 1500 m (Fig. 4.4).

ACCLIMATIZATION TO ALTITUDE

The initial response to altitude is a decrease in plasma volume that results in an increase in haemoglobin concentration over the first few days. As a result, the oxygen content of the blood increases proportionately. On the other hand, the increased haemoconcentration also increases resistance to blood flow. After several weeks at altitude, stroke volume decreases due to the reduction in plasma volume. Red cell volume increases gradually due to the hypoxic stimulus of altitude. At altitudes above 5000 m, smaller increases in haemoglobin concentration have been observed in females compared with those reported for males (Drinkwater *et al.*, 1982). This

may have been due to low iron stores in the females. One recent study found that male and female runners with low ferritin levels, an indication of depleted iron stores, exhibited very little increase in red cell volume during 4 weeks' acclimatization to 2500 m (Stray-Gunderson *et al.*, 1992). Because many female athletes have low ferritin levels (Clarkson & Haymes, 1995), increases in red cell volume may occur more slowly during acclimatization in these athletes.

Following several weeks of acclimatization, subjects are less dependent on muscle glycogen as a source of energy for exercise and are better able to use fatty acids as an energy source (Young *et al.*, 1982). This shift in substrate utilization is a result of several adaptations that occur in muscle tissue during acclimatization, including increases in myoglobin concentration, mitochondria and capillaries (Levine & Stray-Gunderson, 1992).

TRAINING AT ALTITUDE

Prior to the 1968 Olympics in Mexico City, a number of studies were conducted on the effects of training at altitude on performance at altitude. Results from several of these studies suggest improved performance following several weeks of training at altitude (Buskirk *et al.*, 1967; Pugh, 1967; Saltin, 1967). However, performance at altitude in the endurance events was reduced compared with the athletes' performance at sea level. Furthermore, the intensity of training had to be reduced at altitude because of the reduction in $\dot{V}_{O_{2max}}$. Significant reductions in $\dot{V}_{O_{2max}}$ have been observed in trained males at altitudes of 1200 m and above (Squires & Buskirk, 1982) and in competitive athletes at altitudes as low as 900 m (Terrados, 1992).

Some élite athletes train at altitudes of 2000–2500 m for competitive events that will occur near sea level. The advantages of this altitude training have recently been questioned (Levine & Stray-Gunderson, 1992). When male and female runners trained at altitudes of 1200 or 2500 m for 4 weeks, the improvement in 5-km run times at sea level were similar; however, blood lactate levels and heart rate during submaximal exercise decreased more in the runners who trained at 1200 m (Levine & Stray-Gunderson, 1992). This was most probably due to the runners training at a lower percentage of their sea-level $\dot{V}O_{2max}$ and the lower running speeds at 2500 m compared with 1200 m (Stine *et al.*, 1992). On the other hand, when athletes trained at the same absolute intensity at 2300 m and sea level, significant increases in skeletal muscle myoglobin and aerobic enzyme activity and greater increases in endurance were observed after 4 weeks of altitude training (Terrados, 1992). The results of these studies suggest that training at altitudes of 2300–2500 m is more likely to enhance performance at sea level if the athletes can maintain their sea-level training intensity (speed) at altitude.

Recommendations for future research

It is apparent that more research is needed on the effects of different environments on the physiological responses and performance of female subjects. In warm environments, studies involving females should be conducted at higher exercise intensities that simulate competition in various sports (e.g. running, cycling). Although there have been numerous studies that have examined thermoregulatory responses in different phases of the menstrual cycle, most have been conducted during low- and moderate-intensity exercise. Voluntary fluid replacement following exercise should also be examined during different phases of the menstrual cycle. The effects of heat stress on the physiological responses of amenorrhoeic female athletes need to be compared with those of eumenorrhoeic athletes in different phases of the menstrual cycle.

There is very little information available on the exercise responses to cold environments during the different phases of the menstrual cycle. Carbohydrates appear to be the preferred source of energy in cold environments, at least in males. Similar studies should be conducted with female subjects, comparing substrate utilization during the different phases of the menstrual cycle as well as between females and males. Because many female athletes have depleted iron stores, more research is needed on the effects of iron deficiency on performance in the cold. More studies are also needed on acclimatization in female athletes who compete in cold environments (e.g. skiers, speed skaters). For example, it would be interesting to know if performance improves following cold acclimatization.

Although information is available on the effects of different altitudes on $\dot{V}O_{2max}$ in females, more research is needed on the acute and chronic effects of altitude on performance. This information is especially needed in female athletes who are iron depleted. Studies should be conducted also on the effects of iron supplementation during acclimatization. Research on the effects of menstrual status and cycle phase on the physiological responses to altitude is also desirable.

References

American College of Sports Medicine (1996) Position stand: heat and cold illnesses during distance running. *Medicine and Science in Sports and Exercise* **28**(12), i–x.

Araki, T., Matsushita, K., Umeno, K., Tsujino, A. & Toda, Y. (1981) Effect of physical training on exercise-induced sweating in women. *Journal of Applied Physiology* **51**, 1526–1532.

Avellini, B., Kamon, E. & Krajewski, J. (1980) Physiological responses of physically fit men and women to acclimation to humid heat. *Journal of Applied Physiology* **49**, 254–261.

Bergeron, M., Maresh, C., Armstrong, L. *et al.* (1995) Fluid–electrolyte balance associated with tennis match play in a hot environment. *International Journal of Sport Nutrition* **5**, 180–193.

Broad, E., Burke, L., Cox, G., Heeley, P. & Riley, M. (1996) Body weight changes and voluntary fluid intakes during training and competition sessions in team sports. *International Journal of Sport Nutrition* **6**, 307–320.

Buskirk, E., Kollias, J., Picon-Reatigue, E., Akers, R., Prokop, E. & Baker, P. (1967) Physiology and performance of track athletes at various altitudes in the United States and Peru. In R.F. Goddard (ed.) *International Symposium on the Effects of Altitude on Physical Performance*, pp. 65–72. Athletic Institute, Chicago.

Carpenter, A.J. & Nunneley, S.A. (1988) Endogenous

hormones subtly alter women's responses to heat stress. *Journal of Applied Physiology* **65**, 2313–2317.

Clarkson, P. & Haymes, E. (1995) Exercise and mineral status of athletes: calcium, magnesium, phosphorus, and iron. *Medicine and Science in Sports and Exercise* **27**, 831–843.

Cohen, J. & Gisolfi, C. (1982) Effects of interval training on work–heat tolerance of young women. *Medicine and Science in Sports and Exercise* **14**, 46–52.

Drinkwater, B., Denton, J., Kupprat, I., Talag, T. & Horvath, S. (1976) Aerobic power as a factor in women's response to work in hot environments. *Journal of Applied Physiology* **41**, 815–821.

Drinkwater, B., Kupprat, I., Denton, J. & Horvath, S. (1977) Heat tolerance of female distance runners. *Annals of the New York Academy of Sciences* **301**, 777–792.

Drinkwater, B., Folinsbee, L., Bedi, J., Plowman, S., Loucks, A. & Horvath, S. (1979) Response of women mountaineers to maximal exercise during hypoxia. *Aviation, Space and Environmental Medicine* **50**, 657–662.

Drinkwater, B., Kramar, P., Bedi, J. & Folinsbee, L. (1982) Women at altitude: cardiovascular responses to altitude. *Aviation, Space and Environmental Medicine* **53**, 472–477.

Elias, S., Roberts, W. & Thorson, D. (1991) Team sports in hot weather: guidelines for modifying youth soccer. *Physician and Sportsmedicine* **19**, 67–80.

Elliott, P. & Atterbom, H. (1978) Comparison of exercise responses of males and females during acute exposure to hypobaria. *Aviation, Space and Environmental Medicine* **49**, 415–418.

England, A., Fraser, D., Hightower, A. *et al.* (1982) Preventing severe heat injury in runners: suggestions from the 1979 Peachtree road race experience. *Annals of Internal Medicine* **97**, 196–201.

Fein, J., Haymes, E. & Buskirk, E. (1975) Effects of daily intermittent exposures on heat acclimation of women. *International Journal of Biometeorology* **19**, 41–52.

Fortney, S. (1996) Hormonal control of fluid balance in women during exercise. In E.R. Buskirk & S.M. Puhl (eds) *Body Fluid Balance: Exercise and Sport*, pp. 231–258. CRC Press, Boca Raton, Florida.

Fortney, S. & Senay, L. (1979) Effects of training and heat acclimation on exercise responses of sedentary females. *Journal of Applied Physiology* **47**, 978–984.

Frye, A. & Kamon, E. (1981) Responses to dry heat of men and women with similar aerobic capacities. *Journal of Applied Physiology* **50**, 65–70.

Gaebelein, C. & Senay, L. (1982) Vascular volume dynamics during ergometer exercise at different menstrual phases. *European Journal of Applied Physiology* **50**, 1–11.

Graham, T. (1983) Alcohol ingestion and sex differences of the thermal responses to mild exercise in a cold environment. *Human Biology* **55**, 463–476.

Graham, T. & Lougheed, M. (1985) Thermal responses to exercise in the cold: influence of sex differences and alcohol. *Human Biology* **57**, 687–698.

Graham, T., Viswanathan, M., Van Dijk, J., Bonen, A. & George, J. (1989) Thermal and metabolic responses to cold by men and by eumenorrheic and amenorrheic women. *Journal of Applied Physiology* **67**, 282–290.

Haymes, E. & Wells, C. (1986) *Environment and Human Performance*. Human Kinetics Publishers, Champaign, Illinois.

Haymes, E., Dickinson, A., Malville, N. & Ross, R. (1982) Effects of wind on the thermal and metabolic responses to exercise in the cold. *Medicine and Science in Sports and Exercise* **14**, 41–45.

Hessemer, V. & Bruck, K. (1985a) Influence of menstrual cycle on shivering, skin blood flow, and sweating responses measured at night. *Journal of Applied Physiology* **59**, 1902–1910.

Hessemer, V. & Bruck, K. (1985b) Influence of menstrual cycle on thermoregulatory, metabolic, and heart rate responses to exercise at night. *Journal of Applied Physiology* **59**, 1911–1917.

Hong, S., Rennie, D. & Park, Y. (1986) Cold acclimatization and deacclimatization of Korean women divers. *Exercise and Sport Sciences Reviews* **14**, 231–268.

Levine, B. & Stray-Gunderson, J. (1992) A practical approach to altitude training: where to live and train for optimal performance enhancement. *International Journal of Sports Medicine* **13**, S209–S212.

Lukaski, H., Hall, C. & Nielsen, F. (1990) Thermogenesis and thermoregulatory function of iron-deficient women without anemia. *Aviation, Space and Environmental Medicine* **61**, 913–920.

McArdle, W., Magel, J., Spina, R., Gergley, T. & Toner, M. (1984) Thermal adjustment to cold-water exposure in exercising men and women. *Journal of Applied Physiology* **56**, 1572–1577.

Martinez-Torres, C., Cubeddu, L., Dillmann, E. *et al.* (1984) Effect of exposure to low temperature on normal and iron-deficient subjects. *American Journal of Physiology* **246**, R380–R383.

Mathew, L., Purkayastha, S., Jayashankar, A. & Nayar, H. (1981) Physiological characteristics of cold acclimatization in man. *International Journal of Biometeorology* **25**, 191–198.

Maughan, R., McArthur, M. & Shirreffs, S. (1996) Influence of menstrual status on fluid replacement after exercise induced dehydration in healthy young women. *British Journal of Sports Medicine* **30**, 41–47.

Miles, D., Wagner, J., Horvath, S. & Reyburn, J. (1980) Absolute and relative work capacity in women at 758, 586, and 523 torr barometric pressure. *Aviation, Space and Environmental Medicine* **51**, 439–444.

Millard-Stafford, M., Sparling, P., Rosskopf, L., Snow,

T., DiCarlo, L. & Hinson, B. (1995) Fluid intake in male and female runners during a 40-km field run in the heat. *Journal of Sports Sciences* **13**, 257–263.

Nielsen, B. (1996) Olympics in Atlanta: a fight against physics. *Medicine and Science in Sports and Exercise* **28**, 665–668.

Paolone, A., Wells, C. & Kelly, G. (1978) Sexual variations in thermoregulation during heat stress. *Aviation, Space and Environmental Medicine* **49**, 715–719.

Pivarnik, J., Marichal, C., Spillman, T. & Morrow, J. (1992) Menstrual cycle phase affects temperature regulation during endurance exercise. *Journal of Applied Physiology* **72**, 543–548.

Pugh, L. (1966) Accidental hypothermia in walkers, climbers, and campers: report to the medical commissions on accident prevention. *British Medical Journal* **1**, 123–129.

Pugh, L. (1967) Athletes at altitude. *Journal of Physiology* **192**, 619–646.

Rennie, D., Covino, B., Howell, B., Song, S., Kang, B. & Hong, S. (1962) Physical insulation of Korean diving women. *Journal of Applied Physiology* **17**, 961–966.

Roberts, M., Wenger, C., Stolwijk, J. & Nadel, E. (1977) Skin blood flow and sweating changes following exercise training and heat acclimation. *Journal of Applied Physiology* **43**, 133–137.

Saltin, B. (1967) Aerobic and anaerobic work capacity at an altitude of 2250 meters. In R.F. Goddard (ed.) *International Symposium on the Effects of Altitude on Physical Performance*, pp. 97–102. Athletic Institute, Chicago.

Shapiro, Y., Pandolf, K., Avellini, B., Pimental, N. & Goldman, R. (1980a) Physiological responses of men and women to humid and dry heat. *Journal of Applied Physiology* **49**, 1–8.

Shapiro, Y., Pandolf, K. & Goldman, R. (1980b) Sex differences in acclimation to a hot-dry environment. *Ergonomics* **23**, 635–642.

Silami-Garcia, E. & Haymes, E. (1989) Effects of repeated short-term cold exposure on cold induced thermogenesis of women. *International Journal of Biometeorology* **33**, 222–226.

Sloan, R. & Keatinge, W. (1973) Cooling rates of young people swimming in cold water. *Journal of Applied Physiology* **35**, 371–375.

Squires, R. & Buskirk, E. (1982) Aerobic capacity during acute exposure to simulated altitude, 914–2286 meters. *Medicine and Science in Sports and Exercise* **14**, 36–40.

Stephenson, L. & Kolka, M. (1985) Menstrual cycle phase and time of day alter reference signal controlling arm blood flow and sweating. *American Journal of Physiology* **249**, R186–R191.

Stephenson, L. & Kolka, M. (1988) Plasma volume during heat stress and exercise in women. *European Journal of Applied Physiology* **57**, 373–381.

Stevens, G., Graham, T. & Wilson, B. (1987) Gender differences in cardiovascular and metabolic responses to cold and exercise. *Canadian Journal of Physiology and Pharmacology* **65**, 165–171.

Stine, T., Levine, B., Taylor, S., Schultz, W. & Stray-Gunderson, J. (1992) Quantification of altitude training in the field. *Medicine and Science in Sports and Exercise* **24**, S103.

Stray-Gunderson, J., Alexander, C., Hochstein, A., deLemos, D. & Levine, B. (1992) Failure of red cell volume to increase at altitude exposure in iron deficient runners. *Medicine and Science in Sports and Exercise* **24**, S90.

Terrados, N. (1992) Altitude training and muscular metabolism. *International Journal of Sports Medicine* **13**, S206–S209.

Van Loan, M. & Boileau, R. (1996) Age, gender, and fluid balance. In E.R. Buskirk & S.M. Puhl (eds) *Body Fluid Balance: Exercise and Sport*, pp. 215–230. CRC Press, Boca Raton, Florida.

Wagner, J., Miles, D. & Horvath, S. (1980) Physiological adjustments of women to prolonged work during acute hypoxia. *Journal of Applied Physiology* **49**, 367–373.

Walsh, C. & Graham, T. (1986) Male–female responses in various body temperatures during and following exercise in cold air. *Aviation, Space and Environmental Medicine* **57**, 966–973.

Wells, C. (1980) Responses of physically active and acclimatized men and women to exercise in a desert environment. *Medicine and Science in Sports and Exercise* **12**, 9–13.

Young, A., Evans, W., Cymerman, A., Pandolf, K., Knapik, J. & Maher, J. (1982) Sparing effect of chronic high-altitude exposure on muscle glycogen utilization. *Journal of Applied Physiology* **52**, 857–862.

PART 3

TRAINING THE FEMALE ATHLETE

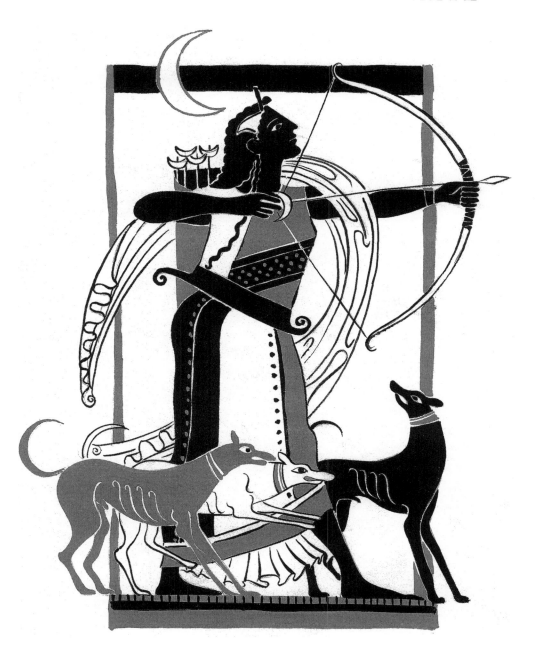

Chapter 5

Physiological Aspects of Training

MARY L. O'TOOLE

Introduction

Women athletes have been competing in Olympic events since the Second Olympiad (1900) of the modern Games. At that time, only a few women contestants participated in just three sports: tennis, golf and yachting. In the 1996 Summer Games, 36% of competing athletes were women. These women athletes were contestants in a broad range of sporting events, most of which were identical to the corresponding men's events. For example, the marathon was a 42.2-km road race, the freestyle swim was 100m long, a basketball game consisted of two 20-min halves, a soccer game two 45-min halves, etc. The physiological demands of the events were therefore the same for women as for men.

The components of success in competition (i.e. winning) for men and women athletes can be summarized succinctly by the motto of the modern Olympic Games: 'Citius, Altius, Fortius' or its translation 'Swifter, Higher, Stronger'. Each of these components is based on capacities of the athlete for cardiorespiratory endurance, muscle endurance, muscle strength, power, flexibility, agility and speed. The extent to which each of these components is important for success depends on an analysis of the requirements of each event. Although a detailed analysis of the components of each of the Olympic events is beyond the scope of this chapter, a general look at what happens during a soccer game serves to illustrate this point. Players are continuously active for two 45-min halves covering distances

ranging from 7 to 12 km. Cardiorespiratory and muscle endurance are of obvious import. Of this total distance, however, up to 12% has been estimated to occur at sprint speed interspersed on the continuous motion (Reilly & Thomas, 1976; Mayhew & Wenger, 1985; Zeederberg *et al.*, 1996). Additionally, accelerations from standing to maximal effort occur 40–62 times per game with pace and/or direction being changed approximately every 5s (Kirkendall, 1985). These bursts require muscular power, reaction time, agility and flexibility.

Understanding the physiological bases for training to become 'Swifter, Higher, Stronger' can help the athlete develop appropriate training programmes aimed at making adaptations to meet the physiological demands of the sport. Thus, the movement requirements of each sporting event (e.g. fast or slow, high intensity or low intensity, short or prolonged) determine the cardiovascular and metabolic requirements for that sport. Training type, intensity and duration should mirror these requirements. Resultant improvement in the capacity for energy transformation (aerobic and anaerobic), aspects of neurophysiological function (e.g. coordination, skill, reaction time) as well as the capacity for strength and power generation are all important for an athlete's performance.

Training for competition fits the same general model as training to improve health or fitness. This can be described as a stimulus–response model, in which the stimulus is the training overload and the response is the physiological adaptation that allows the athlete to go faster, jump higher or be stronger. Although evidence for the adaptive responses of women athletes to training is not as voluminous as that for male athletes, existing evidence does suggest that men and women respond to the same training with the same adaptations (Wells, 1991; Plowman & Smith, 1997). Much is known about the physiological adaptations that occur during the initial stages of exercise training. These are discussed in Chapter 2. Much less is known about the adaptations that occur in athletes to improve performance by very small amounts (often the difference between winning an event and finishing out of medal contention). Since most serious athletes have been training for many years and have made the initial physiological adaptations long ago, training must include stimuli aimed at improving particular aspects of performance in accord with the specific demands of the competitive event. Large amounts of training, while avoiding the pitfalls of overtraining, may be necessary to produce very small improvements in performance. These small improvements are, of necessity, based on some underlying physiological adaptations. The purpose of this chapter is to discuss some of the training techniques commonly used, their physiological bases and the expected adaptations that result in improved performance.

Swifter: training to optimize energy transformation

Most sports events contain some element of swiftness or speed. Speed is ultimately limited by rate of energy transformation. Maximal speed (exercise intensity) sustainable is directly related to the length of time the athlete must be in motion (race or event duration). Table 5.1 shows record times for running races with distances from 100 m to 42.2 km. Quite clearly, exercise intensity (speed) and duration are inversely related. The ultimate source of energy for movement is adenosine triphosphate (ATP). Since only a small amount of ATP is stored in the body, the rate of ATP resynthesis is the limiting factor for

Table 5.1 Women's Olympic track and field records

Distance	Time	Year of record
100 m	10.62 s	1988
200 m	21.34 s	1988
400 m	48.25 s	1996
800 m	1 min 53.43 s	1980
1500 m	3 min 53.96 s	1988
5000 m	14 min 59.88 s	1996
10 000 m	31 min 01.64 s	1996
42.2 km	2 hours 24 min 52 s	1984

all but the shortest of athletic events. For optimal performance, the fastest rates of ATP resynthesis that can be sustained for the length of the race must result from optimal functioning of the energy pathways best equipped to meet these demands. Training methods should be aimed at overloading the energy pathways that will be necessary during competition. For example, a 100-m sprinter needs a very fast rate of energy transformation for a short period of time (9–10 s). She will reach her potential if she can optimize energy transfer via ATP and phosphocreatine systems. An 800-m runner can improve her performance by optimizing ATP, phosphocreatine and anaerobic glycolytic energy transfer. At the other end of the energy spectrum are the needs of a marathon runner. Her main energy requirements must be met with aerobic metabolism with adjuncts from the anaerobic glycolytic system for surges throughout the course of the race and for a finishing kick. These examples are straightforward since the outcome of the race is determined by the swiftness with which the athlete can cover the required distance. Less clear are the swiftness demands of sports events that require some combination of energy transformation pathways for optimal performance. A thorough analysis of the requirements of each sports event is necessary to develop an appropriate training plan for specific events. Such an analysis is beyond the scope of this chapter. The section below reviews some of the commonly used training techniques, as well as their physiological bases, for improving the various types of energy transfer. The translation of this general information into specific training plans is left to the athlete and her coach.

Aerobic energy transformation

Aerobic metabolism is governed by oxygen and nutrient transport as well as by muscle respiratory capacity. According to the training principles of specificity and overload, training to improve aerobic energy transformation should therefore stress the physiological systems involved in transport and use of oxygen and substrate by muscles involved in the tasks specific to the competitive event.

TRAINING METHODS

There are two commonly used methods to train the aerobic energy transformation systems: sustained distance training and aerobic interval training (Wells & Pate, 1988). During sustained distance training, workouts are bouts of continuous rhythmical activity lasting for relatively long periods of time and done at a comfortable pace (also called long slow distance). The specific distance is somewhat arbitrary and may vary considerably depending on the length and type of the competitive event; 8 km of running or at least 30 min of continuous swimming have been reported for rowers and swimmers respectively (Kearney, 1996), while marathon runners have been reported to run for 2–3 hours and cyclists to ride 130–250 km for sustained distance training (Wells & Pate, 1988). The pace of these training sessions should be one that can easily be performed for the specified time. Exercise intensity can be monitored by the athlete during these workouts by using the rating of perceived exertion (RPE) or by monitoring heart rates. RPE during this type of workout should be 'fairly light to light' (RPE = 10–12). If information is available from an incremental exercise test, heart rates representing a pace well below the lactate threshold (see below) can be used to guide pace. Heart rate monitors (on which lower and upper limits can be set) are useful for guiding the athlete to maintain appropriate pace. During sus-

tained distance running, transport (cardiovascular) and utilization (metabolic) systems are stressed. Additional stresses on the athlete include elevation of body temperature, loss of fluid and electrolytes in sweat, repeated microtrauma to joints and muscles, and the need to maintain energy balance.

The second commonly used training technique for improving aerobic metabolism is the use of aerobic interval training. During aerobic interval training, workouts consist of repeated exercise periods (usually lasting 5–15 min) interspersed with short rest periods (5–15 s). With this type of training pattern, more absolute work can be done during a workout session than with sustained distance training. Although neither circulation nor oxygen uptake has time to recover to any appreciable amount during the relatively short recovery intervals, the musculoskeletal system gets brief respites from continuous strain. As with sustained distance training, the specific length of the exercise interval depends on the exercise mode and the length of the competitive event. For example, a 10-km runner might incorporate 800–1600-m repeats into her workout plan. Repetitions may be as few as five per session or as many as 20. The longer the exercise interval in relation to the event length (greater proportion of the whole race), the fewer the repetitions (Costill, 1986). The pace should be slightly below the lactate threshold pace, but faster than the pace for sustained distance training. Intensity can be guided by keeping RPE within the 'somewhat hard to hard' range (RPE = 13–15), with heart rates kept in a range that represents slightly less than lactate threshold. It is commonly recommended that these intervals be done no more than 1–3 days per week because of risk of injury (Costill, 1986). The same benefits to transport and utilization systems occur as with sustained distance training, but additional benefits accrue as well. The movement patterns are more similar to competitive event patterns, thus potentially improving movement economy (see below) and relative proportions of substrate used (fat vs. carbohydrate). Additionally, lactate may increase during the workout, stressing systems involved in tolerating higher lactate levels and those involved in removing lactate.

The physiological adaptations that account for improvement in aerobic energy transformation are reflected in the functional capacities of the cardiovascular and metabolic systems. Adaptations to the cardiovascular system include the variety of cardiac adaptations that allow greater efficiency in the performance of the heart's primary function, that of a muscular pump, as well as those involving more efficient distribution of blood volume (Harrison, 1985). Adaptations to the metabolic system include more efficient utilization of substrate via improved functioning of energy transfer systems.

CARDIOVASCULAR ADAPTATIONS

Initially $\dot{V}_{O_{2max}}$, often used as the 'gold standard' to judge capacity for aerobic energy transfer, increases because of training-induced increases in maximal cardiac output directly attributable to increased stroke volume (Clausen, 1977; Blomqvist & Saltin, 1983). Traditional wisdom has been that during incremental exercise stroke volumes of women as well as men reach maximum at exercise intensities of 40–50% maximal capacity and that training will increase the height of the plateau. Endurance athletes were simply thought to have larger stroke volumes at each exercise intensity and higher plateaus than untrained or less well-trained individuals (Saltin, 1969). Recently, however, Gledhill et al. (1994) confirmed earlier reports (Ekblom & Hermanson, 1968; Vanfraechem, 1979; Crawford et al., 1986) of continued increase in stroke volume throughout an incremental exercise test to maximal effort in highly trained male cyclists. The resultant slower heart rates at submaximal exercise intensities would reduce myocardial oxygen demand. While similar information is not available for female athletes, they have been demonstrated to exhibit many of the physiological changes that could potentially contribute to increased stroke volume.

Several factors can contribute to an increased stroke volume. Increased left ventricular cavity size and left ventricular mass are common findings in female as well as male endurance-trained athletes over a wide age range from a variety of sports (Pollack et al., 1987; Douglas et al., 1988; Douglas & O'Toole, 1992; Pelliccia et al., 1996). The increased wall thickness allows a reduction in the tension applied to each individual fibre, as wall stress is distributed across a greater mass of myocardium (Douglas, 1989). Additionally, preload is increased, in part because of an increase in total blood volume (particularly plasma volume) (Oscai et al., 1968), and results in an increase in stroke volume via the Frank–Starling mechanism. The increased left and right ventricular end-diastolic volumes allow a similar volume of blood to be ejected with less shortening and less friction but with increased tension. Endurance training appears to result also in an increased left ventricular compliance that enhances preload at maximal exercise (Levine et al., 1991). Studies of male and female ultra-endurance triathletes have shown enhanced diastolic function at rest (altered diastolic filling pattern with increased early filling), which presumably would result in increased preload during maximal exercise (Douglas, 1989). Others have also reported enhanced diastolic function, with measured peak filling rates up to 71% greater than control subjects at matched heart rates (Gledhill et al., 1994). In longitudinal studies, training has also been documented to result in improved cardiac filling in younger and older subjects both at rest and during exercise (Levy et al., 1993). Others have reported resting diastolic performance to be an independent determinant of $\dot{V}_{O_{2max}}$ in both sedentary individuals and athletes (Vanoverschelde et al., 1991), although our studies in triathletes have not confirmed this relationship (P.S. Douglas & M.L. O'Toole, unpublished observations).

The effects of endurance training on contractile function are less clear, since contractile function is increased during maximal exercise in untrained as well as highly trained athletes. Gledhill et al. (1994) demonstrated a progressive increase in peak left ventricular emptying rates with maximal exercise testing in cyclists that was not seen in control subjects and a longer left ventricular ejection time, suggesting that augmentation of systolic function during exercise is a mechanism by which athletes are able to enhance performance. It has been postulated that the athlete's ability to enhance systolic function leads to a smaller end-systolic volume which, by virtue of suction, would enhance early diastolic filling.

Peripherally, aerobic training results in increased capillary density; a close correlation has been shown between $\dot{V}O_{2max}$ and number of capillaries per muscle fibre in both women and men athletes (Saltin *et al.*, 1977). Endurance training has also been associated with reduced systolic and diastolic blood pressures and total peripheral resistance, thereby enabling the endurance athlete to achieve high cardiac outputs at maximal exercise with afterload similar to that of sedentary subjects with much lower cardiac outputs. Additionally, a close relationship between submaximal exercise blood pressures and left ventricular mass has been reported for male and female ultra-endurance triathletes (Douglas *et al.*, 1986).

All these findings suggest a more efficiently functioning cardiovascular system in highly trained athletes. Although some of this information, including the work of Gledhill *et al.* (1994), has been derived from studies of male athletes, both Douglas and colleagues and Pelliccia and colleagues have included women athletes and have found no gender-related differences in these responses. The time course of these adaptations in athletes is unknown as are the limits to adaptation in any single athlete.

METABOLIC ADAPTATIONS

Adaptive changes in the muscular system that occur in response to sustained distance or aerobic interval training improve the efficiency of substrate utilization (Saltin & Rowell, 1980; Klausen *et al.*, 1981). These metabolic adaptations (increases in myoglobin, size and number of mitochondria, and levels of various enzymes and transfer agents that enhance aerobic metabolism) can contribute as much as 50% to the initial improvement in the ability to extract and use oxygen during the aerobic resynthesis of ATP (Holloszy, 1975; Clausen, 1977). Gollnick *et al.* (1972) demonstrated that these adaptations in males were specific to the mode of exercise stimulus (e.g. the patterns of enzyme activities in arm and leg muscles of swimmers were clearly different from those of cyclists). Both fat and carbohydrate metabolism is enhanced (Gollnick *et al.*, 1972; Holloszy & Coyle, 1984). The time course of these adaptations appears to be somewhat variable, although Hamel *et al.* (1986) reported adaptation of skeletal muscle enzymes to be near maximal trainability after 15 weeks.

Interindividual differences in movement economy occur in highly trained élite athletes (Daniels, 1985). As has been shown for male runners, Pate *et al.* (1987) demonstrated that élite female runners had lower $\dot{V}O_2$ (better movement economy) at two different submaximal running speeds (230 and 248 m·min^{-1}) compared with non-élite runners. Morgan and Craib (1992) have suggested that these differences are the result of differences in muscle fibre type. However, Williams and Cavanagh (1987) reported no difference in fibre type among trained runners with good, medium and poor running economy. Similarly, Costill *et al.* (1987) confirmed that muscle fibre characteristics and enzyme activities in female runners were directly related to the length of the competitive event but not to skill level. Women marathon runners had a greater percentage of type I fibres than middle distance runners, but muscle enzyme activities were similar in élite and non-élite runners at matched distances (Costill *et al.*, 1987).

Both muscle and liver glycogen reserves are increased with this type of training. Studies have shown that with training, the relative contribution of fat compared with carbohydrate as substrate is increased (Gollnick, 1985). Thus, at the same absolute workload (i.e. same running speed), muscle and liver glycogen are metabolized at a slower rate than before training (Holloszy & Coyle, 1984; Gollnick *et al.*, 1986; Abernathy *et al.*, 1990). The advantage of this is a delay in glycogen depletion, which not only allows activity to proceed at a particular pace for a longer time but also allows brief spurts of higher intensity activity that is reliant on glycolytic energy sources. However, the oxygen cost of burning fat is greater than that of burning carbohydrate. Therefore, one could hypothesize that it would be to the advantage of the successful athlete to be able not only to conserve muscle glycogen but also to oxidize exogenous carbohydrate. No studies have specifically addressed this issue in female athletes.

Sustained distance training and aerobic interval training alter lactate thresholds by decreasing lactate production and/or improving clearance rates at submaximal exercise intensities. Lactate thresholds, when expressed as percentage $\dot{V}_{O_{2max}}$, are similar for equally well-trained men and women athletes. The relationship of lactate threshold to successful performance has been shown to be as important for the woman athlete as the man (O'Toole et al., 1989; Laurenson et al., 1993; O'Toole & Douglas, 1995). Élite marathon runners have been reported to run their races at an average pace equivalent to 86% $\dot{V}_{O_{2max}}$, a pace that represents 93% of their lactate threshold of 4 mmol·l^{-1} (Sjodin & Svedenhag, 1985). Slower marathon runners reportedly run at 65% $\dot{V}_{O_{2max}}$. There is some evidence to suggest that in highly trained male and female athletes who have reached their genetic ceiling for $\dot{V}_{O_{2max}}$ through hard training, continued improvement in performance results from continual improvement in lactate threshold. Kohrt et al. (1989) reported increases of 6% and 10% in lactate thresholds for female as well as male triathletes for cycling and running, respectively, during the course of a triathlon season. No increases in $\dot{V}_{O_{2max}}$ occurred. Neither the time course nor the optimal training stimulus for continual improvement of thresholds in athletes is known.

OTHER CONSIDERATIONS

To derive optimal training benefits from sustained distance and aerobic interval training, energy balance as well as fluid and electrolyte balance must be maintained daily. During sustained distance and aerobic interval training, the athlete metabolizes a combination of fat and carbohydrate for prolonged periods. Since fat stores are essentially unlimited, the focus of energy balance should be on the consumption of adequate calories and enough carbohydrate to keep glycogen stores replete. It is generally accepted that 8–10 g·kg^{-1} (600–650 g) of carbohydrate daily are necessary to maintain maximally full glycogen stores (Sherman & Lamb, 1988). How well female athletes comply with these recommendations may depend on the specific sport for which they are training. For example, caloric intakes of triathletes have been reported to be appropriate for the amount and type of training, with carbohydrate intake quite close to recommended amounts, ranging between 6.7 and 8.8 g·kg^{-1} daily (Burke & Read, 1987; Khoo et al., 1987; Applegate, 1989). Conversely, female cross-country runners, for whom thinness may be perceived as more important, were reported to fall short of both caloric and carbohydrate requirements (Tanaka et al., 1995). The effect on performance of women athletes who do not follow these recommendations is not clear in the light of evidence that women athletes demonstrate greater lipid and less carbohydrate or protein metabolism during moderate-intensity exercise compared with equally trained male athletes (Tarnopolsky et al., 1990).

In addition to daily energy/carbohydrate balance, many endurance athletes also follow carbohydrate-loading regimens before important competitions. During typical carbohydrate loading, dietary carbohydrate is increased to 75% of energy intake for 4 days before competition. Recent research, however, has cast doubt on the usefulness of this practice for female athletes. Tarnopolsky et al. (1995) reported that while men increased muscle glycogen concentration by 41% following such a routine, no change in glycogen concentration was seen in women athletes. In men, this resulted in a 45% improvement in cycling performance at 85% $\dot{V}_{O_{2max}}$, while in women there was no change in performance. Confirmation of these apparent gender differences is needed in larger groups of women athletes and in different exercise modes.

Another major consideration is the maintenance of fluid and electrolyte balance. To maintain body temperature within tolerable limits, the high rate of heat production that occurs with aerobic exercise training and competition must be balanced by a high rate of heat loss. This requires a high sweat rate and therefore loss of both fluids and electrolytes (Nadel, 1988). Both sustained distance training and aerobic interval training, particularly when performed in a hot environment, place large thermoregulatory demands on the female athlete. Tolerance to fluid consumption during endurance exercise appears to be a trainable phenomenon and should be incorporated into sustained distance and aerobic interval training (Sparling *et al.*, 1993) (see Chapter 4 for a more thorough discussion of gender-related differences in thermoregulatory capacities of athletes).

Aerobic and anaerobic energy transformation

Just as the metabolic systems do not operate in isolation, some types of training improve both aerobic and anaerobic metabolism. Pace or tempo training is a perfect example. Pace training is continued for long enough periods of time to stress the oxidative energy systems (see above) but also at a sufficient intensity that there is a large anaerobic component as well.

TRAINING METHODS

Pace training involves exercise performed at a pace slightly faster than lactate threshold pace (Wells & Pate, 1988). Intervals of 3–10 min are interspersed with 30–90 s periods of slower paced activity. The number of intervals performed during any exercise session depends on the exercise mode and the length of the competition. During the exercise intervals, the RPE should represent subjective feelings of 'hard to very hard' exercise (RPE = 15–17). Heart rates that represent an exercise intensity approximately 5% greater than that at lactate threshold

can be used to monitor training (Dwyer & Bybee, 1983; Gilman & Wells, 1993). Since lactate thresholds may vary according to exercise mode, heart rates that have been measured in the particular training mode should be used. For example, in both men and women athletes, lactate thresholds (4 mmol·l^{-1}) have been reported to be 72–88% $\dot{V}O_{2max}$ for cycling but 80–85% $\dot{V}O_{2max}$ for running (Kohrt *et al.*, 1989; O'Toole *et al.*, 1989). Because the pace is above the threshold, lactate accumulates in the muscle during the exercise part of the interval. During the recovery intervals ATP and phosphocreatine are replenished, allowing the athlete to maintain the high intensity at the beginning of the next exercise interval. However, only some of the lactate is removed and metabolized via aerobic metabolism, causing the athlete to try to maintain pace despite a more acidic local muscle environment (Plowman & Smith, 1997). Thus pace training stimulates and causes adaptive responses in both aerobic and anaerobic energy systems. Since many sports require intermittent anaerobic activity over a long period of time, this type of training can be particularly useful. Following a training session, approximately 50% of the lactate is removed with 15–20 min of rest and levels are nearly back to resting levels within 1 hour. Lactate removal can be accelerated by continuous jogging for about 20 min at a comfortable pace just below the lactate threshold. However, the continuous jogging may delay the resynthesis of muscle glycogen and therefore may not be beneficial to all athletes, e.g. one who has repeated heats in a middle-distance event.

PHYSIOLOGICAL BASES AND ADAPTATIONS

The benefits of pace training include many of the adaptations described above for sustained distance and aerobic interval training. Additionally, pace training effectively stimulates an increase in the lactate threshold by increasing the capacity to remove lactate, increasing the tolerance to high levels of lactate, enhancing the capacity for glycolytic energy transfer (increased glycolytic enzymes) and increasing the capacity to store muscle glycogen. Another benefit of pace training is a muscle-fibre recruitment pattern similar to that in competition, thus contributing to improved movement economy. Both male and female athletes respond similarly to lactate and have similar resting levels and similar levels at matched relative intensities (Plowman & Smith, 1997). As with aerobic training, neither the time course nor the upper limits of trainability for female athletes is known.

Anaerobic energy transformation

High-intensity exercise requires a very fast rate of energy transfer. This rate can only be met through anaerobic energy pathways. The limiting factors for continued energy transformation via anaerobic pathways are mainly substrate depletion and the factors associated with accumulation of lactate as described above. Exercise time is severely limited, from seconds to a few minutes, when anaerobic metabolism is the sole energy source. Anaerobic interval training, with intervals of varying lengths, is useful for enhancing power for short events such as the 100-m sprint and for spurts in many game activities. These short intervals, often called speed training, are as effective for women athletes as for men (Weltman et al., 1978).

TRAINING METHODS

Very short exercise intervals are performed at or above the pace associated with $\dot{V}O_{2max}$ (Weltman et al., 1978; Wells & Pate, 1988). Exercise intervals last between 30 s and 4 min with recovery intervals about 2 min long; 5–20 such intervals may be repeated during a training session. Subjective RPE should be 'very, very hard' (RPE=18–20). Heart rates can be monitored but are probably unnecessary for this type of training. ATP and phosphocreatine systems are the main targets for the shorter intervals, with the anaerobic glycolytic system being an additional target during intervals lasting longer than a few seconds. This type of training is very demanding and should be used judiciously and interspersed with training of other energy systems.

PHYSIOLOGICAL BASES AND ADAPTATIONS

For most contests, other than outright sprints, the challenge for the athlete is not to perform only one of these intervals but to recover quickly and perform them repeatedly throughout the course of a game, e.g. basketball, tennis, etc. During the exercise part of the interval, there is marked depletion of phosphagens (ATP and phosphocreatine) along with marked elevations in lactate with the longer intervals. Unlike training with high lactate levels to improve tolerance to low pH, there is no benefit to training with depleted phosphagens. The 2-min recovery interval reflects the time it takes to restore the phosphagens to near resting levels; half-restoration occurs within 30 s (Fox & Mathews, 1974). Although phosphagen recovery is most effective with complete rest, unless the exercise interval has been limited to 10 s or less some lactate has accumulated as well. Low-intensity exercise would then be the most appropriate recovery technique. For most athletes, intervals should have a specific metabolic goal. They should be either very short so as to minimize the contribution of lactate or long enough to include a lactate contribution. The specific combination of intervals should be guided by the competition demands on each athlete. Although the efficiency of splitting ATP is not changed by this or any other type of training (Plowman & Smith, 1997), trained muscle contains more ATP and phosphocreatine as well as enzymes to increase the rate of breakdown. The specific contribution of these increased resting levels to movement and speed in particular is not known.

Higher: training to optimize neurophysiological aspects of movement

In order to soar or jump higher, an athlete needs the capacity for optimal energy transformation (see above) and optimal strength and power (see below). However, these capacities will not produce winning efforts in most sports contests unless neurophysiological aspects of movement are also functioning at optimal levels. There is general agreement that motor skills, including agility, balance, reaction time and quickness, are all important for success in sports. However, there is not general agreement about training methods or underlying physiological changes that contribute to improvement of these parameters. However, since it is known that motor skills are acquired through practice with appropriate feedback (Fox et al., 1996), most athletes train with repetition of the specific movement patterns of the competitive event. Neither the time course for skill development nor the final skill level can be predicted for an individual athlete. It is beyond the scope of this chapter to explore the concepts of motor learning for the athlete.

Stronger: training to optimize strength and power

Most sports contests require a certain element of strength and/or power. As with training for optimal energy utilization and neuromuscular function, strength/power training should be specific to the goals of the individual athlete. A gymnast may require a great deal of strength, long jumpers a great deal of power and athletes in most other sports a combination of these two qualities. As in other types of training, the response of the female athlete is qualitatively similar to that of the male athlete, so that while the male athlete is typically stronger than the female athlete, both will respond to resistance training with similar patterns of strength gains and similar changes in muscle cross-sectional area (Wilmore, 1974; Weltman et al., 1978; Cureton et al., 1988; Tesch, 1992).

As with other types of training, the intensity of the stimulus (amount of weight or resistance) determines the response (strength gain). Therefore near-maximal resistance is used to produce the greatest gains in strength. For the female athlete, strength requirements are a part of the physiological demands necessary for success in a sport or event, rather than a separate event such as weight-lifting for men. Typically, two types of equipment are used to improve strength. 'Fixed-form' equipment includes the various types of weight machines commonly found at fitness clubs. This type of equipment is best for isolating muscles around a particular joint. Because muscle groups are isolated, with little effect on adjacent groups, the athlete must be careful to avoid creating imbalances in strength around a joint. 'Free-form' weights are mainly free weights that require synergistic muscle action to maintain balance and to keep the movement in the appropriate plane. This type of training has the most relevance for sports. As with increasing $\dot{V}_{O_{2max}}$, the main increases in strength should be accomplished before the competitive season; strength training during the season should be used for maintenance. Although some controversy continues to exist regarding concurrent strength and endurance training (Dudley & Djamil, 1985; Callister et al., 1990; Chromiak & Mulvaney, 1990), most of the available studies suggest that concurrent training shows little effect on aerobic capacity but may decrease strength and power. For example, Callister et al. (1990) documented decreases in speed and jumping power following a mixed training regimen. In addition to the resistance applied, the velocity of movement also seems to be important in training for power (Perrin, 1993). Slow-velocity training has been shown to increase torque only at the training velocity. Fast-velocity training seems to have the added advantage of increasing torque at the training velocity and at movement speeds slower than training velocity. Since angular velocities for most sports movements are greater than commonly used isokinetic training velocities, it makes intuitive sense that the athlete should train at the highest velocity possible for a given power requirement.

Training methods

During resistance training, the components that are manipulated to produce the required stimulus are the load, number of repetitions, number of sets and length of rest periods. Of these, load seems to be most important for the development of strength. No single combination of these components has been documented to produce the best results. Research has shown that resistance must be at least 60% of maximum in order to make strength gains. However, most commonly, 80–90% maximal capacity (1 repetition maximum, RM) is lifted for three to six repetitions per set for three to five sets (Fleck & Kramer, 1987). Many athletes quantify and manipulate the volume of training (number of repetitions × set × load) per session to make optimal improvement without undue fatigue (Tesch, 1992). If muscular endurance, i.e. the ability continually to repeat submaximal efforts as in tennis strokes, is the desired outcome, a lower resistance can be used. Gains in muscular endurance have been reported with resistance as low as 30% of maximal capacity if repetitions are continued until the muscle group is fatigued (Cureton et al., 1988). The length of the rest periods is also important. Relatively long rest periods of several minutes between sets are used when the goal is increasing strength. Conversely, shorter rest periods of less than 1 min between sets should be used for training muscular endurance (Fleck & Kramer, 1987). Training 2–4 days a week is thought by weight-lifters to be the most effective. However, they frequently emphasize only one muscle group during a workout. This muscle group is then rested for 48–72 hours before another strength-training session. Whether this is an appropriate way to strength train athletes, other than competitive resistance athletes, is unknown. Once the athlete has achieved the desired level of strength, usually within 1 year of serious training, this level can be maintained with as little as one session per week or multiple sessions with reduced volume as long as the resistance load is maintained.

Training methods to improve power are less clear and not supported by good research studies (Wilmore & Costill, 1994). A given power requirement can be met by training with a high-velocity/low-resistance regimen or a slower-velocity/higher-resistance regimen. Fleck and Kramer (1987) suggest that the load should be similar to that during strength training. However, the choice of exercise equipment may be important in the development of power. One technique that athletes have used is 'speed reps' with free weights. During this type of training,

heavy-resistance free weights are moved as rapidly as possible through the range of motion. The momentum created from the accelerating mass must be decelerated at the end of the range. Newton et al. (1996) have shown this to be counterproductive in the development of power as judged by training-induced decreases, rather than increases, in bench press power. Kraemer and Nindl (1997) suggest that power training would best be done with weights that can be released at the end of the range of motion, e.g. medicine balls. Plyometrics, another technique used by athletes to develop power, is a training technique that employs eccentric contractions immediately followed by concentric contractions. For example, one typical routine involves the athlete trying to rebound and attain greater heights after jumping from a box or platform that is higher than floor or ground level. The quadriceps undergoes rapid eccentric contraction followed immediately by a concentric contraction. This type of training is used by hurdlers, high jumpers and by other athletes, such as basketball players, who must jump higher to improve performance. The role of plyometric training for either male or female athletes has not been clearly proved at this time (Bobbert, 1990).

Physiological bases and adaptations

Strength gains accrue within a few weeks of initiation of a resistance training programme. Initial strength gains are attributed to neural adaptations that include increased neural drive, increased synchronization of motor units and release of the inhibitory effects of Golgi tendon organs (Fleck & Kramer, 1987). These neural adaptations result in improved coordination and increased activation of the prime movers for any muscle action. With continued training, muscle hypertrophy occurs as a result of increased amounts of contractile protein, increased size and number of myofibrils per muscle fibre and an increase in the amount of surrounding connective tissue (Rogers & Evans, 1993). One study of heavy-resistance training in men reported that a 28% increase in strength was accompanied by significant increases in the muscle's resting levels of ATP, phosphocreatine, free creatine and glycogen (MacDougal *et al.*, 1977). Although similar studies using female athletes as subjects have not been reported, there is no reason to believe that their responses would be different.

Speed is a more difficult component than strength to change. In large measure, the physiological changes that allow the athlete to increase her power are much the same as those for increased strength. The physiological mechanisms underlying the improved jumping performance following plyometric training are not well understood. Both the stretch–shortening cycle, which relies on the elastic properties of muscle and connective tissue, and the activation of muscle spindles during the eccentric part of the jump are thought to potentiate the subsequent concentric contraction. However, these mechanisms have not yet been substantiated for either male or female athletes (Bobbert, 1990).

Other considerations for optimal performance

Although winning performances require optimization of the above-mentioned training adaptations, other factors may also contribute to the outcome. Biomechanical aspects of performance are discussed in Chapter 6, psychological aspects in Chapter 7 and nutrition in Chapter 8. However, even in terms of the physiological adaptations, the athlete must optimize these by training sensibly. Periodization and avoidance of overtraining are critical to an athlete's success.

Periodization

Periodization is the purposeful variation in a training programme over the course of time so that the athlete will approach her optimal adaptive potential just before important competitions. A systematic, sequential approach is used to optimize potential for short periods of time by organizing training into blocks of time. In its simplest form, athletes use a hard–easy pattern for daily workouts. In its more complete form, the training year is divided into blocks of time periods ranging from days to weeks to months. During each of these blocks, a particular aspect of training is emphasized.

The longest blocks of time are called macrocycles and usually last 2–4 months; there may be three to four macrocycles per year. Smaller blocks called mesocycles are organized within each macrocycle; a mesocycle typically lasts 8–10 weeks. In turn, microcycles, usually 1 week each, make up each of the mesocycles. Training volumes and intensities are varied by cycle. In its simplest form, volume and intensity are varied inversely. However, the exact make-up of each cycle depends on the specific demands of the competitive event and includes a primary focus and several secondary ones. For example, during the first macrocycle of a training period (frequently referred to as the preparatory phase), high-volume/low-intensity workouts are emphasized as the primary focus. For an endurance athlete, this means that sustained distance and aerobic interval training should make up the bulk of the training, with perhaps some supplemental weight training done with low resistance and medium to high volume. For an athlete whose event demands mainly strength and power, such as a high jumper, resistance training should be emphasized. For this athlete, the primary focus might be high-volume (three to five sets of 8–12 repetitions), low-resistance (50–80% 1 RM) weight training with some sustained distance or aerobic intervals. As the athlete progresses towards competition, training volumes are decreased and intensities increased. The last mesocycle before an important competitive event is typically divided into two parts. During the first part, the emphasis is on maximal intensity, sport-specific training based on the strength, power and endurance requirements for that particular sport and is of very short duration. The second part of the last mesocycle before competition should be the taper. Some form of tapering is universally accepted as a means to optimize performance by allowing adequate recovery from hard training before important competitions (Wells & Pate, 1988). During a taper, some combination of training frequency, intensity and volume is altered to reduce the training stimulus. Most evidence indicates that a rather drastic reduction of up to 85–90% of usual training volume in combination with short intense workouts gives the best result (Shepley *et al.*, 1992; Houmard & Johns, 1994). This type of taper has been shown to result in a performance improvement of about 3% in swimmers and distance runners. Despite this evidence, athletes find the taper a difficult part of training. Typically, athletes undergo tapering (i.e. reduce training volume by at least two-thirds) for about 1 week. This may not be long enough to be optimal. Costill *et al.* (1985) have reported a 3–4% improvement in swim times following a 15-day taper where training yardage was reduced by two-thirds. This work, as well as that of Hickson and Rosenkoetter (1981), shows that training adaptations can be maintained and perhaps potentiated by appropriate use of the taper. Although evaluation of individual periodization routines is difficult, shorter mesocycles can be evaluated to determine the efficacy of specific aspects of training.

Overtraining

Overtraining is a long-term (weeks to months) decrement in performance with or without related physiological and psychological signs or symptoms and can be a serious problem for the competitive athlete (Kreider *et al.*, 1997). To achieve optimal athletic performance, serious athletes devote years to hard training. Knowing that an athlete who does not train hard enough may never reach her full potential, many athletes adopt a 'more is better' philosophy. Unfortunately, training too often and/or too intensely may lead to physiological maladaptations and decreases in performance. Determining the optimal amount of training to optimize performance of individual athletes is difficult. The amount of training that may be optimal for one athlete may undertrain or overtrain others. To complicate the issue further, both undertraining and overtraining may result in

performance plateaus. The usual response to a performance plateau is to increase the amount and intensity of training. If the reason for the plateau is indeed undertraining, additional training may be of benefit. On the other hand, if the reason for the plateau is overtraining, further training will exacerbate the problem and in all likelihood lead to further decrements in performance.

The maladaptations of overtraining are essentially an imbalance between stimulus and recovery. Multiple signs and symptoms have been associated with overtraining. Fry *et al.* (1991) have compiled a list of the major symptoms of overtraining reported in the literature (Table 5.2). These signs and symptoms may be diffuse in nature, presenting as generalized fatigue with or without more specific physiological symptoms. Alternatively, a specific physiological system may break down, e.g. failure of some aspect of the musculoskeletal system may result in an overuse injury such as a stress fracture. Some of these symptoms are seemingly contradictory, e.g. both increased and decreased resting heart rates have been reported in overtrained runners. Multiple symptoms in any combination, any single symptom or even the absence of physiological symptoms characterize an overtrained athlete. The universal finding in overtrained athletes is a decrease in performance ability. However, not all aspects of performance are affected simultaneously or to the same degree. Identification of physiological markers prodromal to the overtraining syndrome is likewise difficult.

Conclusion

The physiological demands of most sporting events are similar for men and women athletes. Likewise, training methods seem to be similar. Although men athletes may be swifter, able to go higher and are stronger than women athletes in absolute terms, women athletes respond to training with many of the same physiological adaptations. Although much is known about the initial responses of women to training and about the

Table 5.2 The major symptoms of overtraining as indicated by their prevalence in the literature. (From Fry *et al.*, 1991 with permission)

Physiological/performance
Decreased performance
Inability to meet previously attained performance standards/criteria
Recovery prolonged
Reduced toleration of loading
Decreased muscular strength
Decreased maximum work capacity
Loss of coordination
Decreased efficiency/decreased amplitude of movement
Reappearance of mistakes already corrected
Reduced capacity of differentiation and correcting technical faults
Increased difference between lying and standing heart rate
Abnormal T-wave pattern in ECG
Heart discomfort on slight exertion
Changes in blood pressure
Changes in heart rate at rest, exercise and recovery
Increased frequency of respiration
Perfuse respiration
Decreased body fat
Increased oxygen consumption at submaximal workloads
Increased ventilation and heart rate at submaximal workloads
Shift of the lactate curve towards the x axis
Decreased evening post-workout weight
Elevated basal metabolic rate
Chronic fatigue
Insomnia with and without night sweats
Feels thirsty
Anorexia nervosa
Loss of appetite
Bulimia
Amenorrhoea/oligomenorrhoea
Headaches
Nausea
Increased aches and pains
Gastrointestinal disturbances
Muscle soreness/tenderness
Tendinostic complaints
Periosteal complaints
Muscle damage
Elevated C-reactive protein
Rhabdomyolysis

Psychological/information processing
Feelings of depression
General apathy

Decreased self-esteem/worsening feelings of self
Emotional instability
Difficulty in concentrating at work and training
Sensitive to environmental and emotional stress
Fear of competition
Changes in personality
Decreased ability to narrow concentration
Increased internal and external distractability
Decreased capacity to deal with large amounts of information
Gives up when the going gets tough

Immunological
Increased susceptibility to and severity of illness/colds/allergies
Flu-like illnesses
Unconfirmed glandular fever
Minor scratches heal slowly
Swelling of lymph glands
One-day colds
Decreased functional activity of neutrophils
Decreased total lymphocyte counts
Reduced response to mitogens
Increased blood eosinophil count
Decreased proportion of null (non-T, non-B) lymphocytes
Bacterial infection
Reactivation of herpes viral infection
Significant variations in CD4:CD8 lymphocytes

Biochemical
Negative nitrogen balance
Hypothalamic dysfunction
Flat glucose tolerance curves
Depressed muscle glycogen concentration
Decreased bone mineral content
Delayed menarche
Decreased haemoglobin
Decreased serum iron
Decreased serum ferritin
Lowered total iron-binding capacity
Mineral depletion (Zn, Co, Al, Mn, Se, Cu, etc.)
Increased urea concentrations
Elevated cortisol levels
Elevated ketosteroids in urine
Low free testosterone
Increased serum hormone-binding globulin
Decreased ratio of free testosterone to cortisol of more than 30%
Increased uric acid production

physiological adaptations (e.g. changes in cardiac structure and function) seen in athletes and attributed to training for many years, much less is known about the small adaptations that occur in athletes throughout their careers allowing them to reach their full potential. This gap in knowledge should be addressed with future studies of women athletes.

References

Abernathy, P.J., Thayer, R. & Taylor, A.W. (1990) Acute and chronic responses of skeletal muscle to endurance and sprint exercise: a review. *Sports Medicine* **10**, 365–389.

Applegate, E. (1989) Nutritional concerns of the ultra-endurance athlete. *Medicine and Science in Sports and Exercise* **21** (Suppl.), S205–S208.

Blomqvist, C.G. & Saltin, B. (1983) Cardiovascular adaptations to physical training. *Annual Review of Physiology* **45**, 169–189.

Bobbert, M.F. (1990) Drop jumping as a training method for jumping ability. *Sports Medicine* **9**, 7–22.

Burke, L.M. & Read, R.S.D. (1987) Diet patterns of elite Australian male triathletes. *Physician and Sportsmedicine* **15**, 140–155.

Callister, R., Callister, R.J., Fleck, S.J. & Dudley, G.A. (1990) Physiological and performance responses to overtraining in elite judo athletes. *Medicine and Science in Sports and Exercise* **22**, 816–824.

Chromiak, J.A. & Mulvaney, D.R. (1990) A review: the effects of combined strength and endurance training on strength development. *Journal of Applied Sport Science Research* **4**, 55–60.

Clausen, J.P. (1977) Effect of physical training on cardiovascular adjustments to exercise in man. *Physiological Reviews* **57**, 779–815.

Costill, D.L. (1986) *Inside Running: Basics of Sport Physiology*. Benchmark Press, Indianapolis.

Costill, D.L., King, D.S., Thomas, R. & Hargreaves, M. (1985) Effects of reduced training on muscular power in swimmers. *Physician and Sportsmedicine* **13**, 94–101.

Costill, D.L., Fink, W.J., Flynn, M. & Kirwan, J. (1987) Muscle fiber composition and enzyme activities in elite female distance runners. *International Journal of Sports Medicine* **8**, 1031–1036.

Crawford, M.H., Petru, M.A. & Rabinowitz, C. (1986) Effect of isotonic exercise training on left ventricular volume during upright exercise. *Circulation* **72**, 1237–1243.

Cureton, K.J., Collins, M.A., Hill, D.W. & McElhannon, F.M. (1988) Muscle hypertrophy in men and women. *Medicine and Science in Sports and Exercise* **20**, 338–344.

Daniels, J.T. (1985) A physiologist's view of running economy. *Medicine and Science in Sports and Exercise* **17**, 332–338.

Douglas, P.S. (1989) Cardiac considerations in the triathlete. *Medicine and Science in Sports and Exercise* **21** (Suppl.), S214–S218.

Douglas, P.S. & O'Toole, M.L. (1992) Aging and physical activity determine cardiac structure and function in the older athlete. *Journal of Applied Physiology* **72**, 1969–1973.

Douglas, P.S., O'Toole, M.L., Hiller, W.D.B. & Reichek, N. (1986) Left ventricular structure and function by echocardiography in ultraendurance athletes. *American Journal of Cardiology* **58**, 805–809.

Douglas, P.S., O'Toole, M.L., Hiller, W.D.B., Hackney, K. & Reichek, N. (1988) Electrocardiographic diagnosis of exercise-induced left ventricular hypertrophy. *American Heart Journal* **116**, 786–790.

Dudley, G.A. & Djamil, R. (1985) Incompatibility of endurance and strength training modes of exercise. *Journal of Applied Physiology* **59**, 1446–1451.

Dwyer, J. & Bybee, R. (1983) Heart rate indices of the anaerobic threshold. *Medicine and Science in Sports and Exercise* **15**, 72–76.

Ekblom, B. & Hermanson, L. (1968) Cardiac output in athletes. *Journal of Applied Physiology* **25**, 619–625.

Fleck, S.J. & Kramer, W.J. (1987) *Designing Resistance Training Programs*. Human Kinetics Publishers, Champaign, Illinois.

Fox, E.L. & Mathews, D.K. (1974) *Interval Training: Conditioning for Sports and General Fitness*. W.B. Saunders, Philadelphia.

Fox, P.W., Hershberger, S.L. & Bouchard, T.J. Jr (1996) Genetic and environmental contributions to the acquisition of a motor skill. *Nature* **384**, 356–358.

Fry, R.W., Morton, A.R. & Keast, D. (1991) Overtraining in athletes. *Sports Medicine* **12**, 32–65.

Gilman, M.B. & Wells, C.L. (1993) The use of heart rates to monitor exercise intensity in relation to metabolic variables. *International Journal of Sports Medicine* **14**, 3334–3339.

Gledhill, N., Cox, D. & Jamink, R. (1994) Endurance athletes' stroke volume does not plateau: major advantage is diastolic function. *Medicine and Science in Sports and Exercise* **26**, 1116–1121.

Gollnick, P.D. (1985) Metabolism of substrates during exercise and as modified by training. *Federation Proceedings* **44**, 353–357.

Gollnick, P.D., Armstrong, R.B., Saubert, C.W., Piehl, K. & Saltin, B. (1972) Enzyme activity and fiber composition in skeletal muscle of untrained and trained men. *Journal of Applied Physiology* **33**, 312–319.

Gollnick, P.D., Bayly, W.M. & Hodgson, D.R. (1986) Exercise intensity, training, diet, and lactate concentration in muscle and blood. *Medicine and Science in Sports and Exercise* **18**, 334–340.

Hamel, P., Simoneau, J.-A., Lortie, G., Boulay, M.R. & Bouchard, C. (1986) Heredity and muscle adaptation to endurance training. *Medicine and Science in Sports and Exercise* **18**, 690–699.

Harrison, M.H. (1985) Effects of thermal stress and exercise on blood volume in humans. *Physiological Reviews* **65**, 149–199.

Hickson, R.C. & Rosenkoetter, M.A. (1981) Reduced training frequencies and maintenance of increased aerobic power. *Medicine and Science in Sports and Exercise* **13**, 13–16.

Holloszy, J.O. (1975) Adaptation of skeletal muscle to endurance exercise. *Medicine and Science in Sports and Exercise* **7**, 155–164.

Holloszy, J.O. & Coyle, E.F. (1984) Adaptations of skeletal muscle to endurance exercise and their metabolic consequences. *Journal of Applied Physiology* **56**, 831–838.

Houmard, J.A. & Johns, R.A. (1994) Effects of taper on swim performance. Practical implications. *Sports Medicine* **17**, 224–232.

Kearney, J.T. (1996) Training the Olympic athlete. *Scientific American* **274**, 52–63.

Khoo, C.S., Rawson, N.E. & Robinson, M.L. (1987) Nutrient intake and eating habits of triathletes. *Annals of Sports Medicine* **3**, 144–150.

Kirkendall, D.T. (1985) The applied sport science of soccer. *Physician and Sportsmedicine* **13**, 53–59.

Klausen, K., Andersen, L.B. & Pelle, I. (1981) Adaptive changes in work capacity, skeletal muscle capilliarization, and enzyme levels during training and detraining. *Acta Physiologica Scandinavica* **113**, 9–16.

Kohrt, W.M., O'Connor, J.S. & Skinner, J.S. (1989) Longitudinal assessment of responses by triathletes to swimming, cycling, and running. *Medicine and Science in Sports and Exercise* **21**, 569–575.

Kraemer, W.J. & Nindl, B.C. (1997) Factors involved in overtraining for strength and power. In R.B. Kreider, A.C. Fry & M.L. O'Toole (eds) *Overtraining in Sport*, pp. 69–86. Human Kinetics Publishers, Champaign, Illinois.

Kreider, R.B., Fry, A.C. & O'Toole, M.L. (eds) (1997) *Overtraining in Sport*. Human Kinetics Publishers, Champaign, Illinois.

Laurenson, N.M., Fulcher, K.Y. & Korkia, P. (1993) Physiological characteristics of elite and club level female triathletes during running. *International Journal of Sports Medicine* **14**, 455–459.

Levine, B.D., Lane, L.D., Buckey, J.C., Friedman, D.B. & Blomqvist, C.G. (1991) Left ventricular pressure–volume and Frank–Starling relations in endurance athletes: implications for orthostatic tolerance and exercise performance. *Circulation* **84**, 1016–1023.

Levy, W.C., Cerqueira, M.D.S., Abrass, I.B., Schwartz, R.S. & Stratton, J.R. (1993) Endurance exercise training augments diastolic filling at rest and during exercise in healthy young and older men. *Circulation* **88**, 116–126.

MacDougall, J.D., Ward, G.R., Sale, D.G. & Sutton, J.R. (1977) Biochemical adaptation of human skeletal muscle to heavy resistance training and immobilization. *Journal of Applied Physiology* **43**, 700–703.

Mayhew, S.R. & Wenger, H.A. (1985) Time–motion analysis of professional soccer. *Journal of Human Movement Studies* **11**, 49–52.

Morgan, D.W. & Craib, M. (1992) Physiological aspects of running economy. *Medicine and Science in Sports and Exercise* **24**, 456–461.

Nadel, E.R. (1988) Temperature regulation and prolonged exercise. In D.R. Lamb & R. Murray (eds) *Perspectives in Exercise Science and Sports Medicine, Vol. 1 Prolonged Exercise*, pp. 25–47. Benchmark Press, Indianapolis.

Newton, R.U., Kraemer, W.J., Hakkinen, K., Humphries, B.J. & Murphy, A.J. (1996) Kinematics, kinetics, muscle activation during explosive upper body movements. *Journal of Applied Biomechanics* **12**, 31–43.

Oscai, L.B., Williams, B.T. & Hertig, B.A. (1968) Effect of exercise on blood volume. *Journal of Applied Physiology* **26**, 622–624.

O'Toole, M.L. & Douglas, P.S. (1995) Applied physiology of triathlon. *Sports Medicine* **19**, 251–267.

O'Toole, M.L., Douglas, P.S. & Hiller, W.D.B. (1989) Lactate, oxygen uptake, and cycling performance in triathletes. *International Journal of Sports Medicine* **10**, 413–418.

Pate, R.R., Sparling, P.B., Wilson, G.E., Cureton, K.J. & Miller, B.J. (1987) Cardiorespiratory and metabolic responses to submaximal and maximal exercise in elite women distance runners. *International Journal of Sports Medicine* **8** (Suppl.), 91–95.

Pelliccia, A., Maron, B.J., Culasso, F., Spataro, A. & Caselli, G. (1996) Athlete's heart in women: echocardiographic characterization of highly trained elite female athletes. *Journal of the American Medical Association* **276**, 211–215.

Perrin, D.H. (1993) *Isokinetic Exercise and Assessment*. Human Kinetics Publishers, Champaign, Illinois.

Plowman, S.A. & Smith, D.L. (1997) *Exercise Physiology for Health, Fitness and Performance*. Allyn & Bacon, Boston.

Pollack, S.J., McMillan, S.T., Mumpower, E. *et al.* (1987) Echocardiographic analysis of elite women distance runners. *International Journal of Sports Medicine* **8** (Suppl.), 81–83.

Reilly, T. & Thomas, V. (1976) A motion analysis of work rate in different positional roles in professional football match play. *Journal of Human Movement Studies* **2**, 87–97.

Rogers, M.A. & Evans, W.J. (1993) Changes in skeletal

muscle with aging: effects of exercise training. *Exercise and Sport Sciences Reviews* **21**, 65–102.

Saltin, B. (1969) Physiological effects of physical conditioning. *Medicine and Science in Sports* **1**, 50–56.

Saltin, B. & Rowell, L.B. (1980) Functional adaptations to physical acitivity and inactivity. *Federation Proceedings* **39**, 1506–1513.

Saltin, B., Henriksson, J., Nygaard, E. & Andersen, P. (1977) Fiber types and metabolic potentials of skeletal muscles in sedentary man and endurance runners. *Annals of the New York Academy of Sciences* **301**, 3–29.

Shepley, B., MacDougall, J.D., Cipriano, N. & Sutton, J.R. (1992) Physiological effects of tapering in highly trained athletes. *Journal of Applied Physiology* **72**, 706–711.

Sherman, W.M. & Lamb, D.R. (1988) Nutrition and prolonged exercise. In D.R. Lamb & R. Murray (eds) *Perspectives in Exercise Science and Sports Medicine, Vol. 1 Prolonged Exercise*, pp. 213–276. Benchmark Press, Indianapolis.

Sjodin, B. & Svedenhag, J. (1985) Applied physiology of marathon running. *Sports Medicine* **2**, 83–99.

Sparling, P.B., Nieman, D.C. & O'Connor, P.J. (1993) Selected scientific aspects of marathon racing. An update on fluid replacement, immune function, psychological factors and the gender difference. *Sports Medicine* **15**, 116–132.

Tanaka, J.A., Tanaka, H. & Landis, W. (1995) An assessment of carbohydrate intake in collegiate distance runners. *International Journal of Sports Nutrition* **5**, 206–214.

Tarnopolsky, L.J., MacDougall, J.D., Atkinson, S.A., Tarnopolsky, M.A. & Sutton, J.R. (1990) Gender differences in substrate for endurance exercise. *Journal of Applied Physiology* **68**, 302–308.

Tarnopolsky, M.A., Atkinson, S.A., Phillips, S.M. & MacDougall, J.D. (1995) Carbohydrate loading and metabolism during exercise in men and women. *Journal of Applied Physiology* **78**, 1360–1368.

Tesch, P.A. (1992) Training for body building. In P.V. Komi (ed.) *Strength and Power in Sport*, pp. 357–369. Blackwell Scientific Publications, Oxford.

Vanfraechem, J.H.P. (1979) Stroke volume and systolic time interval adjustments during bicycle exercise. *Journal of Applied Physiology* **46**, 588–592.

Vanoverschelde, J.L.J., Younis, L.T., Melin, J.A. *et al.* (1991) Prolonged exercise induces left ventricular dysfunction in healthy subjects. *Journal of Applied Physiology* **70**, 1356–1363.

Wells, C.L. (1991) *Women, Sport and Performance: A Physiological Perspective*, 2nd edn. Human Kinetics Publishers, Champaign, Illinois.

Wells, C.L. & Pate, R.R. (1988) Training for performance of prolonged exercise. In D.R. Lamb & R. Murray (eds) *Perspectives in Exercise Science and Sports Medicine, Vol. 1 Prolonged Exercise*, pp. 357–391. Benchmark Press, Indianapolis.

Weltman, A.R., Moffatt, R.J. & Stamford, B.A. (1978) Supramaximal training in females: effects on anaerobic power output, anaerobic capacity, and aerobic power. *Journal of Sports Medicine and Physical Fitness* **18**, 237–244.

Williams, K. & Cavanagh, P. (1987) Relationship between distance running mechanics, running economy and performance. *Journal of Applied Physiology* **63**, 1236–1245.

Wilmore, J.H. (1974) Alterations in strength, body composition, and anthropometric measurements consequent to a 10 week weight training programme. *Medicine and Science in Sports* **6**, 133–138.

Wilmore, J.H. & Costill, D.L. (1994) *Physiology of Sport and Exercise*. Human Kinetics Publishers, Champaign, Illinois.

Zeederberg, C., Leach, L., Lambert, E.V., Noakes, T.D., Dennis, S.C. & Hawley, J.A. (1996) The effect of carbohydrate ingestion on the motor skill proficiency of soccer players. *International Journal of Sports Nutrition* **6**, 348–355.

Chapter 6

Biomechanics

JILL A. CRUSSEMEYER AND JANET S. DUFEK

Introduction

A general definition of biomechanics is the application of mechanical laws to living organisms. In this chapter, the concepts of mechanics are reviewed in order to understand more thoroughly the additional topics covered in this book. Mechanics can be divided into statics and dynamics and both are utilized in the study of biomechanics. Statics deals with the system (athlete, implement or both in combination) under zero acceleration, while dynamics focuses on the accelerating system. Understanding statics and dynamics with respect to the athlete is important in order to improve overall performance and minimize the potential for injury.

The neuromusculoskeletal system is the framework upon which the mechanical laws are applied. A thorough understanding of functional anatomy (structure and function of the body) is crucial when evaluating performances biomechanically. This allows for a general picture of what is happening in the body as well as what could happen if something should suddenly change. Anthropometry, the study and evaluation of body size, also yields vital information when comparing a variety of individuals trying to complete the same task. Kinematics, lever manipulation and force application are important mechanical concepts that one must initially understand prior to completing a biomechanical assessment.

Kinematics or position analyses of movement helps to describe and understand the perfor-

mance more thoroughly and accurately. Generally, kinematic variables measured in biomechanics include both linear and angular position, velocity and acceleration. A coach or teacher knowing the values of these motion descriptors can provide such information to the athlete in order to improve their performance. For example, if a hurdler continuously hits the hurdle with their lead foot, a kinematic analysis may show that they are leaving the ground too close to the hurdle in order to clear it. The coach can explain this to the athlete and together work on a solution so the hurdle can be successfully cleared. The hurdler is constrained by the mechanical laws of parabolic motion. A thorough understanding of the physical laws and mechanical relationships of parabolic motion can lend insight into performance interventions in order to optimize performance.

During any athletic activity the individual utilizes lever systems and attempts to manipulate or maintain the body's centre of mass (COM) throughout the movement. The body itself can be viewed as a series of levers or rigid links that work together to accomplish a goal. Sports equipment such as a diving board can be thought of as an external lever that the athlete must work with in order to achieve the best possible dive. The system's COM is determined relative to the spatial orientation of the levers and the distribution of the performer's segment masses. A simple kinematic analysis of the COM may also yield useful information, such as the relationship of an athlete's COM to the bar during the high jump.

The forces or kinetics that cause motion also need to be addressed. It is important to determine not only the magnitude of the forces acting on the system but also the direction and point of application at which they act. This allows the coach and/or performer to determine if one is applying force appropriately to gain a maximum performance while minimizing the potential for injury. It is important to understand the relationships between kinetics, kinematics and the performer in an attempt to achieve the best possible performance.

Women have been participating in sports for many years, and since the initiation of Title IX Educational Assistance Act of 1972 in the USA the number of female athletes has increased. Coinciding with this increase in number of athletes, there has been an increase in injury and also demand for specialized sporting equipment for the female (Hutchinson & Ireland, 1995). The female athlete is not the same as the male athlete as emphasized throughout this book. Such differences are important to recognize relative to performance potential. This chapter also discusses some of the biomechanical differences and implications of specialized sports equipment.

Anthropometry/structure

Anthropometry consists of body measurements, including height, weight/mass, segment lengths, segment masses and moments of inertia (resistance to change in motion). In studying human body measurements it is apparent that there is a high degree of variability within a certain population and between different populations and genders. The difference in standing height between genders and different populations is given in Fig. 6.1 as an example of the level of structural variability. Therefore, some caution must be exercised when describing the body dimensions of a group of athletes and their associated skill levels since some athletes may lie outside the average for the group but still may be highly skilled performers.

Taking into account that there may be a great deal of structural variability, women tend to

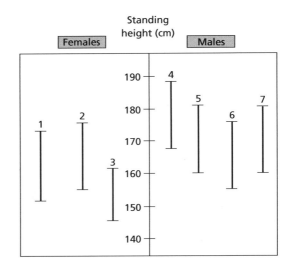

Fig. 6.1 Standing height ranges of variability (5th and 95th percentiles) in males and females of different nationalities: 1, US civilians; 2, Swedish civilians; 3, Japanese civilians; 4, US Air Force fliers; 5, Italian military; 6, Japanese civilians; 7 Turkish military. (Adapted from Pulat, 1992.)

weigh less (less mass), are shorter, and have shorter legs and a wider pelvis compared with men. This leads to a lower COM, which may be desirable in some activities (i.e. judo takedown) and a hindrance in others (high jump). Other general characteristics of women include less muscular development and greater flexibility compared with their male counterparts (Hutchinson & Ireland, 1995).

Specific anatomical differences that seem to be apparent in females include greater genu valgum, increased femoral anteversion, greater external tibial torsion and a greater Q-angle. Genu valgum is defined as the angulation of the tibia away from the midline of the body (Fig. 6.2). This change in angulation may be important when investigating kinematics and forces at the knee joint. In the genu valgum condition, the medial aspect of the knee undergoes greater tensile forces compared with the greater compressive forces on the lateral side (Norkin & Levangie, 1992). The normal angulation of the femoral neck is approximately 15° and any

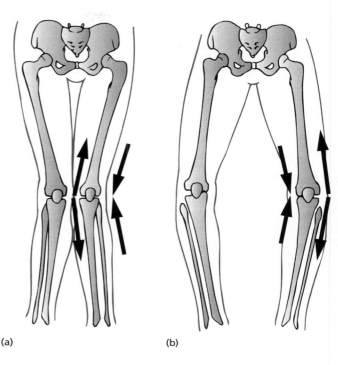

Fig. 6.2 (a) Genu valgum and (b) genu varum. In genu valgum, there is a compressive force on the lateral side and a tensile force on the medial side. In genu varum there is a medial compressive force and a lateral tensile force at the knee joint.

(a)   (b)

anterior deviation from this constitutes femoral anteversion (Hoppenfeld, 1976). An increase in femoral anteversion causes greater internal rotation, which may be seen as a toe-in type of gait. As with genu valgum, the change in angulation may have an effect on kinematics and forces occurring at the hip joint. This also has an effect on the base of support in bipedal sporting activities.

The Q-angle is defined by two lines, one from the anterior superior iliac spine to the midpoint of the patella and one from the midpoint of the patella to the tibial tubercle (Fig. 6.3). The Q-angle is important since it is the angle through which the net force of the quadriceps acts during leg extension. A Q-angle of >20° when measured in the standing position is thought to be abnormal and increases the lateral forces on the patella. As the knee flexes the Q-angle decreases as the tibia internally rotates. Although large Q-angle values may predispose a person to knee problems, individuals with normal alignment are not necessarily excluded from knee problems (Norkin & Levangie, 1992).

As can be gleaned from this brief anthropometric review, the primary structural differences between the genders are most evident in the lower extremity. Due to the predominance of upright bipedal actions in sport, these structural differences can lead to major differences in performance outcomes between males and females. In addition, injury potentials differ due to unique force applications and tissue tolerances.

Kinematics

Kinematics is used to describe motion and includes position, velocity and acceleration in both linear (translation) and angular (movement about a fixed axis) components. Kinematic analyses can be as simple as timing a person running over a marked distance or as complex as using high-speed video or film and taking very sensitive measures from the visual records. More

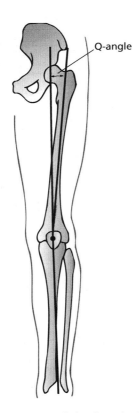

Fig. 6.3 Measurement of the Q-angle. The angle is defined by two lines, one extending from the anterior superior iliac spine to the midpoint of the patella and a vertical line from the midpoint of the patella to the tibial tuberosity.

information can be gained from the example of timing a person across a given distance by dividing the overall distance into smaller and smaller increments. Utilizing film or video, the distance increments are minute and therefore more information about the performance can be obtained. In either case spatial and timing information is gained in order to describe and ultimately understand the motion of the system.

Position

Position is where the object of interest lies in space at any point in time. The position of the athlete with respect to their final goal is one of the

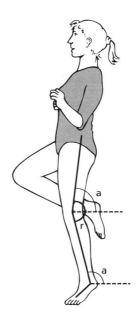

Fig. 6.4 Absolute angle of the thigh and leg (a) and relative angle of the knee (r).

most important factors when analysing performance. A very common and clear example is that of the long jump and foot placement on the take-off board. Since maximum distance is the desired goal and the jump is measured from the end of the board, it is intuitive that the athlete's foot be as close to the end of the board as possible. This maximizes the horizontal distance travelled independent of the distance the COM travels while airborne.

Angular position

Angular position may be described in either absolute or relative terms. An absolute angle (Fig. 6.4) defines a segment's orientation in space, while the relative angle refers to the included angle between two segments. It is important to note that the relative angle refers only to the segment orientations to each other and gives no information as to how the segment is orientated in space. Another method of describing angular position more commonly used in clinical professions is that of 'degrees

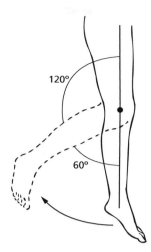

Fig. 6.5 Two different angle measurements: relative knee angle (120°) and 'degrees flexion' (60°).

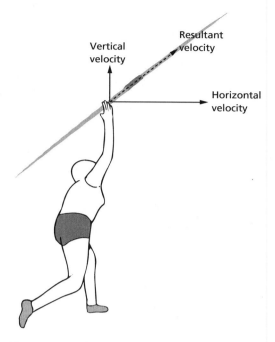

Fig. 6.6 Projectile motion of the javelin, the resultant velocity vector can be broken down into the component vectors (horizontal and vertical).

flexion' or 'degrees extension'. For example, if an athlete had a knee angle at full extension of 180° and then actively flexed the knee by moving the leg 60°, the resulting knee angle could be described as 60° flexion or a knee angle (relative) of 120° (Fig. 6.5).

Angular position of joints is important to ascertain whether or not the athlete is in a potentially injurious situation. One sport activity in which knee angle plays a vital role in injury prevention is landing. Many athletic events incorporate landing from some type of airborne phase, i.e. basketball, gymnastics and volleyball. It has been found that by decreasing the knee angle upon impact a 'softer' landing is obtained (Devita & Skelly, 1992; Dufek *et al.*, 1995). By landing in a softer position it is thought that the injury potential is decreased.

Velocity

Velocity is defined as the time rate of change in position. Velocity is considered a vector quantity, meaning that it has a magnitude and acts in a particular direction. In many instances a velocity vector is broken down into vertical and horizontal components, which yield more information

relative to the performer. The vertical–horizontal resolution of vectors is used because of the vertical orientation of the force of gravity. When an athlete releases a javelin for example, it has a resultant velocity vector. However, that velocity can be broken down into components that may give more meaningful information to the athlete or coach when trying to achieve the longest throw (Fig. 6.6).

Angular velocity

Angular velocity is defined as the time rate of change in angular position or simply the change in angle over a change in time. When investigating performance and injury, the joints are usually a primary focal point because of the rotational nature of motion about the joints; position data alone may not give as much information as one needs. It may be important to understand how quickly the angle is changing and, in combination with knowledge of tissue properties, whether the joint structures may be at risk for damage. From the coach's perspective it may also be beneficial to understand the angular velocity of joints acting in a sequence. For example, determining the velocity and position of the shoulder, elbow and wrist during a shot-put activity may show that the athlete is changing one joint position too quickly compared with the other joints in the system, therefore minimizing total force production potential.

Acceleration

Acceleration is defined as the change in velocity over a change in time, and like position and velocity it has both linear and angular components. Since acceleration is related to velocity, it too is a vector quantity having both magnitude and direction. In sports, frequently a quick change in acceleration is a possible mechanism for injury. A good example is the lower extremity at the end of the swing phase during running just prior to touchdown. The hamstrings must act to slow the leg down and change the direction that the leg is moving. If the acceleration of the leg is too great relative to muscular strength, a hamstring strain is possible.

Projectile motion

Projectile motion occurs whenever a system is thrust into the air. The system can be some type of athletic equipment or the body itself. Some examples of where projectile motion occurs are basketball, discus, diving, high jump, javelin, long jump, shot put, softball and volleyball. In projectile motion once the system is airborne the only forces acting on it are gravity and air resistance. For the most part, air resistance can be neglected because the effects are generally minimal and it simplifies the analysis. Therefore, in this situation the horizontal velocity is constant and the acceleration due to gravity is also constant. When analysing projectile motion it is important to determine whether the vertical

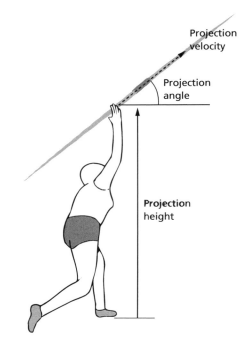

Fig. 6.7 Factors to consider in projectile motion: projection velocity, projection angle and projection height.

(height) or horizontal distance needs to be maximized.

Projection angle, projection velocity and projection height are the three major factors that determine the subsequent path of the projectile once it is airborne (Fig. 6.7) (the fourth factor, aerodynamics, is ignored in this discussion). The projection angle determines the shape of the projectile path and is defined by the angle that the projection velocity vector makes with the horizontal and ranges from 0 to 90°. If the athlete wants to maximize height, the projection angle should be fairly steep (90°); a smaller angle would be desired if horizontal distance is to be maximized. In the high jump, maximum vertical height is desired and the angle of projection ranges from 40 to 48° (Dapena, 1980); in the long jump, where horizontal distance is desired, values range from 18 to 27° (Hay, 1986).

Projection velocity is the resulting velocity at the moment of release or take-off. The projection velocity will influence the height and the horizontal distance of the projectile's path. If the projection angle is 45°, the vertical and horizontal components of the velocity vector will be equal. As the angle increases from 45°, the vertical component increases; similarly with angles <45° the horizontal velocity increases. Therefore, if the object is to gain maximum horizontal distance the angle of projection should be <45°, which is the case for the long jump.

Projection height is the vertical difference between the height at take-off and at landing. If the initial and final heights are equal, the shape of the parabola is symmetrical, the time of ascent and descent are equal and the horizontal distance travelled during the ascent and descent are equal. When the initial position is higher than the final position, the parabola is not symmetrical and the time to the apex is less than the time from the apex to the final position. It is important to realize that all three factors are related and that all must be considered in order to optimize the projectile's path. An example of differences in projection height is the long jump. The COM of the athlete is higher at take-off than at landing and therefore the athlete will travel a greater horizontal distance in the second half of the jump (i.e. on the way down).

Lever systems

All lever systems are comprised of a pivot point or fulcrum, a resistance that is being manipulated (object or body segment) and a force (internal, external or inertial) that is the 'source' of the motion. The distance from the fulcrum to the resistance is termed the resistance arm (RA) and the distance of the force from the fulcrum is termed the force arm (FA). There are three types or classes defined by the orientation of the three parts. Lever systems can be identified within the body, by looking at the musculoskeletal system, and also outside the body, by observing the body interacting with external objects. The functional role of a lever system is to maximize either force production or range of motion. In this regard, it is important to view the lever system and determine its mechanical advantage (MA), which is defined as the ratio of FA to RA. If MA (FA/RA) is >1, then force application is maximized with the lever. If MA is <1, range and velocity of motion are maximized with the lever. Finally, if MA=1, then the lever system offers neither advantage. Figure 6.8 summarizes common lever examples as well as those found in the body.

First-class lever

A first-class lever has the fulcrum positioned between the RA and the FA. The most common example is a see-saw. In this type of system, depending on the position of the fulcrum, either force or range of motion can be maximized. An example of a first-class lever in the body is performing a French press or overhead triceps extension. The elbow is the fulcrum and the insertion site of the triceps is the point of force. The resistance is the mass of the arm acting at the COM of the segment.

Second-class lever

A second-class lever maximizes force because the FA is always longer than the RA by definition (resistance lies between the force and the fulcrum). A common example is the wheelbarrow, where the fulcrum is at the wheel, the RA extends from the wheel to the centre of the load in the wheelbarrow and the FA extends from the wheel to the handle of the wheelbarrow where the person exerts a force. It is easy to understand how force is maximized because a person can lift a much heavier load in a wheelbarrow than by carrying. Very few examples of second-class levers exist in the body, although the jaw can be thought of as such a lever when biting down on an object. Also, if a muscle is working eccentrically many times it is acting as a second-class lever.

Third-class lever

A third-class lever maximizes range of motion because the RA is longer than the FA, yielding an MA <1 (force lies between the fulcrum and the

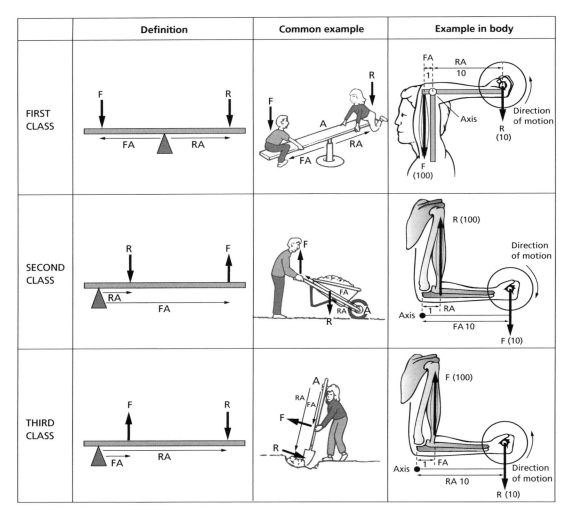

Fig. 6.8 Examples of different lever systems. A, axis; F, force; FA, distance from fulcrum to F arrow; R, resistance force; RA, distance from fulcrum to R arrow.

resistance). A common example is that of a shovel, where the hand at the top acts as the fulcrum, the RA extends from the fulcrum to the load at the end of the shovel and the FA extends from the fulcrum to the other hand. The third-class lever is the most common lever system found in the body and can be illustrated by a biceps curl. The elbow again acts as the fulcrum, the FA is from the elbow to the insertion site of the biceps and the RA is from the elbow to the COM of the arm.

Application of lever systems

Application and manipulation of levers are important concepts to consider when trying to achieve a successful athletic performance. Anatomical lever systems (such as the biceps during execution of elbow flexion) are fixed by definition, but can be functionally modified through training. For example, body mass can be altered and maximum force production can be enhanced. In addition, the line of pull of the muscle changes dynamically, influencing the magnitude of force generated and subsequent movement velocity. Of particular concern for the female athlete are the structural differences between males and females. These differences (e.g. shorter legs) influence the MA of the lever system and can affect performance outcome. However, strength differences produce more obvious deviations with respect to lever applications between men and women. The MA of the lever system and strength differences are important factors to consider when designing and selecting equipment for the female athlete.

Centre of gravity/centre of mass

The centre of gravity (COG) is the point about which all the point masses of the body are balanced and through which the weight vector acts; COM refers only to the even distribution of the masses. Since gravity is always acting on objects on the earth, COM and COG are frequently used interchangeably. The COM can be thought of as a theoretical point that moves in response to the movements of the surrounding segments; if segments are orientated in a particular manner the COM can actually lie outside the boundary of the body.

COG is closely related to stability, which is the resistance to linear and angular acceleration of the system (Hall, 1991). Stability in sports events needs to be minimized, maximized or some combination of both depending on the desired outcome. Stability can be gained by lowering the COG in the vertical direction, by increasing the area of the base of support of the system, by increasing the system's mass, by increasing the friction between the contacting surfaces and by positioning the COG at the edge of the base of support towards an incoming force. Figure 6.9 illustrates different base-of-support configurations that are found in athletic events.

When performing an event, athletes are manipulating their stability from being stable to unstable and usually back again. During either a standing or crouch track start, the 'on your mark' position can be stable. As the starter instructs the

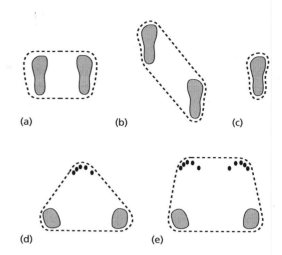

Fig. 6.9 Different types of athletic stances that define the base of support: (a) a square stance; (b) an angled stance; (c) a one foot stance; (d) a three point stance; and (e) a four point stance.

athlete to the 'set' position, the athlete shifts the COG to the edge of the base of support by elevating the hips in the direction of desired motion so that it is easier to accelerate out of the start. Conversely, a volleyball player set to receive a serve is in a very stable position because the COG is low, the base of support is wide, and the COG is positioned forward towards the oncoming force.

Stability and instability are desirable in athletic events; however, being stable at the wrong time can place the athlete in a potentially injurious situation. One of the most common injuries is the unhappy triad, which involves the medial collateral ligament, anterior cruciate ligament and medial meniscus. The injury occurs when the foot is fixed and the femur is forced (usually by an external force) to rotate medially. This is a common injury in skiing but occurs in other activities as well. In this example, the foot is in a stable position by being fixed on a surface; if the foot were not fixed or if it was unstable the injury might be avoided. Therefore, as a coach or athlete it is important to know when it is beneficial to have maximum stability and when instability may be better.

A vivid example of controlling the movement of the COG, along with the role of stability and instability, is the balance beam apparatus in gymnastics. The gymnast must create instability in order to perform the movement patterns, yet must keep the COG positioned directly over the beam. If the COG shifts too far to either side of the beam, the gymnast has to correct for the shift by moving a segment of the body to bring the COG back over the beam; in the worst case the gymnast will fall from the beam.

Determining the path of the COG during a movement can be insightful when analysing sporting events. For example, evaluating the path of the COG of a high jumper will truly identify the 'highest jumper'. It is entirely possible that the high jumper's COG can pass through or even under the bar, yet the jump can be successful. This is achieved by manipulating various body segments in an appropriately timed fashion in order to influence the whole-body COG, which is constrained to projectile motion once the jumper becomes airborne.

Kinetics

Kinetics, either linear or angular, are the forces that act upon a system, where the force is a push or pull between two or more objects that causes motion. Force, like velocity and acceleration, is also a vector quantity, having magnitude and direction. Forces have a point of application, which is the point where the force is applied to the object, and a line of action, which is the line or direction in which the force acts. Newton's laws are a useful starting point when trying to understand the interaction between kinetics and kinematics or the forces and the motion that they cause. Newton's first law of inertia states that an object will remain at rest or in motion unless acted on by some type of force (steady state). Inertia is defined as an object's resistance to change its state and is related to mass. If an object has a large mass then its inertia is greater and it is more difficult to move. Newton's second law of acceleration dictates that the force is equal to the mass of the object multiplied by its acceleration

($F=ma$). Finally, Newton's third law states that for every action there is an equal and opposite reaction (action–reaction).

Generally forces can be divided into two categories: contact and non-contact (Hamill & Knutzen, 1995). As suggested by the name, a contact force occurs between objects that touch each other, while a non-contact force occurs between objects over a distance. The non-contact force always present on the earth is gravity. This force requires that whatever goes up must come down because of gravity's pull towards the centre of the earth. The most common contact forces that must be considered are ground reaction force, friction, joint reaction forces, muscle forces, fluid resistance primarily from air or water, and inertial forces.

Ground reaction force

The ground reaction force (GRF) is the opposing force as an object contacts the ground. However, reaction forces occur between all surfaces and objects in contact. In biomechanics laboratories, GRF is often measured using a device called a force platform. The force platform can measure forces in the vertical, anteroposterior and mediolateral directions. Vertical GRFs have been analysed to illustrate the role of impact forces and the effects on the body during the support phase of walking, running and landing. Vertical GRF is most often studied because of its large magnitude compared with the other two GRF components (anteroposterior and mediolateral).

A characteristic vertical GRF vs. time curve for walking is shown in Fig. 6.10. The curve is bimodal with two peak forces usually ranging from 1.0 to 1.5 body weights. The GRF is most often reported as number of body weights so that comparisons between individuals with different masses can be made. The first peak corresponds to the body lowering after full foot contact with the ground. The second peak represents the phase where the foot is pushing against the ground to prepare for the next step. The anteroposterior GRF for walking has a magnitude much less than that of the vertical component

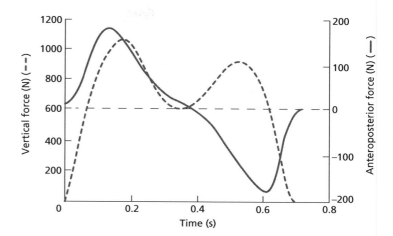

Fig. 6.10 Vertical (---) and anteroposterior (—) GRF curves for walking.

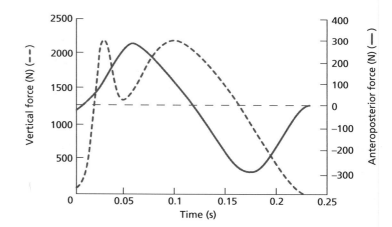

Fig. 6.11 Vertical (---) and anteroposterior (—) GRF curves for running.

(Fig. 6.10). Generally, there is a negative portion of the curve that corresponds to a braking phase followed by a positive portion related to propulsion for the next step. The minimum of the vertical GRF corresponds to the zero point on the anteroposterior curve. As the body is lowered after the initial peak in vertical GRF, the knee joint flexes to decrease the force and the COG of the body is decelerated. As the person prepares for push-off, the COG must be accelerated; therefore, the force increases and changes direction.

Much attention has been given to the impact force that occurs during heel–toe running. A typical vertical GRF curve for a heel–toe runner is shown in Fig. 6.11. The first peak that occurs

rapidly after initial contact is considered the impact peak and may be related to running injuries (James *et al.*, 1978; Nigg, 1986). The second peak, similar to walking, corresponds to the person preparing for push-off. The anteroposterior forces in running are similar to those found during walking but are greater in magnitude. It should be noted that a midfoot striker or toe runner generally does not have an impact peak present on the vertical GRF curve.

The mediolateral GRF has been found to show a great deal of variability between individuals and has not received much attention (Hamill *et al.*, 1983). The variation in mediolateral forces may be attributed to foot placement on the force

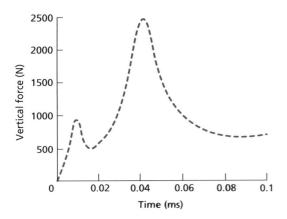

Fig. 6.12 Vertical GRF curve for landing.

platform, variations in foot mechanics between people, or footwear use and accommodating characteristics relative to foot morphology. Another possible reason why mediolateral forces have been neglected is that the magnitude of the forces is very small, approximately 0.01 body weights during walking and 0.1 body weights for running.

Landing is a common activity found in many sports. A typical vertical GRF curve for landing is illustrated in Fig. 6.12. Again the vertical component has been of primary interest due to the potentially high magnitudes. The first peak corresponds to forefoot contact, while the second peak is related to heel contact (opposite to that of heel–toe running). As discussed before, if a person lands with greater knee flexion the second peak can be attenuated and therefore a softer landing occurs. However, some work has shown that previous landing experience or landing on different materials may affect vertical GRF (Dufek *et al.*, 1991; McNitt-Gray *et al.*, 1994). This may be because individuals perceive a softer landing due to the landing surface material and therefore perform in a different fashion.

Friction

Another contact force is the frictional force, which can be either static or dynamic. The fric-

tional force acts parallel to the contacting surfaces between two objects and is equal to the product of the normal or reaction force and the coefficient of friction. The coefficient of friction depends upon the materials found in the interacting surfaces. Static friction occurs when an object undergoes a push or pull from another force yet no movement occurs. At some point the push or pull becomes great enough that limiting friction is overcome and motion occurs; dynamic friction is then present until the object comes back to rest.

Friction is necessary in order for locomotion to occur. If the coefficient of friction is very low it is difficult to walk, such as when attempting to walk on ice with smooth-soled shoes. In some sporting events, such as ice skating and downhill skiing, the coefficient of friction must be minimized in order to gain greater speeds and ease of movement. In other activities, such as soccer and softball, athletes wear shoes with cleats to increase traction and the coefficient of friction. As with most other types of forces, the coefficient of friction needs to be optimized for the particular activity. A slip or fall may occur if the coefficient of friction is too low; conversely, an injury could occur if the coefficient of friction is too high, such as the unhappy triad discussed previously.

Joint reaction forces

Joint reaction forces are the net internal forces acting across the joint at a particular instant in time. It is important to determine joint reaction forces when trying to ascertain if the joint is undergoing forces that may cause injury to the joint or surrounding tissues. Joint reaction forces are calculated from kinematic and kinetic data and are not generally measured directly. The joint reaction force in any single plane consists of a compressive force acting to pull the two adjoining body segments together and a shear force perpendicular to the compressive force. The shear force component is most often studied, since joint and bone structures are least tolerant to forces acting in this direction.

Muscle forces

Muscles create a pull on the insertion site in order to move the body segment through a particular range of motion. Since a muscle can only create a pull on the insertion site, muscles must always work in pairs. The agonist muscle creates the pull and the antagonist muscle resists the agonist in order to maintain a smooth and controlled movement. The net muscle force can be broken down into rotational and stabilizing components in each plane. The stabilizing component acts towards the joint centre. As the angle of muscle pull relative to the insertion site becomes greater, the rotational component is greater than the stabilizing component, up to a maximum of 90°, at which point the rotational component is maximized and the stabilizing component equals zero. As with joint forces, muscle forces *in vivo* are rarely measured, although it can be done by placing a force transducer at the myotendinous junction. Generally, muscle force is estimated by using a mathematical model developed using different assumptions about the system, such as insertion point location and angle of pull.

Fluid resistance

Human movement is affected by air resistance when moving on land and water resistance when swimming. The density and viscosity of air and water are the two properties that have the greatest effect on the body moving through the medium. Fluid resistance, which is the transfer of energy from the body to the medium, consists of two components, drag and lift.

The drag force always acts directly opposite to the velocity vector of the system and is the product of the coefficient of drag, the frontal area of the object, the fluid viscosity and the relative velocity of the object to the fluid. There are three types of drag force: surface, form and wave. Surface drag is related to the surface of the object (texture and shape) interacting with the fluid, while form drag creates a pressure differential from the front of the object to the rear. Wave drag is a reaction force to 'waves' generated as a body

moves through an area where two fluids meet (i.e. air and water). Athletes such as swimmers, cyclists, skiers and sprinters tend to wear form-fitting clothing that helps streamline them and minimize the effects of drag.

The lift force acts perpendicular to the drag force and occurs only if the object is not symmetrical in shape or is spinning. Lift occurs because the air or water on one side of the object moves faster than the medium on the other side, creating a pressure differential. Lift is expressed mathematically as Bernoulli's principle (pressure = 1/velocity). A common example is the wing of an aeroplane, where the air on top of the wing moves faster than the air underneath, creating a high-pressure area below the wing. Since the lift force acts from a high-pressure area to a low-pressure area, the wings of the plane are subjected to the lift force. Similarly swimmers use the lift principle by orienting their hands in different positions relative to the water. This may help the swimmer stay 'on top' of the water and enhance overall speed. Lift force or the Magnus effect also influences the curved path of a spinning object, such as a tennis ball that has topspin. The Magnus effect is also related to a pressure differential and explains why a 'curve ball' curves.

Inertial forces

As with kinematics, kinetics also has angular analogues. However, forces acting about a particular axis cause rotation and the result is termed a torque or moment of force. The torque is equal to the product of the applied force and the perpendicular distance from the line of action to the point of rotation. This perpendicular distance is generally termed the moment arm. All of Newton's laws have angular analogues and may be defined as follows. The first law states that angular momentum is conserved or that an object maintains its current angular motion unless acted on by some external torque. The second law can be stated in angular terms such that torque is equal to the product of the moment of inertia and angular acceleration of the object (T

$=I\alpha$). The moment of inertia is the object's resistance to change in angular motion. It is similar to inertia in that it is dependent on mass, but the moment of inertia also depends on the way the mass is distributed. Recall that the COG is dependent on the mass distribution of the segments, so that the COG can be defined as the point about which the sum of all the torques is equal to zero. Finally, the third law states that for any torque exerted on one object, an equal and opposite torque is applied to the first object.

Torques and momentum (mass×velocity, linear or angular) are principles extensively applied in sports. A diver or gymnast creates angular momentum prior to being airborne by exerting a torque on the ground. Since angular momentum is conserved (Newton's first law), manipulations of the limbs and therefore distribution of masses result in the ability to accomplish complex aerial manoeuvres without having any other forces acting except gravity. Torques or moments occurring at the joints during activities are also calculated to determine if athletes may be at risk for joint injury.

Impulse is defined as the product of a force acting over a time interval and can be thought of as the quantity of force needed in order to change the motion of the object. If the force is applied over time, the momentum of the object is changed and this defines the impulse–momentum relationship (Ft=mass×velocity). An object's momentum can be changed by a large force acting over a short period of time or a smaller force acting over a longer period of time. For example, if a person wanted to jump higher they would try to generate greater impulse against the ground, which would increase the momentum and increase the jump height. Investigating the above equation one can see that if the mass changes, in order to maintain the same impulse value the resulting velocity must also change. More specifically, since women tend to have less mass than men, they must increase their velocity in order to generate the same impulse as a man of larger mass.

Joint moments (torques) are calculated from kinetic, kinematic and anthropometric data and these values provide information about the net forces occurring at the joint. It is important to realize that joint moments represent the net effects of what is happening at the joint. For example, the joint moment includes muscle forces, soft tissue forces, contact forces and any other external force. However, determining a general value of force occurring at the joint and comparing this with failure values measured on cadavers may be of some use when establishing the safety level of an activity.

Equipment interaction

As female participation in sports increases, manufacturers are developing special equipment designed specifically for the female athlete. Most of these design differences are based on the anthropometric variation found between males and females. For example, a woman's basketball is smaller in diameter due to the generally smaller hand size of the female. Women's tennis racquets tend to be shorter because of the strength differences seen between males and females in the upper extremity. When choosing sports or strength equipment it is important to consider the anthropometrics of the individuals using the equipment. However, the laws of physics do not discriminate between genders and a good understanding of how the body acts in the physical world is of utmost importance.

Conclusion

Primary kinematic and kinetic relationships have been discussed relative to sport and/or performance. It is important to recognize that kinematic measures are the outcomes or effects of forces (kinetics) applied to the system. Therefore, if a coach is viewing an effect (i.e. a change in position or velocity), the resulting change is a consequence of an applied force. In order to change a performance outcome, the coach must focus on the cause of motion (force) and how, when and where it is applied. In any situation, we are governed by Newton's three laws of motion in an environment subjected to the forces of gravity and friction. The athlete who best utilizes her mechanical advantages by manipulating the COM and lever systems while understanding how Newton's laws are affecting her is often the best performer in any given event.

References

Dapena, J. (1980) Mechanics of translation in the Fosbury flop. *Medicine and Science in Sports and Exercise* **12**, 37–44.

Devita, P. & Skelly, W.A. (1992) Effect of landing stiffness on joint kinetics and energetics in the lower extremity. *Medicine and Science in Sports and Exercise* **24**, 108–115.

Dufek, J.S., Bates, B.T., Davis, H.P. & Malone, L.A. (1991) Dynamic performance assessment of selected sport shoes on impact forces. *Medicine and Science in Sports and Exercise* **23**, 1062–1067.

Dufek, J.S., Bates, B.T., Stergiou, N. & James, C.R. (1995) Interactive effect between group and single-subject response patterns. *Human Movement Science* **14**, 301–323.

Hall, S.J. (1991) *Basic Biomechanics*. Mosby Year Book, St Louis.

Hamill, J. & Knutzen, K.M. (1995) *Biomechanical Basis of Human Movement*. Williams and Wilkins, Baltimore.

Hamill, J., Bates, B.T. & Knutzen, K.M. (1983) Variations in ground reaction force parameters at different running speeds. *Human Movement Science* **2**, 47–56.

Hay, J.G. (1986) The biomechanics of the long jump. *Exercise and Sports Sciences Reviews* **14**, 401–446.

Hoppenfeld, S. (1976) *Physical Examination of the Spine and Extremities*. Appleton and Lange, Norwalk, Connecticut.

Hutchinson, M.R. & Ireland, M.L. (1995) Knee injuries in female athletes. *Sports Medicine* **19**, 288–302.

James, S.L., Bates, B.T. & Osternig, L.R. (1978) Injuries to runners. *American Journal of Sports Medicine* **6**, 40–50.

McNitt-Gray, J.L., Yokoi, T. & Millward, C. (1994) Landing strategies used by gymnasts on different surfaces. *Journal of Applied Biomechanics* **10**, 237–252.

Nigg, B.M. (1986) *Biomechanics of Running Shoes*. Human Kinetics Publishers, Champaign, Illinois.

Norkin, C.C. & Levangie, P.K. (1992) *Joint Structure and Function: A Comprehensive Analysis*. F.A. Davis, Philadelphia.

Pulat, B.M. (1992) *Fundamentals of Industrial Ergonomics*. Prentice Hall, Englewood Cliffs, New Jersey.

Chapter 7

Psychological Aspects of Training

JOAN L. DUDA

Introduction

Past work on the psychological factors affecting female athletes has been limited. For the most part, the female athlete and/or this dimension of sports involvement has been ignored, or what has been addressed has been restricted in terms of her total athletic experience. Although the physiological aspects of training and performance among female athletes has received some attention (Wells, 1991; Pearl, 1993), less concentrated efforts have targeted psychological factors. For example, in *The Athletic Female* (Pearl, 1993), only one of the 21 chapters deals with psychological aspects. In *Women and Sport: Interdisciplinary Perspectives* (Costa & Guthrie, 1994) several chapters focus on sociological and feminist treatments of the topic, although the majority are concerned with physiological/physical issues, and only two of the 22 chapters centre on the psychology of the female athlete.

With regard to sports psychology texts specifically, the attention given to the sporting female is also confined. Occasionally there is a separate chapter or section on gender and the female athlete (Gill, 1986; Horn, 1992; Singer *et al.*, 1993; Cox, 1994; Weinberg & Gould, 1995). Incredulously, there are even cases where the presentation of information on the psychological facets of sport for females is combined with a discussion of coaching youth sport athletes (Anshel, 1997).

In current textbooks dealing with women in sport, the topics typically addressed include the personality characteristics of female athletes and discussions of the psychological consequences of, and socialization into, the role of athlete (Oglesby, 1978; Boutilier & SanGiovanni, 1983). Other areas that are covered include gender stereotyping in the media portrayal of female athletes; implications of gender role socialization through sport; the frequency of participation of females in the roles of athletes, coaches or sport administrators; and the embodiment of gender in regard to how women experience their bodies, sport and physical activity (see, for example, Oglesby & Hill, 1993; Birrell & Cole, 1994). Moreover, chapters on the psychological aspects of female athletes almost always contain a description of how female athletes characterize themselves in terms of attributes deemed masculine, feminine or androgynous; purported value conflicts between female athletes and a male-created and male-dominated sport system; and gender differences in achievement characteristics. In short, the latter work suggests that she is less competitive and outcome-orientated (Gill & Dzewaltowski, 1988). In general, this literature makes a point of distinguishing between sex differences in sport participation and performance (i.e. the biological differences between males and females) and gender differences (i.e. the social and psychological attributes and behaviours typically observed in males and females within the physical domain) (Gill, 1993).

Although greater coverage is warranted, I am not suggesting that what has been written on the physiology and psychology of women in sport is not pertinent to understanding their involvement or lack of involvement in sports. However, the existent contributions convey little relevant information concerning the psychological dimensions of sport training for girls and women. In this chapter, I tackle this particular topic by summarizing four contemporary areas of investigation: (i) research on female athletes' use of psychological skills in their training and preparation for competition; (ii) studies of the efficacy of mental skills training in female athletes; (iii) work on the psychological factors leading to overtraining in female athletes; and (iv) research concerning the optimal psychological environments for training female competitors. The chapter is biased towards highly trained female athletes.

Use of mental skills

Maximal athletic training and sport performance requires the synchronization and optimization of both the physical and psychological systems. The development of competencies such as vivid and controlled imagery, sound goal-setting, stress management, attentional focusing and positive self-talk are presumed to foster mind–body unison and enhance the execution of athletic skills.

The first major study to examine mental skills and the employment of psychological techniques among athletes was conducted by Mahoney *et al.* (1987). The athletes in this investigation included females and males who varied in competitive level. Specifically, the sample included élite (placed fourth or above in the national championships, the Olympics or world championships; $n=50$), pre-élite (junior national athletes or individuals invited to special camps by national governing bodies from 11 different sports; $n=33$) and non-élite (members of university athletic teams from 21 different sports; $n=185$) competitors.

When Mahoney and his colleagues compared the élite female and male athletes with intercollegiate-level athletes, they found the former group: (i) to be more balanced and moderate in their experience of worry and performance

anxiety; (ii) to be able to deploy their concentration more efficiently before and during competition; (iii) to experience stronger and more stable self-confidence; (iv) to rely more on internally focused and kinaesthetic imagery than on third-person visual forms of mental preparation; and (v) to invest more motivation and personal meaning in doing well in their sport. In total, these findings indicated that female and male élite athletes had more proficient psychological skills than the other athletes. However, it should be noted that, as a group, 14–30% of the male and female élite competitors reported experiencing performance-related anxiety problems and 25–31% of these outstanding athletes indicated that they had concentration and self-confidence problems. These latter results suggest that even the highest-level athletes experience psychological difficulties during sport performances and thus need further to improve their mental skills.

Mahoney *et al.* (1987) observed gender differences among the non-élite athletes only. In particular, non-élite female athletes reported lower self-confidence than their male counterparts. They also used more self-talk and indicated that they experienced more problems with stress. The absence of gender-related distinctions among the élite athletes in the study by Mahoney *et al.* agrees with past research indicating that gender differences in self-confidence dissipate or disappear completely when the task at hand is deemed gender appropriate, feedback is contingent and clear, and the individuals in question have equivalent skill and experience with the activity (Gill, 1993). Their results are also consonant with studies indicating that the confidence of females can be enhanced via physical training (Holloway *et al.*, 1988).

The observed gender difference in anxiety levels among the non-élite athletes in the study by Mahoney *et al.* has also emerged in other investigations. For example, Jones and Cale (1989) administered the multidimensional Competitive State Anxiety Inventory-2 to a sample of male and female university athletes 2 weeks, 1 week, 2 days, 1 day, 2 hours and 30 min before the start of a competition. Results indicated that the female athletes increased their level of cognitive anxiety (or degree of worry) as the competition neared while the males exhibited no such change; 30 min before the competitive event, the females were significantly more cognitively anxious than the males. Although the male athletes increased their degree of somatic anxiety starting on the day of competition, females began to report greater somatic symptoms (e.g. increased heart rate, muscular tension) earlier in the period before competition. Finally, Jones and Cale also found that the male athletes' degree of self-confidence changed little before the contest; in contrast, the female athletes' self-confidence decreased on the day of competition.

Jones et al. (1991) attempted to replicate the findings of Jones and Cale (1989) among 13 male college-level field hockey, 15 female rugby and 13 female netball athletes from the UK. They reported parallel results for cognitive anxiety. In the later investigation, however, both males and females exhibited greater somatic anxiety on the day of the competition. Further, both exhibited decreases in self-confidence, although this decrement was more pronounced among the female athletes. Finally, Jones et al. (1991) found different antecedents of precompetitive anxiety as a function of gender. For females, the perceived threat of not obtaining one's personal goals and perceived readiness for the forthcoming competition were the major predictors of precompetitive stress. For the males, ratings of the competition and expectations concerning a successful outcome contributed to their state anxiety levels.

When predicting the level of sport performance of females (as well as males), we should note that it is not only the level of competitive state anxiety that must be considered but also how athletes interpret their anxiety responses. A study by Jones and Hanton (1996) indicated that if an athlete expects to achieve her/his goal in the forthcoming contest, she or he is more likely to interpret the degree of cognitive anxiety and somatic anxiety as facilitative in terms of performance. The subjects in this investigation were competitive swimmers (46 females and 45 males) aged between 14 and 28 years. No gender differ-

ences were reported in terms of the associations between expectations and the perception that one's stress level was beneficial.

Another study of mental skills usage among élite performers involved 633 of 1200 Olympic hopefuls who were participating in the 1988 US Track and Field Olympic Trials (Ungerleider & Golding, 1992). The sample comprised 52% women and 48% men but the results were not analysed separately by gender. The major findings of the study revolved around the use of imagery: 85% of the athletes reported that they practised imagery, with one-third of these individuals using imagery at least three to six times per week; 99% of the imagery users employed visualization before competing but only one-third employed this strategy during competition. Results also indicated that, in general, those athletes who became Olympians used imagery more than those who did not. Moreover, injured athletes who used imagery to foster the rehabilitation process were more likely to make the team than injured athletes who were not imagers.

Hall et al. (1990) examined imagery use among 381 male and female participants from six sports. This sample varied from recreational level to élite international and/or national competitors. Consistent with the results of Ungerleider and Golding (1992), Hall et al. found that the élite athletes (female and male) reported greater use of imagery in general. It was also found that a high use of imagery was associated with all-time best performance in the case of these female and male athletes.

Past work has also pointed to the relevance of attentional skills with respect to maximizing sport performance. In a qualitative study of 16 former US national champion figure skaters (nine females and seven males), Jackson (1992) examined the characteristics of an optimal skating experience (or *flow* state) and the major contributors to this state. As conceptualized by Csikszentmihalyi (1975), flow results when there is enjoyment and a balance between perceived abilities and demands. When in flow, the athlete feels like she is totally involved in the activity at hand, i.e. there is a merging of action and awareness (Csikszentmihalyi, 1975). Based on extensive interview data, Jackson (1992) found that perceived clarity in, and control of, one's attentional focus were major attributes of an optimal skating experience. Similarly, a factor deemed significant to the athlete attaining the flow state was the ability to maintain one's concentration or appropriate attentional focus. In a follow-up investigation involving 28 (14 female, 14 male) élite Australian athletes from seven sports, Jackson (1995) found that the capacity to focus was important to the facilitation, prevention and disruption of the flow experience.

Another critical facet of mental skill development concerns athletes' responses to the less desirable moments in training or a competitive event. In other words, how does the athlete typically react or cope when performance is not going well? In a sample that included 12 junior female tennis players, Van Raalte *et al.* (1994) found that negative self-talk was associated with losing matches and those players who indicated that they believed in the value of positive self-talk won more points than their counterparts who did not perceive much utility in this performance-enhancement technique.

With regard to athletes' explanations for performance-related problems, Hausenblas and Carron (1996) studied 144 élite female and 101 élite male athletes from a variety of sports. They found that female athletes were more likely than male athletes to indicate that performance disruptions were due to sport problems (e.g. cancelled practice), their physical state and problems with family and friends.

Crocker and Graham (1995) conducted an investigation focused specifically on athletes' coping responses. The subjects were 169 women and 208 men (mean age 20.5±2.5 years) who were involved in a variety of sports. Their competitive level ranged from regional to national competitive experience. Female athletes indicated that they sought out emotional social support and increased their efforts when confronted with stress related to thwarted goals. Contrary to what was expected, no evidence emerged that males used greater problem-solving coping strategies. In fact, both female and male athletes tended to engage in effective coping.

In general, past work suggests that élite female athletes possess stronger mental skills than lower-ranking female athletes. At the highest levels of competition, female athletes are much more similar to their male cohorts with regard to the employment of mental skills. Research indicates that gender differences are more likely to be evident at lower competitive levels. The differences that emerge are typically related to variations in self-confidence and the reported degree of competitive stress experienced. Given that anxiety is likely to result when athletes perceive that their abilities do not match the demands being placed on them, it appears that gender-related distinctions in confidence may also result in the observed differences in anxiety levels between male and female athletes.

Effectiveness of mental skills training

Since sport psychology studies indicate that the possession of strong mental skills is linked to higher competitive level and athletic achievement, it is important to ascertain whether such skills can be learned or enhanced among female athletes. With the aim of exploring the documented effectiveness of mental skills interventions, Greenspan and Feltz (1989) examined results across 19 published studies. They found evidence to suggest that educational-based relaxation interventions and cognitive restructuring techniques with individual athletes produce positive results. Unfortunately in terms of the focus of this chapter, only seven of the studies examined were exclusively based on female athletes. Since this review, female competitors have been subjects in a number of investigations on the effects of mental skills training. Examples of such work are reviewed below.

Burton (1989) conducted a season-long goal-setting training programme with 13 female (and 17 male) collegiate Division I swimmers. The emphasis of this programme was to encourage the swimmers to set personal performance standards rather than outcome goals. In contrast with a control group, trained female athletes reported more accurate performance expectations, exhibited lower cognitive anxiety and witnessed greater performance improvement. The self-confidence of the experimental group was also higher than the control group but this difference was not statistically significant.

In a study involving four female collegiate basketball players, Kendall *et al.* (1990) examined the effectiveness of a 5-day programme during which the athletes received training in the areas of imagery, relaxation and self-talk. A single-subject multiple-baseline design was employed and the behaviour of interest was the defensive skill of cutting an offensive player's move to the baseline/hoop. Based on observational data, questionnaire assessments and personal logs completed by the women, a positive effect for the intervention was demonstrated.

Elko and Ostrow (1991) determined the impact of a rational–emotive programme on the state anxiety and performance of six collegiate Division I gymnasts who were identified as anxiety prone. The focus of this programme was to have the athletes become more attuned to the role of trigger thoughts and irrational beliefs in the stress process. The gymnasts were also taught how to substitute such stress-enhancing irrational statements with positively reinforcing self-statements. Following the cognitive intervention, five of the six gymnasts decreased their cognitive anxiety. However, no effect was observed on the gymnasts' somatic anxiety, performance and reported content of thoughts while they were experiencing competitive-related stressors.

Savoy (1993) examined the effect of a mental training programme on a female intercollegiate Division I basketball player across a season. This athlete was requested to participate in the programme due to her purported problem handling distractions and difficulty in becoming motivated for practices. The techniques employed included imagery, centring, focusing and arousal regulation. The efficacy of the programme was deduced from a lowering of the athlete's anxiety before the game, improvement in performance (as reflected in game statistics) and the coach's overall rating of the athlete.

Daw and Burton (1994) conducted a multi-faceted mental skills training programme for six male and six female collegiate tennis players over the course of a year. The athletes were taught goal-setting, imagery and arousal regulation with the intention of developing an individualized programme. Results based on case-study analyses, a within-team comparison of highly committed and poorly committed players, and a comparison with a control group of tennis players indicated that the programme was effective.

A season-long, multifaceted programme with 14 members of a Division I collegiate women's gymnastics team was evaluated by Cogan and Petrie (1995). The intervention focused on team-building and anxiety-management techniques. In contrast with a control group, the intervention group exhibited higher social cohesion and lower cognitive and somatic anxiety.

Kerr and Goss (1996) examined the effect of a comprehensive, 16-session stress management programme on eight female and 16 male élite gymnasts. The study took place over an 8-month period and the dependent variables of interest included stress levels and perceptions of being injured. With respect to the latter variable, the experimental group (females and males) spent less time injured than the control group but this difference was not statistically significant. From mid-season to peak season, however, the gymnasts trained in stress management reported significantly less negative athletic stress.

Lerner *et al.* (1996) conducted a study of 12 female athletes who were members of a collegiate basketball team. Utilizing a multiple-baseline, single-subject ABA design, subjects were assigned to one of three conditions: (i) goal setting, (ii) imagery or (iii) goal-setting and imagery. Three athletes in the goal-setting condition and one participant in the imagery/goal-setting condition increased their free-throw shooting success. However, three athletes who were in the imagery-alone condition decreased their mean free-throw performance. Shambrook and Bull (1996) in their investigation of the impact of imagery training on the basketball free-throw shooting of four female players also reported mixed results.

In their research on seven female and six male club-level golfers from Australia, Thomas and Fogarty (1997) revealed a beneficial effect of a 2-month imagery and self-talk training on the athletes' imagery skills and psychological responses to competition. Improvements in golf performance were also observed.

In sum, investigations concerning the efficacy of mental skill training suggest that programmes geared towards the development of mental skills are beneficial for female competitors. After learning techniques such as self-talk, goal-setting and stress management, female athletes who participate in a variety of sports have been found to exhibit less anxiety and better performance. Results concerning the effectiveness of imagery training on the execution of sport skills have been more inconsistent.

Psychological factors and overtraining

Overtraining and potential burnout are critical areas of concern regarding the development of contemporary female athletes. As pointed out by Weinberg (1990), 'training in most sports now requires year round workouts with off season becoming shorter and shorter. In fact, in sports such as tennis, gymnastics, and swimming, there is really no "off season" as competitions occur throughout the year.'

Silva (1990) has distinguished between positive and negative training stress. In terms of the former, he refers to the desirable adaptations to training (such as increased strength, skill development, confidence) as a function of the overloads placed on the athlete. The responses to negative training stress are presumed to vary along a continuum from staleness to overtraining to burnout. Such responses generally occur when an imbalance is evident between the demands being placed on the athlete and her ability to meet those demands. Silva defines staleness as an initial failure of the body's adaptive mechanisms to cope with the psychophysiological stress created by training stimuli. When athletes are subjected to chronic training stress and are in a continuous state of staleness, they become overtrained. Overtraining leads to 'detectable psychophysiological malfunctions and is characterized by easily observable changes in the athlete's mental orientation and physical performance' (Silva, 1990). Thus, when an athlete is stale or overtrained, a training plateau or detraining effect is likely to ensue. If such a situation continues over time, burnout and withdrawal from the sport are presumed to be likely consequences. According to Silva, the latter experiences are what characterize the negative training stress syndrome.

Silva's (1990) study of the prevalence and significance of the negative training stress syndrome involved 25 female and 43 male intercollegiate athletes from a variety of sports. Almost 73% of the athletes indicated that they had experienced staleness during their collegiate careers but a little more than half found this experience to be tolerable; 66% of the athletes indicated that they experienced overtraining while participating in college sports. Further, almost half of the athletes reported that they had experienced burnout and over 80% suggested that burnout was the worse response to training stress.

Murphy *et al.* (1990) examined the psychological and performance-related impact of increased training loads among seven female and eight male judo athletes who lived at the US Olympic Training Center in Colorado Springs. Assessments were made on the athletes over a 10-week period and were divided into three phases: a baseline phase (weeks 1–4), an increased conditioning training volume phase (weeks 5–8) and an increased sport-specific training volume phase (weeks 9–10). By week 8, the athletes reported their greatest perceived effort related to training and higher fatigue levels compared with baseline. By week 10, athletes were angrier than at the onset of training and exhibited greater general anxiety, higher somatic anxiety and lower self-confidence. Further, there was a decrease in anaerobic endurance and strength by the conclusion of training. These findings are compatible with the earlier, large-scale work of Morgan *et al.* (1987). They reported greater mood disturbances such as greater anger, depression and fatigue associated with training stimulus increases among a sample of 400 male and female competitive swimmers over a 10-year period.

Recently, Gould *et al.* (1996a,b) have focused specifically on the characteristics of young élite athletes who burn out. Two studies were conducted. The first entailed a quantitative analysis of the psychological and environmental factors that distinguished between a national sample of junior tennis players (26 females, 36 males) who experienced burnout, in contrast to a comparable group of young tennis players. The second investigation involved a qualitative analysis of a subsample of the burned-out tennis players from the first study. The results of the initial study indicated that burned-out tennis players felt they had less influence on their training, competed in too many tournaments and were higher in motivation. This group of athletes also felt that their parents were highly critical and held high expectations for the tennis performance. They had lower personal standards but exhibited a greater fear about making mistakes. Finally, in terms of coping strategies, the burned-out athletes were less likely to employ planning and positive re-interpretation when experiencing stress compared with their healthy cohorts.

In contrast to Silva's (1990) suggestion that burnout is a result of long-term exposure to excessive physical training, Gould *et al.* (1996a) argued that their results were compatible with Smith's (1986) cognitive–affective model of burnout in sport. This framework suggests that burnout is a three-stage process: (i) the athletes perceive that the demands placed on them, both physical and psychological, are overwhelming; (ii) they respond to this appraisal with physiological manifestations of stress; and (iii) they exhibit motivational problems and behavioural

deficits (e.g. decreased performance). This burnout process is presumed to be circular, continuous and reciprocal. Based on the findings of their initial study, Gould *et al.* (1996a) concluded that 'stress-induced burnout appears to be explicitly intertwined with motivation and participant motivation concerns, and burnouts must be studied in a longitudinal process-orientated fashion to understand the interaction between these variables'.

In the second investigation, 10 junior élite tennis players who experienced burnout (six females, four males) engaged in an in-depth interview concerning the characteristics of, and reasons for, burnout (Gould *et al.*, 1996b). With regard to the former, study participants indicated that burnout was accompanied by a lack of motivation, low energy, negative affect, a sense of isolation and concentration problems. The physical symptoms experienced by these athletes were varied and not found to be a significant facet of burnout. The major themes that emerged concerning the perceived contributors to burnout included a dissatisfaction with one's social life, negative parental influences, unfulfilled and/or inappropriate expectations and a lack of enjoyment of tennis.

In summary, the training of female athletes can lead to negative rather than positive effects, i.e. when the physical and psychological training demands placed on female athletes chronically surpass their capacity to meet such demands, there are both physical and psychological costs to pay. She can become physiologically overtrained, emotionally and motivationally burned out, and may quit her athletic activity as a result. Based on the literature, the determinants of this negative training stress syndrome (Silva, 1990) appear to be similar for female and male sport participants.

Adaptive psychological training environments

The fourth and final line of research reviewed in this chapter deals with a theoretically based body of work on the correlates of the motivational climate surrounding athletes. Drawing from goal perspective theories of achievement motivation (Nicholls, 1989; Ames, 1992), it is assumed that these climates are created by the athletes' significant others and tied to those goals emphasized in the athletic environment, namely task or ego goals. In the former, the focus is on personal improvement, task mastery and the exhibition of high effort. Perceptions of one's ability are self-referenced when an athlete is task-involved. When ego goals are evoked, concern is with the demonstration of superior ability and outperforming others. In this case, perceiving oneself to be able stems from favourable social comparisons.

Recent studies of high-level athletes (including female athletes in the competitors sampled) have looked at the achievement-related variables associated with strongly task or ego climates reinforced by coaches. For example, Pensgaard and Roberts (1996) conducted an investigation of the relationship between Norwegian athletes' perceptions of the motivational climate operating on their teams and their reported sources of stress. The athletes in this study were participants in the 1994 Winter Olympics. The results indicated that a perceived ego-involving atmosphere was associated with a stronger emphasis on cognitive factors (e.g. a lack of perceived control) and the coach as contributors to competition-related stress.

Other researchers have examined the links between the situationally emphasized goal structures created by coaches and athletes' appraisals concerning their coaches' leadership style and personal performance and skill development. For example, Balaguer et al. (1996, in press) examined the perceptions of competitive club tennis players of the motivational climate created by the coach in relation to: (i) preference for their present coach and ratings of his or her significance in their tennis training; (ii) satisfaction with their current competitive results, level of play and the overall instruction they received from the coach; (iii) perceptions of their improvement in the technical, tactical, physical and psychological components of their tennis game; and

(iv) preferences for and perceptions of the leadership behaviours exhibited by the coach. The subjects in this study were 219 tennis players (73 females, mean age 15.6±2.1 years) from clubs in Spain. Over 30% of the athletes were at an intermediate level, while more than 60% were advanced or professional level tennis players. Tennis players who perceived that their coaches created a more task-involving environment were more satisfied with their year's results and level of play and reported greater improvement in the psychological and tactical dimensions of their tennis. They also perceived that their coach provided more training, instruction and social support. Satisfaction with the training provided by the coach and the players' indication that their present coach was similar to the coach they would prefer, were negatively related to perceptions of an ego-involving climate and positively associated with perceptions of a task-involving atmosphere. The observed associations did not vary as a function of the gender of the athlete. Extending this study to a team sport, the results reported by Balaguer et al. (1996, in press) were replicated in national-level female handball players from Spain (Balaguer et al., 1997).

Another direction in this area of inquiry focuses on whether the motivational climate created by significant others predicts whether sport is 'health conducive or health compromising' for athletes (Duda, 1996). Pertinent to this issue, the media and popular press have recently raised concerns about the pressures placed on athletes, especially female athletes involved in individual, subjectively scored sports in which the élite competitor is often quite young (Ryan, 1995) (Fig. 7.1). In a series of studies involving élite female gymnasts, Duda and her colleagues (Duda & Benardot, 1997; Duda & Kim, 1997; Duda, in press) have examined the associations between perceptions of the motivational climate operating in the gyms where the gymnasts train and psychological and energy balance precursors to the development of eating disorders and other health and performance-related problems; 70 members of the 1994 USA Gymnastics Talent Opportunity Program National Team (mean age

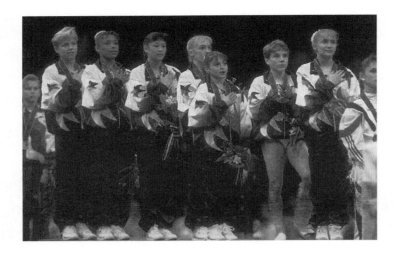

Fig. 7.1 The success of the United States 1996 gymnastics team, which won the Gold Medal in the Atlanta Olympics, raised questions about the pressure on young athletes to perform in spite of injury. (© Allsport.)

10.3 years) participated in the initial investigation (Duda & Benardot, 1997). The sample of junior élite female gymnasts who perceived the training environment created by the coach(es) to be task-involving exhibited higher self-esteem, a more positive body image and enjoyed their sport more. Perceptions of a task-involving gym environment corresponded negatively to the frequency and magnitude of energy deficits during a typical 24-hour training day. Among the older girls in this sample (age 11 years), perceptions of an ego-involving climate were positively correlated with the degree of competitive stress experienced. Duda and Benardot (1997) replicated these findings with a subsequent sample of 15 members of the US international women's artistic team (mean age 15.4 years) and 23 girls of similar age who were on the national artistic team (Duda, in press).

Duda and Kim (1997) extended the studies of Duda and Benardot in three ways. First, the athletes' perceptions of the degree to which their parents create a task- vs. ego-involving climate were determined. Second, we measured another important psychological precursor of the development of eating disorders, namely perfectionism. Third, we assessed disordered eating behaviours and preoccupations with food among more recent members of the Talent Opportunity Program National Team. The results indicated that a perceived ego-involving gym environment corresponded to lower self-esteem and greater dissatisfaction with one's body. When these young gymnasts felt that their coaches emphasized ego goals and their parent-induced motivational climate was ego-involving, they tended to be more perfectionist. Finally, we found that the latter variable mediated the relationship between the two motivational atmospheres surrounding junior élite gymnasts and their attitudes and behaviours concerning food.

The results of the work of Duda and her colleagues is consonant with ethnographic studies of female gymnasts. Krane *et al.* (1997) conducted a qualitative case study of a former élite gymnast involving three unstructured interviews. Through the information gathered, Krane *et al.* found that coaches and parents seemed to create an ego-involving atmosphere which appeared to contribute to the development of the gymnast's strong ego orientation (e.g. she was very concerned with demonstrating her superior competence as a gymnast and was extrinsically motivated). Apparently due to this social environment and her resulting focus on ego-involved goals, the gymnast's athletic experience was marked by overtraining, competing while injured and engaging in disordered eating behaviours.

In summary, the current research on contextually emphasized goal perspectives supports the desirability of task-involving training environments for athletic girls and women. The evidence suggests that such a training climate is conducive to skill development, optimal performance and, most critically, the overall psychological and physical welfare of female athletes.

Conclusion

The research reviewed indicates that the most adaptive and effective training of female athletes must consider the psychological components and consequences of such training. Élite female athletes have been found to possess strong mental skills as well as outstanding physical skills and physiological capacities. Most relevant to sound sport practice, the psychological skills in question, such as maintaining one's confidence and attentional focus, reducing unwanted stress, goal-setting and use of imagery, are trainable. The training of serious female athletes becomes excessive when both the physical and psychological requirements are too great. The implications of overtraining for the athletic female affect the body and the mind and, eventually, her continued involvement in the athletic domain. Conceptually driven investigations are now providing insight into, and guidance concerning the nature of, the training environments most beneficial to the performance and participation of female athletes in sport.

References

Ames, C. (1992) Classroom: Goals, structures, and student motivation. *Journal of Educational Psychology* **84**, 261–271.

Anshel, M.H. (1997) *Sport Psychology: From Theory to Practice*, 3rd edn. Gorsuch Scarisbrick Publishers, Scottsdale, Arizona.

Balaguer, I., Crespo, M. & Duda, J.L. (1996) Dispositional goal perspectives and perceptions of the motivational climate as predictors of coach ratings, satisfaction and perceived improvement among competitive club tennis players. *Journal of Applied Sport Psychology* **8** (Suppl.), S139.

Balaguer, I., Duda, J.L. & Mayo, C. (1997) The relationship of goal orientations and the perceived motivational climate to coaches' leadership style. In R. Lidor & M. Bar-Eli (eds) *Innovations in Sport Psychology: Linking Theory and Practice*. International Society of Sport Psychology, Part 1, pp. 94–96.

Balaguer, I., Duda, J.L. & Crespo, M. (in press) Motivational climate and goal orientations as predictors of perceptions of improvement, satisfaction and coach ratings among tennis players. *Scandinavian Journal of Medicine and Science in Sport*, in press.

Birrell, S. & Cole, C.L. (eds) (1994) *Women, Sport, and Culture*. Human Kinetics Publishers, Champaign, Illinois.

Boutilier, M.A. & SanGiovanni, L. (1983) *The Sporting Woman*. Human Kinetics Publishers, Champaign, Illinois.

Burton, D. (1989) Winning isn't everything: examining the impact of performance goals on collegiate swimmers' cognitions and performance. *Sport Psychologist* **3**, 105–132.

Cogan, K. & Petrie, K. (1995) Sport consultation: an evaluation of a season-long intervention with female collegiate gymnasts. *Sport Psychologist* **9**, 282–296.

Costa, D.M. & Guthrie, S.R. (eds) (1994) *Women and Sport: Interdisciplinary Perspectives*. Human Kinetics Publishers, Champaign, Illinois.

Cox, R.H. (1994) *Sport Psychology: Concepts and Applications*. Brown & Benchmark, Madison, Wisconsin.

Crocker, P.R.E. & Graham, T.R. (1995) Coping by competitive athletes with performance stress: gender differences and relationships with affect. *Sport Psychologist* **9**, 325–338.

Csikszentmihalyi, M. (1975) *Beyond Boredom and Anxiety*. Jossey-Bass, San Francisco.

Daw, J. & Burton, D. (1994) Evaluation of a comprehensive psychological skills training program for collegiate tennis players. *Sport Psychologist* **8**, 37–57.

Duda, J.L. (1996) Fostering motivation in sport and physical education for children and adolescents: the case for greater task involvement. *Quest* **48**, 290–302.

Duda, J.L. (in press) The implications of the motivational climate for motivation, health, and the development of eating disorders in gymnasts. *Revista de Psicologia Social Aplicada*, in press.

Duda, J.L. & Benardot, D. (1997) The motivational climate and psychological and energy balance precursors to the development of eating disorders in female gymnasts. Submitted for publication.

Duda, J.L. & Kim, M. (1997) Parental and gym motivational climates and the development of eating disorders among young elite gymnasts. *Journal of Sport and Exercise Psychology* **19** (Suppl.), S48.

Elko, P.K. & Ostrow, A.C. (1991) Effects of a rational–emotive education program on heightened anxiety levels of female collegiate gymnasts. *Sport Psychologist* **5**, 235–255.

Gill, D.L. (1986) *Psychological Dynamics of Sport*. Human Kinetics Publishers, Champaign, Illinois.

Gill, D.L. (1993) Psychological, sociological, and cultural issues concerning the female athlete. In A.J. Pearl (ed.) *The Athletic Female*, pp. 112–131. Human Kinetics Publishers, Champaign, Illinois.

Gill, D.L. & Dzewaltowski, D.A. (1988) Competitive orientations among intercollegiate athletes: is winning the only thing? *Sport Psychologist* **2**, 212–221.

Gould, D., Udry, E., Tuffey, S. & Loehr, J. (1996a) Burnout in competitive junior tennis players: I. A quantitative psychological assessment. *Sport Psychologist* **10**, 322–340.

Gould, D., Tuffey, S., Udry, E. & Loehr, J. (1996b) **Burnout in competitive junior tennis players:** II. Qualitative analysis. *Sport Psychologist* **10**, 341–366.

Greenspan, M.J. & Feltz, D.L. (1989) Psychological interventions with athletes in competitive situations: a review. *Sport Psychologist* **3**, 219–236.

Hall, C.R., Rodgers, R.M. & Barr, K.A. (1990) The use of imagery by athletes in selected sports. *Sport Psychologist* **4**, 1–10.

Hausenblas, H.A. & Carron, A.V. (1996) Group cohesion and self-handicapping in female and male athletes. *Journal of Sport and Exercise Psychology* **18**, 132–143.

Holloway, J.B., Beuter, A. & Duda, J.L. (1988) Self-efficacy and training for strength in adolescent girls. *Journal of Applied Social Psychology* **18**, 699–719.

Horn, T.S. (ed.) (1992) *Advances in Sport Psychology*. Human Kinetics Publishers, Champaign, Illinois.

Jackson, S. (1992) Athletes in flow: a qualitative investigation of flow states in elite figure skaters. *Journal of Applied Sport Psychology* **4**, 161–180.

Jackson, S. (1995) Factors influencing the occurrence of the flow state in elite athletes. *Journal of Applied Sport Psychology* **7**, 138–166.

Jones, G. & Cale, A. (1989) Precompetition temporal patterning of anxiety and self-confidence in males and females. *Journal of Sport Behavior* **12**, 183–195.

Jones, G. & Hanton, S. (1996) Interpretation of competitive anxiety symptoms and goal attainment expectancies. *Journal of Sport and Exercise Psychology* **18**, 144–157.

Jones, G., Swain, A. & Cale, A. (1991) Gender differences in precompetition temporal patterning and antecedents of anxiety and self-confidence. *Journal of Sport and Exercise Psychology* **13**, 1–15.

Kendall, G., Hrycaiko, D., Martin, G.L. & Kendall, T. (1990) The effects of an imagery rehearsal, relaxation, and self-talk package on basketball game performance. *Journal of Sport and Exercise Psychology* **12**, 157–166.

Kerr, G. & Goss, J. (1996) The effects of a stress management program on injuries and stress levels. *Journal of Applied Sport Psychology* **8**, 109–117.

Krane, V., Greenleaf, C.A. & Snow, J. (1997) Reaching for gold and the price of glory: a motivational case study of an elite gymnast. *Sport Psychologist* **11**, 53–71.

Lerner, B.S., Ostrow, A.C., Yura, M.T. & Eztel, E.F. (1996) The effects of goal-setting and imagery training programs on the free-throw performance of female collegiate basketball players. *Sport Psychologist* **10**, 382–387.

Mahoney, M.J., Gabriel, T.J. & Perkins, T.S. (1987) Psychological skills and exceptional athletic performance. *Sport Psychologist* **1**, 181–199.

Morgan, W.P., Brown, D.R., Raglin, J.S., O'Connor, P.J. & Ellickson, K.A. (1987) Psychological monitoring of overtraining and staleness. *British Journal of Sports Medicine* **21**, 107–114.

Murphy, S.M., Fleck, S.J., Dudley, G. & Calllister, R. (1990) Psychological and performance concomitants of increased volume training in elite athletes. *Journal of Applied Sport Psychology* **2**, 34–50.

Nicholls, J.G. (1989) *The Competitive Ethos and Democratic Education*. Harvard University Press, Cambridge, Massachusetts.

Oglesby, C. (1978) *Women and Sport: From Myth to Reality*. Lea & Febiger, Philadelphia.

Oglesby, C. & Hill, K.L. (1993) Gender and sport. In R. Singer, M. Murphey & L.K. Tennant (eds) *Handbook of Research on Sport Psychology*, pp. 392–413. Macmillan, New York.

Pearl, A.J. (ed.) (1993) *The Athletic Female*. Human Kinetics Publishers, Champaign, Illinois.

Pensgaard, A.M. & Roberts, G.C. (1996) Winter Olympic athletes' perception of the motivational climate and sources of stress. *Journal of Applied Sport Psychology* **8** (Suppl.), S153.

Ryan, J. (1995) *Little Girls in Pretty Boxes: The Making and Breaking of Elite Gymnasts and Figure Skaters*. Doubleday, New York.

Savoy, C. (1993) A yearly mental training program for a college basketball player. *Sport Psychologist* **7**, 173–190.

Shambrook, C.J. & Bull, S.J. (1996) The use of a single-case research design to investigate the efficacy of imagery training. *Journal of Applied Sport Psychology* **8**, 27–43.

Silva, J.M. III (1990) An analysis of the training stress syndrome in competitive athletics. *Journal of Applied Sport Psychology* **2**, 5–20.

Singer, R., Murphey, M. & Tennant, L.K. (eds) (1993) *Handbook of Research on Sport Psychology*. Macmillan, New York.

Smith, R. (1986) Toward a cognitive–affective model of athletic burnout. *Journal of Sport Psychology* **8**, 36–50.

Thomas, P.R. & Fogarty, G.J. (1997) Psychological skills training in golf: the role of individual differences in cognitive preferences. *Sport Psychologist* **11**, 86–106.

Ungerleider, S. & Golding, J.M. (1992) *Beyond Strength: Psychological Profiles of Olympic Athletes*. Brown, Dubuque, Iowa.

Van Raalte, J.L., Brewer, B.W., Rivera, P.M. & Petitpas, A. (1994) The relationship between observable self-talk and competitive junior tennis players' match performances. *Journal of Sport and Exercise Psychology* **16**, 400–415.

Weinberg, R.S. & Gould, D. (1995) *Foundations of Sport and Exercise Psychology*. Human Kinetics Publishers, Champaign, Illinois.

Wells, C.L. (1991) *Women, Sport, and Performance: A Physiological Perspective*, 2nd edn. Human Kinetics Publishers, Champaign, Illinois.

Chapter 8

Nutrition

ANN C. GRANDJEAN, JAIME S. RUUD AND KRISTIN J. REIMERS

Introduction

The past 25 years have seen a dramatic increase in the number of studies examining the physiological, psychological and sociological factors that influence female sports performance. The information acquired from these studies has brought to the forefront many of the nutrition and health-related issues affecting female athletes today. This chapter reviews the most common nutrition-related problems of female athletes, with emphasis on identification and potential interventions.

Inadequate energy intake

Low energy intake is of concern because of the increased risk for illness and injury that can result. Studies have repeatedly shown discrepancies between reported energy intake and estimated energy expenditure among female athletes. (Deuster et al., 1986; Nieman et al., 1989; Dahlström et al., 1990; Wilmore et al., 1992; Edwards et al., 1993; Beidleman et al., 1995; Tanaka et al., 1995). This phenomenon can be explained by at least four different hypotheses: (i) these female athletes have become 'energy efficient', expending fewer kilojoules than estimated by indirect methods; (ii) the athletes are under-reporting food intake; (iii) inexact standards and equations may be the cause, or at least partial cause, of error; and (iv) some female athletes have energy requirements that are truly lower than non-athletic peers. These hypotheses

have been explored and are reviewed here briefly.

ENERGY EFFICIENCY

If the female athlete does indeed become energy efficient, this could be occurring via changes in one or more of the components that constitute total energy expenditure, i.e. resting energy expenditure (REE), the thermic effect of food (TEF) or physical activity. Certainly one explanation for a lower than expected energy expenditure could be a decrease in REE in response to energy restriction (Henson et al., 1987; Leibel et al., 1995). Because REE generally constitutes the largest proportion (60–70%) of total energy expenditure, perturbations in this component could partially explain lower energy requirements. However, in four contemporary studies REE has not been shown to be lower in athletes compared with controls (Schulz et al., 1992; Horton et al., 1994; Beidleman et al., 1995; Fogelholm et al., 1995). In contrast, a study by Thompson et al. (1995) does indicate a lower daily sedentary energy expenditure in a group of male endurance athletes.

The cost of TEF is relatively small, accounting for about 7–10% of total energy needs. Some data have shown that female athletes have a lower TEF than non-athletes, indicating that they may be more energy efficient (LaBlanc et al., 1984). However, other studies have found no differences (Myerson et al., 1991; Wilmore et al., 1992; Beidleman et al., 1995). Of all the components of total energy expenditure, physical activity is the most variable among individuals. It is affected by age, gender, height, weight, body composition, type of activity, physical conditioning, clothing, playing surface, environment in which the activity takes place, genetics, and frequency, intensity and duration of the event or training session. Among well-trained female athletes, energy expended during physical activity can be as high as 36–38% of total energy expenditure (Schulz *et al.*, 1992; Horton *et al.*, 1994). While it is assumed that athletes in training have higher energy expenditure during physical activity compared with non-athletes, this variability may be diminished if non-training physical activity is considered.

UNDER-REPORTING

For years, scientists have questioned the accuracy and reliability of food records. In 1942, Huenemann and Turner compared two different methods of obtaining food intake data. Subjects were interviewed at length regarding food intake (diet history). Following the interview, the subjects recorded food intake for a period of 10–14 days (diet record). Results showed large discrepancies between the two methods. According to the authors, subjects had difficulty estimating the amounts of food they ate. For instance, subjects who thought they drank 1 litre of milk a day actually consumed 0.5 litre. Such errors, which can be significant, have continued to elicit doubts regarding the interpretation of dietary intake data (Guthrie, 1984; Dwyer *et al.*, 1987; Yuhas *et al.*, 1989; Bandini *et al.*, 1990; Dwyer, 1994; Young & Nestle, 1995; Beaton *et al.*, 1997).

While under-reporting is often the conclusion reached by investigators, other factors must be considered. One such factor is inadequate instruction on how to record dietary information; proper instruction may require up to 1 hour per subject to ensure an acceptable degree of accuracy. Another factor is error during computer entry. Human error during this process results from careless coding, miscalculations of amounts (e.g. converting household measurements to metric), unfamiliarity with the foods consumed and entry of generic vs. exact recipes. Precision often requires obtaining recipes from restaurants and to secure food labels in order to verify ingredients. Database limitations (i.e. limited varieties of foods) increase error. With every food substitution made, the potential for error exists even though it may be small; for example entering regular milled white rice instead of long-grain brown rice contributes to error, as does entering pink grapefruit instead of white. Deliberate misreporting (e.g. skimmed milk instead of semi-skimmed) must also be considered.

If small inaccuracies occur throughout the process of estimating energy expenditure and recording and analysing diet records, it is easy to see the potential cumulative effect. For example, if REE and TEF are each overestimated by 2%, activity over a 24-hour period is overestimated by 2%, recorded food intake is underestimated by 2%, and data entry and analysis underestimate actual intake by 2%, a 10% disparity between energy intake and energy expenditure would result when, in reality, small errors in each component account for the disparity.

INEXACTNESS OF STANDARDS

The standards, equations and formulas by which energy requirements/expenditures are estimated use arbitrary 'ideal' heights and weights, body weight, averages, derived values and population data. Even REE is commonly estimated by using any of several empirically derived equations (Food and Nutrition Board, National Research Council, 1989). Therefore, preciseness cannot be expected in many of these calculations.

INDIVIDUALS WITH LOW ENERGY NEEDS

Based on the limited data available, one cannot identify energy efficiency, under-reporting or inexact standards as the conclusive causes of the reported low energy intakes in female athletes. Generally, the accuracy of data becomes an academic discussion, and the perceived problem of low nutrient intake may not be valid. None the less, there undoubtedly are female athletes who have low energy intakes. For discussion purposes, this group can be divided into those who are in energy balance but whose intake is lower than a selected standard and those who are in negative energy balance.

Energy intake below a standard

Athletes participating in sports that require low body weight for performance, such as figure skating, gymnastics, dance, etc., often achieve this body composition by maintaining a low energy intake. An energy intake below an estimated or recommended level in the absence of weight loss does not automatically equate to a nutritional problem. Other criteria must be present. While low energy intake may be accompanied by reduced intake of some nutrients, these can often be corrected without an adjustment in energy intake. However, if indications of energy deficiency are present, even in the absence of weight loss, increased energy intake may be warranted.

Negative energy balance

'Dieting' to decrease or maintain low body fat is often cited by athletes as a reason for low energy intake. While restriction of energy is indicated for some, because they will experience enhanced performance, the necessity of restricting energy intake for others is not as clear. If asked about their purpose in restricting energy intake, quite often these athletes are unable to provide a response. Indeed, in some cases, energy restriction or dieting simply appears to be 'fashionable'.

Although many hypotheses and/or scenarios exist, one theme prevails: female athletes commonly try to achieve a lower energy intake than that indicated to support training. Although certainly not as detrimental to performance as a clinical eating disorder, long-term low energy intake may impede the athlete from reaching her full potential and, moreover, lead to negative consequences, such as inadequate carbohydrate, protein, vitamin and mineral intake, increased risk of injury and increased risk of illness.

Indications

Subjective observations indicative of low energy intake include the following.
- Expressed or displayed concerns about body weight or body composition, even when appropriate for sport.
- Decrease in performance, such as decreased endurance, decreased power or simply decreased enthusiasm.
- Amenorrhoea or oligomenorrhoea: menstrual irregularity caused by negative energy balance may be difficult to distinguish from normal oligomenorrhoea observed in adolescents before the menstrual cycle is established. However, irregular menses combined with the other characteristics listed here can be indicative of an energy shortfall.
- Weight loss may be so gradual that it is very difficult to discern, especially for the coach or trainer who observes the athlete daily.
- Frequent illness: many factors influence frequency of illness, e.g. heavy training, regardless of energy intake, can negatively affect immunity.
- Avoidance of dietary fat: see below for an in-depth discussion of this phenomenon.

Management

Because energy restriction can be a symptom of anorexia nervosa and other eating disorders, ruling out its presence is indicated as an initial step. Discussion with the athlete should elicit whether she is fearful of weight gain, has a distorted body image, or is misinformed about the effect of body weight and body composition on performance. If an eating disorder is suspected, evaluation by a mental health professional and a physician is indicated. If an eating disorder is ruled out, the next step is to assess whether the food restriction is deliberate in order to achieve weight loss or whether the restricted food intake is secondary to other situations, such as problematic relationships, lack of time, lack of money, stress or gastrointestinal pathology.

Discussing problems with the athlete and asking her to record her dietary intake may be effective in increasing dietary intake. It is undeniable that in many cases the athlete achieves a small but noticeable increase in body weight/fat if energy intake is augmented. This can be an obstacle for the athlete who genuinely believes that a lower weight is necessary for good performance. In this case, focusing on performance should be the goal. If performance improves with the increased energy intake and this offsets the change in body composition, the athlete should experience less anxiety. None the less, for other athletes the mental hurdle of gaining weight will not be overcome. In this case, dietary supplementation is a partial solution to an inadequate diet. It is important not to alienate the athlete who is resistant to change, as her readiness to cooperate may alter at a later time.

Excessive restriction of dietary fat

The importance placed on thinness and the health messages that eating a high-fat diet leads to chronic health problems (obesity, cancer, diabetes) have resulted in a trend observed in many people, including female athletes: fat phobia or fear of fat. Weight-conscious athletes often go to extremes to avoid fat. They exclude foods such as meat and dairy products and opt for reduced-fat and fat-free products like rice cakes, pretzels, vegetables and salad with no dressing. Their diets are repetitive, lack variety and are often nutritionally inadequate. The fat-free trend that many athletes perceive as healthy and performance-enhancing is in fact neither. Athletes who consume too little fat can suffer a variety of problems, including low energy levels, menstrual problems and nutrient deficiencies. Extremely low dietary fat intakes are frequently associated with low intakes of vitamins and minerals, such as vitamin B_{12}, folate, vitamin B_6, calcium, iron and zinc.

There is no dietary requirement for fat other than to provide essential fatty acids for phospholipids and cell membranes. The World Health Organization recommends that the total energy from fat is not less than 15% (World Health Organization Study Group, 1990). A prudent level of fat in the diet is 30% of total energy. Low dietary fat intake (15–20%) greatly limits dietary

choices and has been associated with a significant reduction in high-density lipoprotein (HDL) cholesterol levels in women (Denke, 1996). Furthermore, it appears that in endurance athletes with stable weight and body composition, risk factors for coronary heart disease are not adversely affected by increasing dietary fat calories from 30% to 42% (Leddy et al., 1996). In a study of 375 élite athletes, A.C. Grandjean (unpublished data) reported that female athletes (n=110) averaged 33% of total energy from fat with a range of 12–56%. When comparing data from other countries, mean fat intakes of female athletes from the USA are less than those from China (42–49%) (Chen et al., 1989) but comparable to those from The Netherlands (30–35%) (van Erp-Baart et al., 1989).

Just as drastically reducing dietary fat can cause problems, reducing body fat may also negatively affect an athlete's health and performance. Body fat performs many critical functions: it serves as internal padding and surrounds vital organs and protects them from shock and injury. The layer of fat beneath the skin also insulates and protects against the cold. Many female athletes strive to achieve and maintain body weight and body fat at levels much lower than that considered normal or genetically determined. The most usual motivating factor is the desire to be thin. The challenge to the health professional working with such athletes is to help them achieve a body composition that promotes optimal health and performance.

Indications

• Negative attitudes to food: disparaging comments may be made about fried foods, gravies or meats with visible fat. However, more telling are the comments that a food with 1 g of fat is much superior to one with 3 g of fat.
• Decrements in performance: when fat avoidance results in a low energy intake, decrements in performance are likely, as discussed previously.
• Hunger: because dietary fat strongly influences satiety, the athlete who has a restricted dietary fat intake may experience 'always being

hungry'. Our experience with these athletes is that in many cases they are ingesting a relatively high-energy diet from high-carbohydrate sources yet not feeling full after eating. When fat intake is increased, these athletes often reduce their energy intake but feel more satisfied after eating.

• Obvious avoidance of fat in the diet: while omission of entire food groups or specific foods, such as meat, milk, cheese or other dairy products, may be couched in reasons such as vegetarianism, dislike of the food or perception of the food ('it's not healthy'), the true underlying motivation for avoiding some of these foods is, in some cases, simply an effort to avoid fat.

Management

The existence of a very low fat diet by itself is not indicative of dietary risks or impaired performance. Indeed some fastidious athletes achieve balanced varied diets on a low fat intake. On the other hand, some athletes develop a monotonous unvaried diet that leads to inadequate protein, vitamin and mineral intake. Assessing the athlete's dietary intake via computerized diet analysis, checklists, yearly screenings or observation are useful measures for determining whether dietary change is indicated.

When dietary inadequacies have been identified and the culprit appears to be excessive avoidance of fat, it is important to discuss with the athlete the social, emotional, cultural and taste issues leading to fat avoidance in order to elicit faulty perceptions. When misinformation or inaccuracies about the role and function of dietary fat are identified, the first step should be to provide accurate information and dispel misinformation. In some cases the athlete will appear relieved that it is appropriate to increase dietary fat intake. In other cases, perhaps where the athlete has 'grown up' in an environment where fat is thought of as negative, change will be slow or non-existent. Like the situation of low energy intake, if the athlete is resistant to change, dietary supplementation of those vitamins and minerals documented to be inadequate should

be instigated. The nutrients most likely to be inadequate include iron and calcium.

Iron deficiency

The amount of iron absorbed from the diet is determined by multiple factors, with bioavailability being a primary one. Research on the bioavailability of iron allows one to predict, with a degree of confidence, the amount of non-haem iron that will be absorbed from different diets (Monsen *et al.*, 1978; International Nutritional Anemia Consultative Group, 1981) and to classify diets as low, medium or high bioavailability. The amount of available iron that is absorbed by the mucosal cell is inversely related to the iron content of the body. Thus, the total amount of iron in the diet, the bioavailability of that iron and the factors that affect iron requirements and losses in women (e.g. menses, pregnancy, lactation) collectively affect the quantities of iron that must be present in the diet if iron balance is to be maintained.

With median menstrual iron losses of 0.4–0.5 mg daily and basal iron losses of 0.8 mg daily, half the female population would remain in iron balance if 1.3 mg of iron could be absorbed daily; 95% of women would remain in iron balance if 2.8 mg of iron could be absorbed. For women to absorb 2.8 mg of iron when consuming a low-bioavailable diet would require 56 mg of iron in the diet daily (International Nutritional Anemia Consultative Group, 1981). These calculations consider only the bioavailability of diet and become inaccurate in the light of other factors that interfere with the absorption of iron. Compounding factors include pathological bleeding and the malabsorption that occurs with gastrointestinal pathology. Depending on the substance consumed, pica may lead to iron deficiency. Medicinal antacids can also interfere with iron absorption.

It is easy to see why the prevalence of iron deficiency is significant in women. The fact that meat and vitamin C-rich foods (known enhancers of iron absorption) are not available to vast segments of the earth's population is obviously a contributing factor. In developed countries, the problem of decreased energy intake is relevant. With an increasingly sedentary lifestyle, the quantity of food eaten per day has declined significantly and thus iron intake has also declined.

For female athletes, iron deficiency has long been an issue with regard to general health and performance (see Chapter 21). Studies assessing the diets of female athletes show that iron intake is frequently less than the amount recommended by different countries (Manore *et al.*, 1989; Reggiani *et al.*, 1989; Pate *et al.*, 1990; Faber & Spinnler, 1991; Lukaski *et al.*, 1996). Most scientists investigating the iron status of athletes are primarily interested in sports performance, although recent data on cognitive performance should also be recognized. Studies indicate that non-anaemic, low iron levels can impair memory and verbal learning capacity in female adolescents (Bruner *et al.*, 1996).

Indications

- Distinguishing haematological indices (see Chapter 21).
- Fatigue.
- Decreased performance.
- Impairment of temperature regulation.
- Growth retardation.
- Scholastic underachievement.
- Impaired ability to concentrate.
- Impaired cognitive functioning.
- Thin, brittle fingernails and toenails.
- Pallor.

Management

Awareness, early detection and adequate knowledge are important steps in preventing iron deficiency. Ideally, female athletes should be screened once a year to detect the early stages of iron deficiency (International Center for Sports Nutrition and the United States Olympic Committee, 1990). However, this is impractical for many. Therefore, emphasis should be placed on high-risk groups, such as chronic dieters, women with heavy and long menstrual cycles,

endurance athletes in heavy training and vegetarian athletes.

Resistance to taking pills, intolerance of elemental iron and/or the fact that iron supplements are not available, necessitate aggressive dietary strategies in some anaemic female athletes. Information gathered during assessment can be used to estimate dietary iron absorption and indicate appropriate dietary changes.

In the athlete electing for dietary intervention, awareness of good sources of dietary iron is essential. Iron bioavailability depends on several factors, including the form of iron (haem vs. non-haem), the presence of enhancers (e.g. animal tissue, vitamin C) and inhibitors (e.g. polyphenols in tea, phytates, bran), and the athlete's iron status. Including meat, poultry and fish in the diet and foods containing vitamin C will increase iron absorption. In diets where little or no meat is consumed, intake can be increased by including more iron-rich foods such as dried fruits, cooked beans, dark-green leafy vegetables, whole grains and, if available, iron-fortified foods (Table 8.1). The use of iron cookware can significantly increase iron intake.

Athletes who are iron deficient should receive dietary counselling and, when indicated, supplemental iron as described in Chapter 21. However, routine use of iron supplements by all athletes is not warranted and in some cases is contraindicated (see next section).

Precautions

When screening athletes for anaemia, it is imperative that health professionals be aware of haemolytic anaemias/haemolytic disorders. Of the haemolytic disorders, sickle cell anaemia and thalassaemia (major and minor) are more likely to be encountered when working with athletes. The red cell destruction that occurs with the haemolytic disorders increases free iron. Use of iron supplements compounds the problem by further increasing free iron and can result in iron overload. Chronic iron overload is characterized by greater than normal focal or generalized deposition of iron within body tissues

Table 8.1 (a) Dietary haem sources of iron*

Food (85 g, cooked, lean only)	Total iron (mg)	Available iron (mg)
Beef		
Liver, pan fried	5.34	0.60
Chuck, arm pot roast, braised	3.22	0.48
Tenderloin, roasted	3.05	0.46
Sirloin, broiled	2.85	0.42
Roundtip, roasted	2.50	0.38
Top round, broiled	2.45	0.37
Top loin, broiled	2.10	0.31
Ground, lean, broiled	1.79	0.27
Eye round, roasted	1.65	0.25
Pork		
Shoulder, blade, Boston, roasted	1.36	0.15
Tenderloin, roasted	1.31	0.15
Ham, boneless, 5–11% fat	1.19	0.14
Loin chop broiled	0.78	0.09
Loin, roasted	2.07	0.31
Leg, shank half, roasted	1.75	0.26
Lamb		
Loin, roasted	0.93	0.14
Cutlet, pan fried	0.74	0.11
Chicken		
Liver, simmered	7.20	0.81
Leg, roasted	1.11	0.17
Breast, roasted	0.88	0.13
Turkey		
Leg, roasted	2.26	0.34
Breast, roasted	0.99	0.14
Fish		
Tuna, light meat, canned	2.72	0.31
Tuna, white meat, canned	0.51	0.06
Halibut, dry heat	0.91	0.10
Salmon, sockeye, dry heat	0.47	0.06
Flounder/sole, dry heat	0.23	0.03
Seafood		
Oysters, 6 medium, raw	5.63	0.63
Shrimp, moist heat	2.63	0.30
Crab, Alaskan king, moist heat	0.65	0.07

Table 8.1 (b) Dietary non-haem sources of iron*

Food	Portion size	Total iron (mg)	Available iron (mg)
Cereal			
Raisin bran (enrich), dry	28 g	4.5	0.23
Corn flakes (enrich), dry	28 g	1.8	0.09
Shredded wheat, dry	28 g	1.20	0.06
Oatmeal, cooked	117 g	0.80	0.04
Whole wheat hot cereal	121 g	0.75	0.04
Breads and rice			
Bagel	1	1.8	0.09
Bran muffin, home recipe	1	1.4	0.07
Whole wheat bread	1 slice	1.0	0.05
White rice (enrich), cooked	80 g	0.9	0.05
White bread (enrich)	1 slice	0.7	0.04
Brown rice, cooked	98 g	0.5	0.03
Fruit			
Apricots, dried	7 halves	1.16	0.06
Prunes, dried	3 medium	0.84	0.04
Raisins	20 g	0.38	0.02
Banana	1 medium	0.35	0.02
Apple	1 medium	0.25	0.01
Orange	1 medium	0.13	0.01
Vegetables			
Potato, baked with skin	1 medium	2.75	0.14
Peas, cooked	80 g	1.26	0.06
Spinach, raw	15 g	0.76	0.04
Broccoli, raw	44 g	0.39	0.02
Carrots	1 medium	0.36	0.02
Lettuce, iceberg	1/8 head	0.34	0.02
Corn, cooked	82 g	0.25	0.01
Pulses			
Kidney beans, boiled	89 g	2.58	0.13
Kidney beans, canned	128 g	1.57	0.08
Chickpeas, boiled	82 g	2.37	0.12
Chickpeas, canned	120 g	1.62	0.08
Baked beans, canned, plain	127 g	0.37	0.02
Dairy			
Milk, low fat	244 g	0.12	0.01
Yogurt, plain low fat	245 g	0.18	0.01
Cheese, cheddar	28 g	0.19	0.01
Miscellaneous			
Tofu	99 g	2.3	0.12
Egg	1 whole	1.0	0.05
Egg	1 yolk	0.95	0.05
Egg	1 white	trace	–
Peanut butter	32 g	0.6	0.03
Cane, blackstrap	20 g	5.05	0.25

*Source: *Iron in Human Nutrition*. National Live Stock and Meat Board, Chicago, IL, 1990.

(haemosiderosis), which can result in tissue injury (haemochromatosis) and, when left untreated, more severe sequelae.

Inadequate calcium intake

Optimal calcium intake during childhood and adolescence is important for the attainment of peak bone mass and for the prevention of osteoporosis (Matkovic *et al.*, 1990). Although adequate calcium intake is important for all women, it is of extra concern in amenorrhoeic females who are at increased risk of low bone mineral density because of decreased oestrogen levels (Emans *et al.*, 1990). The role of calcium in the prevention and treatment of osteoporosis is covered in Chapter 27. This section briefly presents dietary intake data of female athletes and discusses dietary intervention strategies for women with confirmed inadequate intakes.

The recommended intake for calcium varies among countries, with influencing factors being the composition of the native diet, public health concerns and physiological adaptations. The World Health Organization recommended intake for calcium is 400–500 mg for adults (World Health Organization Study Group, 1990). The recommended intake in Colombia, Hungary, India, Mexico, Philippines, Singapore, Thailand and the UK is 500 mg; in Australia, Brazil, Canada, the former Czechoslovakia, France, Germany, Ireland, Portugal, South Africa and Uruguay it is 800 mg; in Italy it is 1000 mg; and in the USA the current dietary reference intake value is 1300 mg daily for females aged 9–18 and 1000 mg daily for females aged 19–51 years (Food and Nutrition Board, 1997).

Milk and milk products are the richest sources of calcium. In the USA they provide more than half the calcium in a typical diet (Fleming & Heimbach, 1994). Other calcium-rich foods consumed in the USA include dark-green leafy vegetables, canned fish with small bones, and foods fortified with calcium (e.g. juices, bread). Calcium-set tofu (tofu processed with a calcium salt) and calcium-fortified soy milk are important sources of calcium in the diets of many vegans (Weaver & Plawecki, 1994). Calcium from soybeans and green leafy vegetables such as broccoli contain less calcium per serving than milk but are absorbed as well (Weaver & Plawecki, 1994). Lime-processed tortillas, dried fruits, almonds, softened bones of fish and pulverized eggshells added to gruels are also significant sources of calcium for many cultures.

It is important that young female athletes know that dietary and lifestyle factors affect bone health. Although most women are aware of the importance of calcium and think they consume enough, dietary reports from female athletes often reveal less than optimal intakes (Table 8.2). Information provided to athletes on calcium should describe a wide variety of sources, since milk and milk products are often omitted from the diet in an attempt to reduce fat and/or energy intake, or for personal, religious or philosophical reasons.

Indications

Low consumption in otherwise healthy women is indicated by dietary intake analysis, food frequency questionnaire or screening instrument for calcium intake. No biochemical tests to measure status exist. For example, calcium levels in the blood are independent of intake and will be defended during long periods of very low intake by bone resorption.

Management

While there are many reasons for inadequate intake in the presence of adequate supply, three common ones are: (i) the misperception that intake is adequate (e.g. overestimation of consumption); (ii) lack of awareness of calcium requirements (e.g. 1200 mg is equal to almost 1000 ml of fluid milk, 130 g of hard cheese or 640–4200 g of leafy green vegetables); and (iii) avoidance of dairy products because of negative attitudes toward fat and energy. Appropriate education/intervention will be dictated by the contributing factor(s).

Dietary assessment can determine, to a relative

Table 8.2 Summary of calcium intake of female athletes

Reference	No. of subjects	Age*	Sport	Energy†‡ in kJ (kcal)	Calcium‡ (mg)
Cohen *et al.* (1985)	12	24.4 ± 3.8	Dance	6 993 ± 1 881 (1673 ± 450)	821 ± 311
Deuster *et al.* (1986)	51	29.1 ± 0.8	Running	10 019 ± 435 (2397 ± 104)	1227 ± 95
Nowak *et al.* (1988)	10	19.4 ± 0.97	Basketball	7 231 ± 2 395 (1730 ± 573)	903 ± 612
Vallieres *et al.* (1989)	6	22.3 ± 0.5	Swimming	10 333 ± 2 997 (2472 ± 717)	970 ± 369
Barr (1989)	10	16 ± 1.6	Swimming	8 627 ± 1 990 (2064 ± 476)	1354 ± 521
Benardot *et al.* (1989)	22	11–14§	Gymnastics	7 131 ± 1 760 (1706 ± 421)	867 ± 403
Heyward *et al.* (1989)	12	28.7 ± 7.2	Bodybuilding	6 813 ± 2 299 (1630 ± 550)	704 ± 389
Keith *et al.* (1989)	8	22.0 ± 5.0	Cycling	7 445 ± 2 993 (1781 ± 716)	719 ± 369
Reggiani *et al.* (1989)	26	12.3 ± 1.7	Gymnastics	6 487 ± 2 128 (1552 ± 509)	539 ± 291
Tilgner and	19	19	Swimming	10 421 ± 2 270 (2493 ± 543)	1046 ± 404
Schiller (1989)	8	19	Hockey	8 176 ± 1 568 (1956 ± 375)	762 ± 281
Kleiner *et al.* (1990)	8	28 ± 4	Bodybuilding	9 447 ± 11 119 (2260 ± 2660)	293 ± 231
Benson *et al.* (1990)	12	12.5 ± 1.1	Gymnastics	6 454 ± 1 664 (1544 ± 398)	966 ± 339
	18	12.8 ± 0.9	Swimming	7 909 ± 1 864 (1892 ± 446)	764 ± 408
Pate *et al.* (1990)	103	30.6 ± 7.4	Running	6 701 ± 201 (1603 ± 48)	630 ± 23
Worme *et al.* (1990)	21	32 ± 2	Triathlon	9 050 ± 476 (2165 ± 114)	1259 ± 105
Barr (1991)	14	19.8 ± 1.2	Swimming	9 597 ± 1 990 (2296 ± 476)	808 ± 343
Faber and Spinnler (1991)	10	22.3 ± 2.9	Field hockey	9 285 ± 2 013 (2215 ± 479)	739 ± 642
Berning *et al.* (1991)	21	15.0 ± 2.0	Swimming	14 930 ± 614 (3572 ± 147)	1234 ± 96
Bergen-Cico and Short (1992)	44	13.9 ± 1.1	Cross-country running	10 400 ± 1 262 (2488 ± 302)	972 ± 372
Snead *et al.* (1992)	19	31.9 ± 1.3	Running	8 251 ± 607 (1972 ± 145)	948 ± 54
Webster and	32	14.1 ± 1.6	Gymnastics	–	1005 ± 534
Barr (1995)	25	14.3 ± 1.6	Speed skating	–	1527 ± 750
Kirchner *et al.* (1995)	26	19.7 ± 0.2	Gymnastics	5 773 ± 456 (1381 ± 109)	683 ± 58

* Age reported as mean unless otherwise indicated; ± SD given if provided by authors.
† Kilocalories converted to kilojoules (1 kcal = 4.18 kJ).
‡ Mean ± SD (range).
§ Only range reported.

degree of accuracy, the current level of calcium intake. Dietary modification and/or supplementation should then be calculated to obtain the goal level for the athlete while avoiding levels in excess of 2500 mg (Hathcock, 1997).

Some athletes avoid milk and milk products due to actual or perceived lactose intolerance. Many with lactose intolerance can tolerate foods with low lactose, such as yoghurt and hard cheeses such as Swiss, Colby and Cheddar; some can tolerate small amounts of milk. Ingestion of 240 ml of milk twice daily resulted in no change in symptoms in lactose-intolerant individuals in one double-blind crossover study (Suarez *et al.*, 1997). Lactose tablets consumed before meals or

food treated with liquid lactose preparations are other approaches for managing lactose intolerance. Those totally intolerant or who experience increased intolerance during times of stress (e.g. international travel, major competitions) will need to include other sources of calcium (Table 8.3) and/or use calcium supplements.

Conclusion

This chapter has been limited to brief discussions of four significant dietary problems commonly found individually or in combination in female athletes. This is not to imply that nutritional problems are limited to these four. As with all

Table 8.3 Sources of calcium. (Adapted from Weaver & Plawecki, 1994 with permission)

Food	Portion size (g)	Calcium content (mg)	Estimated absorbable calcium per serving (mg)
Almonds, dry roasted	28	80	17.0
Beans, pinto	86	44.7	7.6
Beans, red	172	40.5	6.9
Beans, white	110	113	19.2
Broccoli	71	35	18.4
Brussel sprouts	78	19	12.1
Cabbage, Chinese	85	79	42.5
Cabbage, green	75	25	16.2
Cauliflower	62	17	11.7
Citrus punch with calcium citrate maleate	240	300	150
Fruit punch with calcium citrate maleate	240	300	156
Kale	65	47	27.6
Kohlrabi	82	20	13.4
Milk	240	300	96.3
Mustard greens	72	64	37.0
Radish	50	14	10.4
Rutabaga	85	36	22.1
Sesame seeds, no hulls	28	37	7.7
Soy milk	120	5	1.6
Spinach	90	122	6.2
Tofu, calcium set	126	258	80.0
Turnip greens	72	99	51.1
Watercress	17	20	13.4

athletes, adequate hydration, appropriate training diet, adequate carbohydrate consumption, individualized precompetition meal and managing nutrition when travelling, to name a few, are also nutritional concerns of the female athlete. Although we have identified common characteristics among females, there is a risk in generalizing this population. Each female athlete presents unique nutritional challenges based on her sport, training, environment, genetic predisposition and learned dietary behaviours.

References

Bandini, L.G., Schoeller, D.A., Cyr, H.N. & Dietz, W.H. (1990) Validity of reported energy intake in obese and nonobese adolescents. *American Journal of Clinical Nutrition* **52**, 421–425.

Barr, S.I. (1989) Energy and nutrient intakes of elite adolescent swimmers. *Journal of the Canadian Dietetic Association* **50**, 20–24.

Barr, S.I. (1991) Relationship of eating attitudes to anthropometric variables and dietary intakes of female collegiate swimmers. *Journal of the American Dietetic Association* **91**, 976–977.

Beaton, G.H., Burema, J. & Ritenbaugh, C. (1997) Errors in the interpretation of dietary assessments. *American Journal of Clinical Nutrition* **65**, 1100S–1107S.

Beidleman, B.A., Puhl, J.L. & De Souza, M.J. (1995) Energy balance in female distance runners. *American Journal of Clinical Nutrition* **61**, 303–311.

Benardot, D., Schwarz, M. & Heller, D.W. (1989) Nutrient intake in young, highly competitive gymnasts. *Journal of the American Dietetic Association* **89**, 401–403.

Benson, J.E., Allemann, Y., Theintz, G.E. & Howald, H. (1990) Eating problems and calorie intakes in Swiss adolescent athletes. *International Journal of Sports Medicine* **11**, 249–252.

Bergen-Cico, D.K. & Short, S.H. (1992) Dietary intakes, energy expenditures, and anthropometric characteristics of adolescent female cross-country runners. *Journal of the American Dietetic Association* **92**, 611–612.

Berning, J.R., Troup, J.P., VanHandel, P.J., Daniels, J. & Daniels, N. (1991) The nutritional habits of young adolescent swimmers. *International Journal of Sports Medicine* **1**, 240–248.

Bruner, A.B., Joffee, A., Duggan, A.K., Casella, J.F. & Brandt, J. (1996) Randomised study of cognitive effects of iron supplementation in non-anaemic iron-deficient adolescent girls. *Lancet* **348**, 992–996.

Chen, J.D., Wang, J.F., Li, K.J. *et al.* (1989) Nutritional problems and measures in elite and amateur athletes. *American Journal of Clinical Nutrition* **49**, 1084–1089.

Cohen, J.L., Potosnak, L., Frank, O. & Baker, H.A. (1985) Nutritional and hematologic assessment of elite ballet dancers. *Physician and Sportsmedicine* **13**, 43–54.

Council for Responsible Nutrition (1996) *Vitamin and Mineral Safety*. Washington, DC.

Dahlström, M., Jansson, E., Nordevang, E. & Kaijser, L. (1990) Discrepancy between estimated energy intake and requirement in female dancers. *Clinical Physiology* **10**, 11–25.

Denke, M.A. (1996) Lipids, estrogen status, and coronary heart disease risk in women. *Medicine and Science in Sports and Exercise* **28**, 13–14.

Deuster, P.A., Kyle, S.B., Moser, P.B., Vigersky, R.A., Singh, A. & Schoomaker, E.B. (1986) Nutritional survey of highly trained women runners. *American Journal of Clinical Nutrition* **44**, 954–962.

Dwyer, J.T. (1994) Dietary assessment. In M.E. Shils, J.A. Olson & M. Shike (eds) *Modern Nutrition in Health and Disease*, 8th edn, pp. 842–860. Lea & Febiger, Philadelphia.

Dwyer, J.T., Krall, E.A. & Coleman, K.A. (1987) The problem of memory in nutritional epidemiology research. *Journal of the American Dietetic Association* **87**, 1509–1512.

Edwards, J.E., Lindeman, A.K., Mikesky, A.E. & Stager, J.M. (1993) Energy balance in highly trained female endurance runners. *Medicine and Science in Sports and Exercise* **25**, 1398–1404.

Emans, S.J., Grace, E., Hoffer, F.A., Gundberg, C., Ravnikar, V. & Woods, E.R. (1990) Estrogen deficiency in adolescents and young adults: impact on bone mineral content and effects of estrogen replacement therapy. *Obstetrics and Gynecology* **76**, 585–592.

Faber, M. & Spinnler, A.J. (1991) Mineral and vitamin intake in field athletes (discus-, hammer-, javelin-throwers and shotputters). *International Journal of Sports Medicine* **12**, 324–327.

Fleming, K.H. & Heimbach, J.T. (1994) Consumption of calcium in the U.S.: food sources and intake levels. *Journal of Nutrition* **124**, 1426S–1430S.

Fogelholm, G.M., Kukkonen-Harjula, T.K., Taipale, S.A., Sievänen, H.T., Oja, P. & Vuori, I.M. (1995) Resting metabolic rate and energy intake in female gymnasts, figure-skaters and soccer players. *International Journal of Sports Medicine* **16**, 551–556.

Food and Nutrition Board (1997) *Dietary Reference Intakes for Calcium, Phosphorus, Magnesium, Vitamin D, and Fluoride*. National Academy Press, Washington DC.

Food and Nutrition Board, National Research Council (1989) *Recommended Dietary Allowance*, 10th edn, p. 179. National Academy Press, Washington, DC.

Guthrie, A.H. (1984) Selection and quantification of typical food portions by young adults. *Journal of the American Dietetic Association* **84**, 1440–1444.

Hathcock, J.N. (1997) *Vitamin and Mineral Safety*. Council for Responsible Nutrition, Washington DC.

Henson, L.C., Poole, D.C., Donahoe, C.P. & Heber, D. (1987) Effects of exercise training on resting energy expenditure during caloric restriction. *American Journal of Clinical Nutrition* **46**, 893–899.

Heyward, V.H., Sandoval, W.M. & Colville, B.C. (1989) Anthropometric, body composition and nutritional profiles of bodybuilders during training. *Journal of Applied Sport Science Research* **3**, 22–29.

Horton, T.J., Drougas, H.J., Sharp, T.A., Martinez, L.R., Reed, G.W. & Hill, J.O. (1994) Energy balance in endurance-trained female cyclists and untrained controls. *Journal of Applied Physiology* **76**, 1937–1945.

Huenemann, R.L. & Turner, D. (1942) Methods of dietary investigation. *Journal of the American Dietetic Association* **18**, 562–568.

International Center for Sports Nutrition and the United States Olympic Committee (1990) *Iron and Physical Performance*. ICSN, Omaha.

International Nutritional Anemia Consultative Group (1981) *Iron Deficiency in Women*. Nutrition Foundation, Washington DC.

Keith, R.E., O'Keeffe, K.A., Alt, L.A. & Young, K.L. (1989) Dietary status of trained female cyclists. *Journal of the American Dietetic Association* **89**, 1620–1623.

Kirchner, E.M., Lewis, R.D. & O'Connor, P.J. (1995) Bone mineral density and dietary intake of female college gymnasts. *Medicine and Science in Sports Exercise* **27**, 543–549.

Kleiner, S.M., Bazzarre, T.L. & Litchford, M.D. (1990) Metabolic profiles, diet, and health practices of championship male and female bodybuilders. *Journal of the American Dietetic Association* **90**, 962–967.

LaBlanc, J., Diamond, P., Cote, J. & Labrie, A. (1984) Hormonal factors in reduced postprandial heat production of exercise-trained subjects. *Journal of Applied Physiology* **56**, 772–776.

Leddy, J., Horvath, P., Rowland, J. & Pendergast, D. (1996) Effect of a high or a low fat diet on cardiovascular risk factors in male and female runners. *Medicine and Science in Sports and Exercise* **29**, 17–25.

Leibel, R.L., Rosenbaum, M. & Hirsch, J. (1995) Changes in energy expenditure resulting from altered body weight. *New England Journal of Medicine* **332**, 621–628.

Lukaski, H.C., Siders, W.A., Hoverson, B.S. & Gallagher, S.K. (1996) Iron, copper, magnesium and zinc status as predictors of swimming performance. *International Journal of Sports Medicine* **17**, 535–540.

Manore, M.M., Besenfelder, P.D., Carroll, S.S. & Hooker, S.P. (1989) Nutrient intakes and iron status in female long-distance runners during training. *Journal of the American Dietetic Association* **89**, 257–259.

Matkovic, V., Fontana, D., Tominac, C., Goel, P., Chestnut III, C.H. (1990) Factors that influence peak bone mass formation: a study of calcium balance and the inheritance of bone mass in adolescent females. *American Journal of Clinical Nutrition* **52**, 878–888.

Monsen, E.R., Hallberg, L., Layrisse, M. *et al.* (1978) Estimation of available dietary iron. *American Journal of Clinical Nutrition* **31**, 134–141.

Myerson, M., Gutin, B., Warren, M.P. *et al.* (1991) Resting metabolic rate and energy balance in amenorrheic and eumenorrheic runners. *Medicine and Science in Sports and Exercise* **23**, 15–22.

Nieman, D.C., Butler, J.V., Pollett, L.M., Dietrich, S.J. & Lutz, R.D. (1989) Nutrient intake of marathon runners. *Journal of the American Dietetic Association* **89**, 1273–1278.

Nowak, R.K., Knudsen, K.S. & Schultz, L.O. (1988) Body composition and nutrient intakes of college men and women basketball players. *Journal of the American Dietetic Association* **88**, 575–578.

Pate, R.R., Sargent, R.G., Baldwin, C. & Burgess, M.L. (1990) Dietary intake of women runners. *International Journal of Sports Medicine* **11**, 461–466.

Reggiani, E., Arras, G.B., Trabacca, S., Senarega, D. & Chiodini, G. (1989) Nutrition status and body composition of adolescent female gymnasts. *Journal of Sports Medicine and Physical Fitness* **29**, 285–288.

Schulz, L.O., Alger, S., Harper, I., Wilmore, J.H. & Ravussin, E. (1992) Energy expenditure of elite female runners measured by respiratory chamber and doubly labeled water. *Journal of Applied Physiology* **72**, 23–28.

Snead, D.B., Stubbs, C.C., Weltman, J.Y. *et al.* (1992) Dietary patterns, eating behaviors, and bone mineral density in women runners. *American Journal of Clinical Nutrition* **56**, 705–711.

Suarez, F.L., Savaiano, D., Arbisi, P. & Levitt, M.D. (1997) Tolerance to the daily ingestion of two cups of milk by individuals claiming lactose intolerance. *American Journal of Clinical Nutrition* **65**, 1502–1506.

Tanaka, J.A., Tanaka, H. & Landis, W. (1995) An assessment of carbohydrate intake in collegiate distance runners. *International Journal of Sports Nutrition* **5**, 206–214.

Thompson, J.L., Manore, M.M., Skinner, J.S., Ravussin, E. & Spraul, M. (1995) Daily energy expenditure in male endurance athletes with differing energy intakes. *Medicine and Science in Sports and Exercise* **27**, 347–354.

Tilgner, S.A. & Schiller, M.R. (1989) Dietary intakes of female college athletes: the need for nutrition education. *Journal of the American Dietetic Association* **89**, 967–969.

van Erp-Baart, A.M.J., Saris, W.H.M., Binkhorst, R.A., Vos, J.A. & Elvers, J.W.H. (1989) Nationwide survey on nutritional habits in elite athletes. Part I. Energy, carbohydrate, protein, and fat intake. *International Journal of Sports Medicine* **10**, S3–S10.

Vallieres, F., Tremblay, A. & St-Jean, L. (1989) Study of the energy balance and the nutritional status of highly trained female swimmers. *Nutrition Research* **9**, 699–708.

Weaver, C.M. & Plawecki, K.L. (1994) Dietary calcium: adequacy of a vegetarian diet. *American Journal of Clinical Nutrition* **59**, 1238S–1241S.

Webster, B.I. & Barr, S.I. (1995) Calcium intakes of adolescent female gymnasts and speed skaters: lack of association with dieting behavior. *International Journal of Sport Nutrition* **5**, 2–12.

Wilmore, J.H., Wambsgans, K.C., Brenner, M. *et al.* (1992) Is there energy conservation in amenorrheic compared with eumenorrheic distance runners? *Journal of Applied Physiology* **72**, 15–22.

World Health Organization Study Group (1990) *Diet, Nutrition, and the Prevention of Chronic Diseases*. WHO Technical Report Series 797. WHO, Geneva.

Worme, J.D., Doubt, T.J., Singh, A., Ryan, C.J., Moses, F.M. & Deuster, P.A. (1990) Dietary patterns, gastrointestinal complaints, and nutrition knowledge of recreational triathletes. *American Journal of Clinical Nutrition* **51**, 690–697.

Young, L.R. & Nestle, M. (1995) Portion sizes in dietary assessment: issues and policy implications. *Nutrition Reviews* **53**, 149–158.

Yuhas, J.A., Bolland, J.E. & Bolland, T.W. (1989) The impact of training, food type, gender, and container size on the estimation of food portion sizes. *Journal of the American Dietetic Association* **89**, 1473–1477.

PART 4

THE MASTERS ATHLETE

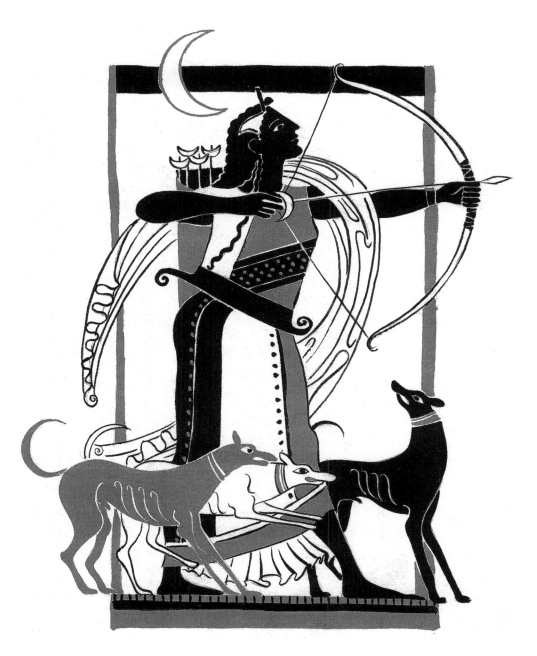

Chapter 9

Cardiorespiratory Function in Masters Athletes

CHRISTINE L. WELLS

Introduction

Sports performance varies with age. Inevitably, at some point following young adulthood, it begins a slow decline. To accommodate all competitors, many sports currently conduct both 'open' competition, in which competitors of any age may compete, and 'masters' competition, events designed for athletes who exceed the age requisite for success in open competition. The minimum age for masters competition varies from sport to sport, but usually reflects the age range at which world records are typically established. In swimming, for example, world records are typically held by very youthful competitors and the minimum age for masters competition is 19 years. In track and field events, world record holders are frequently in their twenties, and the minimum age for masters competition is 40 for men and 35 for women.

People engage in masters competition for numerous reasons. For some, it is a purely recreational activity in which fun and social contacts are the primary goal. For others, it is to maintain levels of fitness attained in youth or to improve their fitness level in order to benefit their health. For an élite few, masters events offer the same intensity of competition as open events, and the primary goal of these athletes is to achieve athletic excellence (Fig. 9.1). Before the 1970s, few women trained vigorously. Due to the relatively recent 'acceptance' of highly competitive sports for women, masters competition may offer the first opportunity many women

have had for challenging and intense athletic competition.

In this chapter, a masters woman athlete is defined as a woman over 30 years of age who enters competitive events for masters athletes at a high level of competence. The chapter describes cardiorespiratory determinants of performance in these women relative to the physiological processes of ageing.

Why study the female masters athlete?

The highly competent masters woman athlete represents an extremely small proportion of her age cohort. She represents 'the extreme end of a distribution that ranges from physical disability and dysfunction at one end to elite athletic accomplishments at the other' (Spirduso, 1995). At the very least, these athletes possess physical and physiological capabilities of value to the scientific understanding of ageing. Their accomplishments and abilities 'raise the ceiling' for everyone at a time when there is a transformation in our thinking about the physical limitations of older adults. And this is particularly true relative to athletic performance by masters *women*. Whereas outstanding physical achievement was previously unusual in women (or at least not recognized due to lack of opportunity and social acceptance), there has been little social or intellectual conceptualization of the physical competence and ability of women as a whole, and of middle-aged or elderly women in particu-

135

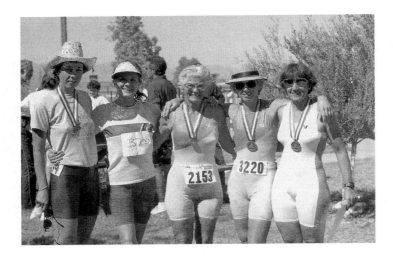

Fig. 9.1 Age-group winners at a duathlon (run–bike) and triathlon (swim–bike–run) event with Olympic distances (1500-m swim, 40-km bike ride and 10-km run).

lar. The outstanding athletic accomplishments of masters women athletes serve to remind us all that physical ability can be maintained, at remarkable levels, for a very long period of one's lifespan and that physical disability is not inevitable. Thus, the study of masters women athletes shatters 'the barriers of expectations' we currently have for the aged (Spirduso, 1995).

Cardiorespiratory determinants of performance

Numerous variables have been identified as important determinants of physical performance. Essentially, athletic performance is limited by the ability of metabolic processes to provide a continuous supply of adenosine triphosphate (ATP) to the contractile mechanisms of active muscle. This requires 'fuelling' by metabolic processes and removal of metabolic end-products to prevent or delay fatigue. These processes function in a highly integrated manner that is impossible to describe fully here. A central feature is an efficient oxygen transport system, characterized by a well-developed heart and vascular system coupled with a healthy lung and adequate blood volume. The performance of masters women athletes in relation to the ageing process is discussed in terms of the following variables:

1 maximum oxygen uptake ($\dot{V}O_{2max}$);
2 maximum cardiac output ($\dot{Q}_{max}$);
3 peripheral blood flow and arteriovenous oxygen (a-vO$_2$) difference;
4 skeletal muscle oxidative capacity;
5 oxygen-carrying capacity and blood volume;
6 pulmonary function;
7 lactate threshold;
8 heat tolerance.

There are very few published studies on masters women athletes. The results published appear to vary considerably with the performance capacity of the subjects studied (very few élite performers), as well as with the intensity and duration (in years) of training in these subjects. Because of this, much of my commentary is based on my general interpretation of the literature obtained from both moderately active and highly trained men *and* women. I will specifically highlight, where available, research published on women, especially masters women athletes. It is my hope that exercise scientists will soon act to fill in the gaps.

Maximum oxygen uptake

$\dot{V}O_{2max}$ is widely accepted as the best single measure of cardiorespiratory fitness and is often referred to as maximal aerobic power. This is due to the strong positive relationships between $\dot{V}O_{2max}$ and variables such as total work output and endurance capacity. $\dot{V}O_{2max}$ represents the upper limit of 'aerobic' performance. Humans can run at speeds that require 79–98% $\dot{V}O_{2max}$ during 10-km races and 68–88% $\dot{V}O_{2max}$ during much longer races (Farrell *et al.*, 1979).

In untrained women, peak values for $\dot{V}O_{2max}$ typically occur before age 20, but in trained athletes $\dot{V}O_{2max}$ continues to increase until age 25 or 30. Élite women athletes often have $\dot{V}O_{2max}$ values exceeding 60 ml·kg^{-1}·min^{-1}. The highest value reported for a woman was 77 ml·kg^{-1}·min^{-1} in a cross-country skier. Table 9.1 presents comparative $\dot{V}O_{2max}$ values for adult women reported by age and physical activity.

The women described in Table 9.1 are very diverse in physical activity. The sedentary women had no regular physical activity. The active women had much higher physical activity

Table 9.1 Comparative $\dot{V}O_{2max}$ values (ml·kg^{-1}·min^{-1}) for adult women reported by age and physical activity. (Adapted from Wells *et al.*, 1992)

Activity level	Age (years)							
	35	40	45	50	55	60	65	70
Sedentary women								
Profant *et al.* (1972)	28.3		25.7		24.5		18.7	
Drinkwater *et al.* (1975)	31.7		29.5		23.7			
Upton *et al.* (1984)	31.4							
Fleg & Lakatta (1988)	28.3		25.7		24.5			
Stevenson *et al.* (1994)					26.5			
Active women								
Profant *et al.* (1972)	31.8		29.0		25.8		27.1	
Drinkwater *et al.* (1975)	41.4		39.2		34.5			
Plowman *et al.* (1979)		33.9		30.4		27.9		
Masters athletes								
Wilmore & Brown (1974) (aged > 31 years)	58.8							
Vaccaro *et al.* (1981a) (swimmers)								37.6
Vaccaro *et al.* (1981b) (distance runners)		43.4						
Upton *et al.* (1984) (10-km runners)	48.5							
Upton *et al.* (1984) (marathon runners)	55.5							
Vaccaro *et al.* (1984) (non-highly trained swimmers)	30.3		27.5		26.0		21.9	
Vaccaro *et al.* (1984) (highly trained swimmers)	42.1		38.3		35.9		32.1	
Wells *et al.* (1992) (distance runners)	54.1	47.4	43.6	41.2	39.5			
Stevenson *et al.* (1994) (distance runners)					48.6			

energy expenditure, but activity was somewhat irregular in nature and did not follow a specific pattern. These women did not 'train' for athletic competition; they were merely physically active in a variety of recreational pursuits, such as hiking, backpacking, tennis and golf. The masters athletes, on the other hand, possessed not only highly active lifestyles but regularly 'trained' for competition and competed in masters events. Descriptions of the physical activity of the masters women athletes are described below.

The subjects in Wilmore and Brown's (1974) study were eight very lean women over the age of 31 years who were national and international-calibre distance runners training at high weekly mileage (not specified by the authors). The two 70-year-old swimmers in the study by Vaccaro et al. (1981a) were members of the 1980 All-American Masters Swimming Team. One, age 71, began training at age 65; the other, age 70, began training at age 67. Both held national age-group records at the time they were tested and were much leaner than typical women their age. The 10 national-calibre distance runners in the study by Vaccaro et al. (1981b) had an average age of 43.8 years and ran between 58 and 106 km·week[-1]. The 84 swimmers studied by Vaccaro et al. (1984) were divided into 'highly trained' and 'non-highly trained' groups. The highly trained swimmers swam a minimum of three times per week for at least 1 hour per session, covering a minimum of 1638 m (range 1638–2275 m). The non-highly trained swimmers swam a minimum of twice per week for at least 30 min per session, covering a minimum of 455 m (range 455–637 m). The $\dot{V}O_{2max}$ of the highly trained swimmers exceeded the non-highly trained swimmers by 30%. The nine middle-aged 10-km runners in the study by Upton et al. (1984) had an average age of 33.1 years and ran an average of 40 km·week[-1]. They had trained for about 3.5 years, and their best times for 10 km averaged 52 min 25 s. The 42 middle-aged marathon runners in the study by Upton et al. (1984) had been running for 5.6 years and averaged 74.2 km·week[-1]. Their mean age was 38.2

years and their average time for a marathon (42 km) was 3 hours 47 min. The 49 runners in the study by Wells et al. (1992) ranged in age from 35 to 70 years and had been training for 8.4 years. Many supplemented their training by swimming ($n=8$) or cycling ($n=18$). They currently were running about 42 km·week[-1] and competed at a high level in regional and local events. The 13 subjects in the study by Stevenson et al. (1994) had an average age of 54.8 years, had been training for 18 ± 2 years (range 10–40 years!) and were currently running 50 km·week[-1] including one or two speed/interval sessions, all at moderate altitude (Colorado, USA). They were consistent age-group winners in national-level competitions.

Performance begins to decline soon after the most frequent age at which open competition records are set. Athletic performance is a function of many factors, and may never be totally explained because there are simply too many confounding variables that remain uncontrolled, perhaps even unidentified. However, $\dot{V}O_{2max}$ is a major determinant of performance in sports with a substantial aerobic component, e.g. middle- and long-distance running, swimming, cycling, skating, cross-country skiing, rowing, etc.

The literature clearly indicates that, after reaching a peak value, $\dot{V}O_{2max}$ declines with advancing age, although the rate of decline and when that decline commences remains controversial. In general, cross-sectional studies suggest that $\dot{V}O_{2max}$ declines at the rate of about 9% per decade beginning at about age 30 in untrained men and women (Heath et al., 1981; Pollock et al., 1992). The rate of decline in data derived from longitudinal studies in men seems to be greater than that determined from cross-sectional studies. This is probably because subjects who volunteer for cross-sectional investigations tend to be more physically fit and disease-free than those who do not volunteer, and thus the subject sample is biased. However, in the most comprehensive review of this topic to date, Buskirk and Hodgson (1987) proclaim that longitudinal studies present a 'picture of inconsistency', with regression slopes of the decline in

$\dot{V}O_{2max}$ with age ranging from $1.04\,ml\cdot kg^{-1}\cdot min^{-1}$ per year to $0.04\,ml\cdot kg^{-1}\cdot min^{-1}$ per year in men. Two longitudinal studies have been completed in women. Astrand et al. (1973) reported a decline of $0.44\,ml\cdot kg^{-1}\cdot min^{-1}$ per year in Swedish physical education teachers aged 22–43 years and Plowman et al. (1979) reported a decline of $0.32\,ml\cdot kg^{-1}\cdot min^{-1}$ per year in nine 'active' women aged 30–49 years. The only cross-sectional study that has examined this question in masters women athletes reported a regression slope of $0.47\,ml\cdot kg^{-1}\cdot min^{-1}$ per year in women aged 35–70 years (Wells et al., 1992). There have been no longitudinal studies of the decline in $\dot{V}O_{2max}$ in masters women athletes.

Of major interest is whether or not the decline in $\dot{V}O_{2max}$ occurs irrespective of the amount of training that an individual undertakes. Some data (Kasch & Wallace, 1976; Heath et al., 1981; Pollock et al., 1987, 1992) suggest that if physical training and body composition are kept constant, deterioration due to ageing is substantially delayed or lessened for a period of about 10–20 years. However, the data are not consistent on this issue, and thus the question of whether a high level of physical training may delay or prevent some of the age-related decline in $\dot{V}O_{2max}$ remains unclear.

Undoubtedly, the suggestion that the physiological ageing process affects all systems, organs and functions equally is an oversimplification at best and misleading at worst. It is far more likely that different rates of decline prevail (whether best described as linear or curvilinear) due to variations in genetic endowment, physical training, body weight gain or loss, 'wear and tear' stress, and disease. Thus, a whole 'family of curves' (Buskirk & Hodgson, 1987) may be necessary to describe variance in $\dot{V}O_{2max}$ and other cardiorespiratory variables relative to age, physical activity level, gender and ethnicity. What is quite clear is that masters athletes, both men and women in their sixties and seventies and irrespective of their rate of decline, have $\dot{V}O_{2max}$ values equivalent to healthy, untrained men and women 20 or more years younger.

Joyner (1993) provides a compelling argument that $\dot{V}O_{2max}$ is limited by central factors that determine oxygen delivery to active cells. These factors include cardiac output (a product of heart rate and stroke volume), the haemoglobin concentration of the blood (a major determinant of oxygen-carrying capacity) and the ability of the lung to oxygenate the blood returned from peripheral tissues (active muscles and other organs). A number of changes have been documented in these variables with increasing age beyond 30 years.

Maximum cardiac output

It is likely that the reduction in $\dot{Q}_{max}$ occurs largely because of a decline in maximum heart rate with age. It appears that highly trained athletes experience a similar decline in maximal heart rate as sedentary people (maximum heart rate=220−age), although this has not been shown in all studies. The decrease in maximum heart rate is mostly mediated by a decrement in sympathetic nervous system reactivity (Pollock et al., 1992). With ageing, the heart and vasculature become less sensitive to β-adrenergic stimulation and thus the heart cannot achieve the maximum heart rate values achieved during youth (Spirduso, 1995). Maximum stroke volume decreases with age at a lesser rate than does maximum heart rate (Saltin, 1986). The Frank–Starling mechanism, in which initial stretching of a muscle fibre yields a more forceful contraction, apparently compensates for the age-related decline in maximum heart rate by causing the ejection of a larger volume of blood during systole following increased ventricular filling during the heart's relaxation phase (end-diastolic volume) during diastole (Spirduso, 1995). This means that healthy, fit older athletes can maintain a high cardiac output even in the face of a lesser increase in heart rate. Aerobic training is well known to increase end-diastolic heart volume and stroke volume even in older subjects. Differences in $\dot{V}O_{2max}$ between sedentary middle-aged men and trained middle-aged men were due almost entirely to a larger stroke volume in the trained subjects (Saltin, 1986).

There is no reason to believe this would be different in women.

Peripheral blood flow and arteriovenous oxygen difference

The ageing cardiovascular system is less able to redirect blood flow from inactive tissues (muscles, viscera, skin) to active tissues. This appears to occur largely because of a decreased number of β-receptors in smooth muscle of arterial walls and results in an imbalance between α- and β-adrenoreceptor function so that the peripheral vasculature leans toward vasoconstriction. Coupled with the increased stiffness of the vascular tree with age (Saltin, 1986), this increases peripheral resistance, decreases limb blood flow during exercise and increases blood pressure. During strenuous exercise, a decreased a-vO_2 difference results. Saltin's (1986) studies of young and middle-aged orienteers led him to conclude that the observed 30% difference in $\dot{V}O_{2max}$ was almost equally related to lower $\dot{Q}_{max}$ and systemic a-vO_2 difference in the older athletes.

Oxygen pulse is a function of stroke volume and a-vO_2 difference. The reduction in oxygen pulse (a measure of cardiorespiratory efficiency) during maximal work in ageing athletes is due to the decline in maximal stroke volume and a reduction in systemic oxygen extraction (a-vO_2 difference), with the latter contributing the most (Saltin, 1986).

Skeletal muscle oxidative capacity

Factors associated with a-vO_2 difference include skeletal muscle blood flow and skeletal muscle oxidative capacity. Cartee (1994) summarized research on old animals and humans and concluded that the evidence supported attenuated blood flow during contractile activity with increasing age. He also concluded that the level of physical training largely determined skeletal muscle oxidative capacity as revealed by enzymatic profiles of muscle biopsies. A few masters athletes train as intensively as younger athletes but, eventually, training intensity declines with age. This would indicate that the lesser training intensity of the masters athlete would eventually result in reduced oxidative capacity in skeletal muscle. These variables need further study, especially in women.

Oxygen-carrying capacity and blood volume

Oxygen-carrying capacity of arterial blood is largely determined by haemoglobin concentration. Daily exercise stimulates a more rapid rate of red blood cell development, and the number of red blood cells may be higher in older athletes than in their age-matched sedentary counterparts. However, in the absence of iron deficiency, the effects of increasing age on oxygen-carrying capacity are probably insignificant.

Endurance training is well known to enhance plasma volume. The net effect is that well-conditioned athletes usually have high blood volume. Nevertheless, pulmonary diffusing capacity for oxygen gradually declines in the elderly and there is a decrease in efficiency of alveolar–arterial gas exchange (Spirduso, 1995). This would result in decreased arterial oxygen saturation in older masters athletes.

Pulmonary function

With increasing age, many minor changes occur in the lung that additively contribute to a reduction in the volume of air that can be breathed per minute ($\dot{V}E$). These changes include degeneration of the elastin and collagen fibres that support alveoli, leading to an increase in the size of alveoli, loss of elastic recoil and, eventually, breakdown of alveolar walls (Jones, 1986). There is a gradual loss of small capillaries in the lung and an increase in resistance to flow through these vessels with age. These changes alter the distribution of blood through the lung and thus the ventilation–perfusion ratios. This most likely leads to higher pressures in the right ventricle and a higher systolic mean pulmonary artery pressure at rest and exercise in older compared with younger subjects.

There are also age-associated changes in the chest cage, including changes in the joints of the ribs where they attach to the vertebral column, changes in the cartilage joining the ribs to the sternum and a gradual loss of strength and metabolic capacity of the muscles of respiration (Jones, 1986). All of this contributes to a stiffening of the chest wall, an increase in the residual volume of the lung (air that cannot be expired) and a shift to the left in the pressure–volume characteristics of the lung. The main effect is an increase in the mechanical work of breathing that is largely expressed in an increased consciousness of respiratory effort or *sense of effort* in breathing during exercise. It is not known what the effect of an increased cost of breathing has on exercise economy–the relationship between a given exercise intensity and oxygen consumption (Joyner, 1993).

Training increases respiratory muscle strength at any age and thus high levels of physical activity may maintain the efficiency of the lungs at a high level for many years. Nevertheless, the older athlete will experience a greater degree of breathlessness or sense of respiratory effort than a similarly well-trained younger athlete. The increased breathlessness during exercise is real. Because $\dot{V}O_{2max}$ is lower, older athletes are exercising at a higher fractional utilization of $\dot{V}O_{2max}$ than younger athletes at a given power output and lactate accumulation may be higher. The resulting elevation in blood acidity results in a strong respiratory drive that, with accumulating years, may not be met adequately. The sensation of breathlessness results.

Lactate threshold

The point at which the rate of lactic acid production significantly exceeds lactic acid removal is called the blood lactate threshold. With ageing, lactic acid production typically declines due to a loss of muscle mass, specifically a disproportionate decrease in the size and number of glycolytic fast-twitch muscle fibres. This is usually accompanied by a gradual loss of strength (0.6–0.9% per year; Green, 1986). The rate of lactic acid

removal may also decline with age due to reductions in intramuscular blood flow. The slower clearing of lactic acid may explain age-related decreases in endurance.

The net effect of these age-related changes is that the onset of blood lactic acid usually occurs at a lower power output in older adults because their $\dot{V}O_{2max}$ has declined and thus older persons perform a given exercise task at a higher percentage of $\dot{V}O_{2max}$. Allen *et al.* (1985) have reported that the lactate threshold may occur at a higher percentage of $\dot{V}O_{2max}$ in older endurance athletes.

Long-term training of the anaerobic system may serve to maintain this metabolic system with advancing age. Reaburn and Mackinnon (1990) found no age-related deterioration in lactic acid accumulation in male masters athletes after a sprint swimming race. The 46–56-year-old swimmers, competitors in the 1988 World Masters Swimming Championships, did not differ from 25–35-year-old swimmers in producing or removing lactic acid. This needs to be confirmed in women masters athletes who are well trained at sprint running and swimming.

Heat tolerance

Heat tolerance is largely a function of cardiorespiratory fitness. If $\dot{V}O_{2max}$ declines, then tolerance to exercise performed in the heat also declines. Thus, heat tolerance or intolerance is largely associated with the decline in $\dot{V}O_{2max}$ with age. Many studies have shown a decrement in heat tolerance with ageing and thus old age is often associated with heat intolerance. Nevertheless, it remains unclear if this simply reflects a decline in cardiorespiratory fitness or is a real impairment of thermoregulatory function.

Women are known to sweat less than men and several studies have shown that older women sweat less than younger women (Shoenfeld *et al.*, 1978; Drinkwater & Horvath, 1979). Because sweating is the primary effector mechanism for dissipating heat during thermal stress, these results may be important in relation to age differences in endurance performance in warm climates.

Decline in physical training with age

Nearly every investigator of age-related decrements in performance or physiological function comments on the decline in habitual physical activity that inevitably seems to accompany ageing. It is clear that physiological functions such as $\dot{V}_{O_{2max}}$, $\dot{Q}_{max}$, $\dot{V}_{E_{max}}$ and maximum heart rate decline eventually irrespective of the amount of training that a masters athlete does, although it is not yet clear whether this inescapable decline is delayed or slowed by maintaining a high level of training. It appears that masters athletes eventually reduce their training intensity, even when they attempt not to do so. When queried, many comment that they currently train at a much slower pace/intensity than they did 10 or 20 years ago or that they have altered their training so that they do more long, slow, distance training and less interval or 'power' training than in their younger years. Many incorporate 'cross-training' into their daily routine in order to maintain their desired level of cardiorespiratory fitness while at the same time easing stress and strain on the musculoskeletal structures used in their primary sport. Many complain of various aches and pains, which they attribute to osteoarthritis from either earlier sports injuries or simply growing older.

It is difficult to distinguish between the effects of ageing and deconditioning when studying lifelong changes in physiological function and performance. Although the factors responsible for age-related decline are interrelated and very complex, decline is inevitable. Nevertheless, it is clear that prolonged intense training throughout life allows masters athletes to surpass the performance capabilities of a majority of the younger population.

Recommendations for future research

As mentioned above, nearly all research available on age-related changes in cardiorespiratory function has been conducted on men. What makes women biologically unique from men, of course, are the endocrine hormones of reproduction. The effects of cyclic oestrogen and progesterone on the cardiorespiratory system are not particularly well understood. Strenuous training in young women often results in menstrual dysfunction characterized by a shortened luteal phase, anovulation or oligomenorrhoea, all conditions distinguished by lowered levels of cyclic oestrogen and/or progesterone. In recent years, research has focused on understanding these issues and on the often consequent lowering of bone mineral density. Concurrent investigations should also be directed to the study of cardiorespiratory function in relation to changing hormonal environments in highly trained women.

Until very recently, most masters women athletes began serious training for competition relatively late in life. A recurring scenario in women that I have worked with is that they began exercising on a regular basis when a husband was diagnosed with heart disease. They began a walking programme to encourage their husbands and later took up jogging and then running or swimming. Upon discovering competition, their 'masters' career began. These women are studied in the exercise physiology laboratory after a few years of competitive training preceded by many years of a basically sedentary lifestyle.

Today, many girls have competitive sport experiences early in life. Some continue their competitive training throughout their lives, often switching to a different sport. Few of these women have yet been studied in the exercise physiology laboratory. What is most needed is a longitudinal study of these well-trained women as they experience menstruation, childbirth, the menopause, hormone replacement therapy and growing old. Such a study has never been attempted and would be difficult to complete for a wide variety of reasons. Nevertheless, lifetime cardiorespiratory function in women should be studied as a function of sports training and changing hormonal environment.

References

Allen, W.K., Seals, D.R., Hurley, B.F., Ehsani, A.A. & Hagberg, J.M. (1985) Lactate threshold and distance-running performance in young and older endurance athletes. *Journal of Applied Physiology* **58**, 1281–1284.

Astrand, I., Åstrand, P.-O., Hallback, I. & Kilbom, A. (1973) Reduction in maximal oxygen intake with age. *Journal of Applied Physiology* **35**, 649–654.

Buskirk, E.R. & Hodgson, J.L. (1987) Age and aerobic power: the rate of change in men and women. *Federation Proceedings* **46**, 1824–1829.

Cartee, G.D. (1994) Aging skeletal muscle: response to exercise. *Exercise and Sport Sciences Reviews* **22**, 91–120.

Drinkwater, B.L. & Horvath, S.M. (1979) Heat tolerance and aging. *Medicine and Science in Sports* **11**, 49–55.

Drinkwater, B.L., Horvath, S.M. & Wells, C.L. (1975) Aerobic power of females, ages 10–68. *Journal of Gerontology* **30**, 385–394.

Farrell, P.A., Wilmore, J.H., Coyle, E.F., Billing, J.E. & Costill, D.L. (1979) Plasma lactate accumulation and distance running performance. *Medicine and Science in Sports* **11**, 338–344.

Fleg, J.L. & Lakatta, E.G. (1988) Role of muscle loss in the age-associated reduction in $\dot{V}O_{2max}$. *Journal of Applied Physiology* **65**, 1147–1151.

Green, H.J. (1986) Characteristics of aging human skeletal muscle. In J.R. Sutton & R.M. Brock (eds) *Sports Medicine for the Mature Athlete*, pp. 17–26. Benchmark Press, Indianapolis.

Heath, G.W., Hagberg, J.M., Ehsani, A.A. & Holloszy, J.O. (1981) A physiological comparison of young and older endurance athletes. *Journal of Applied Physiology* **51**, 634–640.

Jones, N.L. (1986) The lung of the masters athlete. In J.R. Sutton & R.M. Brock (eds) *Sports Medicine for the Mature Athlete*, pp. 319–328. Benchmark Press, Indianapolis.

Joyner, M.J. (1993) Physiological limiting factors and distance running: influence of gender and age on record performances. *Exercise and Sport Sciences Reviews* **21**, 103–133.

Kasch, F. & Wallace, J. (1976) Physiological variables during 10 years of endurance exercise. *Medicine and Science in Sports* **8**, 5–8.

Plowman, S.A., Drinkwater, B.L. & Horvath, S.M. (1979) Age and aerobic power in women: a longitudinal study. *Journal of Gerontology* **34**, 512–520.

Pollock, M.L., Foster, C., Knapp, D., Rod, J.L. & Schmidt, D.H. (1987) Effect of age and training on aerobic capacity and body composition of master athletes. *Journal of Applied Physiology* **62**, 725–731.

Pollock, M.L., Lowenthal, D.T., Graves, J.E. & Carroll, J.F. (1992) The elderly and endurance training. In

R.J. Shephard & P.-O. Åstrand (eds) *Endurance in Sport*, pp. 390–406. Blackwell Scientific Publications, Oxford.

Profant, G.R., Early, R.G., Nilson, K.L., Fusumi, F., Hofer, V. & Bruce, R.A. (1972) Responses to maximal exercise in healthy middle-aged women. *Journal of Applied Physiology* **33**, 595–599.

Reaburn, P.R.J. & Mackinnon, L.T. (1990) Blood lactate responses in older swimmers during active and passive recovery following maximal sprint swimming. *European Journal of Applied Physiology* **61**, 246–250.

Saltin, B. (1986) The aging endurance athlete. In J.R. Sutton & R.M. Brock (eds) *Sports Medicine for the Mature Athlete*, pp. 59–80. Benchmark Press, Indianapolis.

Shoenfeld, Y., Udassin, R., Shapiro, Y., Ohri, A. & Sohar, E. (1978) Age and sex difference in response to short exposure to extreme dry heat. *Journal of Applied Physiology* **44**, 1–4.

Spirduso, W.W. (1995) *Physical Dimensions of Aging*. Human Kinetics Publishers, Champaign, Illinois.

Stevenson, E.T., Davy, K.P. & Seals, D.R. (1994) Maximal aerobic capacity and total blood volume in highly trained middle-aged and older female endurance athletes. *Journal of Applied Physiology* **77**, 1691–1696.

Upton, S.J., Hagan, R.D., Lease, B., Rosentswieg, J., Gettman, L.R. & Duncan, J.J. (1984) Comparative physiological profiles among young and middle-aged female distance runners. *Medicine and Science in Sports and Exercise* **16**, 67–71.

Vaccaro, P., Dummer, G.M. & Clarke, D.H. (1981a) Physiological characteristics of female masters swimmers. *Physician and Sportsmedicine* **9**(12), 75–78.

Vaccaro, P., Morris, A.F. & Clarke, D.H. (1981b) Physiological characteristics of masters female distance runners. *Physician and Sportsmedicine* **9**(7), 105–108.

Vaccaro, P., Ostrove, S.M., Vendervelden, L., Goldfarb, A.H. & Clarke, D.H. (1984) Body composition and physiological responses of masters female swimmers 20–79 years of age. *Research Quarterly for Exercise and Sport* **55**, 278–284.

Wells, C.L., Boorman, M.A. & Riggs, D.M. (1992) Effect of age and menopausal status on cardiorespiratory fitness in masters women runners. *Medicine and Science in Sports and Exercise* **24**, 1147–1154.

Wilmore, J.H. & Brown, C.H. (1974) Physiological profiles of women distance runners. *Medicine and Science in Sports* **6**, 178–181.

Chapter 10

Muscle Function in Masters Athletes

M. ELAINE CRESS

Introduction

Since the 1970s, individual sport has been more accessible to the general population and as a result the number of women regularly participating in sport has increased dramatically. This phenomenon has been called 'mass sport' (Okonek, 1996). In 1972 the USA enacted legislation to require equal opportunities for participation in sports for males and females in federally funded public schools and colleges (Women's Sports Foundation, 1997). Not only in the USA but internationally, competitive skilled women athletes are participating in sport in greater numbers (Dyer, 1989). Legal protection against discrimination in sport was provided for women in Canada in 1982 (Hoffman, 1989) and in Australia in 1984 (Dyer, 1989). As these women bring a greater level of skill and understanding of competition to masters sporting events, performance records are set at a rapid rate, with large increases in performance with each new record (Stefani, 1989). During the period 1990–2000, the first women who played competitive sports in school are qualifying for masters athlete status. The material in this chapter addresses muscle morphology, function and performance in relation to age specifically for women masters athletes.

An athlete is defined as a woman who trains regularly and participates in sport in either a competitive or non-competitive event (Drinkwater, 1984). Unless otherwise designated, in this chapter 'athlete' refers specifically to women. An élite athlete is a woman who ranks as a member of a national or international sports team (Drinkwater, 1984). The qualifying age for masters status varies from sport to sport. For the purposes of this chapter, a masters athlete is a woman competitor aged 35 years or older. 'Active' refers to a woman who engages in a structured exercise regimen of at least 30 min three times per week. 'Sedentary' refers to a woman who does not maintain a structured exercise programme at the level of an active woman. Unless otherwise stated, the data in this chapter were gathered specifically on women and address age effects related to women. In particular, this chapter focuses on women masters athletes and the muscle characteristics altered by age, training, disuse and type of sport. Due to the lack of research data on women masters athletes, data on sedentary and active women are used for comparison. The reader is referred to publications that compare and contrast muscle characteristics of men and women (Wells & Plowman, 1983; Wilmore, 1984; Buskirk & Hodgson, 1987; Wells, 1991).

Body composition

Body composition comprises body fat and fat-free mass, which includes skin, bone, internal organs and muscle mass (Going *et al.*, 1995). The balance of body fat to lean muscle mass shifts with age as the loss of lean mass is exacerbated by increased fat deposition. A cross-sectional comparison of sedentary women indicates that percentage body fat is higher in 50–60-year-old

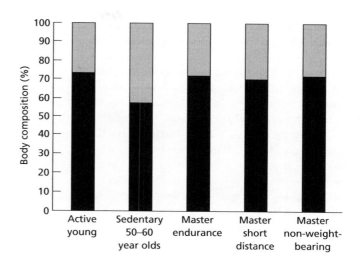

Fig. 10.1 Body composition: lean mass (■) and body fat (□). A comparison of body composition in several categories, including active young, sedentary sixth-decade and masters athletes from several sports (endurance, short distance and non-weight-bearing). (Adapted from Kavanagh & Shephard, 1990.)

women (42.1%) compared with women in their twenties (27.1%) and seventies (36.7%). The absolute quantity of body fat of masters athletes is similar to that of young active women and lower than that of sedentary 50–60-year-old women (Fig. 10.1). Cross-sectional data indicate that the percentage of body fat for masters athletes is relatively constant at about 28% between the ages of 35 and 75 (Kavanagh & Shephard, 1990) (Fig. 10.1). In masters athletes the percentage body fat varies by sport (Fig. 10.1). Athletes participating in weight-bearing endurance sports (e.g. long-distance track) have a lower percentage body fat (23.5%) than those participating in short-distance track (28.8%), racket sports (29.5%) or non-weight-bearing sports such as swimming or canoeing (26.9–28.6%) (Kavanagh & Shephard, 1990).

For the same age span, masters athletes have a lower rate of decline (7.5%) in lean muscle mass than the general population (25–30%) (Grimby & Saltin, 1983; Kavanagh & Shephard, 1990). Due to the small decline in muscle mass, masters athletes have a slightly higher proportion of body fat compared with young athletes (Proctor & Joyner, 1997). Thus masters athletes have a slower increase in body fat and preserve lean mass to a greater extent than the general population. In summary, with respect to body composi-

tion and ageing, masters athletes appear to have two principal advantages over the general population of older adults: (i) a lower rate of decline in lean muscle mass, and (ii) no significant increase in body fat with age.

Basic characteristics of muscle structure, function and capillarization

The basic characteristics of muscle structure and function are described in detail in *The Olympic Book of Sports Medicine* (Komi, 1988). The most important aspects of muscle structure, function and metabolism are provided here to facilitate the understanding of how ageing may affect muscle in athletes and non-athletes. Skeletal muscle is composed of individual muscle cells (fibres) arranged in bundles. Connective tissue, made up largely of collagen, surrounds each muscle and converges at the ends to form the tendon of origin and of insertion. Light microscopy is used to illuminate the striated (striped) appearance of muscle, which is due to the actin and myosin filaments, the primary contractile elements of muscle. Electron microscopy is used to illuminate the ultrastructure of muscle: the dark, anisotropic (A) bands are due to the overlap of the thick (myosin) and thin (actin) myofilaments; the isotropic (I) bands are less dense and therefore appear light. The I-band is divided by a Z-band, which forms the foundation for the molecular mechanism of muscle shortening. The Z-band shows some qualitative changes with age. However, the impact of these changes on muscle function is not well understood (Orlander *et al.*, 1978; Wang *et al.*, 1993).

Muscle fibre types are categorized according to their physiological, ultrastructural and metabolic characteristics (Komi, 1988). Type I (slow-oxidative) muscle fibres have a slow contractile velocity, low actomyosin adenosine triphosphatase (ATPase) activity and a **high mitochondrial** density that parallels the oxidative enzymes of the Krebs cycle and the electron transport chain. Type IIa (fast-oxidative) muscle fibres have a relatively fast contractile velocity, intermediate ATPase activity and mitochondrial density and metabolic characteristics similar to those of type I fibres. Type IIb (fast-glycolytic) muscle fibres have a fast contractile velocity, high ATPase activity, low mitochondrial density and oxidative metabolic characteristics, and high glycolytic metabolic capacity. In young individuals, type I fibres are about 20% smaller than type II fibres and have 15–20% greater blood supply (Rogers & Evans, 1993).

Sarcopenia

Sarcopenia has been defined as the reduction in lean muscle mass often associated with ageing (Evans, 1995). For a full account of the changes in muscle structure and function with age the reader is referred to several comprehensive review articles (Grimby & Saltin, 1983; Vandervoort *et al.*, 1983; Rogers & Evans, 1993). Ageing skeletal muscle undergoes a dramatic loss in mass, approximately 33%, between the ages of 25 and 75 (Grimby & Saltin, 1983). The decline in muscle mass occurs primarily via two mechanisms: (i) decrease in size of individual muscle fibres (atrophy) (Grimby & Saltin, 1983); and (ii) attrition (Lexell, 1995). Because fast-glycolytic fibres (types IIa and IIb) are more labile than slow-oxidative fibres, there is a selective decline in the former (Lexell, 1995). Fast-

glycolytic muscle fibres contribute to strength and speed; since these fibres diminish with age, speed and strength also decline. Women over the age of 60 have an accelerated decline in muscle mass, due in part to loss of fibre number (Sato *et al.*, 1984; Flynn *et al.*, 1989). Loss in fibre number is attributed to the denervation of fast muscle fibres and subsequent reinnervation by axonal nerve sprouting of slow motor neurones (Faulkner *et al.*, 1995). In addition to the loss of fibre number, comparisons of muscle groups in the vastus lateralis indicate a similar selective **diminution** in area with ageing (Lexell, 1995). Slow-twitch fibre cross-sectional area remains constant (3500–4300 μm^2), whereas absolute fast-glycolytic fibre area is reduced (from 3900 to 1500 μm^2). Figure 10.2 illustrates that a larger proportion of high-oxidative fibres (slow-twitch and fast-oxidative) occupy the muscle cross-sectional area of women in their sixties and seventies (Saltin *et al.*, 1977; Essen-Gustavsson & Borges, 1986; Cress *et al.*, 1991). Loss of myofibrillar protein has been identified as one mechanism for muscle atrophy in sedentary older women (Cress *et al.*, 1991, 1996). The shift towards slow-oxidative muscle fibres and the implications for performance are addressed later in the chapter.

Different muscle groups (upper body, lower body) are characterized by a different profile of fibre distribution. The upper body (biceps brachii) has a greater proportion of fast-twitch fibres, whereas the weight-bearing muscles of the lower body (vastus lateralis) have a greater proportion of slow-twitch fibres (Grimby, 1995). Unlike the lower body, no age-associated reduction in fast-twitch fibre cross-sectional area is found in biceps brachii of the general population (Grimby, 1995). This may be because women never have a large fast-twitch fibre cross-sectional area and therefore there is little to lose. An alternative explanation is that the upper body is called upon for short bursts of strength and power for such things as carrying groceries, children, briefcases, books or laundry; stimuli may remain relatively constant across the adult lifespan, accounting for the sustained cross-sectional area of fast-twitch fibres. To understand

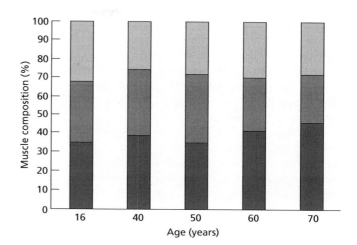

Fig. 10.2 Muscle composition: slow twitch (■), fast oxidative (▦) and fast glycolytic (▨). The percentage contribution of fibre cross-sectional area (μm^2) to total cross-sectional area (μm^2) in sedentary and active women by age is shown. (Adapted from Saltin *et al.*, 1977; Essen-Gustavsson & Borges, 1986; Cress *et al.*, 1991.)

more fully the effects of age, disuse and activity on upper-body muscle fibre morphology will require a longitudinal research study that includes muscle biopsy data.

Sarcopenia has several metabolic and functional consequences. People with hip fractures have a lower muscle and bone mass (Aniansson *et al.*, 1984). Lower muscle mass is associated with a lower resting metabolic rate (Rogers & Evans, 1993). Muscle mass is needed for minimizing the development, and maximizing control, of type 2 (adult-onset) diabetes, hypertension and cardiovascular disease (Roger & Evans, 1993). Adequate muscle mass is essential for physical activity, used as a means to maintain an appropriate level of body fat. Older women with low muscle mass are at risk of institutionalization in later life (Guralnik *et al.*, 1994).

Regular physical activity may prolong independence, maintain quality of life and delay the onset of disability to a time just before death, a phenomenon known as *compression of morbidity* (Fries, 1996). Scientific evidence has clearly demonstrated the ability to reverse the loss in lean muscle mass with age. Male athletes, particularly those that train for power lifting, have a higher muscle mass (Klitgaard *et al.*, 1990). Active adults have lower morbidity and lower risk of death from all causes (US Department of Health and Human Services, 1996). Active men

and women and male élite athletes have lower rates of health-care utilization (Kujala *et al.*, 1996; Buchner *et al.*, 1997).

Capillarization

Energy balance is maintained in part by the tight regulation between mitochondrial oxidative capacity and oxygen delivery via capillarization (Conley, 1994). The absolute number of capillaries is decreased with age, resulting in a decrease in blood flow to the working muscle (Coggan *et al.*, 1992a). However, due to the reduction of fibre size, the overall ratio of capillaries to fibres is not altered (Coggan *et al.*, 1992a). The ability of the muscle to replace the immediate energy stores (ATP) and remove muscle metabolites generated by muscle contraction decreases with age (Chick *et al.*, 1991). Capillarization and oxidative enzymatic activity is generally well maintained in the lower body of older adults; however, it can still be increased with endurance training, by as much as 20% (Coggan *et al.*, 1992a; Grimby, 1995). Insufficient data are available to report on the effect of resistive training on muscle blood flow in women. Muscle blood flow is one determinant of muscle enzymatic activity. In the absence of an adequate supply of oxygen, muscle is dependent upon glycolytic pathways of energy production (Schaufelberger *et al.*, 1997).

Glycolysis

Working muscle derives its energy from a balance between the glycolytic and aerobic pathways. The sympathetic system, important in stimulating glycolysis, is diminished in tandem with reduced fast skeletal muscle fibres (Fagius et al., 1996). Muscle enzymatic activity differs between muscle groups, particularly lower and upper body. Lactate production is blunted during submaximal activity in older compared with younger women (Chick et al., 1991). Male masters athletes with the same performance time for 10 km as young male athletes have a 46% lower activity of lactate dehydrogenase (enzyme of the glycolytic pathway) than their young counterparts (Coggan et al., 1990). Comprehensive and definitive studies on lactate production and utilization in masters and young women athletes could help us understand the effect of sport and training on the balance between the primary pathways of energy production. Yet from the evidence at hand it appears that the diminished ability to produce lactate may be due to a combination of decreased fast-glycolytic fibres and reduced sympathetic stimulation.

Cureton et al. (1988) has suggested that muscle-fibre attrition may be intrinsic whereas atrophy is behaviourally based. The data are clear that at older ages the muscle profile accommodates endurance activity, with a proportional shift toward slow-oxidative fibres and oxidative enzymatic composition. Although there are fewer data on athletes, these suggest that this pattern is consistent in both active and sedentary women (Cureton et al., 1988).

Muscle strength and muscle quality

Muscle force development (strength) is directly related to muscle mass. Muscle quality is the ability of muscle to generate force per unit of muscle mass (Saltin & Gollnick, 1983). Does the quality of muscle change with age? Is there a discrepancy between loss of strength (intrinsic muscle failure) and loss of muscle mass? When fully activated the force generated per square centimetre of muscle (specific force) is lower in old compared with young women (Phillips et al., 1992). Besides a lower specific force, lower strength in older women could be due to partial recruitment of all motor neurones, lower motivation to give a full effort or joint problems.

Isokinetic assessment of muscle strength can be attained at varying limb velocities. Velocities of $30–60°·s^{-1}$ are considered slow while velocities above $300°·s^{-1}$ are considered fast (Davies, 1984). Research studies suggest that the force–velocity relationship in muscle is altered with ageing. Muscle of older women has a lower neural capacity for generating as much force at faster speeds (Harries & Bassey, 1990). Increased time to peak tension and increased time to relaxation has been attributed to the reduced contribution of fast-twitch fibres to muscle performance. The age-related decline in power (force/time) is steeper than the decline in force because of the loss in velocity. Because of the inverse relationship between body fat and lean mass, power relative to body mass (power/body weight) is even more markedly reduced with age (Bassey & Short, 1990; Young & Skeleton, 1994). Older weaker individuals are also slower to develop force and therefore are not operating at the optimum position on the power–velocity curve (Bassey & Short, 1990). Older mice have a 20% decline in specific force and a 30% decline in power compared with that of young mice (Faulkner et al., 1995). Decreased leg power is closely associated ($r=0.83–0.93$) with declines in performance on mobility tasks (Bassey & Short, 1990; Bassey et al., 1992). The lower capacity to generate force and power is not explained by differences in dry-weight mass, extracellular components or intrinsic force-generating capacity of the muscle cross-bridges, excessive connective tissue or interstitial fat falsely elevating the area measurement (Young et al., 1984; Faulkner et al., 1995). By exclusion this suggests that the fault is with the neural stimulation or motivational aspect of performance. However, even highly motivated athletes exhibit performance deficits over time, suggesting that the decline in strength is more than just a reflection of less rigorous training or effort. Contraction-induced microdamage has been hypothesized as one explanation for the failure of well-trained muscle to generate the expected specific force (Faulkner et al., 1995).

Although most studies indicate that resistive training increases fat-free weight, not all studies are in agreement (Cureton et al., 1988). Progressive resistive training increases strength to a greater extent than muscle hypertrophy (Cureton et al., 1988). Increased muscle myofibrillar protein in older women is the underlying basis for increased muscle strength, which in turn is related to muscle performance (Cress et al., 1996). Sufficient studies are not available to address the influence of hormone replacement therapy, menopause, sport or cross-training on muscle strength and quality.

For optimal performance and to minimize injury, a balance of strength between the agonist and antagonist muscles is suggested (Wathen, 1994). In the thigh, it is recommended that the ratio of the strength of the quadriceps to that of the hamstring is 3:2, although this is not without controversy (Wathen, 1994). Women tend to show a more marked loss in concentric strength than eccentric strength with increasing age (Hurley, 1995). Ageing is associated with a disproportionate loss in strength of the knee flexors compared with that of the knee extensors, resulting in an imbalance in agonist and antagonist muscles (Cress et al., 1991; Stanley & Taylor, 1993). In sitting down and descending stairs, the primary action of the quadriceps is eccentric movement. In running or stair climbing, the primary action of the hamstrings is concentric movement (Joseph & Watson, 1967). Previously sedentary older women who train with endurance and stair climbing exhibit a greater gain in strength of the knee flexors compared with that of the knee extensors. The imbalance between the quadriceps and hamstrings may be a combination of intrinsic age-related changes within the muscle and added decline from infrequent use of the muscle in daily function. This imbalance in turn may result in a knee exten-

sor/flexor imbalance that may predispose a woman to injury or early functional decline (see the section Injuries in this chapter).

Muscle endurance and innervation

As described above, the decline in strength with ageing is accompanied by the selective loss of fast muscle fibres, which is more pronounced for fast-glycolytic than fast-oxidative fibres. The ability to sustain power during short bouts of repeated muscle contractions, such as that required for short-distance sprinting events, appears to decay with age (Gerard et al., 1986; Stones & Kozma, 1986). The preservation of endurance performance characteristics has been linked to the greater relative contribution of the slow-twitch fibre population to sustained performance (Harries & Bassey, 1990; Laforest et al., 1990). Long-distance running or rowing relies on the maintenance of an energy balance, which is largely dependent upon the capacity of the muscle to metabolize immediate energy stores (phosphocreatine) and the muscle's capacity for recovery via aerobic metabolism. The phosphocreatine/ATPase buffer system offers a simple feedback mechanism between energy supply and demand. The maximum power output that can be sustained in endurance activity in old mice is 69% of that which can be sustained in adult mice (Faulkner et al., 1990). Age-associated physiological changes seem to affect velocity to a greater extent at short distances than longer distances (Riegel, 1981). Comparing the endurance performance of masters and young athletes, the gap between the two ages is greater for sprint and short distances ($\leq 1500\,m$) that require power than for endurance events ($\geq 15\,km$) (Riegel, 1981).

Twitch and tetanic tension of the soleus and plantaris muscles decrease significantly with age (Klitgaard et al., 1989). In athletes, the slope of the decline in muscular endurance of the knee is more pronounced than that of plantar flexion when using body weight in a partial squat to generate resistance (Nakao et al., 1989). Sustained performance that involves large muscle contractions are similar in older and younger women. However, function in small muscle groups, such as that required for sit-ups and push-ups, deteriorates by as much as 60% (Shephard,1986). Although trained women have greater absolute strength and muscle endurance, the rate of fatigue is similar for the two groups (Huczel & Clark,1993).

In summary, the data suggest that reduced strength with age may result from factors in addition to decline in muscle mass. The loss of power with age is a function of decreased neural ability to generate muscle speed in addition to decreased muscle strength. Preservation of endurance performance is primarily due to the characteristics of slow-oxidative fibres.

Training effects on muscle

The shift in muscle fibre distribution towards greater oxidative potential has implications for performance. Chronic endurance training alters the morphological and metabolic characteristics of muscle. The mitochondria of masters athletes do not show any indication of impairment and respond to training in the same way as in young athletes (Coggan *et al.*, 1992b; Brierly *et al.*, 1997). In male masters athletes with similar 10-km performance times to young athletes, $\dot{V}_{O_{2max}}$ was 11% lower, oxidative enzyme activity was 31% higher and capillary–fibre ratio was greater in the masters athletes due to 34% larger slow-twitch fibres (Coggan *et al.*, 1990). Research is needed to evaluate the performance response of lactate in both young and masters athletes.

Resistive training of sufficient duration, intensity and progression results in metabolic, morphological and functional adaptations. Muscle fibre area, particularly of fast-glycolytic fibres, is increased with a concomitant increase in strength and functional performance (Cress *et al.*, 1991, 1996; Rogers & Evans, 1993). Female athletes aged 66–85 years exhibit a greater cross-sectional muscle area and less fat than their age-matched counterparts (Lexell, 1995). Fibre size is larger in athletes than non-athletes; however, whether this trait is due to a genetic

predisposition or to training is not fully understood. Preservation of muscle mass may occur via inhibition of the loss of muscle fibres, maintenance of individual muscle fibre area, or both (Kavanagh & Shephard, 1990). With proper technique, resistive training results in increases in fibre size whether or not one moves from sedentary to active or active to athlete (Kavanagh & Shephard, 1990). Increases in strength and endurance result in increased function in activities of independent living (Cress, 1997).

The distribution of fibre types is similar for women participating in the same sport (Wilmore, 1984). Endurance athletes have the greatest proportion of slow-twitch fibres followed by short-distance runners, with the lowest in power athletes (Wilmore, 1984). A sport that stimulates slow-twitch oxidative muscle augments the natural course of muscle change. Perhaps endurance masters athletes should engage in cross-training (strength and endurance) to counter the decline in strength with age. Studies in young individuals have suggested that resistive combined with endurance training is counter-productive for optimal performance in endurance athletes (Sale *et al.*, 1990). The impact of the combination of these two training modalities on muscle performance in older women needs further investigation.

Flexibility

Flexibility is the ability of muscle and other soft tissue to yield to a stretch force. Range of motion is the amount of motion allowed between any two bony levers. Muscle shortening alters the length–tension relationship of the muscle, decreasing the peak torque that can be generated, known as tight weakness (Gossman *et al.*, 1986). As discussed earlier, older women are not at the optimum on the force–velocity curve (Bassey & Short, 1990). The inability to generate force rapidly (decreased force–velocity) and tight weakness (decreased length–tension force) are both mechanisms of reduced force in older adults. Soft tissue responds to flexibility training (Bandy & Irion, 1994); however, understanding of the relationship of flexibility and strength and the impact on performance has not been adequately studied.

Sports performance

Records compiled and published as Masters Age Records are approved by the World Association of Veteran Athletes and the Masters Track and Field Records Sub-committee of USA Track and Field (Masters Age Records, 1996). Records are compiled by sex into 5-year categories, with most events beginning at age 35 and no upper age limit. The US National Senior Sports Classic was formed in 1985 to promote health and fitness and competition for athletes from 50 to as high as 100 years of age (US National Senior Sports Classic Web Site). Athletes qualify in their state games to compete at the US National Senior Sports Classic, which includes competition in 18 different sports.

As discussed in earlier sections on muscle characteristics and strength, performance data are mainly from cross-sectional studies. Cross-sectional data are used to predict the athletic performance for different age groups. In general, these predictions overestimate the performance in older age categories because only the most fit older subjects survive or are willing to provide data. However, many other cohort differences may elevate the scores of young compared with masters athletes, e.g. different nutritional, environmental and social exposure. From the mid-1970s to the mid-1980s physical training was characterized by marked philosophical changes in the intensity of training in both men and women, as well as changes in social acceptance of women's competition. With increased openness to competition in the younger age categories (<35 years), women's 10 000m and marathon times improved by about 15% (Joyner, 1993). Mass sport provided a venue for the non-élite athletes to compete. A study of German élite and mass sport athletes found that when using cross-sectional data there was an interaction effect between the cohort category, sports discipline and rate of decline. In longitudinal data, élite ath-

letes, having higher peak performance, show a greater decline than the mass sport athletes, whose lower peak performance shows a gentler and more linear decrease. In addition, the rate of decline is different for different disciplines (1500 m, 3000 m, broad jump) (Okonek, 1996). The following original dataset illustrates the interaction between cohort and performance. E.W. has finished first, second or third in her age-group category in the same 15-km race (River Run, Jacksonville, Florida) for the past 20 years (1978–97). These data are unusual in several ways: (i) data are from the same race course; (ii) E.W. ranked locally allowing for verification of time; (iii) E.W. kept excellent training log records; and (iv) 20 years of data are available. Figure 10.3 shows E.W. on a long training run.

In Fig. 10.4, the filled symbols indicate E.W.'s performance time for a given year as a percent-

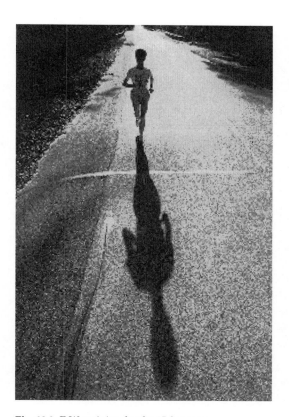

Fig. 10.3 E.W. training for the 15-km race.

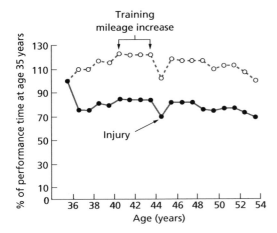

Fig. 10.4 Performance times for E.W. from age 35 to 54 years: ○, performance time for a given year as a percentage of her time at age 35; ●, performance time for a given year as a percentage of the winning time in the 35-year-old category for that same year.

age of her winning time at 35 years of age, 72.83 min or 4.86 min·km⁻¹, for the 15-km race. Her improved performance at age 40–42 coincides with an increase in training mileage by 16 km·week⁻¹ to 64–80 km·week⁻¹. The dip in training to 48–56 km·week⁻¹ and performance at age 43 were due to a hip injury. E.W.'s time improved throughout the 20 years of running, allowing her to exceed her 35-year-old performance, at times by as much as 18%. At age 54, both her training of 56–64 km·week⁻¹ and her race time were the same as at age 35. The 18% improvement in her performance time may be a measure of the improvements in the sport, training strategies, ergonomic aids, shoes and other unknown factors. When her performance is reported in the usual manner as a percentage of the winning time in the 35-year-old category for each year (triangles in Fig. 10.4), her performance dips as low as 70% of the younger athlete's time for the same race. The winner of the 35-year-old category was often an élite athlete of national rank brought in specifically to compete in the race. Depending upon the reporting method,

after 20 years of running E.W. shows a 30% (cross-sectional) or 0% (longitudinal) decline in performance. Performance records are generally surpassed by younger individuals and not by the same aged people, representing a 'sport gain' (Stefani, 1989). To attribute this difference to the effects of ageing is misleading.

When the performance of older athletes is reported relative to the world record performance, factors such as improved training, better nutrition, social attitudes and strategies in competition may all factor into the better performance of the young athlete. Yet this method of reporting attributes the difference to age-related effects. These data also illustrate how comparing people in different age categories can interact with longitudinal data to show different rates of change over the years, as in the cohort interaction effect in the cross-sectional analysis reported by Okonek (1996).

Injuries

The prevalence of athletic injuries was high for women in the late 1970s. This may have been related to the increased number of positions available for women athletes to fill (Hunter, 1988). Often collegiate women played multiple sports, e.g. volleyball, basketball and track. The competitive process screens out individuals who are not anatomically or physiologically suited for optimal performance in a given sport (Francis, 1988). Therefore, the stresses of performance unique to a given sport are the major determinants of injury for élite athletes rather than sex. Training specifically for the unique performance requirements plus general conditioning can reduce sport injuries (Hunter, 1988). However, several anatomical and physiological conditions result in specific injuries for which women are at greater risk (Baker, 1997). In the lower extremities these include bunions and injuries that result from poor knee alignment. Objective screening procedures to test flexibility, strength and gait have been used to address training strategies and prevent injuries in young athletes (Francis, 1988). Unless properly addressed early in the athletic career, a predisposition to injury may result in early retirement from sports. Women who begin their athletic careers later in life may not discover a predisposition to injury until they are in masters events. Participating in sporting events may challenge the anatomical and musculoskeletal system, which may not have otherwise been stressed in daily activities. Screening can provide the necessary direction for preventive conditioning through strengthening and stretching. For example, injuries may be prevented by maintaining an appropriate balance between the quadriceps and hamstrings, which are implicated in anterior cruciate ligament injuries (Baker, 1997). Preventive screening procedures can help direct a woman to the appropriate specialist for further evaluation, proper footwear or in-sole orthotic devices (Francis, 1988).

Effects of anabolic steroids and trophic factors

Natural steroids include testosterone, oestradiol and cortisol; methandienone (Dianabol) is a chemically derived steroid. The muscle-building or 'anabolic' effect of testosterone has been known for over 60 years (Hervy, 1982). The preponderance of evidence, particularly from animal models, is that anabolic steroids increase muscle mass; however, their effect on athletic performance is equivocal (Hervy, 1982). Supplementing the normal levels of these endogenous factors is banned by the International Olympic Committee (De Merode, 1988). As such, the benefits and deleterious side-effects of steroids in general use have not been systematically studied in randomized controlled trials. In spite of the lack of scientific research and a ban on their use, these substances are used widely, particularly in young male athletes (Bamberger & Yaeger, 1997).

Trophic factors include endogenous growth factors such as insulin-like growth factor I, insulin and growth hormone. With ageing there is a gradual reduction in growth hormone, testosterone and oestrogen levels that parallels the decline in muscle mass (Schwartz, 1995). Young growth-hormone-deficient patients have changes in muscle and body composition similar to those associated with the ageing process. These can be reversed with growth hormone replacement therapy (Schwartz, 1995). Preliminary evidence indicates that supplemental growth hormone can reverse the sarcopenia found in healthy older adults (Papadakis *et al.*, 1996), yet growth hormone supplementation has not been shown to enhance performance (Papadakis *et al.*, 1996). A multicentre research trial, funded by the US National Institute on Ageing, is currently underway to determine the ill-effects and efficacy of growth hormone therapy (National Centre for Research Resources Web Site).

The importance of oestrogen in the preservation of bone mass in postmenopausal women has been well established (Cauley *et al.*, 1995). It may also be useful in slowing the increased deposition of fat associated with the menopause (Schwartz, 1995). Oestrogen replacement therapy has been suggested as a method of prevention of loss of muscle mass and strength (Phillips *et al.*, 1993). However, no well-designed, randomized, controlled clinical trials have been published on this important intervention. The use of trophic factors as either a replacement for declining levels or a supplement for normal levels may become standard medical practice. If so, the line between therapeutic and athletic use of these 'muscle-enhancing' substances will be ambiguous.

Recommendations for future research

Studying the physical determinants of peak performance in masters athletes may help decipher some of the mechanisms that contribute to sarcopenia in older, diseased and/or sedentary adults. $\dot{V}_{O_{2max}}$, lactate production and metabolism, strength and economy of performance have been suggested as the primary determinants of performance (Joyner, 1993). Research is needed into the underlying mechanisms such as muscle ultrastructure and the neural and cardiovascular systems that contribute to optimal performance in masters athletes. Flexibility testing has been used to screen for risk of injury (Francis, 1988). Rehabilitation medicine uses flexibility to rehabilitate old injury and prevent new injury (Stanish *et al.*, 1990), yet because of the lack of research the contribution of flexibility training to performance and the prevention of injury is not understood.

Physical activity is an important factor in public health. Many male college athletes decrease their activity dramatically after their competitive career (Paffenbarger *et al.*, 1992). However, this same pattern may not be true for female alumni of collegiate sports. Is there less likelihood for a college athlete to become sedentary in communities in which mass sport is available? Competitive race events are scheduled year-round but they are most commonly held in the summer months. Participation by the community in sponsoring mass sport events provides the opportunity for people to participate in physical sport regardless of age, gender or physical ability. Mass sport gives the community a venue for promoting sport, fund-raising and community activism. It also provides the individual with an increased opportunity for competition outside the customary school setting. What impact will the changing attitudes towards competition have on the overall health of the community? Can competition provide older women with the motivation to train and preserve function? Can sport contribute to the compression of morbidity in a segment of the population with the greatest proportion of disabled individuals?

The opportunity to study women masters athletes comprehensively is dawning as the 'baby boomers', the children born after the Second World War, enter their fifties. World records plateau as athletes perform closer to their maximal physical ability (Joyner, 1993). Older adults have a great capacity for physiological plasticity and the social climate is moving towards acceptance of greater sport participation (Schulz & Curnow, 1988). Peak performance in masters athletes may become the arena for evaluating the potential of the human body in the older years.

Acknowledgements

I am grateful to Val Stewart for her contributions to this chapter. She gathered literature and more performance records than were possible to include, and offered her personal experiences, expertise and friendship during the writing of this chapter. I also want to thank Peter Mundle, National Masters News, and Jana Porter for sending performance records. Elfrieda B. Wyner is a lifetime athlete, dedicated historian and good friend whose devotion to her sport helped to further our understanding of performance over 20 years. I also thank Shannon Manuszewski for preparation of the manuscript.

References

Aniansson, A., Zetterberg, C., Hedberg, M. & Henriksson, K. (1984) Impaired muscle function with aging. A background factor in the incidence of fractures of the proximal end of the femur. *Clinical Orthopaedics and Related Research* **191**, 193–201.

Baker, C.L. (1997) Lower extremity problems in female athletes. *Journal of the Medical Association of Georgia* **86**, 193–196.

Bamberger, M. & Yaeger, D. (1997) Bigger, stronger, faster. *Sports Illustrated* 14 April, 62–70.

Bandy, W.D. & Irion, J.M. (1994) The effect of time on static stretch on the flexibility of the hamstring muscles. *Physical Therapy* **74**, 845–852.

Bassey, E.J. & Short, A.H. (1990) A new method of measuring power output in a single leg extension: feasibility, reliability and validity. *European Journal of Applied Physiology and Occupational Physiology* **60**, 385–390.

Bassey, E.J., Fiatarone, M.A., O'Neill, E.F., Kelly, M., Evans, W.J. & Lipsitz, L.A. (1992) Leg extensor power and functional performance in very old men and women. *Clinical Science* **82**, 321–327.

Brierly, E.J., Johnson, M.A., Bowman, A. *et al.* (1997) Mitochondrial function in muscle from elderly athletes. *Annals of Neurology* **41**, 114–116.

Buchner, D.M., Cress, M.E., de Lateur, B.J. *et al.* (1997) The effect of strength and endurance training on gait, balance, fall risk, and health services use in community-living older adults. *Journal of Gerontology* **52A**, M218–M224.

Buskirk, E.R. & Hodgson, J.L. (1987) Age and aerobic power: the rate of change in men and women. *Federation Proceedings* **46**, 1824–1828.

Cauley, J.A., Seeley, D.G., Ensrud, K., Ettenger, B., Black, D. & Cummings, S.R. (1995) Estrogen replacement therapy and fractures in older women. *Annals of Internal Medicine* **122**, 9–16.

Chick, T.W., Cagle, T.G., Vegas, F.A., Poliner, J.K. & Murata, G.H. (1991) The effects of aging on submaximal exercise performance and recovery. *Journal of Gerontology* **46**(1), B34–B38.

Coggan, A.R., Spina, R.J., King, D.S. *et al.* (1990) Histological and enzymatic characteristics of skeletal muscle in master athletes. *Journal of Applied Physiology* **68**, 1896–1901.

Coggan, A.R., Spina, R.J., King, D.S. *et al.* (1992a) Skeletal muscle adaptations to endurance training in 60–70-year-old men and women. *Journal of Applied Physiology* **72**, 1780–1786.

Coggan, A.R., Spina, R.J., King, D.S. *et al.* (1992b) Histochemical enzymatic comparison on the gastrocnemius muscle of young and elderly men and women. *Journal of Gerontology* **46B**, 71–76.

Conley, K.E. (1994) Cellular energetics during exercise. *Advances in Veterinary Science and Comparative Medicine* **38A**, 1–39.

Cress, M.E. (1997) Quantifying physical functional performance in older adults. *Muscle and Nerve* **77**, 1243–1250.

Cress, M.E., Thomas, D.P., Johnson, J. *et al.* (1991) Effect of training on $\dot{V}o_{2max}$, thigh strength, and muscle morphology in septuagenarian women. *Medicine and Science in Sports and Exercise* **23**, 752–758.

Cress, M.E., Conley, K.E., Balding, S.L., Hansen-Smith, F. & Konczak, J. (1996) Functional training: muscle structure, function, and performance in older women. *Journal of Orthopaedic and Sports Physical Therapy* **24**, 4–10.

Cureton, K.J., Collins, M.A., Hill, D. & McElhannon, F.M. Jr (1988) Muscle hypertrophy in men and women. *Medicine and Science in Sports and Exercise* **20**, 338–344.

Davies, G.J. (1984) *A Compendium of Isokinetics in Clinical Usage.* S & S Publishers, La Crosse, Wisconsin.

De Merode, P.A. (1988) The development, objectives and activities of the IOC Medical Commission. In A. Dirix, H.G. Knuttgen & K. Tittel (eds) *The Olympic Book of Sports Medicine*, pp. 3–6. Blackwell Scientific Publications, Oxford.

Drinkwater, B. (1984) Woman and exercise: physiological aspects. *Exercise and Sport Sciences Reviews* **12**, 21–51.

Dyer, K. (1989) Women's sport and the law: an intro-

duction. In K. Dyer (ed.) *Sportswoman Toward 2000.* Hyde Park Press, Richmond, Australia.

Essen-Gustavsson, B. & Borges, O. (1986) Histochemical and metabolic characteristics of human skeletal muscle in relation to age. *Acta Physiologica Scandinavica* **126**, 107–114.

Evans, W. (1995) What is sarcopenia? *Journal of Gerontology* **50A** (Suppl.), 5–8.

Fagius, J., Ellerfelt, K., Lithell, H. & Berne, C. (1996) Increase in muscle nerve sympathetic activity after glucose intake is blunted in the elderly. *Clinical Autonomic Research* **6**, 195–203.

Faulkner, J.A., Brooks, S.V. & Zebra, E. (1990) Skeletal muscle weakness and fat in old age: underlying mechanisms. *Annual Review of Gerontology and Geriatrics* **10**, 147–166.

Faulkner, J.A., Brooks, S.V. & Zebra, E. (1995) Muscle atrophy and weakness with aging: contraction-induced injury as an underlying mechanism. *Journal of Gerontology* **50A** (Suppl.), 124–129.

Flynn, M.A., Nolph, G.B., Baker, A.S., Martin, W.M. & Krause, G. (1989) Total body potassium in aging humans: a longitudinal study. *American Journal of Clinical Nutrition* **50**, 713–717.

Francis, P.R. (1988) Injury prevention through biomechanical screening: implications for female athletes. In J.L. Puhl, C.H. Brown & R.O. Voy (eds) *Sports Science Perspectives for Women*, pp. 97–100. Human Kinetics Publishers, Champaign, Illinois.

Fries, J.F. (1996) Physical activity, the compression of morbidity, and the health of the elderly. *Journal of the Royal Society of Medicine* **89**, 64–68.

Gerard, E.S., Vaccaro, P., Buckmeyer, P.J., Dummer, G.M. & Vander Velden, L. (1986) Skeletal muscle profiles among elite long, middle, and short distance swimmers. *American Journal of Sports Medicine* **14**, 77–82.

Going, S., Williams, D.P. & Lohman, T.G. (1995) Aging and body composition: biological changes and methodological issues. *Exercise and Sports Medicine Review* **23**, 411–458.

Gossman, M.R., Rose, S.J., Sahrmann, S.A. & Katholi, C.R. (1986) Length and circumference measurements in one-joint and multi-joint muscles in rabbits after immobilization. *Physical Therapy* **66**, 516–520.

Grimby, G. (1995) Muscle performance and structure in the elderly as studied cross-sectionally and longitudinally. *Journal of Gerontology* **50A** (special issue), 17–22.

Grimby, G. & Saltin, B. (1983) The aging muscle. *Clinical Physiology* **3**, 209–218.

Guralnik, J.M., Simonsick, E.M., Ferrucci, L. *et al.* (1994) A short physical performance battery assessing lower extremity function: association with self-reported disability and prediction of mortality and nursing home admission. *Journal of Gerontology* **49**, M85–M94.

Harries, U.J. & Bassey, E.J. (1990) Torque velocity relationships for the knee extensors in women in their 3rd to 7th decades. *European Journal of Applied Physiology and Occupational Physiology* **60**, 187–190.

Hervy, G.R. (1982) What are the effects of anabolic steroids? In B. Davies & G. Thomas (eds) *Science and Sporting Performance: Management or Manipulation*, pp. 120–136. Clarendon Press. Oxford.

Hoffman, A. (1989) Integrating sport: the Canadian experience. In K. Dyer (ed) *Sportswoman Toward 2000*, pp. 25–34. Hyde Park Press, Richmond, Australia.

Huczel, H.A. & Clarke, D.H. (1993) A comparison of strength and muscle endurance in strength trained and untrained women. In R. Shephard, J.A. Anderson, E.R. Eichner, F.J. George, J.R. Sutton & J.S. Torg (eds) *Yearbook of Sports Medicine*, pp. 349–350. Mosby, St Louis.

Hunter, L.Y. (1988) The frequency of injuries in women's sports. In J.L. Puhl, C.H. Brown & R.O. Voy (eds) *Sports Science Perspectives for Women*, pp. 49–58. Human Kinetics Publishers, Champaign, Illinois.

Hurley, B.F. (1995) Age, gender, and muscular strength. *Journal of Gerontology* **50A**, 41–44.

Joseph, J. & Watson, R. (1967) Telemetering electromyography of muscles used in walking up and down stairs. *Journal of Bone and Joint Surgery* **49B**, 774–780.

Joyner, M. (1993) Physiological factors and distance running. *Exercise and Sport Sciences Reviews* **21**, 103–133.

Kavanagh, T. & Shephard, R.J. (1990) Can regular sports participation slow the aging process? Data on masters athletes. *Physician and Sportsmedicine* **18**, 94–104.

Klitgaard, H., Marc, R., Brunet, A., Vanderwall, H. & Monod, H. (1989) Contractile properties of old rat muscles: effects of increased use. *Journal of Applied Physiology* **57**, 684–690.

Klitgaard, H., Mantoni, M., Schiaffino, S. *et al.* (1990) Function, morphology and protein expression of ageing skeletal muscle: a cross-sectional study of elderly men with different training backgrounds. *Acta Physiologica Scandinavica* **140**, 41–54.

Komi, P.V. (1988) The musculoskeletal system. In A. Dirix, H.G. Knuttgen & K. Tittle (eds) *The Olympic Book of Sports Medicine*, pp. 15–39. Blackwell Scientific Publications, Oxford.

Kujala, U.M., Sarna, S., Kaprio, J. & Koskenvuo, M. (1996) Hospital care in later life among former world-class Finnish athletes. *Journal of the American Medical Association* **276**, 216–220.

Laforest, S., St Pierre, D.M., Cyr, J. & Gayton, D. (1990) Effects of age and regular exercise on muscular strength and endurance. *European Journal of Applied Physiology and Occupational Physiology* **60**, 104–111.

Lexell, J. (1995) Human aging, muscle mass, and fiber type composition. *Journal of Gerontology* **50A** (special issue), 11–16.

Masters Age Records (1996) National Masters News, PO Box 16597, North Hollywood, CA 91615-6597, USA.

Nakao, M., Ihoue, Y. & Murakami, H. (1989) Aging process of leg muscular endurance in males and females. *European Journal of Applied Physiology and Occupational Physiology* **59**, 209–214.

National Center for Research Resources, Computer Retrieval of Information on Scientific United States Public Health Service (US-PHS) Web Site. http://www.ncrr.nih.gov/grants/crisp.htm

Okonek, C.C. (1996) Langsschnittanalysen zur sportlichen Leistungsentwicklung von Frauen im alter zwischen 30 und 75 Jahren: ein Vergileich zwischen dem Spitzen und dem Breitensportniveau. *Zeitschrift für Gerontologie und Geriatrie* **29**, 127–135.

Orlander, J., Kiessling, K.H., Larsson, L., Karlsson, J. & Aniansson, A. (1978) Skeletal muscle metabolism and ultrastructure in relation to age in sedentary men. *Acta Physiologica Scandinavica* **104**, 249–261.

Paffenbarger, R.S., Lee, I. & Wing, A.L. (1992) The influence of physical activity on the incidence of site-specific cancers in college alumni. *Advances in Experimental Medicine and Biology* **322**, 7–15.

Papadakis, M.A., Grady, D., Black, D. *et al.* (1996) Growth hormone replacement in healthy older men improves body composition but not functional ability. *Annals of Internal Medicine* **124**, 708–716.

Phillips, S.K., Bruce, S.A., Newton, D. & Woledge, R.C. (1992) The weakness of old age is not due to failure of muscle activation. *Journal of Gerontology* **47**, M45–M49.

Phillips, S.K., Rook, K.M., Siddle, N.C., Bruce, S.A. & Woledge, R.C. (1993) Muscle weakness in women occurs at an earlier age than in men, but strength is preserved by hormone replacement therapy. *Clinical Science* **84**, 95–98.

Proctor, D. & Joyner, M. (1997) Skeletal muscle mass and the reduction of $\dot{V}O_{2max}$ in trained older subjects. *Journal of Applied Physiology* **82**, 1411–1415.

Riegel, P.S. (1981) Athletic records and human endurance. *American Scientist* **69**, 285–290.

Rogers, M.A. & Evans, W.J. (1993) Changes in skeletal muscle with aging: effects of exercise training. *Exercise and Sport Sciences Reviews* **21**, 63–102.

Sale, D.G., MacDougall, J.D., Jacobs, I. & Garner, S. (1990) Interaction between concurrent strength and endurance training. *Journal of Applied Physiology* **68**, 260–270.

Saltin, B. & Gollnick, P.D. (1983) Skeletal muscle adaptability: significance for metabolism and performance. In L.D. Peachy, R.H. Adrian & S.R. Geiger (eds) *Handbook of Physiology, Section 10*, pp. 555–631. Williams & Wilkins, Baltimore.

Saltin, B., Henriksson, J., Nygaard, E., Anderson, P. & Jansson, E. (1977) Part I. Metabolism in prolonged exercise. Fiber types and metabolic potentials of skeletal muscles in sedentary man and endurance runners. *Annals of the New York Academy of Sciences* **301**, 3–29.

Sato, I., Akatsuka, H., Kito, K., Tokoro, Y. & Tauchi, H. (1984) Age changes in size and number of muscle fibers in human minor pectoral muscle. *Mechanisms of Ageing and Development* **28**, 99–109.

Schaufelberger, M., Eriksson, B.O., Grimby, G., Held, P. & Swedberg, K. (1997) Skeletal muscle alterations in patients with chronic heart failure. *European Heart Journal* **18**, 971–980.

Schulz, R. & Curnow, C. (1988) Peak performance and age among superathletes: track and field, swimming, baseball, tennis, and golf. *Journal of Gerontology* **43**, 113–120.

Schwartz, R.S. (1995) Trophic factor supplementation: effects on age-associated changes in body composition. *Journal of Gerontology* **50A** (Suppl.), 151–156.

Shephard, R. (1986) Physiological aspects of sport and physical activity in the middle and later years of life. In B.D. McPherson (ed.) *Sport and Aging*, pp. 221–232. Human Kinetics Publishers, Champaign, Illinois.

Stanish, W.D., Curwin, S.L. & Bryson, G. (1990) The use of flexibility exercises in preventing and treating sports injuries. In W.B. Leadbetter, J.A. Buckwalter & G.L. Gordon (eds) *Sports-induced Inflammation*, pp. 731–745. American Academy of Orthopedic Surgeons, Park Ridge, Illinois.

Stanley, S.N. & Taylor, N.A.S. (1993) Isokinematic muscle mechanics in four groups of women of increasing age. In R. Shephard, J.A. Anderson, B.L. Drinkwater, E.R. Eichner, F.J. George & J.S. Torg (eds) *Yearbook of Sports Medicine*, pp. 264–265. Mosby, St Louis.

Stefani, R.T. (1989) Olympic winning performances: trends and predictions (1952–1992). *Olympic Review* **258**, 157–161.

Stones, M.J. & Kozma, A.C. (1986) Age by distance effects in running and swimming records: a note on methodology. *Experimental Aging Research* **12**, 203–206.

US Department of Health and Human Services (1996) *Physical Activity and Health: A Report of the Surgeon General*. US Department of Health and Human Services, Centers for Disease Control and Prevention, National Center for Chronic Disease Prevention and Health Promotion, Atlanta.

US National Senior Sports Classic Web Site. http://www.fepblue.org/special4.html

Vandervoort, A.A., Hayes, K.C. & Belanger, A.Y. (1983) Strength and endurance of skeletal muscle in the elderly. *Physiotherapy Canada* **8**, 67–73.

Wang, N., Hikida, R.S., Staron, R.S. & Simoneau, J.A. (1993) Muscle fiber types of women after resistance training: quantitative ultrastructure and enzyme activity. *Pflugers Archiv. European Journal of Physiology* **424**, 494–502.

Wathen, D. (1994) Muscle balance. In T.R. Baeckle (ed.) *Essentials of Training and Conditioning*, pp. 424–430. Human Kinetics Publishers, Champaign, Illinois.

Wells, C.L. (1991) *Women Sport and Performance*. Human Kinetics Publishers, Champaign, Illinois.

Wells, C.L. & Plowman, S.A. (1983) Sexual differences in athletic performance: biological or behavioral? *Physician and Sportsmedicine* **11**, 52–63.

Wilmore, J.H. (1984) Morphologic and physiologic differences between men and women relevant to exercise. *International Journal of Sports Medicine* **5** (Suppl.), 193–194.

Women's Sports Foundation Web Site. Women's sports facts 1997. http//www.lifetimetv.com/WoSport/TOPICS/titleIX/descrip.htm

Young, A. & Skeleton, D.A. (1994) Applied physiology of strength and power in older age. *International Journal of Sports Medicine* **15**, 149–151.

Young, A., Stokes, M. & Crowe, M. (1984) Size and strength of the quadriceps muscles of old and young women. *European Journal of Clinical Investigation* **14**, 282–287.

Chapter 11

Hormone Replacement Therapy

WENDY M. EY

Introduction

Competitive sport for older women is a relatively new phenomenon. While large numbers of older men and women have been participating in activities such as lawn bowls and golf for many years, their endeavours in other forms of competitive sport such as athletics, swimming and cycling have not been taken seriously. Although there have been national and international competitions for veteran athletes and masters swimmers, there has been little interest outside those who were directly involved. During the past 10 years, however, there has been a dramatic change in the acknowledgement of competitive sport for older people. Since 1985, when the first multisport World Masters Games was held in Toronto, we have witnessed the rapid growth of organized competitive structures in many sports for those who wish to continue or resume their competitive sport at an older age level. For those who have joined the ranks and become committed athletes there is often a time of frustration when they seek advice or assistance from experts in sports science, sports medicine or sports psychology. Until now there has been very little interest in athletes of this age group by health professionals and as a result almost no research undertaken.

The focus of this chapter is on the female athlete who has reached the stage of life we know as the menopause. This is the time when a significant drop in women's athletic performance occurs. For example, the world record for the 100 m drops by 3.1% in women aged 45 and by 5.1% in women aged 50 and 55 compared with a drop of 1.7% and 3.4% in men of the same age (Table 11.1). The reasons for a general drop in performance can of course be attributed to the ageing process. However, this does not explain the relative difference between men and women. It could be hypothesized that it is due to the impact of the menopause and the changing hormonal status.

Menopause

The last menstrual period for most women occurs between the ages of 48 and 53 years but can happen quite normally five or so years earlier or later than this (Farrell & Westmore, 1993). There are some women who experience an earlier menopause and others who are menopausal through medical intervention, e.g. the surgical removal of the ovaries. The reduction in circulating levels of oestrogen, progesterone and testosterone may be followed by a number of physical and emotional symptoms, such as hot flushes, night sweats, vaginal dryness, depression and mood changes, irritability and forgetfulness, fatigue and loss of strength.

There is convincing evidence that the ovaries continue to play an important role after the menopause because they can still produce small quantities of oestrogen and testosterone for about 12 years. As the ovaries normally are a more potent source of testosterone than the

Table 11.1 Comparison of male and female records in the 100 m event for competitors aged 45, 50 and 55 years

Age	Male	Female
45 years	11.0 s	12.5 s
50 years	11.2 s	12.9 s
55 years	11.6 s	13.6 s

adrenal glands, this continued function, albeit small, will be of particular importance to the sportswoman in maintaining energy levels and muscle strength. In addition, the loss of oestrogen reduces the stimulation of sex hormone-binding globulin (SHBG) in the liver that controls the availability of circulating testosterone. This increases the availability of the testosterone produced from the solid substance of the ovary and the adrenal glands. The production of ovarian testosterone is related to the size of the ovary; as the ovary shrivels, the production of testosterone gradually reduces until it becomes minimal in established menopause, although it continues to be produced by the adrenal glands. If the ovaries are removed, there is not only an abrupt loss of oestrogen but a total loss of testosterone secretion (Jones, 1994). Also, small amounts of oestrogen continue to be produced in the adipose tissue. Heavier women with more fatty tissue have higher total levels of oestrogen than thin women; therefore there is no benefit in being underweight as women pass through the menopausal years (Cabot, 1991; Farrell & Westmore, 1993). As most athletic women are not overweight, they are at greater risk of oestrogen deficiency and the associated symptoms.

After the menopause a woman's total oestrogen production can decrease by 70–80% and androgen production from the ovaries and adrenal glands by as much as 50% and by a further 30% if the ovaries are removed. The current developments and interest in hormone replacement therapy (HRT) have heightened women's awareness of the menopause and alerted women athletes to the potential for better performance. Is it possible that by returning hormonal levels to their premenopausal status that the level of athletic performance can be maintained? A search of the literature reveals that this is an area that has not been investigated. For those women who experience some of the unpleasant symptoms of menopause, the relief resulting from HRT should mean that they will feel better and therefore be more likely to train harder and thus produce better performances. Whether the changed hormonal status *per se* will lead to better performance is another matter.

The implications of HRT for the drug-testing programme are also relevant. The inclusion of androgens in HRT is not routine; however, it is recommended by some physicians in particular circumstances, such as for sexual dysfunction, fatigue and after oophorectomy. There are also some forms of progestogens that have been prepared from androgens. Women athletes who have a legitimate need for these drugs should not be deprived of them simply because of the application of drug-testing rules that have been designed for young athletes in open competition. Variations in the rules need to be made to allow for postmenopausal women taking HRT when drug testing becomes mandatory.

Oestrogen therapy

In the untreated menopause, the ovary continues to produce some testosterone as a result of pituitary hormone stimulation. With the introduction of oestrogen replacement therapy this pituitary hormone is suppressed, which causes a synchronous loss of the production of testosterone from the ovary. The administered oestrogen also increases levels of SHBG and thereby any testosterone that may be produced is largely inactivated. Before the introduction of oestrogen replacement the woman's testosterone level may be quite high or normal, but after the instigation of oestrogen replacement testosterone availability usually falls to zero. This loss of testosterone may be more pronounced in women taking oestrogen by mouth because of enhanced liver stimulation of the binding protein (Jones, 1994). While it could be assumed that a greater availability of testosterone would be an advantage for women athletes, there is no research to demonstrate that this adverse effect of oestrogen replacement on ovarian testosterone production is detrimental to performance.

Oral oestrogens

Studies carried out on the effectiveness of oral oestrogens have indicated that this form of HRT can produce unstable levels of oestrogen, i.e. high concentrations of oestrogen, predominantly oestrone, appear in the systemic circulation within hours of ingestion after which concentrations rapidly decline (Studd & Smith, 1993). In view of these findings sportswomen may find it more beneficial to take oral oestrogens at 12-hour intervals in order to maintain adequate blood levels of oestrogen over a 24-hour period.

Oestrogen patch

Smaller doses of oestrogen can be used in the patch and are far less likely to produce side-effects due to metabolic changes in the liver. The small and relatively constant dose of hormone released from the patch more closely resembles the oestrogen secretions of the body than hormones taken orally, although oestradiol levels may still vary by more than 150% during the 3–4 day lifetime of a single patch.

Although the patch is reported to be waterproof and therefore should remain in place during bathing or showering, some women report that the patch does fall off in water. It may be advisable for sportswomen involved in aquatic activities to remove the patch prior to bathing, apply it to the backing membrane that comes with the patch and reapply it after bathing when the skin is cool and quite dry. Heavily chlorinated water and very hot water may also affect the patch. Women involved in strenuous physi-

cal activity during the summer months may find that perspiration affects the adhesive power of the patch and that body heat may cause a skin irritation.

Sportswomen should also be aware that the site of the patch may affect the rate of hormone absorption into the system, i.e. during intensive exercise expanding blood vessels under the skin increase the rate of absorption. If a patch is placed on a part of the body that is moved frequently, such as the upper arm, the body absorbs the hormone faster than if the patch is attached to the abdomen (Farrell & Westmore, 1993). Women involved in running activities or aerobics may need to consider applying the patch to the buttock or to the upper arm or removing the patch prior to exercise.

Oestrogen implant

The oestrogen implant consists of small pellets of pure crystalline oestradiol and is available in varying strengths to suit individual needs, e.g. 20, 50 or 100 mg. Depending on the strength of the implant it can release oestrogen directly into the bloodstream over a period of 4–12 months. The oestrogen pellet is usually inserted into the fatty tissue of the lower abdomen, buttock or upper thigh under a local anaesthetic. Sportswomen should be mindful of the fact that training may be disrupted for up to 2 days after the insertion of the pellet in order to allow the incision to heal and the implant to settle. According to Farrell and Westmore (1993) the amount of hormone absorbed from the implant varies according to:

- how long it has been in place;
- its position (e.g. in a swimmer more hormone is absorbed if the implant is in the upper arm than if it is placed in the buttock);
- its depth under the skin (the deeper the implant, the greater the absorption);
- physical activity levels (exercise increases blood flow);
- the presence of inflammation or scar tissue around the implant.

The sportswoman who is involved in an intensive training programme that includes regular, deep tissue massage should avoid an implant near a major muscle group. It should be noted that implants can continue to release small amounts of oestrogen for some time after the expected expiration date and it is therefore unwise to discontinue progestogen therapy in those women with an intact uterus for 1–3 years after the last implant is inserted.

Progestins

Progestins differ in the potency of their oestrogenic and androgenic properties and any adverse effects vary with the type of therapy and the dose used. Some women cannot tolerate the progestogen component of HRT and experience side-effects not unlike those of the premenstrual syndrome, e.g. breast tenderness, fluid retention, bloating, backache, abdominal cramps, breakthrough bleeding, mood swings and depression. The sportswoman who finds that any of these symptoms are disruptive to training and competition may find that a progestogen with androgenic properties may have less side-effects.

Androgen therapy

While the current method for treating the menopause with oestrogen and progesterone is widely accepted, there is growing awareness of the significant role of testosterone in the total treatment of some women who have not responded to normal hormone therapies. Despite this, there are still many medical practitioners who doubt the validity of this therapy. However, many specialists in this field do not have any doubts but this standpoint has not always been conveyed to general practitioners. Athletes and coaches should be prepared to seek specialist advice at the highest level.

There is a mistaken view that testosterone is exclusively a male hormone and therefore should not be given to women. Testosterone is secreted by both males and females but obviously at lower levels in the female. While only a small amount is produced in the female, this is of considerable importance to good physiological functioning (Jones, 1994). Barbara Sherwin from McGill University in Montreal, Canada, in an address to the North American Menopause Society in 1992, reported that testosterone had profound effects on several female functions, a fact that has been largely ignored:

> We replaced oestrogen because we always knew what that did, and we totally ignored the fact that one-third of all circulating testosterone in a woman's body comes from the ovary. No one's ever asked what testosterone does in a woman before!

Sherwin (1988) found that when women were given oestrogen plus androgen (testosterone) subsequent to surgical menopause, they reported increased energy levels and feelings of well-being. They also reported fewer bouts of depression, mood swings, irritability and crying than in women who received oestrogen alone. Henry Burger, from Prince Henry's Institute of Medical Research (Melbourne, Australia), supports the therapeutic use of testosterone as part of HRT for postmenopausal women, particularly those who have not responded adequately to oestrogen replacement alone (Burger et al., 1984, 1987).

Effect on sports performance

World records in 5-year age groups, starting from age 35, have been established over a period of 22 years since the first World Veterans Championships were conducted. During that time there has been a dramatic refining of performances to the point now where they are 'tough' records and infrequently reached. Therefore, the relative difference between men and women is well established and unlikely to change markedly (Fig. 11.1). In the 100-m race, in the youngest age group (35 years), the difference between men and women is 0.79 s; this difference increases to 2.51 s at 70 years; at the time of the menopause a noticeable drop of 0.70 s occurs in the women, almost double that seen in the men (0.37 s).

In the absence of any data on athletic performance and HRT that includes an androgen, the following case study is presented as an example of an athlete dealing with surgical menopause and the impact on performance. The athlete received both oestrogen and androgen therapy because of surgical menopause associated with cancer and demonstrated a hormonal profile consistent with the literature (Fig. 11.2). Figure 11.3 shows hormone levels plotted against performance and demonstrates that the best performances occurred when both testosterone and oestradiol levels were high, i.e. at the upper end of the normal range and certainly higher than without the implants. Figure 11.4 illustrates the change in performance as a result of HRT and supports the theory that returning hormone levels to premenopausal values reduces the dramatic drop in performance that occurs around menopause.

There are many 'older women' who take their competitive sport seriously and train as hard as younger athletes. These women and their coaches are keen to obtain information relating to their training and performances and how to reach their full potential. While many of the principles of coaching apply to all athletes regardless of age, there are specific issues relating to the postmenopausal woman. To determine how physiological changes following the menopause affect individual performance a specific training diary (Daly & Ey, 1993) was devised (Fig. 11.5). This diary, which can be used both by women who have elected not to use HRT and those who have, was developed for the daily recording of physical activities alongside a measure of body weight, temperature, heart rate and menopausal symptoms (recorded by the usual method, i.e. 0 indicates no problem, 1 mild problems, 2 moderate problems and 3 severe problems). At the end of each month a graph can be drawn where the fluctuations in performance are compared with the menopausal symptoms and physiological measures. The athlete and coach can then make appropriate adjustments to the training and competition programmes and seek medical assistance if the hormonal fluctuations are of concern. The athlete should be encouraged not to emphasize the negative aspects of the hormonal fluctuations and, by recording the positive times, should be able to determine the 'strongest' days each month. Athletes who have used this diary

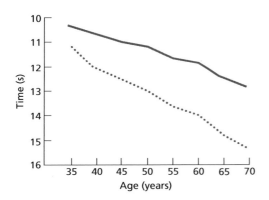

Fig. 11.1 Comparison of male (—) and female (····) world 100-m veteran records for competitors aged 35–70 years.

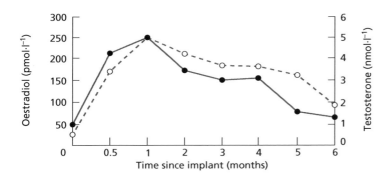

Fig. 11.2 Hormone profile following oestradiol (○) and testosterone (●) implants of 50 and 100 mg, respectively. (From Thom *et al.*, 1981 with permission.)

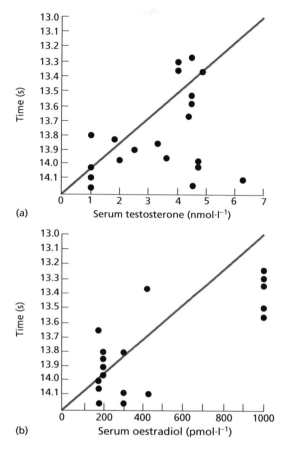

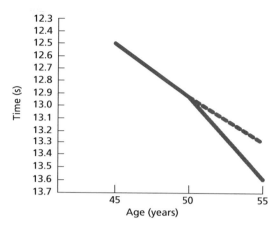

Fig. 11.4 Effect of oestrogen/androgen therapy on 100-m sprint times for veteran women. —, current records; ---, androgen therapy.

Fig. 11.3 (a) Relationship between serum testosterone concentration and 100-m sprint times in a 55-year-old menopausal athlete. (b) Relationship between serum oestradiol concentration and 100-m sprint times in a 55-year-old menopausal athlete.

have found it to be most helpful in identifying the relationship between their hormone levels and athletic performance. It has enabled them to adjust their HRT and ensure optimum levels for athletic performance.

At this stage, there is a paucity of reliable information on the impact of HRT on athletic performance. There is still much to be learnt, much research to be done and some very real pioneering work to be undertaken by the present athletes and their coaches.

Drug testing

The application of drug testing to masters sport is a new concept. Occasional reference has been made in events such as swimming, athletics and weight-lifting, where the world games are conducted under the rules of their respective international sports federations, that competitors are liable to be subjected to drug testing, although this has occurred infrequently. However, at the World Masters Games in 1994 and the World Veterans Track and Field Championships in 1995, drug testing did take place. It is now assumed that this will continue in the future. Competitors on medication were advised to present a medical certificate giving details of the medication, including dosage and the condition for which it was prescribed, should they be selected for testing. No reports have been released and there have been no public statements concerning the tests.

Drug-testing rules designed and intended for élite athletes in open competition are not appropriate for masters competitors. The organizers of masters sport have adopted the rulings of the International Olympic Committee rather than devise their own. Many older athletes, women and men, have legitimate reasons to take medica-

Month:..................... Year:.......................

Date	Menopausal symptoms								BPR	Weight	Medication	Injury/ illness	Daily training notes	Comments
	Hot flushes, night sweats	Insomnia	Anxiety	Mood changes	Muscle joint pain	Fatigue	Positive, strong	Other						
													a.m.	
													p.m.	
													a.m.	
													p.m.	
													a.m.	
													p.m.	
													a.m.	
													p.m.	
													a.m.	
													p.m.	
													a.m.	
													p.m.	
													a.m.	
													p.m.	

Fig. 11.5 Training diary for menopausal athletes. BPR, basal pulse rate.

tion including drugs from the banned list. This matter needs to be addressed before decisions are made to apply the present rules without careful analysis of the implications.

For women athletes on androgen therapy the current rules relating to drug testing and testosterone are as follows:

The presence of a testosterone (T) to epitestosterone (E) ratio greater than six (6) to one (1) in the urine of a competitor constitutes an offence unless there is evidence that this ratio is due to a physiological or pathological condition.

In order to assist in this evaluation the IOC accredited laboratories shall report every case to the proper authorities in accordance with the following criteria:

A. Negative, if the ratio is less than 6, or

B. T:E greater than 6.

In the case of B, it is mandatory that additional studies be carried out under the guidance of the responsible authority before considering the case as positive or negative. A full report will be written and will include, at a minimum, a review of previous tests and results of endocrine investigations. 'In the event that previous tests are not available, the athlete should be tested unannounced at least once per month for three months. The results of these investigations should be included in the report' (IOC Web Site, Medical Code, article I, (c) 1.b).

The concern about the rules governing testosterone in relation to postmenopausal athletes is twofold: (i) it is a banned substance that no athlete should be receiving; and (ii) the test is designed to detect any exogenous testosterone regardless of the overall level, so a menopausal athlete on HRT may have very low levels but would still test positive.

Even though drug-testing procedures are improving all the time, there are still concerns over the legitimacy of the tests, particularly in the light of the devastating effect it can have on an athlete's career. Consequently, new tests and new definitions are continually being sought. In relation to the concern over the situation for older women athletes on androgen therapy, it is significant that the International Amateur Athletic Federation (IAAF) has recently adopted new definitions of testosterone, dihydrotestosterone and human chorionic gonadotrophin as follows:

> Testosterone—a sample will be deemed to be positive for testosterone if the concentration of testosterone in urine so exceeds the range of values normally found in humans as not to be consistent with normal endogenous production.

The feature of this new definition is that the concentration of testosterone will be considered in relation to the normal range, and menopausal women receiving androgen therapy as replacement to restore their levels to normal should have no problem. The question is how and who will determine the normal range. In addition there is a clause in the IAAF 'Procedural Guidelines for Doping Control' to grant an exemption, as follows:

> An athlete may request the Doping Commission to grant prior exemption allowing him to take a substance normally prohibited under IAAF rules. Such an exemption will only be granted in cases of clear and compelling clinical need. Details of the procedure for such an application are to be found in the 'Procedural Guidelines for Doping Control'.

IAAF legal adviser Mark Gay was unable to comment upon the implications for masters athletes but did say that 'Cases concerning hormone replacement therapy in veteran women athletes will, I think, be viewed sympathetically'.

It has been suggested that the use of hormone replacement that includes androgen therapy in some older women athletes who are very serious about their training and competition could present them with the opportunity to cheat, using an 'overdose' in order to produce a better performance. There will always be some athletes who will abuse the system; however, unlike young athletes, older women tend to be cautious about drugs and more interested in good health than short-term athletic performance.

This issue is now being addressed by a task force of WomenSport International, who are taking it up on a global basis. They believe that 'women should be encouraged to participate in sport at all levels and all ages. Masters athletes should not have to choose between sport and their health when they reach the menopause'. The outcome of the work of the task force, the support of eminent scientists in the field of menopause and lobbying by women athletes to keep this on the agenda should see it brought to a successful conclusion.

Conclusion

With athletes continually seeking ways to improve their performances, it is of some surprise to realize that the potential impact of hormones on the performance of postmenopausal masters athletes has been ignored. It seems extraordinary that in the days of sophisticated training programmes, nutritional supplements, scientific technology, sports medicine and any number of other means to improve performance that the fundamental issue of how the menopause and HRT affect athletic performance has not been addressed.

References

Burger, H.G., Hailes, J., Menelaus, M., Nelson, J., Hudson, B. & Balazs, N. (1984) The management of persistent menopausal symptoms with oestradiol–testosterone implants: clinical, lipid and hormonal results. *Maturitas* **6**, 351–358.

Burger, H.G. *et al.* (1987) Effect of combined implants of oestradiol and testosterone on libido in postmenopausal women.

Cabot, S. (1991) *Menopause: You Can Give It a Miss.* Australian Print Group, Melbourne, Australia.

Daly, J. & Ey, W. (1993) *Training Diary for Women.* Department of Recreation and Sport, Adelaide, Australia.

Farrell, E. & Westmore, A. (1993) *The HRT Handbook: How to Decide if HRT is Right for You.* Anne O'Donovan P/L, Australia.

Jones, R.A. (1994) *Testosterone: An Information Leaflet for Women.* Adelaide Private Menopause Clinic, Memorial Hospital, Adelaide, Australia.

Sherwin, B.B. (1988) Affective changes with oestrogen

and androgen replacement therapy in surgically menopausal women. *Journal of Affective Disorders* **14**, 177–187.

Sherwin, B. (1992) Researcher backs androgen for women. *Australian Doctor Weekly*, 28 February.

Studd, J.W.W. & Smith, R.N.J. (1993) Oestradiol and testosterone implants in menopause management. In H.G. Burger (ed.) *The Menopause.*

Thom, M.H., Collins, W.P. & Studd, T.W. (1981) Hormonal profiles in postmenopausal women after therapy with subcutaneous implants. *British Journal of Obstetrics and Gynaecology* **88**, 426–433.

PART 5

MEDICAL ISSUES

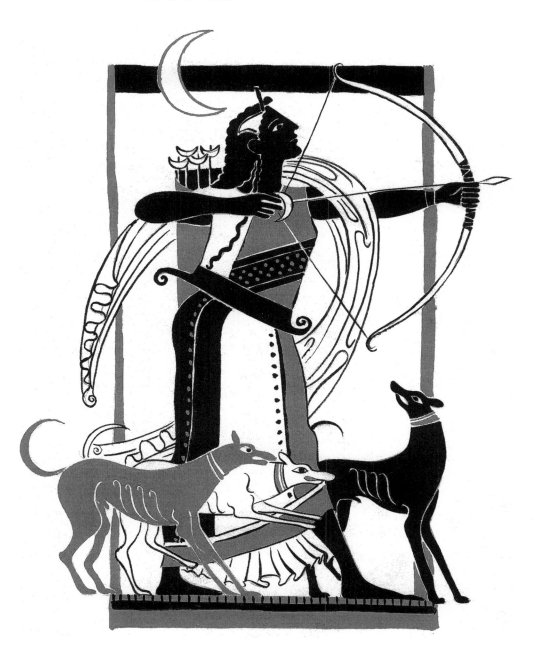

Chapter 12

Preparticipation Examination

MIMI D. JOHNSON

Introduction

Over the last decade, the number of female athletes participating in organized sports has risen exponentially. As a result, physicians and other healthcare providers are being asked to perform preparticipation examinations on an increasing number of female athletes in the junior high, high school and college age groups. Although the basics of this examination are the same for both male and female athletes, there are some special issues that require consideration when dealing with the female athlete.

The objectives of the preparticipation examination (PPE) are: (i) to determine the general health of the athlete; (ii) to detect any medical or musculoskeletal conditions that may limit sports participation or predispose the athlete to injury or illness during participation; (iii) to institute treatment that will bring the athlete to the optimal level of performance before the season begins; and (iv) to meet legal and insurance requirements (Allman, 1974; Shaffer, 1978; Linder *et al.*, 1981; Lombardo, 1984). Although the PPE is not intended to substitute for an athlete's regular health maintenance examination, studies show that for over 78% of athletes the PPE is their only periodic contact with a physician (Goldberg *et al.*, 1980; Risser *et al.*, 1985). Therefore, depending on the setting and available time, the PPE may also be used as an opportunity to counsel the athlete on health and personal issues. Topics of discussion may include healthy eating patterns, tobacco use, drug and alcohol use, seat belt use, birth control and the prevention of sexually transmitted diseases.

Timing and setting of the preparticipation examination

Ideally, the PPE should take place 6 weeks prior to the beginning of the sports season. This allows time to evaluate abnormal or questionable findings further and to correct most musculoskeletal problems. There are differing opinions as to how often the school-age athlete should be evaluated. Some feel that the health maintenance examination should be performed every year. Others recommend that a full physical examination be performed at each school entry level (junior high, high school, college), with an interim history and limited examination (as indicated by the history) to be performed annually (Lombardo, 1984; McKeag, 1985). The annual visits provide an opportunity for guidance and counselling.

The two most common settings for performing the PPE are the station-based screening environment and the physician's office (Lombardo, 1984; McKeag, 1985; American Academy of Family Physicians *et al.*, 1997). The station-based mass examination can be a time- and cost-effective method of screening athletes. However, the office-based examination provides the opportunity to counsel the athlete and answer questions about health and personal issues.

Growth and development considerations

Changes that occur during the growth and pubertal development of the adolescent athlete may affect injury patterns (Micheli, 1983) and alter expectations of sports participation (e.g. puberty in the élite gymnast, height concerns in the basketball player). With an understanding of these changes, the physician is able to explain the aetiology and prevention of some growth-related injuries, and counsel the young athlete on future growth and developmental expectations.

Pubertal growth accounts for 20–25% of final adult height. Pubertal weight gain accounts for 50% of an individual's ideal adult body weight (Barnes, 1975). Peak weight velocity occurs approximately 6 months after peak height velocity in girls (Tanner, 1962). Menarche occurs at about the time of maximum deceleration of linear growth following peak height velocity (Barnes, 1975). Growth after menarche is limited, with a median height gain of 7.4 cm (Roche & Davila, 1972). Figure 12.1 demonstrates the interrelationship of pubertal stage, height spurt and menarche in the female adolescent. Although pubertal staging is not a necessary part of the PPE, it can be helpful in determining an athlete's stage of growth and maturation and its appropriateness as well as the need to address nutritional issues.

Growth can result in decreased flexibility and increased strength that may not be uniform in distribution. This results in muscle–tendon imbalances that can place the athlete at risk for injury. In addition, the epiphyseal plate, the articular cartilage of the joint surface and the apophyseal insertions of the major muscle–tendon units are at increased risk for injury (Micheli, 1983). Repetitive forces at the epiphyseal plate may result in damage, such as the irregularity, widening and premature closure of the distal radial physis in the young gymnast (Roy et al., 1985; Albanese et al., 1989). Osteochondritis dissecans may be associated with repetitive forces at the joint surface (Adams, 1965). Traction apophysitis, such as that occurring at the tibial tubercle (Osgood–Schlatter disease) (Ogden & Southwick, 1976) or the os calcis (Sever's disease) (Micheli, 1983), may be exacerbated by tight muscle–tendon units at these sites. The physician performing the PPE can assess flexibility and strength in the growing athlete, check for signs of growth-related injuries and counsel the athlete on preventative measures such as stretching.

Female athlete triad

The young female athlete, desiring a thin physique or driven to excel in her sport, may attempt to lose weight or body fat by developing patterns of disordered eating. These may include

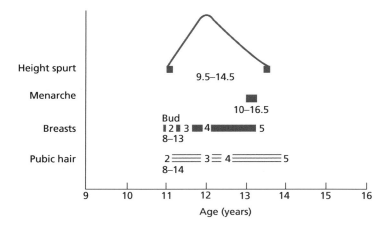

Fig. 12.1 Biological maturity in girls. (From Tanner, 1962 with permission.)

food restriction, bingeing and/or purging, and compulsive overexercise. The caloric deprivation resulting from disordered eating behaviour may lead to menstrual dysfunction (Loucks & Heath, 1994a) and subsequent premature bone loss or osteoporosis (Drinkwater *et al.*, 1984; White *et al.*, 1992). These three conditions—disordered eating, amenorrhoea and osteoporosis—form what has been termed the female athlete triad (Yeager *et al.*, 1993). The practitioner performing the PPE should be watchful for physical signs and symptoms of these conditions (Johnson, 1992, 1994).

Medical history

The medical history is considered to be the most important component of the PPE and can identify up to 75% of all problems (Goldberg *et al.*, 1980; Risser *et al.*, 1985). There is evidence that the information obtained is more accurate when both parent and athlete provide the history (Risser *et al.*, 1985). The history can be obtained from a questionnaire similar to the one shown in Fig. 12.2. The general history should address general health, past hospitalization and surgery, chronic disease, medication use, immunization status, allergies, missing organs and family history of cardiovascular disease. A more specific history concerned with conditions that most commonly affect, or are affected by, sports activity should also be obtained. These conditions typically involve the respiratory, cardiovascular, neurological, dermatological and musculoskeletal systems. Further, the athlete is questioned about heat-related illness, eyewear and the use of protective equipment. The female athlete should also be questioned about menstrual and gynaecological history in addition to nutritional history (Johnson, 1992). A supplemental history for the female athlete can be used to obtain this information (Table 12.1).

Table 12.1 Health history for the female athlete

Name: Age:
Directions: please answer the following questions to the best of your ability.
1 How old were you when you had your first menstrual period?
2 How long do your periods last?
3 How many periods have you had in the last year?
4 Have you ever gone for 3 or more months without having a period?
5 When was your last period?
6 Do you ever have trouble with heavy menstrual bleeding?
7 Do you ever experience cramps during your period?
8 If so, how do you treat them?
9 Have you ever been on birth control pills or hormones?
10 When was your last pelvic examination?
11 Have you ever been treated for anaemia?
12 How many meals do you eat each day? How many snacks?
13 What have you eaten in the last 24 hours?
14 Are there certain food groups you do not eat (i.e., meats, sweets)?
15 Have you ever been on a diet?
16 What is the highest your weight has ever been?
17 What has been your lowest weight in the last year?
18 What is your present weight?
19 Are you happy with this weight? If not, what would you like to weigh?
20 Have you ever tried to lose weight by vomiting/using laxatives/diuretics/diet pills?
21 Have you ever been diagnosed as having an eating disorder?
22 Do you have questions about healthy ways to control weight?

HISTORY

Date of exam _____

Name _____ Sex _____ Age _____ Date of birth _____

Class ___ School _____ Sport(s) _____

Address _____ Phone _____

Personal doctor _____

In case of emergency, contact:

Name _____ Relationship _____ Phone (H) _____ (W) _____

Explain 'Yes' answers below.
Circle questions you don't know the answers to.

Yes No

1. Have you had a medical illness or injury since your last check up or sports physical? ☐ ☐
   Do you have an ongoing or chronic illness? ☐ ☐
2. Have you ever been hospitalized overnight? ☐ ☐
   Have you ever had surgery? ☐ ☐
3. Are you currently taking any prescription or non-prescription (over-the-counter) medications or pills or using an inhaler? ☐ ☐
   Have you ever taken any supplements or vitamins to help you gain or lose weight or improve your performance? ☐ ☐
4. Do you have any allergies (e.g. to pollen, medicine, food or stinging insects)? ☐ ☐
   Have you ever had a rash or hives develop during or after exercise? ☐ ☐
5. Have you ever passed out during or after exercise? ☐ ☐
   Have you ever been dizzy during or after exercise? ☐ ☐
   Have you ever had chest pain during or after exercise? ☐ ☐
   Do you get tired more quickly than your friends do during exercise? ☐ ☐
   Have you ever had racing of your heart or skipped heartbeats? ☐ ☐
   Have you had high blood pressure or high cholesterol? ☐ ☐
   Have you ever been told you have a heart murmur? ☐ ☐
   Has any family member or relative died of heart problems or of sudden death before age 50? ☐ ☐
   Have you had a severe viral infection (e.g. myocarditis or mononucleosis) within the last month? ☐ ☐
   Has a doctor ever denied or restricted your participation in sports for any heart problems? ☐ ☐
6. Do you have any current skin problems (e.g. itching, rashes, acne, warts, fungus or blisters)? ☐ ☐
7. Have you ever had a head injury or concussion? ☐ ☐
   Have you ever been knocked out, become unconscious or lost your memory? ☐ ☐
   Have you ever had a seizure? ☐ ☐
   Do you have frequent or severe headaches? ☐ ☐
   Have you ever had numbness or tingling in you arms, hands, legs or feet? ☐ ☐
   Have you ever had a stinger, burner or pinched nerve? ☐ ☐
8. Have you ever become ill from exercising in the heat? ☐ ☐
9. Do you cough, wheeze or have trouble breathing during or after activity? ☐ ☐
   Do you have asthma? ☐ ☐
   Do you have seasonal allergies that require medical treatment? ☐ ☐

Yes No

10. Do you use any special protective or corrective equipment or devices that aren't usually used for your sport or position (e.g. knee brace, special neck roll, foot orthotics, brace on your teeth, hearing aid)? ☐ ☐
11. Have you had any problems with your eyes or vision? ☐ ☐
    Do you wear glasses, contact or protective eyewear? ☐ ☐
12. Have you ever had a sprain, strain or swelling after injury? ☐ ☐
    Have you broken or fractured any bones or dislocated any joints? ☐ ☐
    Have you had any other problems with pain or swelling in muscles, tendons, bones or joints? ☐ ☐
    If yes, check appropriate box and explain below.
    ☐ Head   ☐ Elbow   ☐ Hip
    ☐ Neck   ☐ Forearm   ☐ Thigh
    ☐ Back   ☐ Wrist   ☐ Knee
    ☐ Chest   ☐ Hand   ☐ Shin/calf
    ☐ Shoulder   ☐ Finger   ☐ Ankle
    ☐ Upper arm   ☐ Foot
13. Do you want to weigh more or less than you do now? ☐ ☐
    Do you lose weight regularly to meet weight requirements for your sport? ☐ ☐
14. Do you feel stressed? ☐ ☐
15. Record the dates of your most recent immunizations (shots) for:
    Tetanus _____ Measles _____
    Hepatitus B _____ Chickenpox _____

Females only

16. When was your first menstrual period?_____
    When was your most recent menstrual period?_____
    How much time do you usually have from the start of one period to the start of another? _____
    How many periods have you had in the last year?_____
    What was the longest time between periods in the last year?__

Explain 'Yes' answers here:_____
_____
_____
_____
_____
_____
_____
_____
_____
_____

I hereby state that, to the best of my knowledge, my answers to the above questions are complete and correct
Signature of athlete _____ Signature of parent/guardian _____ Date _____

Fig. 12.2 History questionnaire for the preparticipation examination. (From American Academy of Family Physicians *et al.*, 1997 with permission.)

Respiratory history

During the PPE an attempt should be made to identify athletes who have asthma or exercise-induced bronchospasm. These athletes often need medication prior to exercise, particularly during cold weather or allergy seasons.

Cardiovascular history

Although the risk of sudden death is lower for women than for men, over 95% of sudden deaths in athletes under the age of 30 are due to cardiac conditions (Van Camp, 1988). Therefore, careful attention must be paid to the cardiac history. Family cardiac history is important because several causes of sudden cardiac death may be familial (i.e. hypertrophic cardiomyopathy, Marfan syndrome, lipid abnormalities). Syncope or near-syncopal episodes, chest pain on exertion, palpitations, or dyspnoea on exertion all warrant further evaluation.

Neurological history

History of neurological conditions or injuries, such as concussion, seizures, 'burners', severe or recurrent headaches, transient quadriplegia or 'pinched nerves' warrant thorough review and possible further evaluation.

Dermatological history

History of infectious conditions, such as herpes simplex, scabies and molluscum contagiosum, can be important for athletes involved in contact/collision sports or in sports that share mats, towels, etc. Acne can also be potentiated from sweating and wearing constrictive clothing.

Heat-related illness

Heat-related illness is often recurrent and therefore information should be obtained about hydration and medications that may increase the risk for heat-related disorders (e.g. antihistamines, caffeine).

Eyewear

An athlete requiring correction of vision needs to have lenses and frames that are safe for sports. A history of eye injury or surgery is important.

Protective equipment

This question can often alert the examiner to a musculoskeletal problem that the athlete may have failed to remember. Status of the current equipment can be evaluated for efficacy. Although mouth-guards are currently required in most collision sports, they are also recommended for all athletes wearing braces on their teeth.

Musculoskeletal history

The history alone has been shown to be 92% sensitive in detecting significant musculoskeletal injuries (Gomez *et al.*, 1993). A history of previous musculoskeletal injuries that limited sports participation should be obtained, in addition to treatment received and adequacy of rehabilitation. Unrehabilitated previous injuries are strong predictors of subsequent injuries. Previous stress fractures should prompt inquiries about biomechanical evaluation as well as menstrual dysfunction. A history of scoliosis, which is more common in females than males, should be obtained. Finally, history of a recent growth spurt may alert the physician to possible growth-related injuries.

Menstrual and gynaecological history

Menstrual and gynaecological history should include age of menarche, length and frequency of periods, date of the last period and use of hormonal therapy. Past history of amenorrhoea or oligomenorrhoea should be obtained.

Athletes with menstrual irregularity require further evaluation. If the athlete is aged 14 and prepubertal, or 16 and premenarcheal, she should be evaluated for primary amenorrhoea. If she is menarcheal and has missed three consecutive menstrual periods or has not had a period in 6 months, she should be evaluated for secondary amenorrhoea (Speroff *et al.*, 1989). The athlete should also be evaluated if she has irregular menses or is bleeding more frequently than once every 25 days or less frequently than once every 35 days (Shangold, 1986). Athletes with primary amenorrhoea, oligomenorrhoea and secondary amenorrhoea may be in 'energy deficit' (exercise calorie expenditure is greater than dietary calorie intake), although other medical causes of these conditions need to be ruled out (Loucks & Callister, 1993; Loucks & Heath 1994a,b).

The amount of menstrual flow should be ascertained. If it is unusually heavy, one should ask about symptoms of, and previous treatment for, anaemia. Dysmenorrhoea, which can interfere with sports activities, can usually be treated successfully with antiprostaglandin therapy. Young athletes may have questions about tampon use during sports activities. If the athlete is 18 years of age or older or has been sexually active, she should be encouraged to undergo a pelvic examination if one has not been previously performed. It is also appropriate to ask about frequency of urinary tract infections; some athletes restrict fluids, which could aggravate such an infection.

Adequate breast support should be encouraged, especially in running and jumping activities. Women can be advised to obtain a sport bra that is firm, made mostly of non-elastic material and has good absorptive qualities.

Nutritional history

All female athletes should be questioned about their eating patterns. Disordered eating patterns have been reported in up to 32% of female college athletes (Rosen *et al.*, 1986) and are seen in younger athletes as well (Benson *et al.*, 1985; Loosli *et al.*, 1986; Dummer *et al.*, 1987). Athletes from all sports can develop eating disorders, but those involved in sports that emphasize a lean appearance (gymnastics, diving, ballet, ice skating), body leanness for optimal performance (long-distance running, swimming) or weight classifications (rowing, martial arts) may be at

highest risk. The athlete requires further evaluation if she is normal or underweight and wants to lose weight, her caloric intake is lower than her caloric expenditure, she avoids groups of food (i.e. all fats or all meats) or admits to disordered eating behaviour. If an eating disorder is suspected, referral to a physician, nutritionist and therapist trained in the management of eating disorders is appropriate. If the athlete has questions regarding weight control, guidelines about appropriate nutrition and weight management may dissuade her from developing disordered eating behaviours.

Health habits

In the physician's office setting, the health habits of the athlete can be assessed in a non-judgemental way. Topics such as alcohol, tobacco and drug use, safe sex and birth control, seat belt and helmet use, gun control and use of ergogenic aids can be addressed. The athlete can be asked if she feels stressed, if she has an adequate support system to deal with stressors and if there are other topics she would like to address (American Academy of Family Physicians *et al.*, 1997).

Physical examination

The physical examination emphasizes the areas of greatest concern with regard to the athlete's particular sport and areas identified as problems in the athlete's history. Ideally, the athlete should be dressed in a T-shirt or gown and shorts.

General assessment

During the assessment of body habitus, the physician has an opportunity to make an initial estimation of maturity, nutritional status, body fat and the presence of any syndromic features. Evidence for an eating disorder or exogenous hormone use may be seen.

Vital signs

Height and weight measurements are useful for evaluating overall growth and development and nutritional status. Most athletes should weigh between the 25th and 50th percentiles for height and age because of the presence of increased muscle mass, compared with the non-athletic population. Resting heart rate may be elevated in anaemia and may be abnormally low (30–50 beats·min^{-1}) in anorexia nervosa. Hypertension in the 10–12 year old is defined as a blood pressure of $\geq 126/82$ mmHg (16.8/10.9 kPa); in the 13–15 year old as a blood pressure of $\geq 136/86$ mmHg (18.1/11.4 kPa); and in the 16–18 year old as a blood pressure of $\geq 142/92$ mmHg (18.9/12.2 kPa) (Task Force on Blood Pressure Control in Children, 1987). To confirm elevated blood pressure, abnormal measurements should be found on three different occasions.

Head, eyes, ears, nose and throat examination

Visual acuity should be 20/40 or better in each eye, with or without corrective lenses. Pupils should be examined for anisocoria (unequal pupil size). The swimmer should be evaluated for otitis externa and tympanic membrane perforation. Decreased tooth enamel may be seen in the athlete with longstanding bulimia. The remainder of this examination should assess for the general health of these areas.

Respiratory examination

Respiratory examination should reveal clear breath sounds. A normal examination does not exclude exercise-induced bronchospasm.

Cardiovascular examination

Palpation of the radial and femoral pulses and auscultation of the heart should be performed. Auscultation should be carried out with the athlete in supine and sitting or standing positions (the murmur of hypertrophic cardiomyopathy may be louder in the standing position). Murmurs are commonly heard in the adolescent. Deep inspiration and Valsalva's manoeuvre can help differentiate a functional murmur from a pathological murmur (Lembo et al., 1988). Any systolic murmur greater than II/VI in severity, any diastolic murmur or any murmur that gets louder with a Valsalva manoeuvre should be further evaluated (American Academy of Family Physicians et al., 1997).

Abdominal examination

In addition to the general assessment, enlargement of the liver and spleen should be evaluated in the athlete with recent history of Epstein–Barr virus infection, viral illness or haematological disorder.

Dermatological examination

The athlete should be examined for rashes, infections and infestations.

Neurological examination

In the athlete with a history of concussion, severe or recurrent headaches, or nerve impairment, a thorough neurological evaluation is appropriate.

Pubertal staging and gynaecological examination

Pubertal staging may be appropriate in the pubescent female athlete, not only to evaluate development but also to educate the athlete on future developmental expectations (Table 12.2). If the physical examination is part of the health maintenance examination, a breast inspection with instructions on self-examination is appropriate. A pelvic examination can be performed if warranted.

Musculoskeletal examination

The musculoskeletal examination may include a general screen (Table 12.3). It should also include joint-specific testing of those areas of previous injury, pain, swelling, locking, weakness, atrophy or joint instability that may have been detected in the history or on the general screen. Joint-specific testing of those areas at increased risk of injury in the athlete's specific sport can also be performed (Table 12.4) . The joint-specific

Table 12.2 Classification of pubertal staging in girls. (Adapted from Tanner, 1962)

Stage	Pubic hair	Breasts
1	None	Prepubertal, no glandular tissue
2	Sparse, long, straight, lightly pigmented on labia majora	Breast bud, small amount of glandular tissue
3	Darker, beginning to curl, extend laterally	Breast mound and areola enlarge, no contour separation
4	Coarse, curly, abundant, less than adult	Breast enlarged, areola and papilla form mound projecting from breast contour
5	Adult type and quantity, extending to medial thigh	Mature, areola part of breast contour

Table 12.3 General musculoskeletal screen. (Adapted from American Academy of Pediatrics Committee on Sports Medicine and Fitness, 1991 and American Academy of Family Physicians *et al.*, 1997)

Instructions	Points of observation
Stand facing examiner	General habitus, trunk and upper extremity symmetry
Look at ceiling, floor, over both shoulders; touch ears to shoulders	Cervical spine motion
Shrug shoulders (examiner resists)	Trapezius strength
Abduct shoulders 90° (examiner resists)	Deltoid strength
Full external and internal rotation of arms	Shoulder motion
Flex and extend elbows	Elbow motion
Arms at sides, elbows 90° flexed; pronate and supinate wrists	Elbow and wrist motion
Spread fingers; make fist	Hand or finger motion and deformities
Contract/relax quadriceps	Inspect lower extremities for symmetry, alignment
'Duck walk' four steps (away from examiner with buttocks on heels)	Hip, knee and ankle motion; strength and balance
Back to examiner	Upper extremity and trunk symmetry
Knees straight, touch toes	Back and hip motion, spine curvature, hamstring tightness
Extend back toward examiner	Lumber spine for spondylolysis/spondylolisthesis
Raise up on toes, raise heels	Calf symmetry, leg strength, balance

Table 12.4 Sport-specific areas of increased risk

Ballet	Feet, ankles, knees, hips, lumbar spine
Basketball	Feet, ankles, knees, shoulders
Gymnastics	Ankles, knees, lumbar spine, wrists, elbows, shoulders
Ice skating	Feet, ankles, shins, lumbar spine
Racquet sports	Shoulders, elbows, wrists, knees, ankles, feet
Rowing	Spine, Achilles tendon, knees, hands, shoulders, elbows, wrists
Soccer	Feet, ankles, shins, knees, thighs, pelvis, lumbar spine, neck
Softball	Shoulders, elbows, ankles, knees
Swimming	Shoulders, lumbar spine
Track/cross-country	Shoulders, feet, ankles, shins, knees, thighs, hips
Volleyball	Ankles, knees, shoulders, hands

examination includes inspection and range of motion of the indicated joint(s) (i.e. neck, spine, shoulders, elbows, wrists, fingers, hips, knees, ankles and feet). Stability of the shoulders, elbows, knees and ankles can also be assessed. Symmetry of joint appearance and motion is noted, and general strength and flexibility around the joint(s) should be assessed.

Laboratory assessment

Routine screening laboratory tests in the asymptomatic athlete are not recommended for the PPE (Goldberg et al., 1980; American Academy of Pediatrics Committee on Sports Medicine and Fitness, 1991; American Academy of Family Physicians et al., 1997). However, findings from the history or physical examination may indicate a need for specific diagnostic tests. For example, if the athlete has a history of anaemia, fatigue, poor dietary intake or increased menstrual flow, a haematological profile and ferritin level would be appropriate. A urinalysis may be diagnostic if she complains of dysuria, urgency or frequency.

Rehabilitation, evaluation and treatment of abnormal findings

The athlete with musculoskeletal conditions requiring rehabilitation can be instructed in the appropriate exercise programme by the physician knowledgeable in sports medicine, or by a physical therapist or athletic trainer. The athlete with medical conditions requiring treatment should be started on therapy or referred for further evaluation. A follow-up visit should be planned to ensure that appropriate treatment was received and to give clearance for sports participation.

The female athlete with disordered eating behaviour often requires an additional office visit to allow the physician to assess whether her behaviour can be changed with nutritional education alone or whether she requires psychological intervention as well (Johnson, 1994). The athlete with an eating disorder may need to be withheld from sports participation when there is evidence or concern that continued participation could cause injury or increased morbidity.

The athlete with exercise-associated amenorrhoea will usually experience a resumption of menses with increased caloric intake (Loucks & Callister, 1993). She can be counselled on this at the time of the PPE or at a subsequent visit. If she has difficulty changing her eating patterns, despite nutritional and psychological counselling, hormone replacement therapy may be considered, depending on her age, in order to preserve her bone mineral density (Emans & Goldstein, 1990; Marshall, 1994; Hergenroeder, 1995).

Clearance for sports participation

Clearance can be divided into three categories: (i) unrestricted clearance; (ii) clearance after completion of further evaluation or rehabilitation; and (iii) not cleared for certain types of sport or for all sports. Clearance for a particular sport may be based on guidelines established by the American Academy of Pediatrics Committee on Sports Medicine and Fitness (1994) (Table 12.5)

Table 12.5 Medical conditions affecting sports participation. (From American Academy of Pediatrics Committee on Sports Medicine and Fitness, 1994 with permission)

Condition	May participate?
Atlantoaxial instability (instability of the joint between cervical vertebrae 1 and 2) *Explanation*: athlete needs evaluation to assess risk of spinal cord injury during sports participation	Qualified yes
Bleeding disorder *Explanation*: athlete needs evaluation	Qualified yes
Cardiovascular diseases Carditis (inflammation of the heart) *Explanation*: carditis may result in sudden death with exertion	No
Hypertension (high blood pressure) *Explanation*: those with significant essential (unexplained) hypertension should avoid weight and power lifting, body building and strength training. Those with secondary hypertension (hypertension caused by a previously identified disease), or severe essential hypertension, need evaluation	Qualified yes
Congenital heart disease (structural heart defects present at birth) *Explanation*: those with mild forms may participate fully; those with moderate or severe forms, or who have undergone surgery, need evaluation	Qualified yes
Dysrhythmia (irregular heart rhythm) *Explanation*: athlete needs evaluation because some types require therapy or make certain sports dangerous, or both	Qualified yes
Mitral valve prolapse (abnormal heart valve) *Explanation*: those with symptoms (chest pain, symptoms of possible dysrhythmia) or evidence of mitral regurgitation (leaking) on physical examination need evaluation. All others may participate fully	Qualified yes
Heart murmur *Explanation*: if the murmur is innocent (does not indicate heart disease), full participation is permitted. Otherwise the athlete needs evaluation (see congenital heart disease and mitral valve prolapse above)	Qualified yes
Cerebral palsy *Explanation*: athlete needs evaluation	Qualified yes
Diabetes mellitus *Explanation*: all sports can be played with proper attention to diet, hydration and insulin therapy. Particular attention is needed for activities that last 30 min or more	Yes
Diarrhoea *Explanation*: Unless disease is mild, no participation is permitted, because diarrhoea may increase the risk of dehydration and heat illness. See Fever	Qualified no
Eating disorders Anorexia nervosa Bulimia nervosa *Explanation*: these patients need both medical and psychiatric assessment before participation	Qualified yes
Eyes Functionally one-eyed athlete Loss of an eye Detached retina Previous eye surgery or serious eye injury *Explanation*: a functionally one-eyed athlete has a best corrected visual acuity of < 20/40 in	Qualified yes

Continued

Table 12.5 (*Continued*)

Condition	May participate?
the worse eye. These athletes would suffer significant disability if the better eye was seriously injured as would those with loss of an eye. Some athletes who have previously undergone eye surgery or had a serious eye injury may have an increased risk of injury because of weakened eye tissue. Availability of eye-guards approved by the American Society for Testing Materials and other protective equipment may allow participation in most sports, but this must be judged on an individual basis	
Fever *Explanation*: fever can increase cardiopulmonary effort, reduce maximum exercise capacity, make heat illness more likely and increase orthostatic hypotension during exercise. Fever may rarely accompany myocarditis or other infections that may make exercise dangerous	No
Heat illness, history of *Explanation*: because of the increased likelihood of recurrence, the athlete needs individual assessment to determine the presence of predisposing conditions and to arrange a prevention strategy	Qualified yes
HIV infection *Explanation*: because of the apparent minimal risk to others, all sports may be played that the state of health allows. In all athletes, skin lesions should be properly covered, and athletic personnel should use universal precautions when handling blood or body fluids with visible blood	Yes
Kidney: absence of one *Explanation*: athlete needs individual assessment for contact/collision and limited contact sports	Qualified yes
Liver: enlarged *Explanation*: if the liver is acutely enlarged, participation should be avoided because of risk of rupture. If the liver is chronically enlarged, individual assessment is needed before collision/contact or limited contact sports are played	Qualified yes
Malignancy *Explanation*: athlete needs individual assessment	Qualified yes
Musculoskeletal disorders *Explanation*: athlete needs individual assessment	Qualified yes
Neurological History of serious head or spine trauma, severe or repeated concussions, or craniotomy *Explanation*: athlete needs individual assessment for collision/contact or limited contact sports, and also for non-contact sports if there are deficits in judgement or cognition. Recent research supports a conservative approach to management of concussion	Qualified yes
Convulsive disorder, well controlled *Explanation*: risk of convulsion during participation is minimal	Yes
Convulsive disorder, poorly controlled *Explanation*: athlete needs individual assessment for collision/contact or limited contact sports. Avoid the following non-contact sports: archery, riflery, swimming, weight or power lifting, strength training, or sports involving heights. In these sports, occurrence of a convulsion may be a risk to self or others	Qualified yes

Continued p. 180

Table 12.5 (*Continued*)

Condition	May participate?
Obesity *Explanation*: because of the risk of heat illness, obese persons need careful acclimatization and hydration	Qualified yes
Organ transplant recipient *Explanation*: athlete needs individual assessment	Qualified yes
Ovary: absence of one *Explanation*: risk of severe injury to the remaining ovary is minimal	Yes
Respiratory Pulmonary compromise including cystic fibrosis *Explanation*: athlete needs individual assessment, but generally all sports may be played if oxygenation remains satisfactory during a graded exercise test. Patients with cystic fibrosis need acclimatization and good hydration to reduce the risk of heat illness	Qualified yes
Asthma *Explanation*: with proper medication and education, only athletes with the most severe asthma will have to modify their participation	Yes
Acute upper respiratory infection *Explanation*: upper respiratory obstruction may affect pulmonary function. Athlete needs individual assessment for all but mild disease. See Fever	Qualified yes
Sickle cell disease *Explanation*: athlete needs individual assessment. In general, if status of the illness permits, all but high-exertion, collision/contact sports may be played. Overheating, dehydration and chilling must be avoided	Qualified yes
Sickle cell trait *Explanation*: it is unlikely that individuals with sickle cell trait (AS) have an increased risk of sudden death or other medical problems during athletic participation except under the most extreme conditions of heat, humidity and possibly increased altitude. These individuals, like all athletes, should be carefully conditioned, acclimatized and hydrated to reduce any possible risk	Yes
Skin: boils, herpes simplex, impetigo, scabies, molluscum contagiosum *Explanation*: while the patient is contagious, participation in gymnastics with mats, martial arts, wrestling or other collision/contact or limited contact sports is not allowed. Herpes simplex virus probably is not transmitted via mats	Qualified yes
Spleen, enlarged *Explanation*: patients with acutely enlarged spleens should avoid all sports because of risk of rupture. Those with chronically enlarged spleens need individual assessment before playing collision/contact or limited contact sports	Qualified yes
Testicle: absent or undescended *Explanation*: certain sports may require a protective cup	Yes

This table is designed to be understood by medical and non-medical personnel. In the Explanation section, 'needs evaluation' means that a physician with appropriate knowledge and experience should assess the safety of a given sport for an athlete with the listed medical condition. Unless otherwise noted, this is because of the variability of the severity of the disease or of the risk of injury among the specific sports or both.

or, for cardiovascular abnormalities, on the 26th Bethesda Conference (1994). Occasionally, an athlete will wish to participate despite medical recommendations to the contrary. In this situation, the athlete, parents, coach and school/programme administrators should all understand the potential long-term consequences of participation and the appropriate legal documentation should be prepared.

Conclusion

When performing a PPE on the female athlete it is helpful to keep in mind her developmental stage, so that appropriate guidance can be given about expectations for growth and maturation and the avoidance of growth-related injuries. The female athlete striving to attain a thin physique is at risk for the development of disordered eating patterns, menstrual dysfunction and potential loss of bone mineral density. Careful evaluation for, and treatment and prevention of, these and other conditions that may affect sport participation will result in a healthier athlete on and off the field.

References

Adams, J. (1965) Injury to the throwing arm: a study of traumatic changes in the elbow joints of boy baseball players. *California Medicine* **102**, 127–132.

Albanese, S., Palmer, A., Kerr, D., Carpenter, C., Lisi, D. & Levinsohn, M. (1989) Wrist pain and distal growth plate closure of the radius in gymnasts. *Journal of Pediatric Orthopedics* **9**, 23–28.

Allman, F. (1974) Medical qualification for sports participation. In A. Ryan & F.L. Allman (eds) *Sports Medicine*, pp. 86–111. Academic Press, New York.

American Academy of Family Physicians, American Academy of Pediatrics, American Medical Society for Sports Medicine, American Orthopaedic Society for Sports Medicine & American Osteopathic Academy of Sports Medicine (1997) *Preparticipation Physical Evaluation*, 2nd edn. McGraw-Hill Healthcare, Minneapolis.

American Academy of Pediatrics Committee on Sports Medicine and Fitness (1991) *Sports Medicine: Health Care for Young Athletes*, 2nd edn. American Academy of Pediatrics, Elk Grove Village, Illinois.

American Academy of Pediatrics Committee on Sports Medicine and Fitness (1994) Medical conditions affecting sports participation. *Pediatrics* **94**, 757–760.

Barnes, H. (1975) Physical growth and development during puberty. *Medical Clinics of North America* **59**, 1305–1317.

Benson, J., Gillien, D., Bourdet, K. & Loosli, A. (1985) Inadequate nutrition and chronic calorie restriction in adolescent ballerinas. *Physician and Sportsmedicine* **13**, 79–90.

Bethesda Conference, 26th (1994) Recommendations for determining eligibility for competition in athletes with cardiovascular abnormalities. *Medicine and Science in Sports and Exercise* **26** (Suppl.), S223–S283.

Drinkwater, B., Nilson, K., Chesnut, C., Bremner, W., Shamholtz, S. & Southworth, M. (1984) Bone mineral content of amenorrheic and eumenorrheic athletes. *New England Journal of Medicine* **311**, 277–280.

Dummer, G., Rosen, L., Heusner, W., Roberts, P. & Counsilman, J. (1987) Pathogenic weight control behaviors of young competitive swimmers. *Physician and Sportsmedicine* **15**, 75–86.

Emans, S. & Goldstein, D. (1990) *Pediatric and Adolescent Gynecology*. Little, Brown, Boston.

Goldberg, B., Saraniti, A., Witman, P., Gavin, M. & Nicholas, J. (1980) Pre-participation sports assessment: an objective evaluation. *Pediatrics* **66**, 736–745.

Gomez, J., Landry, G. & Bernhardt, D. (1993) Critical evaluation of the 2-minute orthopedic screening examination. *American Journal of Diseases of Children* **147**, 1109–1113.

Hergenroeder, A. (1995) Bone mineralization, hypothalamic amenorrhea, and sex steroid therapy in female adolescents and young adults. *Journal of Pediatrics* **126**, 683–689.

Johnson, M. (1992) Tailoring the preparticipation examination to female athletes. *Physician and Sportsmedicine* **20**, 61–72.

Johnson, M. (1994) Disordered eating in active and athletic women. *Clinics in Sports Medicine* **13**, 355–369.

Lembo, N., Dell'Italia, L., Crawford, M. & O'Rourke, R. (1988) Bedside diagnosis of systolic murmurs. *New England Journal of Medicine* **318**, 1572–1578.

Linder, C., DuRant, R., Seklecki, R. & Strong, W. (1981) Preparticipation health screening of young athletes. *American Journal of Sports Medicine* **9**, 187–193.

Lombardo, J. (1984) Pre-participation physical evaluation. *Primary Care Clinics* **11**, 3–21.

Loosli, A., Benson, J., Gillien, D. & Bourdet, K. (1986) Nutrition habits and knowledge in competitive adolescent female gymnasts. *Physician and Sportsmedicine* **14**, 118–130.

Loucks, A. & Callister, R. (1993) Induction and prevention of low-T3 syndrome in exercising women. *American Journal of Physiology* **264**, R924–R930.

Loucks, A. & Heath, E. (1994a) Induction of low-T3 syndrome in exercising women occurs at a threshold of energy availability. *American Journal of Physiology* **266**, R817–R823.

Loucks, A. & Heath, E. (1994b) Dietary restriction reduces luteinizing hormone (LH) pulse frequency during waking hours and increases LH pulse amplitude during sleep in young menstruating women. *Journal of Clinical Endocrinology and Metabolism* **78**, 910–915.

McKeag, D. (1985) Preseason physical examination for the prevention of sports injuries. *Sports Medicine* **2**, 413–431.

Marshall, L. (1994) Clinical evaluation of amenorrhea in active and athletic women. *Clinics in Sports Medicine* **13**, 371–387.

Micheli, L. (1983) **Overuse injuries in children's sports:** the growth factor. *Orthopedic Clinics of North America* **14**, 337–360.

Ogden, J. & Southwick, W. (1976) Osgood–Schlatter's disease and tibial tuberosity development. *Clinical Orthopedics* **116**, 180–189.

Risser, W., Hoffman, H. & Bellah, G. (1985) Frequency of preparticipation sports examinations in secondary school athletes: are the University Interscholastic League guidelines appropriate? *Texas Medicine* **81**, 35–39.

Roche, A. & Davila, G. (1972) Late adolescent growth in stature. *Pediatrics* **50**, 874–880.

Rosen, L., McKeag, D., Hough, D. & Curley, V. (1986) Pathogenic weight-control behavior in female athletes. *Physician and Sportsmedicine* **14**, 79–86.

Roy, S., Caine, D. & Singer, K. (1985) Stress changes of the distal radial epiphysis in young gymnasts. *American Journal of Sports Medicine* **13**, 301–308.

Shaffer, T. (1978) The health examination for participation in sports. *Pediatric Annals* **7**, 666–675.

Shangold, M. (1986) How I manage exercise-related menstrual disturbances. *Physician and Sportsmedicine* **14**, 113–120.

Speroff, L., Glass, R. & Kase, N. (eds) (1989) *Clinical Gynecologic Endocrinology and Infertility*, 4th edn. Williams & Wilkins, Baltimore.

Tanner, J. (1962) *Growth at Adolescence*, 2nd edn. Blackwell Scientific Publications, Oxford.

Task Force on Blood Pressure Control in Children (1987) **Report of the Second Task Force on Blood Pressure Control in Children 1987**. *Pediatrics* **79**, 1–25.

Van Camp, S. (1988) Sudden death in athletes. In W.A. Grana & J.A. Lombardo (eds) *Advances in Sports Medicine and Fitness*. Year Book Medical Publishers, Chicago.

White, C., Hergenroeder, A. & Klish, W. (1992) Bone mineral density in 15 to 21 year old eumenorrheic and amenorrheic subjects. *American Journal of Diseases of Children* **146**, 31–35.

Yeager, K., Agostini, R., Nattiv, A. & Drinkwater, B. (1993) The female athlete triad: disordered eating, amenorrhea, osteoporosis. *Medicine and Science in Sports and Exercise* **25**, 775–777.

Chapter 13

Gender Verification

ARNE LJUNGQVIST

Introduction

Competitive sport was created by men for men. However, once sport for women became recognized it developed rapidly. In many sports, women's competitions at the world élite level, such as the Olympic Games, are as prestigious as men's competitions and meet with the same degree of interest.

Sports achievements are to a large extent, although not in all sports, based on the physical capacity and muscular strength, and also aggressiveness, of the individual. Because these characteristics are usually considerably more developed in men than women, due to the effects of the androgenic steroids (testosterone) secreted by the testes, it is important to be certain that no men compete in women's competitions. This does not seem to have been an issue in earlier days (i.e. before the Second World War). In the postwar years, however, success in high-level international sports competitions became increasingly important and prestigious for the individual athlete as well as for the country he or she represented. In our time, international élite sport is also growing more professional and many successful athletes earn their living and/or make great fortunes from their sport. Therefore, the authorities who govern sport feel very strongly the responsibilities they have to make sure that fair play prevails, that rules are adhered to and that any unfair advantage sought be identified and counteracted. To prevent men from participating in women's competitions is one such responsibility. It may seem an easy problem to solve, but this chapter shows that it is a complicated matter.

Methods for gender verification

Historical background

A number of cases are known of athletes with testes who have competed as women. One famous case from the 1930s was revealed in 1980 when an autopsy was performed on the women's 100m sprint champion of the 1932 Olympic Games. The autopsy was said to show the existence of testes, the coroner's report stating that 'the problem is a subtle one which requires chromosome tests to settle once and for all the questions of her gender' (Anon., 1981, cited in Ferguson-Smith & Ferris, 1991).

In 1957 a German athlete confessed openly to having been forced during the Nazi era in Germany to compete as a woman. The athlete actually broke the world record in women's high jump in 1938. It seems never to have been clarified whether this was a case of true hermaphroditism (both male and female sex organs) as claimed by Donohoe and Johnson (1986) or a male imposter as claimed by Ryan (1976). The person was later disqualified from female competition by the German Athletic Federation.

There are also examples in which successful athletes in women's events have later undergone sex-change operations to become men. Such examples include a runner who was the

183

women's 800 m world record holder in 1931 (Tachezy, 1969). Furthermore, two members of a women's relay team that finished second in the European Athletics Championships in 1946 also underwent sex-change operations later and one of these individuals even became a father (Ryan, 1976; Donohoe & Johnson, 1986). The most famous case in this context would probably be the winner of the 1966 women's world downhill skiing title who retired after medical examination in 1967. Later, after surgery this athlete married a woman and became a father (Ryan, 1976). There are also reports of transsexual individuals who were brought up as boys or young men but later competed in women's competitions after sex reassignment to female (Ryan, 1976; Higdon, 1992).

All the above-mentioned individual cases fuelled the rumours that men actually did compete in women's events in the early postwar era. Means were sought to prevent this from happening in the future.

Physical examination

The first attempt to make sure that only women participate in women's competition seems to have been made by the British Women's Amateur Athletic Association. In 1948 they decided to require a doctor's certificate from athletes who entered women's athletics competitions. This measure was soon recognized as insufficient and abandoned. Due to persistent rumours in the 1950s and 1960s a new attempt was made at the European Athletics Championships in Budapest in 1966. Female participants were required to undergo physical inspection. Reportedly this meant that the 243 female participants had to parade more or less nude in front of a panel of female doctors (Larned, 1976). All participants were reported to have passed this test successfully, but the resulting humiliation was widely resented. However, it is of some interest to know that no less than five or six athletes (information varies), who until 1966 had participated in women's athletics events at the world élite level, did not show up

at the test. It was widely speculated that these athletes withdrew knowing that they would have problems in passing the test, speculations which have remained unproven (Larned, 1976; Donohoe & Johnson, 1986). Despite the experience in Budapest, physical examination was again conducted on the female athletes at the Commonwealth Games in Kingston, Jamaica in 1966 and at the Pan American Games in Winnipeg in 1967. On the former occasion manual examination of the external genitalia was conducted on all women athletes by a gynaecologist (Turnbull, 1988).

The experience with physical examination as a method for verification of female gender at sports competitions was not encouraging. The humiliation inflicted on the individuals involved was widely resented and less humiliating methods had to be found in order to verify eligibility for women's competitions.

Sex chromatin testing

At the European Athletics Cup in Kiev in 1967 attempts were first made to determine the gender of the female athletes on the basis of chromosome constitution. This type of investigation is based on the assumption that cells from men normally carry 46 chromosomes including one X and one Y sex chromosome (46,XY individuals); the sex chromosomes in cells from women comprise two X chromosomes (46,XX individuals).

In Kiev one individual was found with a chromosomal abnormality that was judged to render her ineligible for participation in women's competitions. This happened to be a high-profile athlete, namely the Polish world record holder for 100 m. She had also won one gold and one bronze medal in the Tokyo Olympic Games 3 years earlier and had successfully passed the examination in Budapest in 1966. When the result of the investigation in Kiev was officially announced, major unrest developed. In 1970 the results were annulled by the International Amateur Athletic Federation (IAAF) (Krawczynski, 1978; Turnbull, 1988). This particular athlete was found to have 'one chromosome too many'

(Larned, 1976), probably a case of 46,XX/47,XXY mosaicism. There is no evidence that this would afford her any physical advantage over normal XX females. The athlete is reported by friends to be still suffering from the incident both mentally and socially.

After some years of preparatory work (Hay, 1972), the International Olympic Committee (IOC) tentatively introduced genetic tests for gender verification at the Winter Olympic Games in Grenoble in 1968 and made it compulsory for all female athletes at the Games in Mexico City later the same year. The laboratory investigation performed (the so-called *sex chromatin test*) was again based on the difference between male and female sex chromosome patterns. The test involves staining interphase cells to detect sex chromatin, which is located in the nucleus (Fig. 13.1). The presence of sex chromatin reflects the inactivation of one of the X chromosomes. This requires the presence of two X chromosomes in the cell, one of which remains active. Therefore in XY individuals no chromatin body will be identifiable. For this reason the test will be positive (present) in XX individuals and negative (absent) in XY individuals. Cells for this test are most easily obtained by scraping epithelial cells from the inside of the cheek (the buccal area) with a spatula (Fig. 13.2). The test is therefore often also

referred to as the *buccal smear test*. Obtaining a smear of cells from the buccal mucosa is extremely simple and non-invasive; thus the test seemed to have raised no major objection amongst female athletes when it was introduced. It was therefore quickly adopted by other international sports organizations, becoming the principal gender verification test in sport for a long period of time.

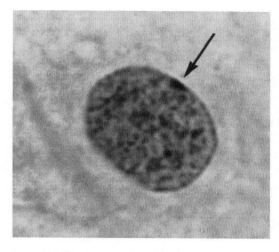

Fig. 13.1 X-chromatin (arrow). (From Simpson & Golbus, 1976 with permission of W.B. Saunders.)

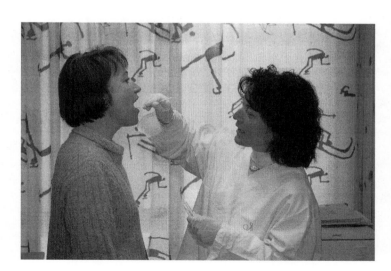

Fig. 13.2 Obtaining a sample of epithelial cells from the buccal area inside the cheek for gender verification. (© CIO / Jean-Paul Maeder.)

Gender verification as developed and practised by the IOC thus included the sex chromatin test as a screening procedure. Should this be negative or inconclusive a full chromosome analysis on a blood sample (determination of the karyotype) would follow. Should this also be inconclusive the athlete would be subjected to a gynaecological examination before a final decision. Once an athlete passed the test, whether the screening procedure only or the full three-stage investigation, she would be issued with a *sex certificate*. A carrier of such a certificate would not be required to undergo the gender verification test again. This approach has remained essentially unchanged and only the screening procedure has been modified, as explained below (Comité International Olympic, 1995).

However, as the science of medical genetics developed it became obvious that chromosomal aberrations occur in otherwise healthy men and women. Thus, individuals with a male phenotype (physical appearance of a man) may well have two X chromosomes, whereas individuals with a female phenotype (physical appearance of a woman) may have only one X chromosome and may even carry a Y chromosome. Both false-positive and false-negative results may thus occur in the sex chromatin test. Furthermore, quite complex aberrations in the sex chromosome pattern have been identified, e.g. mosaicism, where cells with either XX or XY sex chromosome complements are found in the same individual (de la Chapelle, 1986; Ferguson-Smith & Ferris, 1991; Simpson *et al.*, 1993). Ironically, it would seem that in retrospect the Polish sprinter disqualified in 1967 would in all probability have passed the gender verification test employed in Mexico City.

It should be borne in mind that in a buccal-smear specimen not all cells will stain favourably or show a clear picture. Usually some 30% of the cells will be positive and thus judged as 'female'. Therefore, a certain subjectivity on the part of the examiner is inevitable. This is exemplified by the well-known case of the Spanish hurdler Maria José Martinez Patiño, which was widely publicized in the media (Fig. 13.3). In the World

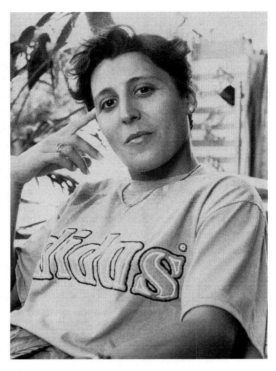

Fig. 13.3 The Spanish hurdler Maria José Martinez Patiño, who publicly challenged the sex test procedures in sport after having tested 'male' (46,XY). (Courtesy of Maria José Martinez Patiño.)

University Games in Kobe in 1985, this athlete was found to have a negative sex chromatin test. Therefore she was judged ineligible for female competition. This was particularly frustrating for the athlete since she had already passed the same test 2 years earlier at the World Championships in Helsinki. Unfortunately, she had left her sex certificate from that test at home in Spain and was therefore tested again in Kobe. The athlete then suffered extreme hardship both socially and financially. She courageously challenged the system publicly and later had her female gender re-established. In fact, she is an example of a 46,XY female with testicular feminization syndrome or androgen insensitivity syndrome. Although these individuals carry the typical chromosome pattern of normal men, they are actually physically women (Ferguson-Smith,

1998). Moreover, they are resistant to androgenic hormones and therefore cannot benefit from the administration (doping) or endogenous presence of such hormones. Although data from previous Olympic Games are incomplete, Ferguson-Smith and Ferris (1991) estimated the frequency of such female athletes to be at least 1 in 500 at high-level international competitions.

The inadequacy of the sex chromatin test, and indeed genetic tests as screening methods, raised growing and serious objections within the scientific community, particularly in the USA but also in Europe (de la Chapelle, 1986; Simpson, 1986). Others defended the procedure despite its shortcomings (Bassis, 1987). Today the sex chromatin test is no longer conducted in genetics laboratories. However, numerous petitions were delivered to sports organizations, including the IOC, urging abandonment of genetic gender verification tests in sport.

Identification of the Y determinant gene by polymerase chain reaction

Under pressure from the scientific community, sports organizations attempted to find alternative ways for gender verification. Believing that screening for female gender is important for the integrity of the Olympic Games but recognizing the shortcomings of the sex chromatin test, the IOC adopted a new method for determination of the presence of the Y chromosome (Fig. 13.4). Using the polymerase chain reaction (PCR), minute amounts of DNA material (e.g. from buccal cells) can be amplified for a specific sequence, in this case one on the Y chromosome. This method was used in the Olympic Games in Albertville in 1992 to identify the sex-determining region on the Y chromosome (SRY) (Dingeon et al., 1992), the main candidate for the testis-determining gene (Sinclair et al., 1990). This screening procedure has since been used in the Olympic Games in Barcelona (1992), Lillehammer (1994), Atlanta (1996) and Nagano (1998). If laboratory results are abnormal, a gynaecological examination is performed.

The International Skiing Federation (FIS) went

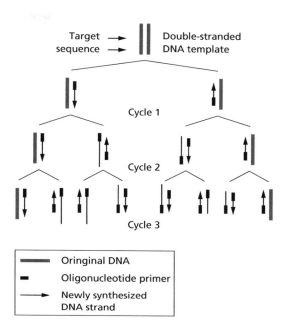

Fig. 13.4 Polymerase chain reaction. Addition of the DNA in question, unique primers and *Taq* polymerase results in amplification (cycle 1). When the temperature is raised, denaturation into single-stranded DNA occurs. On cooling, a second amplification cycle occurs. Continued amplification increases the DNA between primers in logarithmic fashion. (From Simpson, 1996 with permission of Churchill Livingstone.)

even further. In addition to genetic tests, FIS included both physical inspection and determination of serum sex hormone levels. These procedures are supposed to be conducted at the national level, following which a sex certificate is issued. Should a female athlete appear at the FIS world championships without a sex certificate, the organizing committee would arrange for the tests to be conducted.

The IAAF went in the opposite direction from the IOC and FIS. After having conducted gender verification tests in accordance with the IOC protocol, the IAAF convened a conference composed of scientists, sports leaders and athletes. This conference was held in 1990 in Monaco, where recommendations were issued. Member federations of IAAF who enter athletes for international competitions should have both men and women checked before the competition for general health; health certificates should be issued by the authorized national doctor (Ljungqvist & Simpson, 1992). This check would automatically include a determination of gender and thus no specific screening for female gender would be required. This approach was regarded as a step in the right direction (Wilson, 1992) and was tentatively used at the major IAAF competitions in 1991, including the World Athletics Championships in Tokyo. However, the protocol proved unworkable due to insufficient administrative infrastructure in many member federations. Therefore, another conference was convened in London in May 1992, at which a new recommendation called for the IAAF to abandon sex testing at their competitions. This was agreed by the IAAF Council later that month, and since that time no gender verification tests have taken place at IAAF competitions. Should suspect cases occur, however, the medical committee (or medical delegate) is authorized to intervene. Health checks are recommended but no longer compulsory.

The 1990 IAAF conference also addressed the delicate question of sex reassignment and issued the following recommendations, which were adopted by the IAAF Council: (i) individuals undergoing a sex reassignment of male to female before puberty should be regarded as girls and women; and (ii) sex reassignment of transsexuals who change from male to female after puberty should be decided upon by the relevant medical body within the sports organization concerned and after consultation with experts in the field, should such persons not be available within the sports body itself.

Discussion

Controversy exists concerning gender verification tests in sport. Different sports organizations have taken different standpoints and the international sports community is not united in this respect. This raises five fundamental questions.
1 How is male and female gender defined?
2 Is gender verification in sport necessary?
3 What is the view of the female athletes?
4 What is the view of the scientific and legal authorities?
5 Are there any alternative procedures for gender verification?

Gender definition

The identification of female and male individuals would seem to be an easy matter. However, on delving more deeply into the question, it becomes evident that determining gender is quite complex. In fact, the medical community has agreed that eight criteria determine a person's sexual status (Fastiff, 1992): (i) sex chromosome constitution; (ii) sex hormonal pattern; (iii) gonadal sex, i.e. testes or ovaries; (iv) internal sex organs; (v) external genitalia; (vi) secondary sexual characteristics; (vii) apparent sex, as presumed by others and consequently the role in which a person is reared; (viii) psychological sex or gender identity, i.e. that which a person presumes himself or herself to be.

For most of the population the above criteria pose no difficulties; their sexual identity (man or woman) is quite clear. For certain individuals, however, one or more of the criteria may be vague and the assigned sex therefore questionable. Although no single criterion should be regarded as more important than any other, courts have been reported to state that criterion (viii), i.e. the individual's perception of his/her gender identity, may be of greatest importance (Fastiff, 1992).

Because most sports organizations that conduct gender testing base their screening procedure on only one of the eight criteria (i.e. the chromosome pattern), the actual purpose of gender testing has to be clarified. In 1991 the IOC convened a working group that met twice. Although no major conclusions were reached, it emerges from the minutes of both meetings that the sole purpose of gender testing in Olympic Games is to ensure that men do not masquerade as women. Thus, the purpose of gender testing is *not* to identify ambiguous cases.

Is gender testing at sports competitions needed?

With reference to the purpose of gender testing, what is the likelihood that men would masquerade as women in high-level competition? Some feel that today there is no realistic reason to fear that men will try to compete as women. However, others feel that abolition of gender testing in sport would open the door for such misuse. Fastiff (1992) states that the IOC has to evaluate whether gender testing is deemed necessary and, if necessary, whether all eight criteria for gender identity should be tested. This is, of course, not practically possible. The IOC, on the other hand, has defended its position by making clear that the chromosome analysis only serves as a screening procedure and that any case that produces a pathological result (i.e. presence of a Y chromosome) will be subjected to further investigations including clinical/gynaecological examination. Therefore the IOC feels that the most important of the eight criteria are met, enabling it to establish whether the competitor is a man or a woman. FIS has taken a different standpoint, requiring an assessment of the anatomical, hormonal and chromosomal sex. Most federations seem to have found that gender testing is not needed or will serve no purpose: of the 34 international federations with their sport on the Olympic programme only five still conduct gender verification tests at their own world championships (Ljungqvist, 1997). Gender verification tests have recently been abolished at the World University Games and Commonwealth Games.

As discussed above, different screening methods have been tried and, with the exception of physical examination (which met with great resistance and could not be further conducted), have been based on analysis of the chromosome pattern of the individual. The IOC screening procedure, which identifies a DNA sequence from the Y chromosome, will not eliminate the possibility of phenotypic men participating in women's competitions. Moreover, females with a Y chromosome will be singled out as if they were

men. Admittedly this would result in further investigations but many claim that such screening is ethically unacceptable and can inflict persistent harm on the individual (de la Chapelle, 1986; Simpson et al., 1993). The case of the Spanish athlete referred to earlier is just one such example. Moreover, there is evidence that female athletes have silently withdrawn after having been informed about an adverse screening result (Ferguson-Smith & Ferris, 1991). It was on the basis of these arguments that a resolution passed at the first IOC World Conference on Women and Sport in October 1996 urged the IOC 'to discontinue the current process of gender verification during the Olympic Games' (Mascagni, 1996/97). Should the IOC decide accordingly it can be assumed that the five remaining Olympic federations still conducting gender verification tests at their own world championships will follow. (See 'Note added in proof', p. 192.)

View of the female athletes

The attitude of the female athletes themselves to the gender verification procedure is, of course, of central interest in the ongoing discussion. As mentioned earlier the test does not seem to have raised any spontaneous opposition from this group. Furthermore, enquetes performed during both the Albertville Games in 1992 and the Atlanta Games in 1996 showed great support for the test from those who were subjected to it (Dingeon, 1993; Elsas et al., 1997).

On the other hand, there has been practically no request from female athletes to introduce (or reintroduce) such testing in the many Olympic sports that do not conduct gender verification tests at their own world championships. This has only happened once. In 1994, a group of female road runners urged the IAAF to reintroduce gender tests in high-stakes competitions and road races with prize money (Heinonen, 1994a). Because of the inadequacy of the usual screening procedure a different protocol was proposed, with blood analysis for hormone and chromosome assessments (Heinonen, 1994b). The subsequent debate showed that the athletes had not understood the procedure or had not received correct information. The trigger for their request was the sudden success of Chinese female runners, particularly at the World Athletics Championships in Stuttgart in 1993. Moreover, the frequently expressed suspicion regarding these athletes never concerned questions of gender but rather of new performance-enhancing substances. This suspicion was not addressed.

The silence of female athletes and the support from this group when questioned is due in all probability to the fact that the test is very simple and that the athletes believe that it protects their sport. This is supported by the detailed interviews conducted by the Norwegian Sports University on behalf of the IOC at the Lillehammer Games in 1994 (B. Skirstad, unpublished observations). It was confirmed that, in general, athletes supported the tests, although this basically reflected lack of information and knowledge. The more informed the athletes were, the more likely they were to object to the test. There is an obvious need for education of female athletes, and their entourage of sports physicians, team leaders and coaches also need education in this field.

Any education programme should include the information that female athletes may look quite masculine for genetic or endocrinological reasons. It is highly probable that most of the female athletes who caused rumours in the past were in fact women with varying degrees of congenital adrenal hyperplasia. This disorder is far from uncommon in its milder forms (New & Levine, 1984; Speiser et al., 1985), the most common being due to 21-hydroxylase deficiency. In an attempt to overcome the enzyme defect, increased production of adrenocorticotrophic hormone occurs, leading to increased androgenic hormones. Affected women tend to develop hirsutism and a muscular and male body habitus. Alternatively, some of the masculine-looking female athletes from the 1950s, 1960s and 1970s may well have been users of anabolic steroids (which were banned in 1974). To attribute their

physical appearance and sports achievements to a questionable or male sex seems far-fetched.

View of scientific and legal authorities

The commendable efforts of sports organizations to protect women's sport from male imposters and the unfortunate fact that there is no such thing as a simple laboratory method for gender screening are the main reasons for the present controversy. While support has been expressed for the gender verification procedures (Dingeon, 1993; Heinonen, 1994a), most scientists in the field who have participated in the recent debate oppose genetic screening (e.g. de la Chapelle, 1986; Ferguson-Smith et al., 1992; Wilson, 1992; Simpson et al., 1993; McDonald, 1996; Stephenson, 1996). Before the Albertville Games a group of 20 French scientists issued a public statement in which they protested against the test being conducted in France with reference to the Comité Consultif National d'Ethique. In Spain, scientific and ethical arguments were raised against the test before the Barcelona Games (Anderson, 1991).

At the Lillehammer Games in 1994 this controversy came to a head. The Norwegian scientific community simply refused to conduct the screening procedure required by the IOC. Instead, the IOC brought the Albertville team into Norway to conduct the testing. At the junior world championships in alpine skiing in Voss, Norway in 1995 the controversy continued and it was argued that genetic gender testing for sports purposes is against Norwegian law. After further study an amendment to the current law was proposed to the Norwegian parliament in January 1997 in which it was clarified that this type of testing is indeed illegal in Norway. Under these circumstances FIS decided not to insist on gender testing at the world championships in Nordic skiing in Trondheim in February 1997. The amended law was passed by the Norwegian parliament in April 1997. To my knowledge, the legality of this has not been tested in other countries; however, the group of French scientists who protested before the Albertville Games also questioned whether the test is in accordance with the French constitution.

Since it has been clarified scientifically that genetic testing for the sex chromosomes will not fulfil the aims of gender testing in sport, such testing is also considered by many as unethical (de la Chapelle, 1986; Fastiff, 1992; Simpson *et al.*, 1993) and therefore not acceptable. If sports organizations feel that there is need for gender testing, other methods for screening should be found. It has been argued generally that the easiest and most scientifically acceptable way to prevent men from masquerading as women would be by means of clinical examination and not genetic laboratory tests. This view was endorsed by the American Medical Association, whose House of Delegates adopted such a resolution in December 1992. From the practical point of view, however, this solution has proved impossible to implement. Sport has, therefore, been in a dilemma.

Alternative solutions

Based on the experience at the Olympic Games in Atlanta in 1996, Elsas *et al.* (1997) suggested that the present protocol for gender verification be abandoned. They proposed the institution of a protocol in which female entries are selected at random before the Games and subjected to a medical examination by an IOC-recognized medical organization. This would obviously eliminate the criticism against the present procedures. Although the protocol is based on random selection and a central medical body, in principle it is not very different from the system that the IAAF tried in 1991 and found unworkable. Moreover, there would be organizational problems since the examinations would have to be conducted within the short period between the entry of athletes for the Games and the actual competition. Despite these reservations, the suggested protocol may be worth trying if the IOC still feels that there is a need for a special gender verification procedure.

However, there are acceptable procedures already available to deter men from entering women's competitions, at least at the élite level where this would be most likely to occur (Simpson *et al.*, 1993). The present procedure for drug testing requires that large numbers of athletes, particularly those who are finalists or medallists at Olympic Games, be selected for drug testing. According to the rules, the athletes must provide a sample of urine under the supervision of officials. This means that male competitors have to present themselves at the men's doping station and female competitors at the women's doping station. There they will be asked to provide a urine sample under the supervision of a male or a female observant. According to the rules these observants have to make sure that the urine actually derives from the athlete. This, together with the close coverage of élite sport by the media, would seem to make special screening for gender unnecessary.

Conclusion

- There is past evidence that intersex individuals (with testes) have participated in women's sports competitions, but none in recent decades.
- It is agreed by the IOC that the sole reason for gender verification tests is to prevent men from participating in women's events.
- There is no current evidence that males are masquerading as females.
- Gender should not be confused with genetic sex as determined by chromosomal tests.
- There is no evidence that females with a Y chromosome have any advantage over chromosomally normal (46,XX) females in sport.
- 46,XX true hermaphrodites (external genitalia and sex of rearing predominantly male) usually pass genetic tests as females, as will some 20% of 46,XX males.
- Female athletes with a Y chromosome will be singled out as if they were men by the current screening method.
- For the above reasons, genetic tests (chromosomal analysis) will not fulfil the aims of gender

verification in sport, not even as screening methods.

• There is no single and adequate laboratory method for screening for gender.

• Although physical examination has been proposed as the only adequate method for gender verification in sport, it has proved unworkable.

• It is suggested that the close media coverage of today's élite sport and the current drug-control procedures when properly followed will together serve as a sufficient deterrent to attempts by males to masquerade as female athletes.

Note added in proof

In June 1999, the IOC decided to abandon the genetic-based screening for female gender of the female participants at the Olympic Games and to replace it with a system that allows the IOC Medical Commission to arrange for a scientifically and ethically proper investigation of any suspect individual case.

References

Anderson, C. (1991) Olympic row over sex testing. *Nature* **353**, 784.

Anonymous (1981) Athlete's sex secret. *Guardian*, 26 January 1981.

Bassis, L.M. (1987) Sex chromatin screening of female athletes. *Journal of the American Medical Association* **257**, 1896–1897.

Comité International Olympic (1995) *Code Medical du CIO*. Comité International Olympic.

de la Chapelle, A. (1986) The use and misuse of sex chromatin screening for gender identification of female athletes. *Journal of the American Medical Association* **256**, 1920–1923.

Dingeon, B. (1993) Gender verification and the next Olympic Games. *Journal of the American Medical Association* **269**, 357–358.

Dingeon, B., Harnon, P., Robert, M., Schamash, P. & Pugeat, M. (1992) Sex testing at the Olympics. *Nature* **358**, 447.

Donohoe, T. & Johnson, N. (1986) Drugs and the female athlete. In *Foul Play*, pp. 66–79. Basil Blackwell, Oxford.

Elsas, L.J., Hayes, R.P. & Muralidharan, K. (1997) Gender verification at the Centennial Olympic Games. *Journal of the Medical Association of Georgia* **86**, 50–54.

Fastiff, P.B. (1992) Gender verification testing: balancing the rights of female athletes with a scandal-free Olympic Games. *Hastings. Constitutional Law Quarterly* **19**, 937–961.

Ferguson-Smith, M.A. (1998) Gender verification and the place of XY females in sport. In M. Harries, C. Williams, W.D. Stanish & L.J. Mitchell (eds) *Oxford Textbook of Sports Medicine*, 2nd edn, pp. 355–365. Oxford University Press, Oxford.

Ferguson-Smith, M.A. & Ferris, E.A. (1991) Gender verification in sport: the need for a change? *British Journal of Sports Medicine* **25**, 17–21.

Ferguson-Smith, M.A., Carlson, A., de la Chapelle, A. et al. (1992) Olympic row over sex testing. *Nature* **355**, 10.

Hay, E. (1972) Sex determination in putative female athletes. *Journal of the American Medical Association* **221**, 998–999.

Heinonen, J. (1994a) A decent proposal. *Keeping Track. International Track and Field Newsletter* no. 24 (March).

Heinonen, J. (1994b) Give-and-take on gender verification. *Keeping Track. International Track and Field Newsletter* no. 26 (May).

Higdon, H. (1992) Is she or isn't she? *Runners World* **27**, 54–59.

Krawczynsky, M. (1978) Zagadnienie intersekusulizmu w sporcie kwalifokwanum. *Wiadomoski Lekarskie* **3**, 189–191.

Larned, D. (1976) The femininity test: a woman's first Olympic hurdle. *Women Sports* **3**, 8–11.

Ljungqvist, A. (1997) Gender verification in sport: the so called 'femininity test'. *The Starting Line. WomenSports International Newsletter* no. 3.

Ljungqvist, A. & Simpson, J.L. (1992) Medical examination for health of all athletes replacing the need for gender verification in international sport. *Journal of the American Medical Association* **267**, 850–852.

McDonald, K.A. (1996) Olympics pose difficult questions for sports-medicine experts. *Chronicle of Higher Education* **43**, A23–A24.

Mascagni, K. (1996/97) World conference on women and sport. *Olympic Review* **XXVI-12**, 23–31.

New, M. & Levine, L.S. (1984) Recent advances in 21-hydroxylase deficiency. *Annual Review of Medicine* **35**, 649–653.

Ryan, A.J. (1976) Sex and the singles player. *Physician and Sportsmedicine* **4**, 39–41.

Simpson, J.L. (1986) Gender testing in the Olympics. *Journal of the American Medical Association* **256**, 1938.

Simpson, J.L. (1996) Genetic counseling and prenatal diagnosis. In S.G. Gabbe, J.R Niebyl & J.L. Simpson (eds) *Obstetrics, Normal and Problem Pregnancies*, 3rd edn, p. 236. Churchill Livingstone, Edinburgh.

Simpson, J.L. & Golbus, M.S. (1976) Disorders of sexual differentiation: etiology and clinical delineation. In J.L. Simpson & M.S. Golbus (eds) *Genetics in Obstetrics and Gynaecology*, 2nd edn, p. 10. W.B. Saunders Company, New York.

Simpson, J.L., Ljungqvist, A., de la Chapelle, A. *et al.* (1993) Gender verification in competitive sport. *Sports Medicine* **16**, 305–315.

Sinclair, A.H., Besta, P., Plamer, M.S., Hawkins, J.R. & Griffiths, B.L. (1990) A gene from the human sex determining region encodes a protein with known homology to a conserved DNA-binding motif. *Nature* **346**, 240–244.

Speiser, P.W., Dupont, B. & Rubinstein, P. (1985) High frequency nonclassical steroid 21-hydroxylase deficiency. *American Journal of Human Genetics* **37**, 650–667.

Stephenson, J. (1996) Female olympian's sex tests outmoded. *Journal of the American Medical Association* **276**, 177–178.

Tachezy, R. (1969) Pseudohermaphroditism and physical efficiency. *Journal of Sports Medicine and Physical Fitness* **9**, 119–122.

Turnbull, A. (1988) Woman enough for the Games? *New Scientist* **119**(1630), 61–64.

Wilson, J. (1992) Sex testing in athletics: a small step forward. *Journal of the American Medical Association* **267**, 853.

Chapter 14

The Pregnant Athlete

MICHELLE F. MOTTOLA AND LARRY A. WOLFE

Introduction

In the past, during pregnancy the medical advice for women was to rest (Wolfe *et al.*, 1994a). However, this outdated medical opinion does not address the increasing population of women actively engaged in sports and recreational activities. Pregnancy is a unique process in which almost all the control systems of the body are modified in an attempt to maintain both maternal and fetal homeostasis. In theory, the addition of exercise may represent a significant challenge to maternal and fetal well-being, especially at higher intensities of physical work (Wolfe *et al.*, 1994a). Several potential risks have been identified in the literature and each appears to have a dose–response relationship to the intensity of maternal exercise, i.e. as the intensity of maternal exercise increases, the risk of hypothetical effects also increases. Wolfe *et al.* (1989, 1994a), Clapp (1996a) and Stevenson (1997) provide excellent reviews on the effects of maternal exercise on maternal and fetal well-being.

Figure 14.1 is a flow diagram of three hypothetical risks to the fetus during maternal exercise, for which three different mechanisms have been proposed (Wolfe *et al.* 1989, 1994a). The first hypothetical effect results from an increase in the utilization of maternal blood glucose as a metabolic fuel by the muscles of the mother during exercise. Strenuous maternal exercise, especially in the third trimester, may lead to maternal hypoglycaemia after exercise, which would decrease fetal glucose availability. Recent studies have shown that maternal exercise, especially in late pregnancy, may decrease maternal blood glucose values (Clapp *et al.*, 1987; Bonen *et al.*, 1992; Soultanakis *et al.*, 1996). Soultanakis *et al.* (1996) evaluated late gestational women and non-pregnant women in response to 1 hour of prolonged moderate-intensity exercise (55% $\dot{V}_{O_{2max}}$). Blood glucose values in the pregnant women decreased at a faster rate and to a significantly lower level after exercise compared with the non-pregnant women. Since the fetus utilizes maternal blood glucose as the main energy source for growth and development, regular exposure to reduced maternal blood glucose levels may lead to fetal malnutrition, intrauterine growth restriction and reduced birth weight (Clapp *et al.*, 1987).

The fetus may be protected to some extent from low maternal blood glucose levels because the placenta can utilize alternate fuels in times of maternal hypoglycaemia (Hay *et al.*, 1983). The placenta has been shown to use maternal blood lactate as an energy source; it can also produce lactate from glucose metabolism and this may enter the fetal circulation for use as a fuel in times of glucose deficiency (Sparks *et al.*, 1982; Hay *et al.*, 1983). Placental lactate may be an important fetal fuel, second only to glucose (Burd *et al.*, 1975; Hay *et al.*, 1983).

The second hypothetical risk (Fig. 14.1) is due to increased catecholamine release into the maternal blood as a result of exercise. This causes a redistribution of maternal blood flow from the gut and uterus to the working muscles (Lotgering *et al.*, 1983a). Maternal blood flow

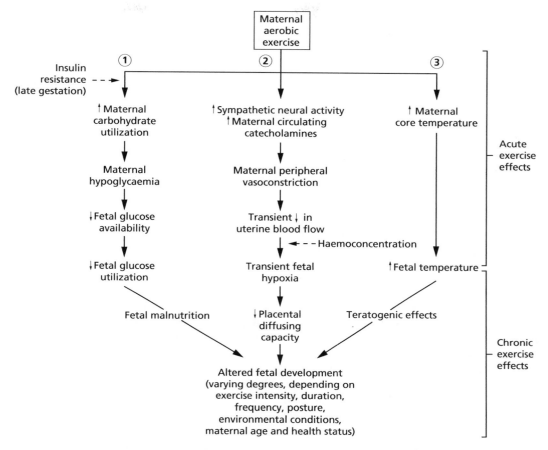

Fig. 14.1 Hypothetical effects of aerobic exercise on fetal development. (From Wolfe *et al.*, 1989 with permission of Williams & Wilkins.)

redistribution during exercise appears to obey a dose–response relationship. As the intensity and duration of maternal exercise increases, the amount of blood shunted from the uteroplacental area to the working muscles of the mother is also augmented (Jones *et al.*, 1991). Maternal training does not seem to alter this phenomenon. Jones *et al.* (1990) showed that chronic maternal exercise in rats did not change the amount of blood shunted from the gut to the working muscles of the mother during acute maternal exercise compared with sedentary control animals. However, in the trained state at any given absolute work rate there may be less blood flow redistributed because the trained individual

is not working as hard. Webb *et al.* (1994) demonstrated that physically conditioned pregnant women can perform at a higher exercise work rate than sedentary pregnant women to achieve the same absolute heart rate.

The amount of blood flowing to the placenta and fetus is important because oxygen delivery to the uteroplacental area is directly proportional to uterine blood flow (Mostello *et al.*, 1991). In an experiment using pregnant sheep, a hydraulic occluder was placed on the uterine vasculature. Quantitative assessments of acute placental blood flow and fetal responses showed that the changes in fetal P_{O_2} and oxygen content were directly related to the magnitude of vascular occlusion. Fetal β-endorphin (a marker for fetal distress) was not released until uteroplacental blood flow was reduced by 65% (Skillman & Clark, 1987). Equating this to a specific maternal exercise intensity must be verified through scientific study; however, it appears to occur at about 80% $\dot{V}_{O_{2max}}$ in the exercising pregnant sheep (Jones et al., 1991). With a reduced uteroplacental blood flow, there may be a reduction in fetal oxygenation and decreased placental oxygen diffusion capacity, which may lead to altered fetal growth and development (Wolfe et al., 1994a). Several studies have shown that women who exercise at higher intensities and who exercise past 28 weeks of gestation give birth to smaller babies (Clapp & Dickstein, 1984; Clapp & Capeless, 1991; Bell et al., 1995; Clapp, 1996b). In contrast, Hatch et al. (1993) analysed a cohort of 800 pregnant women and found that, with heavy exercise, there was an increase of 300 g in birth weight in women who expended about 8400 kJ·week^{-1} (2000 kcal·week^{-1}).

The fetus may be somewhat protected during moderate maternal exercise because fetal blood has a higher affinity for oxygen, which would promote oxygen transfer across the placental barrier from maternal to fetal blood (Gilbert et al., 1985). The fetal oxygen–haemoglobin dissociation curve (i.e. the relationship between percentage saturation of haemoglobin with oxygen and the partial pressure of oxygen) lies to the left of the maternal curve, which promotes better extraction of oxygen from haemoglobin at a given partial pressure (Gilbert et al., 1985). The fetal curve lies to the left of the maternal curve because of the differential effect of 2,3-diphosphoglycerate on the oxygen-binding characteristics of fetal haemoglobin compared with adult haemoglobin. In addition, other protective fetomaternal adaptive mechanisms are in place to ensure oxygen transfer. These include haemoconcentration of maternal blood during exercise (Webb et al., 1994; Wolfe et al., 1994a) and the redistribution of uterine blood flow so that the placenta is favoured over the myometrial vasculature (Webb et al., 1994; Wolfe et al., 1994a).

The final hypothetical risk, an increase in maternal body core temperature (Fig. 14.1), may occur with maternal exercise. As the intensity and duration increases, maternal body core temperature may increase in proportion to the intensity of exercise. At rest, fetal body core temperature is normally about 0.6°C higher than maternal body temperature because of the increase in fetal metabolic rate due to fetal growth and development (Lotgering et al., 1983b). This maintains the normal heat gradient and ensures that heat dissipation is from higher to lower, namely fetal to maternal heat dissipation. As maternal body temperature increases, maternal body core temperature becomes higher than that in the fetus. This reverses the normal temperature gradient between fetus and mother so that the fetus may now receive heat from the mother (Lotgering et al., 1983b). The reversal in the normal heat gradient may delay fetal body heat dissipation and may alter fetal development, especially if the exposure to heat occurs during early fetal life (Bell et al., 1983; Mottola et al., 1993; Sasaki et al., 1995). However, Clapp et al. (1987), after analysing 10 fit recreationally active women before pregnancy and during the second and third trimesters, suggested that the efficiency of heat dissipation may be increased during pregnancy because of pregnancy-induced increases in blood volume and skin blood flow. These changes occur because of vasodilation of peripheral vessels and may promote a thermoneutral environment in exercising pregnant women as long as the mother is well hydrated and exercises in a cool environment.

The hypothetical effects of maternal exercise illustrated in Fig. 14.1 may be offset by many protective mechanisms during pregnancy, as discussed above. These protective mechanisms are summarized in Fig. 14.2. Unfortunately, no threshold has been determined for intensity and duration of maternal exercise above which problems may occur and, because of this, it is important that medical screening take place to ensure a healthy pregnancy. The literature on animal

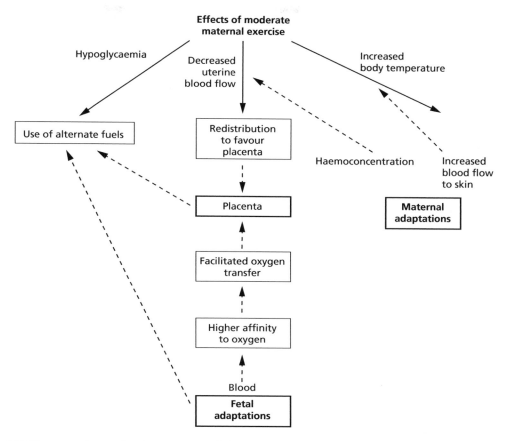

Fig. 14.2 Fetoprotective mechanisms to counterbalance the effects of moderate-intensity exercise. The dashed arrows indicate the protective mechanisms and the solid arrows the hypothetical risks to the fetus as a result of maternal exercise.

studies suggests that the higher the intensity and duration of maternal exercise, the greater the risk of these potential effects occurring. Current guidelines recommend exercise intensities of about 60–70% $\dot{V}o_{2max}$ (moderate exercise) and these guidelines are well accepted as safe for most healthy pregnant women. Scientific data are lacking for pregnant women who wish to engage in strenuous exercise above the accepted guidelines and for pregnant athletes participating in various sports. Regardless of the exercise intensity, it is important for all pregnant women to be medically screened before engaging in any exercise programme.

Medical prescreening

An important medical screening tool that physicians can use to monitor patients performing exercise during pregnancy is the *Physical Activity Readiness Medical Examination for Pregnancy* (*PARmed-X for Pregnancy*) document. This was developed by Dr Larry Wolfe of Queen's University, Kingston, Ontario and Dr Michelle Mottola of the University of Western Ontario. The Canadian Society for Exercise Physiologists (CSEP) now holds the copyright for this document, which is also endorsed by Health Canada. It includes a prescreening questionnaire to identify contraindications to exercise during pregnancy, a list of safety considerations, and aerobic and muscle conditioning guidelines. This document can be ordered from CSEP, 185 Somerset St. West, Suite 202, Ottawa, Ontario, Canada K2P OJ2 (tel. (613) 234 3755; fax (613) 234 3565). In addition, the Canadian Academy of Sports Medicine published a position paper on exercise during pregnancy in the summer of 1999 and this includes the *PARmed-X for Pregnancy* document.

Contraindications for exercise and safety considerations

Table 14.1 shows the contraindications to exercise during pregnancy, Table 14.2 indicates safety considerations for maternal exercise and Table 14.3 shows reasons to discontinue exercise and consult a physician.

Table 14.1 Contraindications to exercise in pregnant women. (Modified from *PARmed-X for Pregnancy* document, 1996 with permission of the Canadian Society for Exercise Physiology)

Absolute contraindications
Ruptured membranes, premature labour
Persistent second- or third-trimester bleeding/ placenta praevia
Pregnancy-induced hypertension, pre-eclampsia or toxaemia
Incompetent cervix
Evidence of intrauterine growth restriction
Multiple pregnancy (e.g. triplets)
Uncontrolled type 1 diabetes, hypertension or thyroid disease; other serious cardiovascular, respiratory or systemic disorder

Relative contraindications
History of spontaneous abortion or premature labour in previous pregnancies
Mild/moderate cardiovascular or respiratory disease (e.g. chronic hypertension, asthma)
Anaemia or iron deficiency (haemoglobin < $10\,g\cdot dl^{-1}$)
Very low body fat, eating disorder (anorexia, bulimia)
Twin pregnancy after 28th week
Other significant medical condition

Note: Risk may exceed benefits of regular physical activity. The decision to be physically active or not should be made with qualified medical advice.

The contraindications to exercise are divided into conditions in which no exercise should occur (absolute contraindications) and relative contraindications. With regard to relative contraindications, the risk of regular exercise may exceed the benefits. The conditions listed under relative contraindications may change with medical treatment, at which point exercise may be encouraged. The decision to engage in exercise or not should be made with qualified medical advice.

In Table 14.2, the safety considerations listed are common sense. The American College of Obstetricians and Gynecologists (1994) has recommended avoidance of exercise in the supine position past 4 months of pregnancy because of possible blocking of the inferior vena cava and/or the abdominal aorta by the gravid uterus. Symptoms associated with blockage of the inferior vena cava are light-headedness and dizziness; there are no symptoms for blockage of the abdominal aorta, which may decrease blood flow to the uteroplacental area. The footnote to Table 14.2 suggests that the temperature of heated pools be monitored. This is based on an

Table 14.2 Safety considerations for pregnant women performing exercise. (Modified from *PARmed-X for Pregnancy* document, 1996 with permission of the Canadian Society for Exercise Physiology)

Avoid prolonged or strenuous exertion during the first trimester
Avoid isometric exercise or straining while holding your breath
Maintain adequate nutrition and hydration: drink liquids before and after exercise
Avoid exercising in warm/humid environments
Avoid exercise while lying on your back past the fourth month of pregnancy
Avoid activities that involve physical contact or danger of falling
Periodic rest periods may help to minimize possible low-oxygen or temperature stress to the fetus
Know the reasons to stop exercise and consult a qualified physician immediately if they occur
It is important to monitor the temperature of heated pools. During exercise, maternal body temperature may be increased more by exercising in a warm environment

Table 14.3 Reasons for pregnant women to discontinue exercise and consult a physician. (Modified from *PARmed-X for Pregnancy* document, 1996 with permission of the Canadian Society for Exercise Physiology)

Persistent uterine contractions (more than six to eight per hour)
Bloody discharge from vagina
Any 'gush' of fluid from vagina (suggesting premature rupture of the membranes)
Unexplained pain in abdomen
Sudden swelling of extremities (ankles, hands, face)
Swelling, pain and redness in the calf of one leg (suggesting phlebitis)
Persistent headaches or disturbances of vision
Unexplained dizziness or faintness
Marked fatigue, heart palpitations or chest pain
Failure to gain weight (less than 1 kg per month during last two trimesters)
Absence of usual fetal movement

animal study (Mottola *et al.*, 1993) that found an increase in teratogenic problems in animals exercised (swim-trained) in warm water (37.4°C). In Table 14.3, the reasons for consulting a physician are also based on common sense.

Exercise prescription

Healthy sedentary pregnant women who wish to start an exercise programme should be treated differently from the recreational athlete or the well-conditioned pregnant athlete. Aerobic and muscular conditioning exercises for the previously sedentary pregnant woman are described in the *PARmed-X for Pregnancy* document. Exercise prescription for sedentary women is not discussed here. Women who have been exercising prior to pregnancy have been advised by the medical profession to continue exercise during pregnancy. However, it is necessary to determine the frequency, intensity, duration and type of exercise before advising pregnant women to continue exercising. In addition, medical prescreening must occur to rule out contraindications. The following guidelines for aerobic and muscular conditioning are suggested for active healthy pregnant women (taken from *PARmed-X for Pregnancy*).

Aerobic guidelines

Pregnant women who have been exercising about three times per week may increase to a

Table 14.4 Target heart rate zones for healthy pregnant women. (Modified from *PARmed-X for Pregnancy* document, 1996 with permission of the Canadian Society for Exercise Physiology)

Age (years)	Heart rate zone (beats·min^{-1})
< 20	140–155
20–29	135–150
30–39	130–145
≥ 40	125–140

maximum of five times per week in the second trimester. Increasing frequency, intensity or duration of exercise is not recommended in the first or the third trimester because of fatigue and because the risks may outweigh the benefits of exercise. The intensity of exercise should be monitored by heart rate (pulse rate), which should be targeted within specific heart rate zones based on age (Table 14.4). These target heart rate zones are approximately 60–70% $\dot{V}o_{2max}$ based on age (Wolfe & Mottola, 1993). At the start of a new exercise programme and in late pregnancy, exercise intensity should be targeted at the lower end of the heart rate zone. The rating of perceived exertion (Borg, 1962) should be used in conjunction with the heart rate target zones. On a scale of 20, pregnant women should be exercising at an intensity of between 12 and 14 ('somewhat hard'). On the 10-point scale, an intensity between 3 and 4 is recommended (Wolfe &

Mottola, 1993). In addition, one final check of intensity is the 'talk test': if the pregnant woman is out of breath while talking during exercise, she should reduce the intensity.

The duration of exercise should be a minimum of about 15 min per session at the target heart rate to a maximum of about 30 min per session at the target heart rate. Intensity or duration of exercise should not be increased past week 28 of gestation (Wolfe & Mottola, 1993) due to fatigue; again, the risks may exceed the benefits of exercise.

Each exercise session should start with 5–15 min of warm-up and 5–15 min of cooling down at a lower intensity. Recommended aerobic exercise modalities include walking, low-impact aerobics and exercise where body weight is supported, such as cycling and swimming. However, if a woman has been jogging before pregnancy, she may continue within the aerobic exercise guidelines, unless she develops joint problems or is uncomfortable with this mode of exercise. Switching to stair climbing (with no jarring movements) or to body weight-supported exercise would be recommended. All pregnant women should know the safety signs and consult a physician should any contraindications to exercise occur (see Tables 14.2 & 14.3).

Precautions for muscle conditioning exercise

The precautions listed in Table 14.5 for muscular conditioning exercise suggest modifications during pregnancy. It is important to avoid exercise in the supine position past 4 months of pregnancy as has been suggested previously (American College of Obstetricians and Gynecologists, 1994). Abdominal exercises should be performed lying on one side or in a standing position.

Joint laxity may occur during pregnancy. Schauberger *et al.* (1996) suggested that joint laxity was found in five of the seven peripheral joints studied over the course of pregnancy and after birth but there was no correlation with serum relaxin values. Joint laxity was not altered by maternal age, parity or prenatal exercise

Table 14.5 Precautions for muscular conditioning during pregnancy. (Modified from *PARmed-X for Pregnancy* document, 1996 with permission of the Canadian Society for Exercise Physiology)

Variable	Effects of pregnancy	Exercise modifications
Body position	In the supine position (lying on the back), the enlarged uterus may decrease the flow of blood returning from the lower half of the body as it presses on a major vein (inferior vena cava)	Past 4 months of gestation, exercises normally done in the supine position should be done lying on one side or standing
Joint laxity	Ligaments become relaxed due to increasing hormone levels Joints may be prone to injury	Avoid rapid changes in direction and bouncing during exercises Stretching should be performed with controlled movements
Abdominal muscles	Presence of a rippling (bulging) of connective tissue along the midline of the pregnant abdomen (diastasis recti) may be seen during abdominal exercise	Abdominal exercises are not recommended if diastasis recti develops
Posture	Increasing weight of enlarged breasts and uterus may cause a forward shift in the centre of gravity and may increase the arch in the lower back This may also cause shoulders to slump forward	Emphasis on correct posture

levels (Schauberger *et al.*, 1996). Thus, it is important to avoid ballistic movements and rapid changes in direction. In addition, stretching should be controlled.

If diastasis recti develops during pregnancy, abdominal exercises are not recommended. Tearing of the linea alba (connective tissue) occurs with this condition, which causes the bulging or rippling along the midline. Continuing to strengthen the rectus abdominis muscles through abdominal exercises may worsen this condition as the pregnant abdomen continues to protrude, because tearing will occur at the weakest point, i.e. along the connective tissue.

Posture is important and a 'neutral' pelvic alignment is suggested rather than the pelvic tilt position. The use of the pelvic tilt is controversial because this position may decrease the normal lordotic curvature in the spine, which may place excessive stress on the vertebral ligaments in the lumbar region. To find the neutral pelvic position, it is suggested that women over-accentuate the lordotic curve, then push the pelvis into an exaggerated pelvic tilt position and find the neutral pelvic position midway between these two postures.

Weight-lifting or resistance exercise is another area that sparks controversy. Weight-lifting performed while lying on the back should be modified to either a sitting, standing or side-lying position. The use of a resistive tool such as low-weight free weights or a Dynaband are recommended. Low-resistance weight and high repetitions are also recommended for free weights and weight machines. Correct breathing should be emphasized, with exhalation on exertion and inhalation on relaxation. The Valsalva manoeuvre (breath-holding while working against a resistance) causes an increase in blood pressure and therefore should be avoided. Table 14.6 describes examples of exercises for muscular conditioning.

The well-conditioned athlete

Pregnancy is not the time for engaging in sports competition or strenuous activity that would place the mother at risk for bodily injury. In addition, there are no known benefits to the fetus during maternal exercise $>80\%$ $\dot{V}_{O_{2max}}$. In fact, studies on animals, as previously discussed, indicate that beyond this intensity the fetus may be stressed and uteroplacental blood flow may

Table 14.6 Exercise prescription for muscular conditioning. (Modified from *PARmed-X for Pregnancy* document, 1996 with permission of the Canadian Society for Exercise Physiology)

Category	Purpose	Example
Upper back	Promotion of good posture	Shoulder shrugs, shoulder blade pinch
Lower back	Promotion of good posture	Modified standing opposite leg and arm lifts
Abdomen	Promotion of good posture, prevention of low-back pain, prevention of diastasis recti, strengthen muscles of labour	Abdominal tightening, abdominal curl-ups, head raises, lying on side or standing position
Pelvic floor ('Kegels')	Promotion of good bladder control, prevention of urinary incontinence	'Wave', 'elevator'
Upper body	Improve muscular support for breasts	Shoulder rotations, modified push-ups against a wall
Buttocks, lower limbs	Facilitation of weight-bearing, prevention of varicose veins	Buttocks squeeze, standing leg lifts, heel raises

be reduced by 65% (Skillman & Clark, 1987). The physician must ask the athlete why she wants to pursue such high-intensity training while pregnant. In this situation, the risks to the fetus far outweigh any maternal benefits and reduction in intensity and duration would be highly recommended. The physician or exercise professional can utilize the 'talk test' for a highly motivated athlete, as this may be a safe way to prescribe exercise to an individual who may not fall within the guidelines suggested above for aerobic exercise. For the well-conditioned athlete the precautions for muscle conditioning are the same as above.

The literature describing the effects of high-intensity exercise on mother and fetus are limited. Historically, most of the data presented are from case studies of women athletes or retrospective reports, not randomly designed trials. Pregnancy outcome in athletic women has been reviewed by Wolfe et al. (1989). Briefly, Zaharieva (1972) studied pregnancy outcome in women who participated in the Olympic Games between 1952 and 1972 ($n=27$), women who were masters of sport ($n=59$) and those who were 'first-grade' athletes ($n=64$); the percentage of women who continued to train during pregnancy was 63%, 76% and 77%, respectively. Of the Olympic athletes, 70% had no pregnancy complications and the remainder had only 'mild complaints'. The masters of sport athletes had somewhat higher rates of birth complications. Erdelyi (1962) found shorter labour times on average and lower frequencies of toxaemia, Caesarean section and threatened abortion in 172 Hungarian athletes compared with 150 sedentary women. Two-thirds of the athletes continued to exercise during the first 3–4 months of pregnancy, but the average level of intensity and the number of women who continued to exercise for the remainder of pregnancy were not reported (Erdelyi, 1962). A more recent retrospective study (also not randomly controlled) assessed the effects of a vigorous exercise programme into late pregnancy on birth weight. The results indicated that women who exercised vigorously more than four sessions per week past 25 weeks

of gestation gave birth to babies weighing 315 g lower than control patients (Bell et al., 1995).

Maternal physiological responses to strenuous exercise

As described above, it is well established that healthy pregnant women experiencing a normal pregnancy can participate safely in regular, moderate aerobic and muscular conditioning programmes. Unfortunately, very little information exists on the effects of strenuous physical conditioning involving competitive and recreational female athletes (Wolfe et al., 1994a; Hale & Milne, 1996).

In recent years, a number of studies have been published that describe maternal and fetal responses to single bouts of maximal or near-maximal exercise. The effects of pregnancy on maximal aerobic power remain controversial and results may depend on whether or not women change their level of habitual exercise (Wolfe et al., 1989). The results of Clapp and Capeless (1991), who studied active women before pregnancy and 6–8, 12–20 and 36–44 weeks after giving birth, indicated that continuation of moderate training throughout pregnancy and the early postpartum period may result in small but significant increases in $\dot{V}O_{2max}$ in the postpartum period compared with before pregnancy. Anecdotal reports have also shown that élite endurance athletes may enhance their personal best performances after childbirth.

Other studies of performance during strenuous exercise suggest that maximal exercise heart rate is moderately attenuated in mid to late gestation (Lotgering et al., 1991, 1992). Since resting heart rate is already augmented, heart rate increases at a slower rate in response to increases in $\dot{V}O_{2max}$ (Sady et al., 1989; Pivarnik et al., 1990; Wolfe et al., 1990; Lotgering et al., 1992) and maximal heart rate reserve is reduced (Wolfe & Mottola, 1993) in late gestation compared with the non-pregnant state.

Important pregnancy-induced changes in lactate metabolism have also been described. Two laboratories have recently reported that the ventilatory anaerobic threshold (an indicator of the onset of blood lactate accumulation) is not significantly altered by pregnancy (Wolfe *et al.*, 1994b; Lotgering *et al.*, 1995). However, peak values for the respiratory exchange ratio (RER) (Lotgering *et al.*, 1991, 1995; Wolfe *et al.*, 1994b) during maximal exercise tests and peak post-exercise blood lactate concentrations (Clapp *et al.*, 1987; McMurray *et al.*, 1988; Wolfe *et al.*, 1994b; Spinnewijn *et al.*, 1996) appear to be blunted. Presumably, the blunted peak RER values reflect a reduced need for respiratory compensation for lactic acidosis (Wolfe *et al.*, 1994b; Lotgering *et al.*, 1995). Reduced blood lactate levels following strenuous exercise in late gestation may result from dilution of lactate produced in an expanded maternal blood volume (McMurray *et al.*, 1988), fetal use of lactate as a metabolic fuel (Burd *et al.*, 1975) or increased maternal peripheral insulin resistance which appears in late pregnancy. Some evidence also suggests that aerobic conditioning may help to preserve the ability to exercise anaerobically and produce lactate in late gestation (Wolfe *et al.*, 1994b). Finally, the recent findings of Kemp *et al.* (1997) confirm that pregnant women are able to maintain lower blood hydrogen ion concentrations both at rest and following maximal exercise stress compared with the non-pregnant state.

Fetal responses to strenuous maternal exercise

As described in a recent review on maternal exercise, fetal well-being and pregnancy outcome (Wolfe *et al.*, 1994a), a substantial body of evidence exists to confirm that the most common fetal response to sustained aerobic exercise is a transient increase in fetal heart rate (FHR) from baseline. The findings of Clapp *et al.* (1993) suggest that the degree of elevation of FHR is related directly to the intensity and duration of exercise and becomes more pronounced with advancing gestational age. Increased FHR during and following such exercise may be the result of increased fetal temperature, transfer of maternal catecholamines across the placenta, an increased state of fetal wakefulness or activity,

mild fetal hypoxia or a combination of these factors. Fetal deceleratory responses (bradycardia, increased FHR decelerations that may indicate significant fetal hypoxia) appear to be rare during moderate maternal exercise where maternal heart rate does not exceed about 150 beats·min^{-1}.

Recent studies suggest that FHR responses to maximal exercise testing may differ in sedentary vs. athletic populations. For example, Carpenter *et al.* (1988) reported fetal bradycardia (defined as FHR <110 beats·min^{-1} for ≥10 s) following 15 of 79 maximal cycling tests (16.2%). Subjects were healthy sedentary women studied at 25±3 weeks' gestation using two-dimensional echocardiography. Similarly, Watson *et al.* (1991) studied the FHR responses of 13 healthy inactive women (gestational ages 25 and 35 weeks) to maximal cycling and tethered swimming tests. Transient fetal bradycardia (defined as a decrease in FHR ≥20 beats·min^{-1} from pre-exercise baseline) was observed following about 15% of these tests and was more frequent during cycling than swimming and at 35 vs. 25 weeks' gestation. Three more recent studies that involved maximal cycle ergometer testing of moderately active pregnant subjects (Lotgering *et al.*, 1992; Spinnewijn *et al.*, 1996; Kemp *et al.*, 1997) have reported transient exercise-induced increases in FHR baseline but no incidences of fetal bradycardia. In our experience, such tests are also accompanied by a transient postexercise reduction in FHR reactivity.

Some evidence exists to support the concept that maternal physical conditioning may cause beneficial fetal and placental effects. For example, Webb *et al.* (1994) employed a controlled longitudinal study design to examine the effects of moderate aerobic conditioning on FHR responses to exercise in healthy, previously sedentary women. During steady-state exercise tests (maternal heart rate target 145 beats·min^{-1}) conducted in late gestation, FHR responses to exercise (gradual increase in FHR normal variability and reactivity) were similar even though the conditioned subjects were exercising at significantly higher work rates. Clapp and Rizk

(1992) have also reported that increases in placental volume during the first 24 weeks of pregnancy were significantly greater in recreational athletes ($n=18$) who continued to exercise regularly compared with previously active women ($n=16$) who discontinued regular exercise during pregnancy. Although much more research is needed, these studies suggest that maternal and/or placental responses to physical conditioning may have important fetoprotective effects.

Postpartum exercise

Many women are concerned about when they can safely return to exercise after the baby is born. The interval before returning to an aerobic exercise regimen depends upon the number of complications during labour and delivery. If labour and delivery are uncomplicated, a woman can usually return to aerobic exercise after vaginal bleeding from delivery has stopped and/or her postpartum check-up from her physician is normal. It is recommended that she begin her exercise programme by aiming for the same target heart rate zone (Table 14.4) and by following the same guidelines as if she were pregnant. Avoiding unnecessary fatigue is an important consideration for any new mother and returning to exercise too quickly and exercising too intensely are not recommended. If the woman has had a Caesarean section or complications during labour and delivery, it is suggested that she wait at least 10 weeks or until labour and delivery complications have healed or returned to normal.

Muscular conditioning exercises are also recommended after birth. It is suggested that these exercises be resumed after the first postpartum check-up and vaginal bleeding due to delivery has stopped. Kegel exercises for the pelvic floor are important and can be continued as soon as the woman feels well enough to start them. These exercises may help to strengthen pelvic floor muscles weakened during a vaginal delivery and may help postpartum incontinence. Abdominal exercises can also be started and may be performed in the supine position. Women who have experienced diastasis recti during pregnancy are advised to proceed with extra care and start abdominal exercise slowly, gradually building up the number of repetitions.

Lactation and the athlete

Altemus et al. (1995) studied the responses of 10 lactating and 10 non-lactating women between 7 and 18 weeks after birth to 20 min of graded treadmill exercise; the last 5 min of exercise was to elicit 90% $\dot{V}O_{2max}$ for each subject. The lactating women had attenuated responses for plasma adrenocorticotrophic hormone, cortisol and glucose due to the exercise. Basal noradrenaline levels were also decreased in the lactating women. The authors suggested that lactating women may have neurohormonal systems that are restrained during stress-responsive tasks such as treadmill exercise (Altemus et al., 1995). This may explain why mild to moderate exercise has little adverse effect on milk quality or quantity or on infant weight gain (Dewey et al., 1994).

Infants are able to detect sweet and sour tastes (Wallace et al., 1992). The literature has suggested that after exercise infants may refuse to nurse or may fuss during a feeding because of an increase in the lactic acid content of the milk, producing a sour taste (Wallace et al., 1992). Maximal exercise has been shown to increase the amount of lactic acid in breast milk, which leads to diminished acceptance of the milk after exercise (Wallace et al., 1992). In addition, animal studies have suggested that strenuous exercise continued through lactation exaggerated further the growth restriction seen in the offspring (Pinto & Shetty, 1995). However, aerobic exercise at 60–70% $\dot{V}O_{2max}$ performed four or five times per week beginning at 6–8 weeks after birth had no adverse effect on lactation (Dewey et al., 1994), nor did an aerobic programme ($\dot{V}O_{2max}$ improved 25%) performed for 45 min, 5 days per week for 12 weeks (Lovelady et al., 1995). It seems that mild to moderate exercise is well tolerated in lactating women (Dewey & McCrory, 1994; Prentice, 1994; Spaaij et al., 1994), although strenuous (near-maximum) aerobic activity should be avoided until lactation is terminated.

Conclusion

Healthy pregnant women with no contraindications to exercise may perform mild- to moderate-intensity activity safely within the current guidelines with no adverse effects on fetal growth and development. There are limited scientific data on the effects of high-intensity training on pregnancy and fetal outcome. Studies examining the effects of maximal and peak exercise on maternal and fetal well-being are few in number but are becoming more common. At present, with limited information, it would seem that the healthy pregnant woman and the fetus appear to tolerate the effects of an acute bout of peak to maximal exercise satisfactorily, although more studies must be completed. The effects of high-intensity endurance training on pregnancy and fetal outcome are largely unknown and must be determined before advice can be given to the pregnant athlete. Common sense suggests that women athletes should not compete while pregnant, especially in sports where bodily injury or contact may occur. In addition, the intensity of exercise training should be reduced to moderate because the effects of strenuous exercise on the pregnant athlete and on fetal outcome are largely unknown.

Acknowledgement

The authors have received financial support for exercise/pregnancy research from the US Army Medical Research and Material Command Contract #DAMD-17–96-C-6112.

References

Altemus, M., Deuster, P.A., Galliven, E., Carter, C.S. & Gold, P.W. (1995) Suppression of hypothalamic–pituitary–adrenal axis responses to stress in lactating women. *Journal of Clinical Endocrinology and Metabolism* **80**, 2954–2959.

American College of Obstetricians and Gynecologists (1994) Exercise during pregnancy and the post partum period. *ACOG Technical Bulletin* **189**, 2–7.

Bell, A.W., Hales, J.R.S., King, R.B. & Fawcett, A.A. (1983) Influence of heat stress on exercise-induced changes in regional blood flow in sheep. *Journal of Applied Physiology* **55**, 1916–1923.

Bell, R.J., Palma, S.M. & Lumley, J.M. (1995) The effect of vigorous exercise during pregnancy on birth-weight. *Australian and New Zealand Journal of Obstetrics and Gynaecology* **35**, 46–51.

Bonen, A., Campagna, P., Gilchrist, L., Young, D.C. & Beresford, P. (1992) Substrate and endocrine responses during exercise at selected stages of pregnancy. *Journal of Applied Physiology* **73**, 134–142.

Borg, G. (1962) A category scale with ratio properties for intermodal and interindividual comparision. In H.G. Geissler and P. Petzold (eds) *Psychophysical Judgement and the Process of Perception.* Deutscher Verlag der Wissenschaften, Berlin.

Burd, L.I., Jones, M.D., Simmons, M.A., Makowski, E.L., Meschia, G. & Battaglia, F.C. (1975) Placental production and foetal utilisation of lactate and pyruvate. *Nature* **254**, 710–711.

Canadian Society for Exercise Physiology (1996) *PARmed-X for Pregnancy.* CSEP, Health Canada, Ottawa, Ontario, Canada.

Carpenter, M.W., Sady, S.P., Hoegsborg, B. *et al.* (1988) Fetal heart rate response to maternal exertion. *Journal of the American Medical Association* **259**, 3006–3009.

Clapp, J.F. III (1996a) Pregnancy outcome: physical activities inside vs. outside the workplace. *Seminars in Perinatology* **20**, 70–76.

Clapp, J.F. III (1996b) Morphometric and neurodevelopmental outcome at age five years of the offspring of women who continued to exercise regularly throughout pregnancy. *Journal of Pediatrics* **129**, 856–863.

Clapp, J.F. III & Capeless, E. (1991) The $\dot{V}o_{2max}$ of recreational athletes before and after pregnancy. *Medicine and Science in Sports and Exercise* **23**, 1128–1133.

Clapp, J.F. III & Dickstein, S. (1984) Endurance exercise and pregnancy outcome. *Medicine and Science in Sports and Exercise* **16**, 556–562.

Clapp, J.F. III & Rizk, K.D. (1992) Effect of recreational exercise on midtrimester placental growth. *American Journal of Obstetrics and Gynecology* **167**, 1518–1521.

Clapp, J.F. III, Wesley, M. & Sleamaker, R.H. (1987) Thermoregulatory and metabolic responses to jogging prior to and during pregnancy. *Medicine and Science in Sports and Exercise* **19**, 124–130.

Clapp, J.F. III, Little, K.D. & Capeless, E.L. (1993) Fetal heart rate response to sustained recreational exercise. *American Journal of Obstetrics and Gynecology* **168**, 198–206.

Dewey, K.G. & McCrory, M.A. (1994) Effects of dieting

and physical activity on pregnancy and lactation. *American Journal of Clinical Nutrition* **59**, 446S–452S.

Dewey, K.G., Lovelady, C.A., Nommsen-Rivers, L.A., McCrory, M.A. & Lonnerdal, B. (1994) A randomized study of the effects of aerobic exercise by lactating women on breast-milk volume and composition. *New England Journal of Medicine* **330**, 449–453.

Erdelyi, G.J. (1962) Gynecological survey of female athletes. *Journal of Sports Medicine and Physical Fitness* **2**, 174–179.

Gilbert, R.D., Lis, L. & Longo, L.D. (1985) Temperature effects on oxygen affinity of human fetal blood. *Journal of Developmental Physiology* **7**, 299–304.

Hale, R.W. & Milne, L. (1996) The elite athlete and exercise in pregnancy. *Seminars in Perinatology* **20**, 277–284.

Hatch, M.C., Shu, X., McLean, D.E. *et al.* (1993) Maternal exercise during pregnancy, physical fitness and fetal growth. *American Journal of Epidemiology* **137**, 1105–1114.

Hay, W.W., Myers, S.A., Sparks, J.W., Wilkening, R.B., Meschia, G. & Battaglia, F.C. (1983) Glucose and lactate oxidation rates in the fetal lamb. *Proceedings of the Society for Experimental Biology and Medicine* **173**, 553–563.

Jones, M.T., Norton, K.I., Dengel, D.R. & Armstrong, R.B. (1990) Effects of training on reproductive tissue blood flow in exercising pregnant rats. *Journal of Applied Physiology* **69**, 2097–2103.

Jones, M.T., Rawson, R.E., Riplog, S. & Robertshaw, D. (1991) Oxygen consumption and uterine blood flow in exercising pregnant sheep (Abstract). *Medicine and Science in Sports and Exercise* **23**, S169.

Kemp, J.G., Greer, F.A. & Wolfe, L.A. (1997) Acid–base regulation following maximal exercise testing in late gestation. *Journal of Applied Physiology* **83**, 644–651.

Lotgering, F.K., Gilbert, R.D. & Longo, L.D. (1983a) Exercise responses in pregnant sheep: oxygen consumption, uterine blood flow and blood volume. *Journal of Applied Physiology* **55**, 834–841.

Lotgering, F.K., Gilbert, R.D. & Longo, L.D. (1983b) Exercise responses in pregnant sheep: blood gases, temperatures and fetal cardiovascular responses. *Journal of Applied Physiology* **55**, 842–850.

Lotgering, F.K., Van Doorn, M.K., Struijk, P.C., Pool, J. & Wallenberg, H.C.S. (1991) Maximal aerobic exercise in pregnant women: heart rate, O_2 consumption, CO_2 production, and ventilation. *Journal of Applied Physiology* **70**, 1016–1023.

Lotgering, F.K., Struijk, P.C., Van Doorn, M.B. & Wallenberg, H.C.S. (1992) Errors in predicting maximal oxygen consumption in pregnant women. *Journal of Applied Physiology* **72**, 562–567.

Lotgering, F.K., Struijk, P.C., Van Doorn, M.B., Spinnewijn, W.E.M. & Wallenberg, H.C.S. (1995) Anaerobic threshold and respiratory compensation in pregnant women. *Journal of Applied Physiology* **78**, 1772–1777.

Lovelady, C.A., Nommsen-Rivers, L.A., McCrory, M.A. & Dewey, K.G. (1995) Effects of exercise on plasma lipids and metabolism of lactating women. *Medicine and Science in Sports and Exercise* **27**, 22–28.

McMurray, R.G., Katz, V.L., Berry, M.J. & Cefalo, R.C. (1988) The effect of pregnancy on metabolic responses during rest, immersion and aerobic exercise in the water. *American Journal of Obstetrics and Gynecology* **158**, 481–486.

Mostello, D., Chalk, C. & Khoury, J. (1991) Chronic anemia in pregnant ewes: maternal and fetal effects. *American Journal of Physiology* **261**, R1075–R1083.

Mottola, M.F., Fitzgerald, H.M., Wilson, N.C. & Taylor, A.W. (1993) Effect of water temperature on exercise-induced maternal hyperthermia on fetal development in rats. *International Journal of Sports Medicine* **14**, 248–251.

Pinto, M.L. & Shetty, P.S. (1995) Influence of exercise-induced maternal stress on fetal outcome in Wistar rats: inter-generational effects. *British Journal of Nutrition* **73**, 645–653.

Pivarnik, J.M., Lee, W., Clark, S.L., Cotton, D.B., Spillman, H.T. & Miller, J.F. (1990) Cardiac output responses of primigravid women during exercise determined by the direct Fick technique. *Obstetrics and Gynecology* **75**, 954–959.

Prentice, A. (1994) Should lactating women exercise? *Nutrition Reviews* **52**, 358–360.

Sady, S.P., Carpenter, M.W., Thompson, P.D., Sady, M.A., Haydon, B. & Coustan, D.R. (1989) Cardiovascular response to cycle exercise during and after pregnancy. *Journal of Applied Physiology* **66**, 336–341.

Sasaki, J., Yamaguchi, A., Nabeshima, Y., Shigemitsu, S., Mesaki, N. & Kubo, T. (1995) Exercise at high temperature causes maternal hyperthermia and fetal anomalies in rats. *Teratology* **51**, 233–236.

Schauberger, C.W., Rooney, B.L., Goldsmith, L., Shenton, D., Silva, P.D. & Schaper, A. (1996) Peripheral joint laxity increases in pregnancy but does not correlate with serum relaxin levels. *American Journal of Obstetrics and Gynecology* **174**, 667–671.

Skillman, C.A. & Clark, K.E. (1987) Fetal beta-endorphin levels in response to reductions in uterine blood flow. *Biology of the Neonate* **51**, 217–223.

Soultanakis, H.N., Artal., R. & Wiswell, R.A. (1996) Prolonged exercise in pregnancy: glucose homeostasis, ventilatory and cardiovascular responses. *Seminars in Perinatology* **20**, 315–327.

Spaaij, C.J., van Raaij, J.M., deGroot, L.C., vander Heijden, L.J., Boekholt, H.A. & Hautvast, J.G. (1994) Effect of lactation on resting metabolic rate and on diet- and work-induced thermogenesis. *American Journal of Clinical Nutrition* **59**, 42–47.

Sparks, J.W., Hay, W.W., Bonds, D., Meschia, G. &

Battaglia, F.C. (1982) Simultaneous measurements of lactate turnover rate and umbilical lactate uptake in the fetal lamb. *Journal of Clinical Investigation* **70**, 179–192.

Spinnewijn, W.E.M., Wallenberg, H.C.S., Struijk, P.C. & Lotgering, F.K. (1996) Peak ventilatory responses during cycling and swimming in pregnant and non-pregnant women. *Journal of Applied Physiology* **81**, 738–742.

Stevenson, L. (1997) Exercise in pregnancy. Part 1: update on pathophysiology. *Canadian Family Physician* **43**, 97–104.

Wallace, J.P., Inbar, G. & Ernsthausen, K. (1992) Infant acceptance of postexercise breast milk. *Pediatrics* **89**, 1245–1247.

Watson, W.J., Katz, V.L., Hackney, A.C., Gall, M.M. & McMurray, R.G. (1991) Fetal responses to maximal swimming and cycling exercise during pregnancy. *Obstetrics and Gynecology* **77**, 382–386.

Webb, K.A., Wolfe, L.A. & McGrath, M.J. (1994) Effects of acute and chronic maternal exercise on fetal heart rate. *Journal of Applied Physiology* **97**, 2207–2213.

Wolfe, L.A. & Mottola, M.F. (1993) Aerobic exercise in pregnancy: an update. *Canadian Journal of Applied Physiology* **18**, 119–147.

Wolfe, L.A., Ohtake, P.J., Mottola, M.F. & McGrath, M.J. (1989) Physiological interactions between pregnancy and aerobic exercise. *Exercise and Sport Sciences Reviews* **17**, 295–351.

Wolfe, L.A., Ohtake, P.J., George, K.A. & McGrath, M.J. (1990) Aerobic training effects on exercise hemodynamics during pregnancy (Abstract). *Medicine and Science in Sports and Exercise* **22**, S28.

Wolfe, L.A., Brenner, I.K.M. & Mottola, M.F. (1994a) Maternal exercise, fetal well-being and pregnancy outcome. *Exercise and Sport Sciences Reviews* **22**, 145–194.

Wolfe, L.A., Walker, R.M.C., Bonen, A. & McGrath, M.J. (1994b) Effects of pregnancy and chronic exercise on respiratory responses to graded exercise. *Journal of Applied Physiology* **76**, 1928–1934.

Zaharieva, E. (1972) Olympic participation by women. Effects on pregnancy and child birth. *Journal of the American Medical Association* **221**, 992–995.

Chapter 15

Musculoskeletal Injuries

ELIZABETH ARENDT AND LETHA GRIFFIN

Introduction

The musculoskeletal system is composed of bones and their articulated surfaces (joints) and surrounding soft tissues, including ligaments, muscles and tendons. Acute and overuse injuries to the periarticular soft tissues are the most common sports injuries. The pertinent anatomy and physiology of these structures are discussed as these concepts provide a central and recurrent theme in evaluation of acute and overuse injuries of soft-tissue musculoskeletal structures.

Pathophysiology of injured musculoskeletal tissue

An acute injury is created by a single episode of force that results in damage to musculoskeletal tissue. This force can be external, such as a direct blow to a limb, or internal, such as a non-contact rotational injury of a limb. An acute injury is typically characterized by immediate onset of pain and dysfunction of varying degrees. Swelling is typically present immediately or within several hours of the injury. An acute injury to the knee joint is a common sports experience; the approach to and evaluation of this complex joint can be directed towards individual intra-articular structures (Arendt, 1995).

Treatment for an acute injury to the musculoskeletal system varies with the magnitude of the injury, the location and the structure injured. However, the acronym PRICE is useful for remembering *p*rotection of the injured part, *r*est or relative rest of the injured part, *i*ce, compression and *e*levation. In general, acute injuries to the musculoskeletal system should be evaluated by trained personnel who understand the magnitude of the injury before return to activity is advised.

An overuse injury is characterized by the absence of a specific injury, or at least no injury significant enough to explain the current clinical situation. An overuse injury is repetitive submaximal/subclinical trauma that results in macroscopic or microscopic damage to an area. This is thought to result from damage to a structural unit and/or its blood supply. This injury is characterized by a *change* of circumstance. The transitional athlete (an athlete with a change in her internal or external environment) is at high risk for the development of overuse injuries (Table 15.1).

Treatment of overuse injuries typically requires time for healing. Rest or relative rest of the injured part by reducing activities, substituting activities and/or protecting the injured part during activities is advised Further treatment recommendations are reviewed in Table 15.2. Important elements in the treatment of overuse injuries are education of the athlete in the causative factors of injury, understanding of the progression from injury to health including activity modification, and implementation of a paced return to activity. Education is also the best treatment for prevention of future overuse injuries.

Table 15.1 Characterization of the transitional athlete

Change in training
    Intensity (distance/time, frequency, duration)
    Footwear changes
    Surface changes, including material composition
        and slope
Change in competitive climate
Weather conditions
Life-cycle changes
    Puberty
    Ageing
    Pregnancy and after birth
    Menopause

Table 15.2 Treatment of overuse injuries

Reduce inflammation/pain
Non-steroidal anti-inflammatory drugs
Physical therapy modalities
Relative rest of injured part
Ice
Compression if swelling is present

Correct anatomical problems when possible
Patella sleeve
Orthotics to control foot overpronation
Surgery (rare)

Correct biomechanical errors
Training sequence
Sports style and form
Stretching and strengthening of musculoskeletal units
    (agonist/antagonist)

Correct environmental concerns when possible
Shoes and equipment concerns
Environmental concerns including running surface
Adequate clothing in the cold

Sports-specific rehabilitation
Recovery of strength (emphasis on
    closed-chain/eccentric strengthening)
Maintenance of endurance and aerobic fitness
Maintenance of flexibility of the kinematics (motion)
    linkage system

Tendons

Tendons are strong, closely packed collagen bundles that attach muscle to bone. Tendons are some of the strongest soft-tissue structures in the body and their nutrition is primarily provided by the vascular system. However, in heavily sheathed regions where the tendon is avascular, nutrition can come from diffusion of synovial fluid. Tendons are connected to muscles and due to their strength most can withstand tensile forces greater than those exerted by their muscles. Therefore, it is uncommon to have a mid-substance rupture of tendons. When a mid-substance tendon rupture occurs, most physicians feel it requires a pre-existing pathological condition. This is seen in chronic overuse injuries where there is intersubstance weakening of that tendon. Exercise has a positive long-term effect on the mechanical properties of tendons, increasing stiffness, ultimate force and weight. Age can alter these mechanical properties by increasing collagen cross-linkage and other factors that adversely affect the ultimate biomechanical strength of tendons. These biomechanical and material changes occur by the third decade of life and may contribute to chronic overuse tendon injuries. The role of unique cyclical hormones in women and their effect on the biology of musculoskeletal soft tissues is not well understood. The decline in oestrogen levels that occurs in the fourth and fifth decades of a woman's life may negatively affect the health of tendons and increase the frequency and severity of overuse injuries in this age group.

After an acute injury to a tendon, inflammatory products brought to the area by blood vessels invade the area around the injured tendon. Collagen and fibroblast production increase significantly in the first several weeks. Secondary remodelling begins approximately 3–4 weeks after injury. This remodelling can continue up to 4–5 months after injury, when the vascularity and cellularity of the healing tendon are minimally different from that of normal tendon.

Overuse injuries to tendons are common in sport. Few data exist concerning the healing response in soft tissues exposed to repetitive overuse or overload. This is an area of intense investigation since such injuries commonly occur in the workplace as well as in sport. There is currently no well-defined animal or cellular model for the study of overuse or overload syndromes. Chronic tendon overload and injury occur at sites of high exposure to repetitive tensile load. Common sites are the rotator cuff tendons of the shoulders, Achilles tendon complex of the calf muscles, and medial and lateral epicondylar regions of the elbows. Although traditionally overuse and overload injuries were seen in middle-aged recreational athletes and thought to be related to the ageing process, overuse injuries are now documented in virtually every age group, particularly young élite athletes exposed to high levels of repetitive load and young athletes involved in programmes that emphasize an intense training schedule.

Tendon overuse injuries near the bony end of the tendon insertion, i.e. the tendo-osseus junction, are attributed to tendinitis or a low-grade inflammatory condition. Tendinitis is rare at the musculotendinous junction, the junction where muscle meets tendon. It is in this region that muscle strain is most common (see section on Muscle, p. 211). Despite the fact that these tendon injuries are called tendinitis, the role that inflammation plays is not clear. Chronic degenerative changes and the absence of inflammation are typically found on pathological review of surgical cases of these tendon injuries. These chronic degenerative changes and the absence of inflammation are more appropriately termed 'tendinosis'. Tendinosis is frequently observed in cases of spontaneous tendon rupture and may be clinically silent until rupture occurs. The causes of tendon failure remain speculative. It is probable that a focal microscopic tendon injury occurs or perhaps a microscopic tear. Incomplete healing follows. The physiological range of load necessary for maintenance of normal tendon function is not known. Similarly, the threshold and conditions responsible for tendon injury are not known. The kind of environment that might be pertinent to a sports-related injury cannot be completely duplicated. Such an environment involves a complex interaction between temperature, hormonal factors secondary to excitement

and competition, and the role each individual tendon plays in the complex orchestration of other muscle tendon units in the limb. A number of other factors, including anatomical location, vascular supply of the tissue, magnitude of the applied force and position of the limb at the time of the applied force, all come together to create an injury. Alterations in the vascular supply to the tendon due to age or repetitive load may affect the capacity for a tendon to heal in minor repetitive injuries, instituting the development of chronic degenerative change. Intrinsic repair may be affected by growth or hormonal factors, including oestrogen, although these changes are not well understood.

The vast majority of tendon overuse injuries respond to a combination of rest or relative rest of the injured part, stretching, passive physical therapy modalities and intermittent use of non-steroidal anti-inflammatory medication. Selective strengthening of the muscle, particularly eccentric strengthening, is thought to be helpful in the repair process. A grading system of sports-induced inflammation is provided in Table 15.3. This grading scheme is useful for the clinician as it is designed to quantify subjective symptoms and relate them to physical findings, with a strategy for relevant therapeutic measures. However, little pathological or scientific documentation exists for this grading system.

Of patients with an overuse injury, 15–20% may present with multiple sites of tendinopathy and have been classified as having a mesenchymal syndrome. Rheumatological evaluation typically shows no abnormality. The cause of this mesenchymal syndrome is not known at present. This syndrome is more common in women and usually presents in the third to fourth decade of life (Griffin, 1994).

Ligaments

Ligaments are short bands of fibrous connective tissue that connect and stabilize bones at their articulated surfaces (joints). Ligaments and tendons are biomechanically and structurally different: ligaments contain a lower percentage

Table 15.3 Grading of sports-induced inflammation. (From Leadbetter, 1990 with permission)

Grade	Pain pattern	Physical signs	Relevant therapeutic measures
I	Pain only after activity; duration of symptoms < 2 weeks	Generalized soreness	Proper warm-up and conditioning; avoidance of abrupt transition in activity level
II	Pain during and after activity; no significant functional disability	Localized pain; minimal or no other signs of inflammation	Analysis of technique and efficiency; decrease in abusive training; improved conditioning
III	Pain during and after activity; significant functional disability; duration of symptoms > 6 weeks	Intense point tenderness with prominent inflammation (oedema, effusion, erythema, crepitus, etc.)	Structural vulnerability; protected activity with sports modification; substitutions of sports activity to avoid excessive load
IV	Constant pain; significant functional disability; unable to train or compete; impending tissue failure	Grade III symptoms plus tissue breakdown, atrophy, etc.	Surgery (fibrogenesis, repair, structural alteration); possible permanent withdrawal from activity (as in degenerative joint disease)

of collagen and a higher percentage of extracellular matrix with a more random collagen alignment. Ligaments rely on diffusion as well as a vascular supply for adequate nutrition.

Healing of an acute ligament injury is a complex process and is influenced by both local and systemic factors. However, it appears that healing of extra-articular ligaments more closely parallels that of tendons. This includes ligament injuries around the finger and ankle, as well as collateral ligament injuries around the knee, in particular the medial collateral ligament. Healing of intra-articular ligaments is less well understood. However, it is known that prolonged immobilization of a ligament results in significant compromise of ligament properties. Resumption of joint motion and load application results in a slow, progressive recovery of the material properties of ligaments. This process, the recovery of normal ultimate force and energy absorbed to failure, can take 8–12 months for ligaments. The alterations in ligament properties are reversible if immobilization is not prolonged. Most treatment protocols for injured ligaments try to incorporate mobilization and exercise into the repair process. Reapplication of the load necessary for recovery of normal function and the

minimal amount of load necessary to increase the strength of the ligament without compromising its length or function is not well understood. Recovery of normal function is affected by age and other local and systemic factors, including hormonal influences. The role of oestrogen in normal and pathological states of ligament function is currently being investigated (Hart *et al.*, 1996; Sciore *et al.*, 1997; Slaughterbeck *et al.*, 1997).

Muscle

Muscle strain injuries account for more than half the injuries occurring in some sports. The most common type of muscle injury is a muscle strain. If the magnitude of force and its direction of application is greater than a musculoskeletal unit can resist, an acute injury occurs. Certain muscles have several features in common that predispose them to acute strain injuries. These include muscles that cross two joints, a configuration that may facilitate passive restraint of one joint by the position of its adjacent joint (hamstring muscle, rectus femoris muscle, groin muscles, gastrocnemius muscle). These muscles tend to be composed of a large percentage of type IIB fibres that work primarily during eccentric contractions. Ultrastructurally, eccentric muscle contractions have been shown to cause severe myofibrillar disorganization and cytoskeletal segregation, commonly associated with 'delayed muscle soreness'. Forceful eccentric contractions, particularly against a limb that is trying to elongate, can place stresses on the muscle. The weakest component of the muscle–tendon unit is typically the musculotendinous junction. Clinical and experimental observations suggest that most of these strains do occur at the muscle–tendon junction, although the reasons for this are poorly understood.

An acute muscle strain initiates a complex sequence of cellular mechanisms. These can be divided into inflammatory, proliferative and maturation phases. The inflammatory phase begins immediately after injury with an influx of blood and/or plasma into the injury site and formation of a fibrin clot. Muscle maturation and regeneration is complete approximately 6 months after injury in humans. Although individual muscle fibres may contract normally after regeneration, whole-muscle contractile function rarely is normal after gross skeletal muscle injury and repair. After a muscle strain has healed, there can be stiffness and initial flexibility can be limited in the muscle–tendon unit. Keeping the area warm, e.g. use of a thigh sleeve after a hamstring strain, and emphasis on warm-up before intense play are critical in order to reduce the risk of further muscle injury.

Muscle strengthening is thought to decrease the likelihood of a strain injury by increasing the energy-absorbing capacity of the muscle–tendon unit. Additionally, strain injury increases with muscle fatigue. Muscle strengthening, in particular endurance strengthening, will decrease muscle fatigue. Cyclic stretching of the muscle–tendon unit increases tissue compliance. Any stretching that causes direct tissue damage must be avoided. Stretching should not be done 'cold', but rather after the body has warmed up. Stretching to pain sends a signal to the brain to contract the muscle; the muscle is trying to resist the pain. Therefore, the athlete should stretch just to the point of discomfort, back off a bit and then

hold this position for a count of 10. Increased intramuscular temperature, i.e. warm-up, benefits the biomechanical properties of muscle by decreasing the stiffness of the musculotendinous unit (Garrett, 1990). Within physiological range, stretch is resisted largely by myofibril interaction. Beyond that range, most of the tension is taken up by connective tissue elements, particularly at the musculotendinous junction.

Sports injuries

Sports injury results from a complex interaction of risk factors. Risk factors can be classified into two categories: (i) extrinsic factors, which are related to the type of sports activity, the manner in which a sport is practised, environmental conditions and the equipment used to play a sport; and (ii) intrinsic factors, which are individual, physical and psychosocial characteristics (Lysens et al., 1984) (Table 15.4).

Increasing numbers of women and girls began participating in sports in the 1970s. In the USA, this increased participation in sports at the secondary school and college levels paralleled the passage of Title IX. However, passage of Title IX coincided with a more universal women's movement, which in turn led to increased recognition for, and acceptance of, the talent and skill levels of women both inside and outside the athletic arena.

Early studies maintained that sports injuries sustained by female athletes were no different from those of men (Calvert, 1975/1976; Haycock & Gillette, 1976). Whiteside (1980) and Clarke and Buckley (1980) independently concluded that, with regard to injury, there was a greater difference *between* different sports than between the injuries of men and women within the same sport. Thus, it was felt that sports injury was largely dictated by the type of sport and was not necessarily influenced by gender. Early studies of the first female military cadets helped establish women's physiological capabilities in conditioned and non-conditioned states, suggesting that many performance variables resulted from improper conditioning for young

Table 15.4 Risk factors for sports injury

Extrinsic factors
Equipment
  Equipment worn, including protective equipment
  Footwear
  Free-standing equipment (e.g. the uneven parallel
    bars in gymnastics, the high jump apparatus and
    pit in track and field)
Environment
  Type and condition of playing surface
  Weather conditions
  Time of day
Exposure
  Playing time
  Position on the team
  Knowledge of sport and its rules
Training

Intrinsic factors
Physical characteristics
  Age
  Sex
  Somatotype
  Previous injuries
  Joint instability
  Joint hypermobility (tissue-laxity factors)
  History of previous injuries
  Alignment of the lower extremity
Psychosocial characteristics

women (Tomasi *et al.*, 1977; Lenz, 1979; Protzman, 1979).

The continuing challenge in sports medicine is injury prevention. Attempts to identify key risk factors involved in the pathogenesis of sports injuries have been sought in both past research (Lysens *et al.*, 1984) and more recent studies (Milgrom *et al.*, 1991). There appears to be agreement that the history of previous injury is a strong risk factor for recurrent injury. There have been few studies that have examined risk factors in relationship to specific sports injuries, probably due to the difficulty of controlling studies with numerous variables and poor understanding of the interrelatedness of such variables. However, studies support the following observations.

• There are significant differences in upper body strength, power and endurance of women, and lesser but significant differences in their lower body strength, power and endurance, compared with men (Hoffman *et al.*, 1979).

• Men accomplish tasks with fewer injuries and diseases and less apparent stress (Protzman, 1979).

• Women may be capable of equal efficiency in aerobic metabolism (Protzman, 1979).

• Women may report injuries differently from men (Jones *et al.*, 1993).

In the early 1980s, studies began to report a greater number of knee injuries among women participating in sports compared with men (Shively *et al.*, 1981; Zelisko *et al.*, 1982). Gray *et al.* (1985) were among the first to focus on an apparently higher incidence of anterior cruciate ligament (ACL) injury among women basketball players. Recent studies continue to reveal the differences in the total number of injuries (Engstrom *et al.*, 1991; Zillmer *et al.*, 1991; de Loës, 1995) and the incidence of serious knee injuries (Ireland & Wall, 1990; Ferretti *et al.*, 1992; Lindenfeld *et al.*, 1994) among men and women who participate in jumping and pivoting sports. In particular, there are increasing epidemiological data that support an increased incidence of non-contact ACL injury in women (Ireland & Wall, 1990; Arendt & Dick, 1995).

Non-contact ACL injury in women has come under extensive review. Numerous theories concerning this injury have been discussed, with no conclusive evidence to support a reason for the increased injury rate. Examining injury risk factors is complex, particularly as these relate to gender. The role that certain factors may play in acute and overuse injuries is discussed below, emphasizing possible relationships to gender variables.

Examining risk factors for gender-specific injury

Much of the information concerning risk factors and injury has come from the military population. The risk factors for increased injury prevalence that have been identified include gender (Kowal, 1980), age (Gardner *et al.*, 1988), level of past physical activity (Kowal, 1980; Gardner *et al.*, 1988) and race. In non-military studies, the positive risk factors for exercise-related injuries that have been identified include higher amounts of training (Koplan *et al.*, 1982, 1985; Blair *et al.*, 1987; Macera *et al.*, 1989a), past injuries and body mass index (Macera *et al.*, 1989b).

A recent well-designed study that investigated the risk factors for exercise-related injuries among male and female military trainees concluded that female gender and lower aerobic fitness measured by run times are positive risk factors for training injuries (Jones *et al.*, 1993). The author suggested that prior activity levels and height may affect men and women differently. The authors further suggested that gender *per se* may not be an independent risk factor for injury, but rather that the underlying risk factor may be physical fitness. Their data further indicated that women are more likely than men to report to the clinic for injury when both sexes are engaged in the same types of activities under similar conditions for the same amount of time. This suggests that there may be some societal differences in the way men and women seek help with regard to their injuries, adding yet another variable to epidemiological studies of injury occurrence. Indeed, psychosocial factors have rarely been included as a variable in studies of risk factors and injury identification.

A review of specific extrinsic and intrinsic risk factors is discussed below, with particular emphasis on non-contact ACL injury.

EXTRINSIC FACTORS

Shoe–surface interface, in particular increased friction between shoe and playing surface, has been suggested as a cause of injury to both knees and ankles (Heidt *et al.*, 1996). More specifically, a study of team handball players in Norway revealed that the friction rate of certain shoes on certain materials, particularly a court shoe on green turf, showed a higher friction rate. This increased friction rate correlated with a higher incidence of non-contact ACL injury (Myklebust *et al.*, 1997). Although one could theorize that the shoe–floor interface accounts for some non-contact ACL injuries, it is apparent that it only accounts for a small number of these injuries, particularly when the diversity of sports that report a high incidence of female non-contact ACL injuries is considered, e.g. gymnastics (Jackson *et al.*, 1980; de Loës, 1995), team handball (de Loës, 1995; Myklebust *et al.*, 1997), volleyball (Ferretti *et al.*, 1992; de Loës, 1995) and alpine skiing (de Loës, 1995; Ettinger *et al.*, 1995). The largest epidemiological study to date used the National Collegiate Athletic Association Injury Surveillance System to review two sports, basketball and soccer (Arendt & Dick, 1995). This study showed that non-contact ACL injury in women was twice as likely in soccer and three times more likely in basketball compared with non-contact ACL injury in men over a 5-year period (1989–93). These sports demand similar body mechanics (deceleration, plant and pivot) with widely different shoe–surface requirements (field surface with a cleated shoe vs. court surface with an uncleated shoe).

The literature strongly supports the view that the primary mechanism of ACL injury is non-contact in nature (Noyes *et al.*, 1983; Strand *et al.*, 1990; Arendt & Dick, 1995), with the injuries often occurring on landing from a jump, cutting/pivoting or with sudden deceleration. Indeed, a single prospective study identified three 'no hit' mechanisms as being responsible for ACL injury (Griffis *et al.*, 1989): planting and cutting, straight knee landing and one-step landing with a hyperextended knee. When a modification of these techniques was prospectively taught to female basketball teams, the incidence of ACL injury was reduced by 89% during a 2-year period.

This strongly suggests that muscle function, muscle recruitment or some aspect of training is an important component in knee function and injury risk (Moore & Wade, 1989). Earlier studies looking at the role of quadriceps and hamstring muscle strength in relationship to injury were inconclusive (Grace *et al.*, 1984; Colosimo *et al.*, 1991). However, a recent, more sophisticated study that investigated tibiofemoral laxity as well as lower extremity muscle strength, endurance, reaction time and muscle recruitment suggests differences between female athletes and male athletes as well as between female athletes and non-athletic male and female controls (Huston & Wojtys, 1996). The authors of this study hypothesized that the female athlete has a 'quadriceps-dominant' knee. This might be responsible for increased anterior translation in certain activities, thus increasing the risk of ACL stress and injury. It has been previously documented in studies of ligament failure that ligaments acting alone would not be able to withstand the levels of loading commonly seen with sport. The quadriceps muscles can produce forces in excess of those needed for ligament failure (Wojtys & Huston, 1994). Studies have found that there are sex differences in the rate of muscle force production (Komi & Karlsson, 1978; Bell & Jacobs, 1986; Häkkinen, 1991; Winter & Brookes, 1991). In particular, women require more time than men to produce the same relative muscle force levels. Some authors have suggested that this lower rate of force development in women is the result of structural differences in the series elastic component of muscle (Komi & Karlsson, 1978; Winter & Brookes, 1991). This strongly suggests a prominent role for muscle strength and the pattern of muscle recruitment in coordinated and safe knee function. The role that training may play in changing muscle pattern recruitment has come under recent review. For example, women volleyball players have been shown to have decreased adduction moments on jump landings after 6 weeks of intense training emphasizing plyometrics (Hewett *et al.*, 1996).

Skill level continues to be implicated as a causative factor in injuries in both men and women. This concern is highlighted due to the recent increase in sport participation by women. Some feel that this has created an influx of players into a sport, potentially decreasing the average skill level of those playing. Studies comparing the rate of injuries over time suggest that skill level is a reason for a decrease in the injury rate (Engebretsen, 1985). Collection of further injury data over time, with emphasis on more direct measurement of skill level of the partici-

pants, history of sports participation, quality and quantity of coaching instruction, and participants matched for skill levels, will help to support or dispel this belief.

INTRINSIC FACTORS

In the orthopaedic literature, the most discussed reason for ACL failure has been the dimensions of the intercondylar notch of the knee (the Y-shaped space in the middle of the knee through which the ACL runs). The intercondylar notch has been implicated as a reason for ACL failure in both newly injured and ACL-reconstructed knees (Table 15.5) (Arendt & Dick, 1995). The exact role that a small notch plays in creating an ACL tear remains speculative. However, some researchers theorize that a smaller notch creates increased stress on the ACL in certain positions, most particularly internal rotation and hyperextension of the knee. Others theorize that a small notch houses a small ACL, with concomitant decrease in ligament strength (Shelbourne *et al.*, 1998). In looking for a gender difference in the size of the notch, two prospective studies in large groups have agreed that athletes with smaller notch width indices (the ratio of the femoral bicondylar width to the width of the intercondylar notch) are at risk for a non-contact ACL injury (Souryal & Freeman, 1993; LaPrade & Burnett, 1994). However, one study found no sex differences in notch width index or rate of ACL injury (LaPrade & Burnett, 1994), while the second study found the notch width index in women to be less than that in men (Souryal & Freeman, 1993). The role that the notch plays in causing non-contact ACL injury (Muneta *et al.*, 1997; Shelbourne *et al.*, 1998) and whether size or gender is the determining factor in such injury needs further study before answers are known.

The role of the unique cyclical hormones in women and their possible effects on ligaments are being increasingly investigated. The effect of hormones, particularly oestrogen, on soft tissues is not well understood. However, it is well known that the hormone relaxin, found in women during pregnancy, is largely responsible

Table 15.5 Intercondylar notch (ICN) vs. anterior cruciate ligament (ACL) injury

Reference	Population	Measurement technique	Conclusion	Gender differences
Anderson *et al.* (1987)	Patients with bilateral ACL injury, unilateral injury and no known knee injury. Retrospective study	CT scan	An association exists between anterior outlet stenosis of the ICN and ACL rupture	
Houseworth *et al.* (1987)	Patients with acute ACL injury and no known knee injury. Retrospective study	Computer graphic study	A narrow posterior notch may predispose to ACL failure	
Souryal *et al.* (1998)	Patients with bilateral ACL injury, acute ACL injury and normal knees. Retrospective study	Notch radiographic view: defines notch width index (NWI) as ratio of width of ICN to width of femoral condyle, using radiographic landmarks	NWI of bilateral ACL injury < NWI of acute ACL injury and normal knees. NWI of acute injuries equals NWI of normal knees	No gender difference though population largely male
Good *et al.* (1991)	Patients with acute and chronic unilateral ACL injury. Normal measured from cadaver knees. Retrospective study	Direct measurement of anterior notch opening using a calliper technique	Normal notch width 18.1–20.4 mm. Acute ACL injury had narrower notch measurements	
Souyral & Freeman (1993)	902 high-school athletes. Prospective study	Notch radiographic view: measurement of NWI	Athletes with no contact ACL injury have smaller notches	NWI in females < NWI in males
Schickdatz & Weiker (1993)	Patients with unilateral and bilateral ACL injury, and normal knees. Retrospective study	Eight different mathematical measurements from notch radiographic view	ICN measurements from X-rays may not be reliable predictors of ACL injury	
Lund-Hassen *et al.* (1994)	Female Norwegian national team handball players. Retrospective study	Notch radiographic view: direct measurement of notch width	Notch width < 17 mm are at high risk of injury	Only females studied
LaPrade & Burnett (1994)	213 Division I athletes. Prospective study	Notch radiographic view: measurement of NWI	Athletes with stenotic notches playing certain sports are at high risk for ACL injury	No significant difference between sex and average NWI or rate of ACL tears

for the ligamentous relaxation of the pelvis during childbirth. Several recent studies have tried to uncover the relationship between ligament biology and hormones. A role for the hormonal effects on ligament function continues to be investigated (Hart *et al.*, 1996; Sciore *et al.*, 1997; Slaughterbeck *et al.*, 1997).

Knee joint laxity, defined as an increase in anterior–posterior motion of the tibia and femur, is most commonly measured using an instrumented arthrometer (Fig. 15.1). Arthrometer measurements of anterior–posterior motion have been reviewed in the knees of normal male and female basketball players (Weesner *et al.*, 1986), normal knees in the population (Daniel *et al.*, 1983), athletic knees before and after exercise (Skinner *et al.*, 1986; Steiner *et al.*, 1986), ACL-intact and ACL-deficient knees (Grana & Muse, 1988) and in athletes across different sports (Steiner *et al.*, 1986), all revealing no apparent relationship between knee laxity, gender and injury. A more sophisticated review of knee laxity has been performed recently by Huston and Wojtys (1996). This is the first study to show a difference in knee laxity between men and women and women athletes.

Multiple joint laxity, or hypermobility, has been implicated as a risk factor for injury. The most common way to define hypermobility is by specific tests of joint motion. A range of articular movements of defined joints, i.e. knees, elbows, wrists, fingers, is measured. A 'laxity scale' is defined giving each joint motion a certain numerical value (Carter & Wilkinson, 1964; Breighton *et al.*, 1973) (Table 15.6). Hypermobility syndrome is said to be present if an individual has three or more positive laxity tests, together with joint or muscle symptoms (Biro *et al.*, 1983; Gedalia *et al.*, 1985). A consistent relationship

Table 15.6 Laxity scale for defining hypermobility. (From Bird, 1993 with permission)

1	Passive dorsiflexion of the little fingers beyond 90° (one point for each hand)	2 points
2	Passive apposition of the thumbs to the flexor aspects of the forearm (one point for each thumb)	2 points
3	Hyperextension of the elbows beyond 10° (one point for each knee	2 points
4	Hyperextension of the knees beyond 10° (one point for each knee)	2 points
5	Forward flexion of the trunk with knees extended so that the palms of the hands rest on the floor	1 point
	Total	9 points

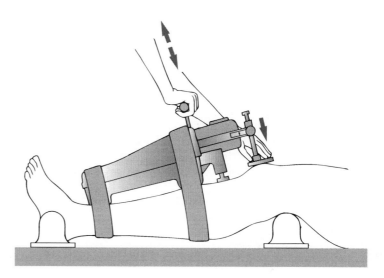

Fig. 15.1 A KT-1000 arthrometer, a portable device which is capable of measuring anterior tibial translation in millimetres when fixed loads of 6.75, 9 and 13.5 kg force are applied.

between hypermobility of the knee joint and injury has not been found. Nicholas (1970) reported that 28 of 39 football players (72%) with knee injuries had hypermobility. This incidence has yet to be substantiated in further studies. Other studies, using various modified laxity scales, have found no correlation between knee ligament injuries and laxity scores in college football players (Godshall, 1975; Kalenak & Morehouse, 1975; Moretz *et al.*, 1982; Grana & Muse, 1988) or between knee and ankle ligament injuries and laxity scores in high-school athletes (Godshall, 1975; Grana & Moretz, 1978).

Looking at musculoskeletal injuries in general, Diaz *et al.* (1993) studied 23 military recruits, correlating injury with a modified laxity scale. These authors concluded that lax individuals (those with three of five laxity tests positive) had more musculotendinous injuries than those who were not lax. Hypermobile joints, or an increased laxity scale, have been implicated principally in the creation of overuse injuries. However, their role in patellofemoral pain, overuse injuries about the foot and ankle, and shoulder laxity syndromes has been poorly defined. Breighton *et al.* (1973) felt that musculoskeletal symptoms, as judged by laxity scales, are positively related to mobility scores. This relationship is most evident for females. The fact that, using laxity scales, women demonstrate more joint laxity than men has been confirmed by others (Klemp *et al.*, 1984; Larsson *et al.*, 1987; Diaz *et al.*, 1993; Wiesler *et al.*, 1996).

Anatomical limb variation has been suggested as being responsible for the increased rate of non-contact ACL injury in women. There are few data to support this. A single retrospective study reviewing the experience of one sports medicine clinic concluded that there is no apparent relationship between standing tibiofemoral alignment, Q-angle (the angle formed by the intersection of a line parallel to the long axis of the femur and a line drawn through the centre of the patella tendon) and knee injuries (particularly ACL injury) in a series of female basketball players (Gray *et al.*, 1985).

Anatomical limb variation is perhaps most

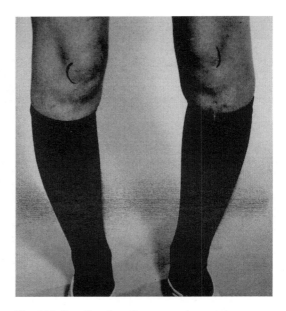

Fig. 15.2 Standing leg alignment of a young woman with an extreme case of the typical features of miserable malalignment syndrome, including increased femoral anteversion (resulting in a standing posture of increased internal rotation of the hip), high Q-angle, tibial vara, external tibial torsion and pronated flat feet.

often quoted as a reason for overuse injuries of the lower extremity in females. A variation in limb alignment has been termed 'miserable malalignment syndrome' (Fig. 15.2), which is a combination of lower extremity features that include increased anteversion of the femoral head, external rotation of the tibia and a pronated foot. Other features can include an increased Q-angle, tibiofemoral valgus, tibial varus and a hypermobile patella. These anatomical features, alone or in combination, have been blamed for a variety of overuse syndromes in the lower legs of active people, particularly women. This type of limb alignment is seen more commonly in the female population but is not limited to women. The exact prevalence of miserable malalignment syndrome in population studies has not been elicited. However, limb alignment, particularly femoral anteversion, has been reviewed (Huid & Anderson, 1982; Staheli, 1987, 1993).

A pronated flat foot, frequently associated with miserable malalignment syndrome, has been implicated as a factor in non-contact ACL injury (Canavan, 1996). Biomechanical studies have verified that internal rotation of the tibia places greater force on the ACL ligament than external rotation of the tibia (Markolf *et al.*, 1990). Therefore, one can theorize that the pronated foot, which obligates a linked system of tibial internal rotation, may place more stress on the ACL. In this theory shoe wear, with or without the addition of a prefabricated orthotic, would obviously play a moderating role.

Other gender-specific injury concerns

Dislocation of the patella is an acute injury of the knee in which the kneecap is forced out of the trochlear groove of the femur by a strong valgus or external rotation force, creating an injury in the medial patella and retinacular restraints. A few studies (Larsen & Lauridsen, 1982; Halbrecht & Jackson, 1993), supported by many physicians' personal impressions, report that recurrent dislocations of the patella occur more frequently in females. However, most studies on acute dislocations of the patella continue to show a male preponderance (Cofield & Bryan, 1977; Hawkins *et al.*, 1986; Vainiopaa *et al.*, 1990). It is difficult to interpret these findings, as most studies reporting acute dislocations of the patella in men are not prevalence studies and date from a time when men constituted the majority of athletes. However, collective review of studies does suggest that women have a higher incidence of recurrent dislocation of the patella. Further analysis of this potential gender difference would need to address issues similar to those discussed previously under ACL injury. In addition, outcome studies of dislocations of the patella would need to examine morphology of the bony patella, degree of soft-tissue damage and treatment protocols after injury in order to assess whether gender is a risk factor for recurrent dislocations.

Ankle sprains have not undergone much analysis with regard to possible gender differences. However, at least one study suggests that ankle sprains are more prevalent in women and girls (Harrer *et al.*, 1996). Again, rigid analysis of risk factors needs to be undertaken to evaluate whether this gender difference is real and whether intrinsic and/or extrinsic factors are responsible.

Although not classified in an injury category, arthritic disorders (arthritis and arthralgias) include more than 100 different illnesses and are the most frequent reason for decreasing physical activity in the ageing population. Most patients with arthritis are women. Arthritic disorders are 60–80% more common in women (Heiwick *et al.*, 1995; Gabiel, 1996; Lawta, 1996). Osteoarthritis (typically referred to as age-related joint wear and tear) is more prevalent among women than men (1.5–4.0 times more common); this prevalence increases with age. A subcollection of arthritides commonly known as connective tissue diseases includes, but is not limited to, rheumatoid arthritis, systemic lupus erythematosus (SLE) and fibromyalgia. Rheumatoid arthritis is two to three times more common in women of all ages, while 90% of patients with SLE are women and it is three times more common among African Americans. Fibromyalgia is perhaps the most poorly defined condition of this group. It is a chronic musculoskeletal syndrome characterized by diffuse pain at specific tender points; about 90% of all identified cases of fibromyalgia are women. Arthritis has been identified as a major women's health issue. Currently, most preventative and palliative measures are aimed at patient education, weight loss and appropriately directed exercise.

Overuse injuries of the lower extremities

Overuse injuries are common in athletic and active populations. The most common injuries facing the female athlete are detailed below, with strategies for diagnosis, treatment and prevention.

Patellofemoral pain syndrome

Patellofemoral pain syndrome (PFPS) is a global term used to describe anterior knee pain that originates in the extensor mechanism. The extensor mechanism includes the bony patella and its femoral groove, quadriceps muscle, quadriceps and patella tendon, and retinacular structures that surround the patella. PFPS is pain in the patellofemoral joint without documented joint instability and can be further classified as occurring with or without malalignment. Malalignment refers to an abnormal relationship between the patella and the trochlear groove; this can lead to asymmetry as the patella tracks in its groove. Malalignment syndromes are typically revealed on axial X-rays (Fig. 15.3) (Carson *et al.*, 1984; Fulkerson & Cautilli, 1993). The vast majority of cases of PFPS do not fall into a malalignment category. This is perhaps because the spectrum of malalignment is not clearly defined. Typically, X-rays are taken in a static view

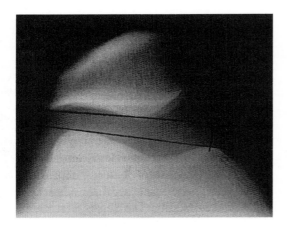

Fig. 15.3 A 20° axial view (Laurin's view) of the knee of a patient who sustained an acute dislocation of the patella. Radiographic lines drawn along the lateral patella facet and across the highest point of the medial and lateral femoral condyles reveal converging lines that represent continued tilt of this kneecap. A perpendicular line drawn from the highest point of the medial femoral condyle reveals more than 3 mm lateral displacement of the patella from this perpendicular line, indicating continued subluxation of this kneecap.

without contractions of the quadriceps muscle and in a single arc of motion. PFPS without X-ray demonstration of malalignment may represent subtle malalignment not detectable with current static imaging techniques. This subtle malalignment may be a result of an imbalance of the quadriceps muscles, either in recruitment or strength. Alternatively, it may be an imbalance secondary to laxity or tightness in the peripatellar structures, including laterally (iliotibial muscle and lateral retinaculum) or medially (vastus medialis muscle and medial retinaculum). Normal medial–lateral translation of the patella allows the examiner to move the patella medially about one-quarter the diameter of the patella and laterally about one-half the diameter of the patella (Arendt & Teitz, 1997). Normal tilt can be assessed on physical examination by the ability to bring the lateral border of the patella to the level of the horizontal plane or greater. This examination is done in the supine position with the knee in extension and muscle relaxed. Abnormal tightness or laxity, as demonstrated by translation and tilt tests, can lead to imbalance in motion of the patella during active use of the knee. This imbalance can lead to pain.

Important features regarding the treatment of PFPS are listed below.

• Central in the treatment of PFPS is balancing the movement of the patella as it tracks in the trochlear groove. Rehabilitation, particularly quadriceps strengthening, is widely recognized as useful for treating patellofemoral disorders (Bennett & Stauber, 1986; O'Neill *et al.*, 1992; Molnar, 1993; Steinkamp *et al.*, 1993).

• The entire lower kinematic change in PFPS should be assessed for gait characteristics, flexibility and strength of the proximal and distal portions. Decreased rotation or weakness of external rotators of the hips, hamstring tightness, quadriceps tightness and Achilles tendon tightness are frequently associated with PFPS. These should be assessed and treated with appropriately directed rehabilitation.

• Retinacular tightness of the patella should be examined by translation and tilt, with referral to physical therapy for mobilization of the patella if tight restraints are identified.

• A quadriceps strengthening programme should be started, emphasizing those activities that do not irritate patellofemoral pain. Isometric exercises, advancing to closed-chain isotonic exercises, are preferred as tolerated by the patient's pain symptoms. Closed-chain kinetic exercises are more functional and result in lower contact stresses to the patella in mid-arc motion (Hungerford & Lennox, 1983; Steinkamp et al., 1993). Eccentric quadriceps strengthening is emphasized (Bennett & Stauber, 1986) as the quadriceps muscle is an important decelerator.

• Control of overpronation of the foot with a semirigid orthosis is popular, although there are few controlled studies that have demonstrated success using acceptable outcome measures (Tria et al., 1992).

• The McConnell tape technique (McConnell, 1986) is based on assessment and tape correction of patellar position, including glide, tilt and rotation. This may be useful for select patients but must be an adjunct to full treatment. The use of patellar braces in patients with PFPS remains controversial (Podesta & Sherman, 1988; Molnar, 1993).

• Recognition of our incomplete knowledge of the aetiology of PFPS is appropriate. Athletes need to be instructed to acknowledge painful activities and decrease or avoid them if possible. Posture and exercise modification, including repetitive squatting and habitual hyperextension of the limb in the standing position, may be employed with a positive effect on chronic patellofemoral pain.

When planning a patellofemoral rehabilitation programme for women, particular attention needs to be paid to the woman's typically shorter stature and decreased strength. Strength-training equipment needs to be sized to an individual to be effective and safe.

PFPS is frequently seen in adolescent females. During adolescence, the female body undergoes significant changes, including increase in height, widening of the pelvis and deposition of sex-specific fat stores. The period of time in which these changes take place is shorter than the growth period in adolescent boys (Tanner, 1962). This period of accelerated body changes can produce changes in sports-specific performance as girls accommodate to their new body shapes.

Miserable malalignment syndrome

Miserable malalignment syndrome has been blamed for a variety of overuse syndromes of the lower extremity. An overpronated foot necessitates more foot motion in the stance phase. Pronation of the foot necessitates internal rotation of the tibia, which forces a similar rotational sequence up the lower extremity. Therefore, in the person with an overpronated stance there is greater rotation of the limb in accomplishing the stance phase of gait. Running aggravates this problem because the stance phase occupies a shorter period of time. One can think of this as a 'windscreen wiper' effect, with a wider arc of motion for the 'windscreen wiper' in the overpronated foot. Progression from walking to running causes overpronation of the limb to occur at a faster pace. This can lead to a variety of overuse syndromes, including plantar fasciitis, Achilles tendinitis, medial overload of the ankle (including posterior tibial tendinitis and shin splints), distal iliotibial band syndrome, proximal iliotibial band syndrome and PFPS. Treatment directed at reduction of pain and inflammation in the painful area, along with review of the entire alignment and function, as outlined for PFPS, can be useful.

Distal and proximal iliotibial band tendinitis can also be seen when a tight iliotibial band and lateral retinacular structures of the patella are present. Relief of this syndrome should be attempted with physical therapy modalities directed at the painful site and stretching of the iliotibial band and lateral retinacular structures of the patella (patellar mobilization). At times, a cortisone injection directed at the bursal site with subsequent reduction of bent knee activities for 5–7 days following the injection can be useful.

Stress fractures

Stress fractures can be thought of as an overuse injury of bone. Historically, stress fractures have been defined on the basis of the X-ray appearance of a fracture line and/or the bone's healing response as interpreted by traditional roentgenographic images (Savola, 1971). With the advent of newer techniques for investigating stress phenomena of bone, particularly scintigraphic analysis (Roub *et al.*, 1979) and magnetic resonance imaging (Arendt & Clohisy, 1995), bone stress is now regarded as a continuum from normal remodelling to fatigue and bone exhaustion. Bone can successfully accommodate stress or undergo failure in response to increasing load. The ultimate result of increasing load would be a frank stress fracture on X-ray.

Special attention must be given to irregularities of the menstrual cycle when considering stress fractures and stress phenomena of bone. The effect of oestrogens on vertebral and cancellous bone is well documented (Cann *et al.*, 1988; Drinkwater *et al.*, 1990; Arendt, 1993). An association between stress fractures and menstrual irregularities has been observed (Warren *et al.*, 1986; Barrow *et al.*, 1988). Stress injury to bone and stress fractures have been noted to occur more commonly in females, especially in the presence of disordered eating, amenorrhoea and low bone density. There is probably a complex interaction between mechanical (limb alignment and training factors), nutritional and hormonal factors on bone health. A careful menstrual history is mandatory for the complete evaluation of any stress fracture or stress phenomenon in women. Any change in intensity, duration or frequency of the menstrual cycle associated with increased training should be a cause of concern (Shangold *et al.*, 1990).

Posterior tibial tendinitis

The posterior tibial tendon contributes to the maintenance of the longitudinal arch of the foot and functions to invert the hind foot during heel strike and in initiating the stance phase of the gait cycle. Stress is put on the posterior tibial tendon during the pronation phase of stance, stabilizing the foot in pronation. The posterior tibial muscle also fires during the push-off phase of walking and running. Tendinitis and rupture of this tendon are more prevalent in women, especially in those over age 40 (Frey & Shereff, 1988). Whether this increased prevalence in women is secondary to an increased incidence of pronation related to shoe wear or to the hormonal environment remains speculative.

In more severe cases of posterior tibial tendinitis, particularly in the middle-aged athlete, detailed attention to management is paramount due to the potential for rupture (Johnson, 1989). Typical features on physical examination include a flattened or pronated foot and inability to perform a toe raise. In the younger female athlete, posterior tibial tendinitis is frequently missed as a cause of medial ankle discomfort. Typically, the posterior tibial tendon is inflamed but functionally intact. Typical examination features include pain to direct palpation of the tendon and discomfort when single-leg toe raising is attempted. Rest, ice and occasional non-steroidal anti-inflammatory medications are used in the early phase. Immobilization may be required to reduce this inflammation.

After the acute inflammation has subsided, attention is given to strengthening the posterior tibial muscle and stretching of the Achilles tendon complex if tight; use of a semirigid orthotic for control of overpronation is recommended. When performing Achilles tendon strengthening and closed-chain partial squats, the appropriate technique should be followed carefully. Often patients will perform an Achilles tendon stretch or a partial squat by placing increased valgus on the knee in such a way that a plumb-line from the knee falls medial to the ankle (Fig. 15.4). This places increased stretch on the posterior tibial tendon.

Flexor halluxus tendinitis

Flexor halluxus longus tendinitis is most common in the female ballerina who dances

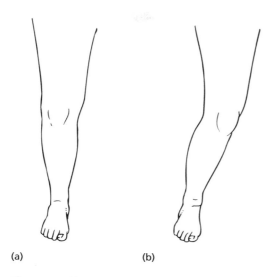

Fig. 15.4 Athlete performing squats and duck walks. Note full hip, knee and ankle flexion or any weakness: (a) normal; (b) asymmetrical hip, knee and ankle flexion.

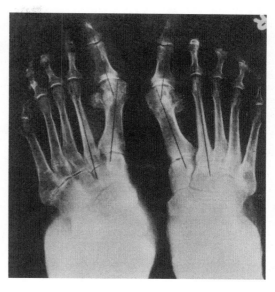

Fig. 15.5 A 44-year-old woman with bilateral hallux valgus. The patient also has arthritic changes at the first metatarsal phalangeal joints as well as medial subluxation of the first phalanx bilaterally.

enpointe (on the tips of her toes). In this position the flexor halluxus acts as an accessory push-off muscle. Athletes such as high jumpers or gymnasts who may use this muscle for accessory push-off can also suffer from this type of tendinitis. There is frequently pain in the muscle belly superior to the medial malleolus just medial to the Achilles tendon. This has been confused with Achilles tendinitis but can be easily distinguished by careful examination. Pain is aggravated by maximum passive dorsiflexion of the great toe or resisted plantar flexion of the great toe. Despite the fact that the pain is medial and superior to the ankle, attention should be given to limiting great toe motion with review of sports-specific techniques for its treatment.

Foot concerns

A bunion is inflammation of the bursa over the medial prominence of the first metatarsal (Fig. 15.5). Bunions are nine times more common in women than in men. This is thought to be due to a combination of hereditary predisposition,

poorly fitting shoes, ligamentous laxity and overpronation (Hunter-Griffin, 1991; Frey *et al.*, 1993). Women's shoes may aggravate bunions and other toe deformities. Frequently, women's shoes, particularly sports shoes, are smaller adaptations of men's shoes. In general, the female foot has a different shape from that of the male foot, being narrower relative to length with a narrower heel compared with the forefoot. As foot length increases, forefoot width increases somewhat but heel width rarely increases significantly. However, most shoe manufacturers typically scale their shoes by enlarging all key internal dimensions in fixed proportions. This often results in shoes that are too loose in the hind foot, particularly for women with bigger feet (US size 8 or larger). Women who have a wide forefoot and a narrow hind foot may have a difficult time finding shoes that fit. If feet are forced into a bigger shoe to fit the forefoot but not the hind foot, this creates a sloppy shoe that allows the foot to move back and forth during activities. This can cause posterior heel pain and lesser toe deformities. If the shoe is a snug fit on the hind foot, it can create undue pressure on the forefoot, creating increased symptoms over a bunion (medial aspect of the first toe) or bunionette (lateral aspect of the fifth toe). Careful attention to sports shoe selection will help a woman avoid injury and minimize the forces that can complicate foot problems (Frey, 1997). Variable eyelet patterns exist in sports shoes that allow for adjustable lacing. This can create variable width for a narrow foot or a wide foot, particularly in a high-arched foot. Current sports shoe design has variation in the type of last (outline of the sole of a shoe), typically each shoe company having a slightly different last. The type of last helps determine the stability of the shoe and the 'fit' of a shoe to a particular foot. Motion control vs. shock absorbency is another important consideration when selecting a sports shoe.

Overuse injuries of the upper extremities

Shoulder pain

The shoulder is a joint of extreme mobility that sacrifices bony stability. Anatomically, the humeral head is held in its bony socket, the glenoid, by ligaments that reinforce the joint capsule and by the muscles of the rotator cuff that surround the joint. These muscles serve to rotate the shoulder internally and externally. The tendons of four distinct muscles, the subscapularis (anteriorly), the supraspinatus (superiorly), the infraspinatus and teres minor (posteriorly), form a supportive cuff about the humeral head (Fig. 15.6). The scapular stabilizing muscles, i.e. the trapezius, the rhomboids and the serratus anterior, are also important in glenohumeral stability since proper positioning of the scapula is needed for normal rotator cuff muscle function.

Shoulder pain in women athletes may be a result of: (i) laxity with secondary impingement; (ii) laxity with recurrent subluxation; or (iii) impingement secondary to a compromised subacromial space. Contributing factors to the prevalence of these conditions in women include poor upper body strength, shorter upper extremities and faulty technical skills. Whether ligamentous laxity is a contributing factor in shoulder problems in women remains speculative.

As previously discussed in this chapter, liga-

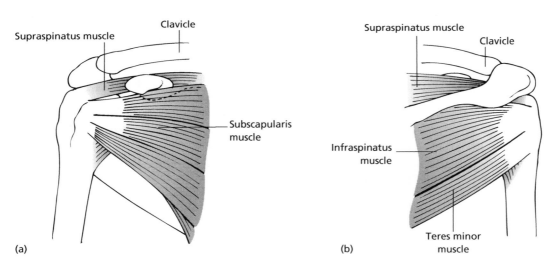

Fig. 15.6 The anterior ligaments of the shoulder that lend stability to the capsule include the superior glenohumeral ligament, the middle glenohumeral ligament and the inferior glenohumeral ligament. (a) Anterior aspect, and (b) posterior aspect.

mentous laxity is common in women. In the majority of studies, this increased ligamentous laxity has not been found to be directly related to an increase in sports injuries (Godshall, 1975; Kalenak & Morehouse, 1975). However, in the shoulder, glenohumeral laxity has been directly related to one type of shoulder problem, recurrent atraumatic instability or AMBRI (*a*traumatic *m*ultidirectional *b*ilateral treated by *r*ehabilitation *i*nstability). This type of shoulder instability occurs atraumatically, i.e. with little or no abnormal force on the joint. Typically, no damage to tissue occurs. Ligaments and tissue are so lax that the shoulder can dislocate or sublux without trauma. AMBRI was so termed to differentiate it from traumatic shoulder dislocation. With traumatic shoulder dislocation, injury to bone and soft tissue occurs, including damage to the humeral head that results in an impaction fracture (Hill–Sachs lesion) and/or damage to the glenoid by disruption of the labrum. This decreases the bony and ligamentous stability of the shoulder joint. This latter type of instability has been termed *t*raumatic *u*nilateral instability with a *B*ankart lesion (TUB) (Matsen *et al.*, 1993). Treatment for these shoulder problems is very different.

TUB responds favourably to operative treatment, i.e. repair of the bony glenoid and tightening of the stretched capsular restraints. The AMBRI type of instability implies a genetic predisposition for tissue laxity. Laxity in other joints (i.e. knees, fingers, elbows) is typically present in the athlete with AMBRI. This type of shoulder instability should initially be treated with a prolonged rehabilitation programme to strengthen the muscles about the shoulder and avoidance, if possible, of positions that could sublux or dislocate the shoulder. Surgical intervention is rarely advised, for failure is common secondary to poor quality tissue (Jobe *et al.*, 1990d; Matsen *et al.*, 1993).

The presenting history of athletes with symptomatic multidirectional instability of the shoulder is variable. Some athletes, when participating in sports requiring repetitive overhead motion such as swimming, gymnastics, weight-lifting or volleyball, may describe pain coupled with a sense of apprehension when raising their arm overhead, especially in an abducted position (Pink & Jobe, 1991). They may even experience an episode where the shoulder 'slips out' and stays out for a few seconds before being easily reduced by the athlete or a friend (Jobe & Kvitne, 1989). On physical examination, those with multidirectional instability of the shoulder demonstrate laxity with anterior, posterior and inferior translation of the humeral head in the glenoid. Inferior translation of the humeral head is noted by a positive sulcus sign (Fig. 15.7) (Silliman & Hawkins, 1994).

Treatment of athletes with multidirectional shoulder instability is aimed at strengthening the rotator cuff, deltoid and scapular stabilizing

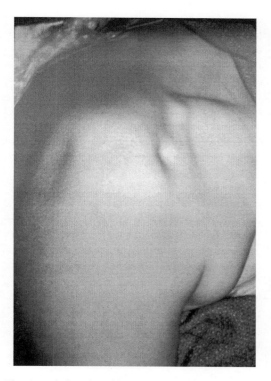

Fig. 15.7 A female athlete with multiple directional instability of the shoulder. Note the positive sulcus sign, which is produced by downward traction on the arm pulling the humeral head inferiorly in its bony socket.

muscles. Initially, such exercises should be performed below shoulder height. Anti-inflammatory drugs may be useful at the beginning of the exercise programme to decrease inflammation and its associated discomfort. Sport-specific technique, e.g. swimming style, racquet strokes or throwing motions of the athlete, needs to be examined and improper technical skills corrected.

The athlete with an unstable shoulder may not complain of instability but have shoulder pain with overhead activities. Shoulder pain can result from a humeral head that is not firmly seated in the glenoid and therefore displaces superiorly with overhead motion, causing impingement of the structures (tendons and bursa) in the subacromial space (Jobe *et al.*, 1990a). This leads to an impingement syndrome. On examination, these athletes have a positive impingement sign, as well as multidirectional shoulder laxity. Weakness of the rotator cuff is typically present. Treatment is similar to that prescribed for multidirectional instability with symptomatic subluxation, centring on rehabilitation of the rotator cuff and scapular stabilizing muscles. It is important to recognize this pain syndrome as an instability problem, not as impingement. Surgical treatment directed at impingement alone, without recognizing the underlying instability, will fail.

The symptom of impingement with underlying instability is also associated with unilateral anterior instability. Features on physical examination include unilateral anterior shoulder laxity with a positive impingement sign. Internal rotation of the shoulder joint is frequently reduced, aggravating this symptom complex. In addition to rotator cuff strengthening exercises, stretching and strengthening of the soft tissues of the posterior shoulder are also important. Surgical stabilization of the unidirectional unstable shoulder can be considered after failure of conservative treatment (Jobe *et al.*, 1990b).

Impingement without instability generally occurs in the older athlete and results from a weak rotator cuff and a compromised subacro-mial space that may be narrowed by degenerative subacromial spurring. The subacromial space may be genetically small secondary to a hooked or beaked acromion (Hawkins & Kennedy, 1980). On physical examination, athletes with impingement without instability have a positive impingement sign (pain when the shoulder is abducted and internally rotated) and weakness of the rotator cuff. They may have associated biceps tendon irritability, since this tendon can also be traumatized from repetitive impingement against the bony acromion (Hawkins & Kennedy, 1980; Keirns, 1994).

Treatment for impingement without instability is aimed at reducing inflammation of the tendons and bursa in the subacromial space. This can involve anti-inflammatory drugs and reduction of aggravating activities (typically overhead activities). Exercises to strengthen the cuff and the scapular stabilizing muscles are recommended in order to improve shoulder mechanics (Wilk *et al.*, 1994). Intermittent judicious use of injections of cortisone into the subacromial bursa can be useful. Technical considerations, including proper throwing mechanics, body rolling with breathing and stroking in swimming and position of the shoulder in relationship to the body during the golf swing, need to be examined. The surgical approach is used when conservative treatment has failed. This involves arthroscopic or open débridement of the undersurface of a beaked acromion or resection of degenerative spurs and débridement of a thickened bursa. This may improve shoulder mechanics by increasing the size of the subacromial space (Hawkins & Kennedy, 1980).

Frozen shoulder

Frozen shoulder syndrome (also termed adhesive capsulitis) is inflammation of the periarticular shoulder structures that results in marked limitation of forward and side elevation and internal rotation of the shoulder (Parker *et al.*, 1989). A repetitive activity can be the precipitating event, although why the activity results in such severe secondary inflammation and pain with marked limitation of motion is not well understood. The frozen shoulder syndrome is most common in women between the ages of 40 and 60 years (Ott *et al.*, 1994). Some researchers feel that it represents a type of dystrophy. It is often associated with medical conditions such as arteriosclerotic heart disease, epilepsy, pulmonary disorders, thyroid disorders, diabetes mellitus and gastrointestinal disorders (Ozaki *et al.*, 1989). The onset can be quite insidious. Even though this condition has been termed 'adhesive capsulitis', adhesions have been found outside and inside the joint and in the subacromial bursa. Some subscapular bursal irritation may be present, and increased vascularization around the cuff and biceps tendon has been described (Duralde *et al.*, 1993).

Anti-inflammatory medication administered orally and injected into the joint, combined with exercises to increase flexibility and strength in the muscles about the shoulder, comprise the recommended treatment. Some physicians feel that manipulation of the shoulder under anaesthesia is helpful to break up scar tissue and improve shoulder function. Such manipulation must be done with great care to avoid fracturing the proximal humerus (Duralde *et al.*, 1993). This is a greater risk in older individuals who have been restricting the use of their arm secondary to pain and hence have weaker bones due to osteoporosis and disuse. Frozen shoulder syndrome typically improves with time, although its duration can last 6–12 months.

Lateral epicondylitis of the elbow

Repetitive stress to the wrist extensor muscles can result in inflammation in the origins of these muscles as they arise from their bony origin, the lateral epicondyle of the elbow. Lateral epicondylitis is five times more common than medial epicondylitis and generally occurs in those 21–65 years of age (Rettig & Patel, 1995).

One might assume that the lower upper body strength of women would predispose them to a greater incidence of lateral epicondylitis. However, the incidence of lateral epicondylitis is similar for both men and women, whereas medial epicondylitis (inflammation of the origin of the wrist flexors at the medial epicondyle) occurs more commonly in men (Rettig & Patel, 1995). The greater use of the two-handed backhand by women playing racquet sports may contribute to their lower incidence of lateral epicondylitis.

Figure 15.8 illustrates the origin of the wrist extensors on the lateral epicondyle of the humerus. The extensor brevis muscle has been the muscle cited as the primary injury site. A rapid rise in repetitive wrist flexion–extension activities and/or poor mechanics in performing such activities has been implicated in the development of lateral epicondylitis. Although this overuse syndrome was originally observed in tennis players, frequently other activities are implicated in its development and include other wrist-intensive sports, especially those that emphasize wrist extensors. These include rac-

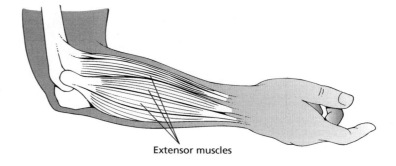

Fig. 15.8 The pain in lateral epicondylitis is thought to be due to chronic inflammation secondary to micro tears at the site of origin of the wrist extensor muscles on the lateral epicondyle.

Extensor muscles

quetball and volleyball, household tasks such as wallpapering or painting, or job-related activities such as paper thumbing, keyboarding, hammering and tightening screws.

Diagnosis is made on the basis of the history of pain with repetitive wrist extension, combined with a clinical examination revealing pain to palpation in the muscles originating on the lateral epicondyle. This pain will increase with resisted wrist extension.

Treatment of lateral epicondylitis consists of the following strategies.

- **Increasing the strength** and flexibility of the wrist extensor muscles and balancing them with strong, flexible wrist flexors.
- Evaluating and correcting improper technique used in performing the sport or work activity. For example in tennis, if the racquet handle size is inappropriate for a player's palm size it should be changed, or if the racquet is strung too tightly it should be adjusted. If a carpenter's hammer is too long or if it is improperly weighted, this needs to be corrected. In the case of the ticket counter's repetitive thumbing of stubs during a work day, one needs to consider if this activity could be changed or reduced (counting is done using a rubber-tipped knob).
- Use of oral anti-inflammatory drugs and analgesic creams.
- Use of a brace reportedly can influence the amount of tension created at the muscle origin and hence minimize continued stress on the irritated condyle.

Medial tension/lateral compartment overload syndrome to the elbow

A woman's increased valgus angle of the elbow, combined with her naturally occurring ligamentous laxity and lower upper body strength, can predispose her to compressive injuries around the lateral side of the elbow, termed lateral compressive overload syndrome or traction injury to the medial elbow structures (Kibler, 1995; Johnston *et al.*, 1996). Since there are less women participating in baseball than men, these injuries occur more commonly in field sports (javelin or

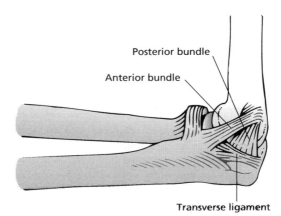

Fig. 15.9 The stabilizing ligaments of the medial side of the elbow.

shot put) as well as in gymnastics, where the gymnast uses her elbow as a weight-bearing post (Griffin, 1991).

The elbow is stabilized medially by thickening of the elbow joint capsular (medial collateral ligament) (Fig. 15.9). Of these, the anterior oblique bundle is the prime stabilizer of valgus load (Jacobson, 1995). The lateral collateral ligament complex of the elbow is not as well defined, although varus stress is far less common due to the normal valgus position of the elbow. In throwing sports, the acceleration and cocking phase places significant tensile stresses on the medial side of the elbow, as well as compressive forces on the lateral structures. This can result in sprains of the medial collateral ligament and/or sprains of the flexor pronator muscles, which arise on the medial epicondyle; in the case of growing bones, there is tension on the medial epicondylar physis as well as compressive forces laterally on the radial capitellar joint. Additionally, valgus overload can result in abnormal tracking of the olecranon process if, as it travels in its groove in the distal humerus, it tracks 'off centre'. The distal humerus olecranon 'hits' sideways in the fossa instead of centring within it, resulting in spur formation (Wilson *et al.*, 1983; Rettig & Patel, 1995; Johnston *et al.*, 1996). These spurs can cause pain during the act

Table 15.7 Possible sites of involvement in lateral compressive overload syndrome of the elbow

---

Medial collateral ligament sprain
Avulsion fracture of medial epicondyle (seen in youngsters with open physes)
Sprain of flexor pronator muscles where they arise on medial epicondyle
Osteochondritis dissecans of the lateral humeral condyle or radial head secondary to high compressive loads

---

of throwing, as well as with activities of daily living that require elbow extension. Fractures through a spur may result in a loose body.

This entity of lateral compressive overload syndrome may simply present as a painful elbow after or during participation in sport. Therefore, careful physical examination is needed to define whether an athlete's elbow pain is due to the tensile forces on the medial side of the elbow, the compressive forces laterally or abnormal forces within the trochlear groove (Table 15.7).

Treatment involves not only strengthening the muscles of the upper extremity, especially the wrist extensors and flexors, but also the elbow power flexors (biceps and brachioradialis) and extensors (triceps). Sport techniques should be examined to correct inadequacies. For example, is the gymnast 'locking her elbow', i.e. jamming it to make it carry her body weight rather than carrying her weight through the muscles about the elbow? Moreover, during her routine, is her body centred over the elbow such that the load is distributed equally throughout her elbow joint rather than merely concentrated laterally?

Wrist impingement syndrome

The wrist joint is a complex entity held together by an elaborate network of ligaments that articulate with the distal radius and ulna proximally and the metacarpals distally. Injuries to the hand and wrist are the most common types sustained during athletic competition (McCue *et al.*, 1998). The majority of these injuries are sprains and strains; however, overuse injuries to the wrist are common in sports where the wrist is used as a weight-bearing joint (principally gymnastics) and in sports requiring repetitive flexion–extension of the wrist (fast-pitch softball, volleyball and weight-lifting). Other sports where the wrist is used intensively include golf, basketball and racquet sports.

Dorsal wrist pain from capsular impingement is seen in the gymnast or tennis player who stabilizes her wrist by locking it in dorsiflexion instead of stabilizing the joint by tightening the muscles about it. Whether the pain of dorsal wrist impingement is due to bony impingement or impinging synovium in the joint is not clearly understood. Treatment consists of initial rest combined with anti-inflammatory drugs and modalities to decrease inflammation, followed by an exercise programme to strengthen the muscles about the wrist (Griffin, 1991; Mattov *et al.*, 1996). A thorough evaluation of technique is also warranted, so that modifications can be made to prevent recurrent impingement. A thick wrist band or multiple layers of tape can be used to block hyperextension of the wrist in the symptomatic athlete when she returns to competition.

Stress injuries of the radial physis

Stress reaction of the distal radius (radial stress syndrome) is most common in gymnasts and is a source of wrist pain during the early teenage years (Roy *et al.*, 1985; Carek & Fumich, 1992; DeSmet *et al.*, 1994). Diagnosis is made on physical examination. Symptomatic athletes have pain to palpation over the physeal growth area. In more advanced cases the stress reaction can be confirmed radiographically, with widening and haziness of the epiphyseal plate, fragmentation and cystic changes in the metaphyseal portion of the plate and a beaked defect of the distal aspect of the epiphysis (Carek & Fumich, 1992). In one study, 10% of the gymnasts studied had evidence of stress-related changes, either the acute changes described above or chronic changes as noted by a widened and shortened distal radius (Fig. 15.10) (DeSmet *et al.*, 1994).

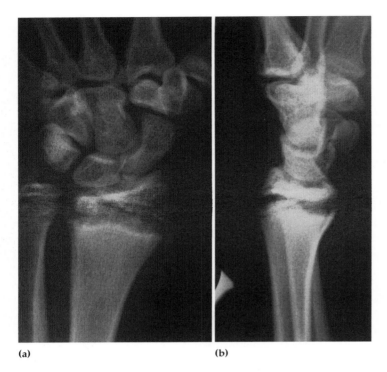

(a)   (b)

Fig. 15.10 (a) Anteroposterior and (b) lateral view of the wrist of a 14-year-old gymnast, demonstrating stress-related changes.

The dowel grip in both female and male gymnasts has been implicated in the development of radial stress syndrome because it transfers forces from the hand to the wrist. Also thought to be predisposing factors are weak upper body strength, poor technique, jamming the wrist into the so-called fixed hand–wrist position to improve stability, the use of very soft mats and multiple repetitions of manoeuvres involving single-arm weight-bearing (Carek & Fumich, 1992). Others blame the rotational forces suffered on impact during performance of the vault as a prime cause of this stress reaction (Roy *et al.*, 1985).

In most instances of symptomatic radial stress syndrome, rest relieves symptoms without sequelae if initiated prior to the development of bony changes. Recovery generally takes 3–4 weeks. However, if treatment is delayed until after radiographic changes appear, symptoms may be prolonged for up to 4–6 months (Roy *et al.*, 1985; DeSmet *et al.*, 1994).

Overuse tendinitis of the hand and wrist

Tenosynovitis of the hand and wrist can commonly occur from the repetitive microtrauma experienced during upper-extremity intensive sports, such as racquetball, golf, volleyball and basketball. The left thumb of a right-handed golfer can develop de Quervain's syndrome from being hyperabducted during the swing. In this overuse syndrome, there is pain and swelling in the long abductor and short extensor tendons of the thumb, the two tendons that occupy a common sheath in the first dorsal wrist compartment (Fig. 15.11). This swelling leads to impingement within the sheath. The smaller hand of the woman may predispose her to this condition, especially if she uses clubs with grips that are too large. De Quervain's syndrome may also be seen in new mothers caused by the repetitive peeling and tightening of nappy tape closures. It has been conjectured that hormonal influences, particularly during the early postpartum period,

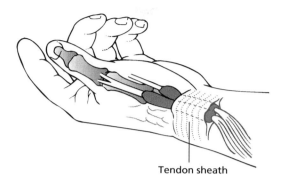

Fig. 15.11 The first dorsal compartment of the wrist houses the long abductor and short extensor tendons of the thumb.

Tendon sheath

may result in increased joint laxity and hence greater stress on the extensor tendons and stabilizing ligaments about the metacarpophalangeal joint. However, this has not been proved.

Initial treatment consists of the use of anti-inflammatory creams, oral anti-inflammatory drugs and splinting of the thumb to decrease continued irritation of the tendons. This should be followed by an exercise programme for the involved tendons, as well as activity modification to decrease abduction forces on the metacarpophalangeal joint and on the thumb extensor tendons (Sailer & Lewis, 1995). If such conservative measures fail to relieve symptoms, the careful injection of steroids into the tendon sheath is an appropriate and often successful manoeuvre. In recalcitrant cases, operative release of the sheath is recommended.

Carpal tunnel syndrome

Carpal tunnel syndrome, which is characterized by pain, numbness and/or tingling in the distribution of the medial nerve, results from compression of this nerve as it passes through the wrist in the carpal canal. It has been reported in cyclists and weight-lifters, as well as in athletes participating in other sports requiring wrist flexion with a strong grasp. Symptomatic athletes may have symptoms only after their sport or at night following a day of sport activity. The

incidence of carpal tunnel syndrome in athletes is slightly higher than the 1% reported in the general population. This condition is more frequent in women, particularly women greater than 50 years of age and especially those with predisposing factors, such as diabetes, alcoholism or inflammatory arthritis (Steyers & Schelkun, 1995). Treatment consists of rest from repetitive wrist activity (often a wrist splint is used) combined with oral anti-inflammatory drugs. In severe cases, the injection of steroids into the canal to decrease inflammation is required. The athlete should be screened for medical conditions such as hypothyroidism or diabetes. In recalcitrant cases or cases with severe nerve impingement, surgical release of the carpal canal is required.

Overuse injuries of the lumbar spine

Muscle strains and ligament sprains

Back pain has been reported to occur in 75% of high-performance athletes (Gerbino & Micheli, 1995). The back pain experienced by most children and adults during or following sport activity is the result of inflammation of the vertebral or sacral ligaments or of the paravertebral muscles, i.e. sprains and strains. For example, lightweight rowers have pain from the stress on muscles and ligaments caused by the increased flexion of their lower back that occurs with sitting bent forward in the catch position. Weight-lifters frequently strain paravertebral muscles due to improper lifting techniques. Low back strain has also been reported in what has been termed the 'cosmetic' athlete, i.e. those improving their physique through exercise (Goodman, 1987). Exercises implicated are bilateral leg lifts, donkey kicks, sitting double toe touches and the Yoga plough position. These activities are particularly irritating to those with poor posture, deficient muscle strength and inflexibility of the paravertebral and abdominal muscles; they should be done only by those with strong and flexible paravertebral and abdominal muscles.

Generally in children, back pain caused by sprains and strains resolves in 4–6 weeks with conservative care, i.e. rest from the aggravating activity, back strengthening exercises, oral anti-inflammatory drugs and, if indicated, braces for support. Pain that persists longer merits further evaluation (Gerbino & Micheli, 1995).

Spondylolysis and spondylolisthesis

Gymnasts, skaters and dancers who repetitively place their spine in hyperextension are prone to develop stress reactions of the pars interarticularis, the area of the posterior arch linking the lamina to the superior articular facet (Fig. 15.12). In fact, it has been reported that 20% of female gymnasts have pars lesions (Jackson *et al.*, 1976). Unlike other stress fractures, this stress reaction of bone has not been directly related to low bone mineral density in women. Its occurrence is almost equal in males and females participating intensely in sports requiring repetitive hyperextension and/or flexion of the lumbar spine (Jackson *et al.*, 1976). Football linemen seem to be as predisposed as female gymnasts if the hours of play and practice of these two sport participants are equalized.

Although this defect is found in 5% of randomly selected adults, implying a congenital aetiology to its development, in an athletic population it is felt to occur also as a stress reaction (Jackson *et al.*, 1976; Gerbino & Micheli, 1995). Studies have documented its development in symptomatic athletes who present with normal appearance on X-ray but who have increased bony uptake in the region of the pars on bone scan. Follow-up X-ray evaluation may show the defect, verifying that in these individuals the defect is not a congenital variant but a true stress reaction of bone leading to a fracture.

The recommended treatment of the athlete with normal appearance on X-ray and a positive bone scan is rest from sport with brace protection using a lumbar orthosis for approximately 3 months. It is felt that time is needed to diminish inflammation and for the bone to repair itself (Micheli *et al.*, 1980; Gerbino & Micheli, 1995). This is followed by a rehabilitation programme to increase strength and flexibility of back and abdominal muscles prior to returning to sport. Though it is important to strengthen back extensor muscles, the hyperextended position should be avoided. Extension exercises to the neutral position only, if pain free, are encouraged.

In the symptomatic athlete with a radiographic defect already present, it is important to

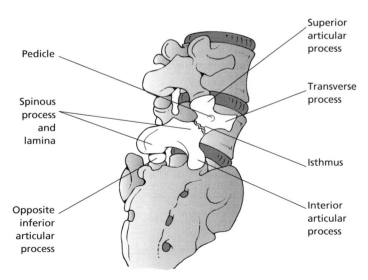

Pedicle

Spinous process and lamina

Opposite inferior articular process

Superior articular process

Transverse process

Isthmus

Interior articular process

Fig. 15.12 Spondylolysis is a defect in the pars interarticularis and may occur as a stress fracture.

distinguish between a new and a chronic lesion. Long-standing lesions are treated symptomatically, i.e. a period of rest until acute symptoms subside. A brace may be useful in this time period for intermittent symptomatic treatment only, not continuous use. This is coupled with a rehabilitation programme and a paced return to sport as pain allows (Jackson *et al.*, 1976; Johnson, 1993; Yu & Garfin, 1994). Bone sclerosis at the margin of the fracture indicates a chronic lesion. This can be seen on plain X-rays or, if necessary, thin-slice axial tomographic views of the lumbar region. A fracture is felt to be new if there is a positive bone scan, no previous X-ray evidence of a fracture and no widening or sclerosis at fracture margins. There is debate on how aggressively new fractures should be treated, although these fractures do have the potential to heal. Aggressive conservative treatment includes 3–6 months away from a sport with use of a low-back orthosis for the first 3 months. Whether this lesion heals with bony or fibrous union, more aggressive treatment is often successful at reaching a pain-free state.

If a pars defect is present on both sides of a vertebral body, the spine loses its posterior integrity and can slip forward (ventral) on the vertebra below. This forward slipping is called spondylolisthesis (Fig. 15.13). There is a difference of opinion on continued sport participation with this problem. Most orthopaedic experts agree that if slippage is less than 25% of the width of the vertebrae, i.e. a grade 1 spondylolisthesis (Fig. 15.14), and the athlete is asymptomatic, she can participate in sports, including contact sports. If the slippage progresses, activity must be stopped. This is most common during the period of rapid growth in early teenage years. Some physicians recommend that an athlete with a slip of grade 2 or greater should not participate in contact sports. If the athlete with a slip of grade 2 or greater is symptomatic despite sport modification, surgical fusion of the involved vertebrae may need to be considered. Generally, individuals with a significant spondylolisthesis have decreased lumbar flexibility and marked hamstring tightness. This combination typically

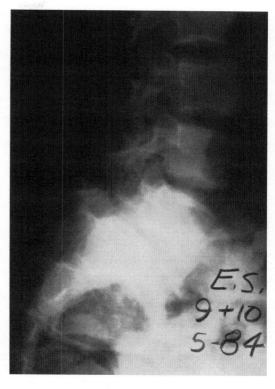

Fig. 15.13 Radiograph demonstrating spondylolysis of L5 with a spondylolisthesis of L5 on S1.

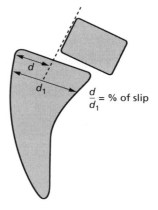

$$\frac{d}{d_1} = \% \text{ of slip}$$

Fig. 15.14 The amount of anterior displacement of L5 on S1 is calculated by the ratio of the distance L5 has moved on the sacrum (d) to the anterior–posterior diameter of the sacrum (d_1), i.e. d/d_1.

decreases their ability to be highly competitive athletes. Following fusion, return to competitive sports is reasonable as long as the athlete completes an adequate rehabilitation programme to strengthen the muscles of the paravertebral and abdominal area and axial tomography of the spine does not reveal any compromise of the neural foramina or neural canal (Micheli, 1985). For the athlete with a slip, rehabilitation programmes involve not only developing strong and flexible paravertebral and abdominal muscles but also increasing hamstring flexibility.

Lumbar apophysitis

In the growing athlete, repetitive hyperextension or hyperflexion of the spine, such as occurs in gymnastics, dancing and skating, can result in irritation of the vertebral growth centres, i.e. the superior and inferior vertebral apophyses. It is theorized that a tight anterior longitudinal ligament, perhaps inadequately balanced by strong vertebral and abdominal muscles and further stressed by repetitive extension of the spine, causes irritation of the vertebral apophyses that can result in back pain. X-rays of these symptomatic youngsters demonstrate the irregular growth centres (Fig. 15.15). Lumbar apophysitis will generally improve in 4–6 weeks when treated with a programme of exercise and rest from strenuous activity. Some athletes also find that a back brace used during activity provides additional support when they are symptomatic.

Idiopathic scoliosis

Adolescent idiopathic scoliosis is a structural curvature of the spine presenting at or about the onset of puberty. It accounts for about 8% of all cases of idiopathic scoliosis, the others being juvenile and infantile. It has a prevalence of 2–3% in the general population, with a female to male distribution of 3.6:1 for curves greater than 10° (Weinstein & Buckwalter, 1994). Of athletes with scoliosis, 8% have a relative who suffered from scoliosis. Like spondylolisthesis, curves are

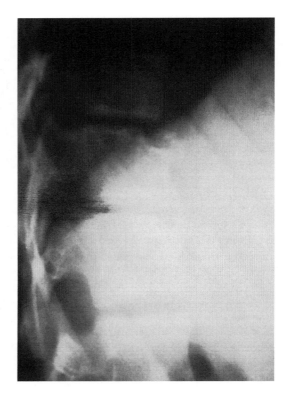

Fig. 15.15 A 13-year-old figure skater with apophysitis. Note the irregular vertebral growth centres.

progressive during the rapid growth of early teenage years.

Curves less than 20° are usually no obstacle to full athletic participation. It is a myth that athletic activity causes progression of the curve. In fact, participation in sports that develop lumbar and thoracic spine strength is probably advantageous to those with scoliosis. Bracing is often recommended for those with curves between 20 and 40°, although 'brace-free' time for athletic participation is usually permitted (Benson et al., 1977). Those with more severe curves, i.e. >50–60°, often require surgical intervention. Typically these patients do not have the spinal flexibility or balance required for competitive participation in sports such as basketball, volleyball, gymnastics, dance, skating and hockey.

References

Anderson, A.E., Lipscomb, A.B., Liudahl, K.J. *et al.* (1987) Analysis of the intercondylar notch by computed tomography. *American Journal of Sports Medicine* **15**(6), 547–552.

Arendt, E.A. (1993) Osteoporosis in the athletic female: amenorrhea and amenorrheic osteoporosis. In A.J. Pearl (ed.) *The Athletic Female*, pp. 41–59. Human Kinetics Publishers, Champaign, Illinois.

Arendt, E.A. (1995) Assessment of the athlete with an acutely injured knee. In L.Y. Griffin (ed.) *Rehabilitation of the Injured Knee*, pp. 20–33. Mosby, St Louis.

Arendt, E.A. & Clohisy, D.R. (1995) Stress injuries of bone. In J.A. Nicholas & E.B. Hershman (eds) *The Lower Extremity and Spine*, 2nd edn, pp. 65–79. Mosby, St Louis.

Arendt, E.A. & Dick, R. (1995) Knee injury patterns among men and women in collegiate basketball and soccer. *American Journal of Sports Medicine* **23**, 694–701.

Arendt, E.A. & Teitz, C.C. (1997) The lower extremities. In C.C. Teitz (ed.) *The Female Athlete*, pp. 45–59. American Academy of Orthopaedic Surgeons, Rosemont, Illinois.

Barrow, G.S. & Saba, S. (1988) Menstrual irregularities: stress fractures in collegiate distance runners. *American Journal of Sports Medicine* **16**, 209–216.

Bell, D.G. & Jacobs, I. (1986) Electro-mechanical response times and rate of force development in males and females. *Medicine and Science in Sports and Exercise* **18**, 31–36.

Bennett, J.G. & Stauber, W.T. (1986) Evaluation and treatment of anterior knee pain using eccentric exercise. *Medicine and Science in Sports and Exercise* **18**, 526–530.

Benson, D., Wolf, A. & Shoji, H. (1977) Can the Milwaukee brace patient participate in competitive athletics. *American Journal of Sports Medicine* **5**, 7–12.

Bird, H.A. (1993) Joint hyperlaxity and its long-term effects on joints. *Journal of the Royal Society of Health* **113**(6), 327–329.

Biro, F., Gewanter, H.L. & Baum, J. (1983) The hypermobility syndrome. *Pediatrics* **72**, 701–706.

Blair, S.N., Kohl, H.W. & Goodyear, N.N. (1987) Rates, and risks for running and exercise injuries: studies in three populations. *Research Quarterly for Exercise and Sport* **58**, 221–228.

Breighton, P., Solomon, L. & Soskolne, C.L. (1973) Articular mobility in an African population. *Annals of the Rheumatic Diseases* **32**, 413–418.

Calvert, R. (1975/1976) *Athletic Injuries and Deaths in Secondary School and Colleges, 1975–1976*. National Center for Education Statistics, Department of Health, Education and Welfare, US Government Printing Office, Washington, DC.

Canavan, P.K. (1996) Pronation and ACL injuries: what's the link? *Advance/Rehabilitation* **5**(9), 39–41.

Cann, C.E., Cavanaugh, D.J. & Schurpfiel, K. (1988) Menstrual history is the primary determinant of trabecular bone density in women. *Medicine and Science in Sports and Exercise* **20**, 559.

Carek, P. & Fumich, R. (1992) Stress fracture of the distal radius. *Physician and Sportsmedicine* **20**, 115–118.

Carson, W.G. Jr, James, S.L., Larson, R.L., Singer, K.M. & Winternitz, W.W. (1984) Patellofemoral disorders: physical and radiographical evaluation. Part II: radiographic examination. *Clinical Orthopaedics and Related Research* **185**, 165–167.

Carter, C. & Wilkinson, J. (1964) Persistent joint laxity and congenital dislocation of the hip. *Journal of Bone and Joint Surgery* **46B**, 40–45.

Clarke, K.S. & Buckley, W. (1980) Women's injuries in collegiate sports. *American Journal of Sports Medicine* **8**, 187–191.

Cofield, R.H. & Bryan, R.S. (1977) Acute dislocation of the patella: result of conservative treatment. *Journal of Trauma* **17**, 526–531.

Colosimo, A.J., Ireland, M.L. & Horn, T. (1991) Isokinetic peak torque and knee joint laxity comparison in female basketball and volleyball college athletes (Abstract). *Medicine and Science in Sports and Exercise* **23**, S135.

Daniel, D., Malcom, L. & Losse, G. (1983) Instrumented measurement of ACL disruption (Abstract). *Orthopaedic Transactions* **7**, 585–586.

de Loës, M. (1995) Epidemiology of sports injuries in the Swiss organization 'Youth and Sports' 1987–1989. *International Journal of Sports Medicine* **16**, 134–138.

DeSmet, L., Claessens, A., Lefebre, J. & Beunen, G. (1994) Gymnast's wrist: an epidemiology survey of ulnar variance and stress changes of the radial physis in elite female gymnasts. *American Journal of Sports Medicine* **22**, 846–850.

Diaz, M.A., Estevez, E.C. & Guijo, P.S. (1993) Joint hyperlaxity and musculoligamentous lesions: study of a population of homogeneous age, sex, and physical exertion. *British Journal of Rheumatology* **32**, 120–122.

Drinkwater, B.L., Bruemner, B. & Chestnut, C.H. (1990) Menstrual history as a determinant of current bone density in young athletes. *Journal of the American Medical Association* **263**, 545–548.

Duralde, X., Pollock, R., Flatow, E. & Bigliani, L. (1993) Frozen shoulder: prevention, diagnosis, and management. *Journal of Musculoskeletal Medicine* **10**, 64–72.

Engebretsen, L. (1985) Soccer injuries in Norway.

Journal of the Norwegian Medical Association **105**, 1766–1769.

Engstrom, B., Johansson, C. & Tornkvist, H. (1991) Soccer injuries among elite female players. *American Journal of Sports Medicine* **19**, 372–375.

Ettinger, C.F., Johnson, R.J. & Shealy, J.E. (1995) A method to help reduce the risk of serious knee sprains incurred in alpine skiing. *American Journal of Sports Medicine* **23**, 531–537.

Ferretti, A., Papandrea, P., Conteduca, F. & Mariani, P.P. (1992) Knee ligament injuries in volleyball players. *American Journal of Sports Medicine* **20**, 203–207.

Frey, C. (1997) Shoes. In C.C. Teitz (ed.) *The Female Athlete*, pp. 63–73. American Academy of Orthopedic Surgeons, Rosemont, Illinois.

Frey, C.C. & Shereff, M.J. (1988) Tendon injuries about the ankle in athletes. *Clinics in Sports Medicine* **7**, 103–118.

Frey, C., Thompson, F., Smith, J., Sanders, M. & Horstman, H. (1993) American Orthopaedic Foot and Ankle Society women's shoe survey. *Foot and Ankle* **14**, 78–81.

Fulkerson, J.P. & Cautilli, R.A. (1993) Chronic patellar instability, subluxation and dislocation. In J.M. Fox & W. Del Pizzo (eds) *The Patellofemoral Joint*, pp. 135–148. McGraw-Hill, New York.

Gabiel, S.E. (1996) Update on the epidemiology of the rheumatic diseases. *Current Opinion in Rheumatology* **8**, 96–100.

Gardner, L.I., Dzaidos, J.E., Jones, B.H. *et al.* (1988) Prevention of lower extremity stress fractures: a controlled trial of a shock-absorbent insole. *American Journal of Public Health* **78**, 1563–1567.

Garrett, W.E. Jr (1990) Muscle strain injuries. *Medicine and Science in Sports and Exercise* **22**, 436–443.

Gedalia, A., Person, D.A., Brewer, E.J., Jr. & Giannini, E.H. (1985) Hypermobility of the joints in juvenile episodic arthritis/arthralgia. *Journal of Pediatrics* **107**, 873–876.

Gerbino, P. & Micheli, L. (1995) Back injuries in the young athlete. *Clinics in Sports Medicine* **14**, 571–590.

Godshall, R.W. (1975) The predictability of athletic injuries: an eight-year study. *Journal of Sports Medicine* **3**, 50–54.

Good, L., Odensten, M. & Gillquist, J. (1991) Intercondylar notch measurements with special reference to anterior cruciate ligament surgery. *Clinical Orthopaedics and Related Research* **263**, 185–189.

Goodman, C. (1987) Low back pain in a cosmetic athlete. *Physician and Sportsmedicine* **15**, 97–103.

Grace, T.G., Sweetser, E.R., Nelson, M.A., Yedens, L.R. & Skipper, B.J. (1984) Isokinetic muscle imbalance and knee-joint injuries. *Journal of Bone and Joint Surgery* **66A**, 734–740.

Grana, W.A. & Moretz, J.A. (1978) Ligamentous laxity in secondary school athletes. *Journal of the American Medical Association* **240**, 1975–1976.

Grana, W.A. & Muse, G. (1988) The effect of exercise on laxity in the anterior cruciate ligament deficient knee. *American Journal of Sports Medicine* **16**, 586–588.

Gray, J., Taunton, J.E., McKenzie, D.C., Clement, D.B., McConckey, J.P. & Davidson, R.G. (1985) A survey of injuries to the anterior cruciate ligament of the knee in female basketball players. *International Journal of Sports Medicine* **6**, 314–316.

Griffin, L. (1991) Upper extremity injuries. In A. Pearl (ed.) *The Athletic Female*, pp. 235–250. Human Kinetics Publishers, Champaign, Illinois.

Griffin, L. (1994) Pathophysiology and healing of musculoskeletal tissues. In L.Y. Griffin (ed.) *AAOS Orthopedic Knowledge Update: Sports Medicine*, pp. 17–33. American Academy of Orthopaedic Surgeons, Rosemont, Illinois.

Griffis, N.D., Vequist, S.W. & Yearout, K.M. (1989) Injury prevention of the anterior cruciate ligament (Abstract). Paper presented at the 1989 AOSSM Annual Meeting, Traverse City, Michigan.

Häkkinen, K. (1991) Force production characteristics of leg extensor, trunk flexor and extensor muscles in male and female basketball players. *Journal of Sports Medicine and Physical Fitness* **31**, 325–331.

Halbrecht, J.L. & Jackson, D.W. (1993) Acute dislocation of the patella. In J.M. Fox. & W. Del Pizzo (eds). *The Patellofemoral Joint*, pp. 123–156. McGraw-Hill, New York.

Harrer, M.F., Berson, L., Hosea, T.M., Cody, R.P. & Leddy, T.P. (1996) Lower extremity injuries: females vs. males in the sport of basketball (Abstract). Paper presented at the 1996 AOSSM Annual Meeting, Orlando, Florida.

Hart, D.A., Roux, L., Frank, C. & Shrive, N. (1996) Sex hormone influences on rabbit ligaments *in vivo* and *in vitro*. *Transactions of the Orthopaedic Research Society* **21**, 792.

Hawkins, R. & Kennedy, J. (1980) Impingement syndrome in athletes. *American Journal of Sports Medicine* **8**, 151–158.

Hawkins, R.J., Bell, R.H. & Anisette, G. (1986) Acute patella dislocations: the natural history. *American Journal of Sports Medicine* **14**, 117–120.

Haycock, C.E. & Gillette, J.V. (1976) Susceptibility of women athletes to injury: myths vs. reality. *Journal of the American Medical Association* **236**, 163–165.

Heidt, R.S. Jr, Dormer, S.G., Cawley, P.W., Scranton, P.E., Losse, G. & Howard, M. (1996) Differences in friction and torsional resistance in athletic shoe–turf surface interfaces. *American Journal of Sports Medicine* **24**, 834–842.

Heiwick, C.G., Lawrence, R.C., Pollar, R.A., Lloyd, E. & Heyses, S.P. (1995) Arthritis and other rheumatic conditions: who is affected now, who will be affected later. *Arthritis Care Research* **8**, 203–211.

Hewett, T.E., Stoupe, A.L., Nance, T.A. & Noyes, F.R.

(1996) Plyometric training in female athletes. *American Journal of Sports Medicine* **24**, 765–773.

Hoffman, T., Stauffer, R.W. & Jackson, A.S. (1979) Sex difference in strength. *American Journal of Sports Medicine* **7**, 265–267.

Houseworth, S.W., Mauro, V.J., Mellon, B.A. *et al.* (1987) The intercondylar notch in acute tears of the anterior cruciate ligament: a computer graphic study. *American Journal of Sports Medicine* **15**, 221–229.

Huid, J. & Anderson, L. (1982) The quadriceps angle and its relation to femoral torsion. *Acta Orthopaedica Scandinavica* **53**, 577–579.

Hungerford, D.S. & Lennox, D.W. (1983) Rehabilitation of the knee in disorders of the patellofemoral joint: relevant biomechanics. *Orthopedic Clinics of North America* **14**, 397–402.

Hunter-Griffin, L.Y. (1991) Female athletes. In L.Y. Hunter-Griffin (ed.) *Athletic Training and Sports Medicine*, 2nd edn, pp. 921–932. American Academy of Orthopedic Surgeons, Rosemont, Illinois.

Huston, L.J. & Wojtys, E.M. (1996) Neuromuscular performance characteristics in the elite female athletes. *American Journal of Sports Medicine* **24**, 427–435.

Ireland, M.L. & Wall, C. (1990) Epidemiology and comparison of knee injuries in elite male and female United States basketball athletes (Abstract). *Medicine and Science in Sports and Exercise* **22**, S82.

Jackson, D., Wiltse, L. & Circione, R. (1976) Spondylolysis in the female gymnast. *Clinical Orthopaedics and Related Research* **117**, 68–73.

Jackson, D.S., Furman, W.K. & Berson, B.L. (1980) Patterns of injuries in college athletes: a retrospective study of injuries sustained in intercollegiate athletics in two colleges over a two-year period. *Mount Sinai Journal of Medicine* **47**, 423–426.

Jacobson, K. (1995) Functional anatomy in biomechanics of the elbow. In C. Baker (ed.) *Hughston Clinic Sports Medicine Book*, pp. 299–305. Williams and Wilkins, Baltimore.

Jobe, F. & Kvitne, R. (1989) Shoulder pain in the overhead or throwing athletes. *Orthopaedic Review* **28**, 963–975.

Jobe, F.W., Bradley, J.P. & Pink, M. (1990a) Impingement syndrome in overhand athletes, Part 1. *Surgical Rounds For Orthopaedics* August, 19–24.

Jobe, F.W., Bradley, J.P. & Pink, M. (1990b) Impingement syndrome in overhand athletes, Part II. *Surgical Rounds For Orthopaedics* September, 39–41.

Jobe, F.W., Bradley, J.P. & Pink, M. (1990c) Impingement syndrome in overhand athletes, Part III. *Surgical Rounds For Orthopaedics* October, 24–26.

Jobe, F., Tibone, J., Jobe, C. & Kvitne, R. (1990d) The shoulder in sports. In C.A. Rockwood & F.A. Matsen (eds) *The Shoulder*, pp. 961–990. W.B. Saunders, Philadelphia.

Johnson, K.A. (1989) Tibialis posterior tendon dysfunc-

tion. In *Surgery of the Foot and Ankle*, pp. 221–244. Raven Press, New York.

Johnson, R. (1993) Low back pain in sports: managing spondylolysis in young patients. *Physician and Sportsmedicine* **21**, 53–59.

Johnston, J., Plancher, K. & Hawkins, R. (1996) Elbow injuries to the throwing athlete. *Clinics in Sports Medicine* **15**, 307–328.

Jones, B.H., Bovee, M.W., Harris, J. III & Cowan, D.N. (1993) Intrinsic risk factors for exercise-related injuries among male and female army trainees. *American Journal of Sports Medicine* **21**, 705–710.

Kalenak, A. & Morehouse, C.A. (1975) Knee stability and knee ligament injuries. *Journal of the American Medical Association* **234**, 1143–1145.

Keirns, M. (1994) Conservative management of shoulder impingement. In J. Andrew & K. Wilk (eds) *The Athlete's Shoulder*, pp. 603–622. Churchill Livingstone, New York.

Kibler, W.B. (1995) Pathophysiology of overload injuries around the elbow. *Clinics in Sports Medicine* **14**, 447–458.

Klemp, P., Stevens, J.E. & Isaacs, S. (1984) A hypermobility study in ballet dancers. *Journal of Rheumatology* **11**, 692–696.

Komi, P.V. & Karlsson, J. (1978) Skeletal muscle fibre types, enzyme activities and physical performance in young males and females. *Acta Physiologica Scandinavica* **103**, 210–218.

Koplan, J.P., Powell, K.E. & Sikes, R.K. (1982) An epidemiologic study of the benefits and risks of running. *Journal of the American Medical Association* **248**, 3118–3121.

Koplan, J.P., Siscovick, D.S. & Goldbaum, G.M. (1985) The risks of exercise: a public health view of injuries and hazards. *Public Health Report* **100**, 189–195.

Kowal, D.M. (1980) Nature and causes of injuries in women resulting from an endurance training program. *American Journal of Sports Medicine* **8**, 265–269.

LaPrade, R.F. & Burnett, Q.M. II (1994) Femoral intercondylar notch stenosis and correlation to anterior cruciate ligament injury. A prospective study. *American Journal of Sports Medicine* **22**, 198–203.

Larsen, E. & Lauridsen, F. (1982) Conservative treatment of patellar dislocations: influence of evident factors on the tendency to redislocation and the therapeutic results. *Clinical Orthopaedics and Related Research* **171**, 131–136.

Larsson, L.-G., Baum, J. & Mudholkar, S. (1987) Hypermobility: features and differential incidence between the sexes. *Arthritis and Rheumatism* **30**, 1426–1430.

Lawta, R.G. (1996) The connective tissue diseases and the overall influence of gender. *International Journal of Fertility and Menopausal Studies* **41**, 156–165.

Leadbetter, W.B. (1990) Clinical staging concepts in

sports trauma. In W.B. Leadbetter, J.A. Buckwalter & S.L. Gordon (eds) *Sports-Induced Inflammation*, pp. 587–595. American Academy of Orthopaedic Surgeons, Rosemont, Illinois.

Lenz, H.W. (1979) Women's sports and fitness programs at the US Naval Academy. *Physician and Sportsmedicine* 7, 41–50.

Lindenfeld, T.N., Schmitt, D.J., Hendy, M.P., Mangine, R.E. & Noyes, F.R. (1994) Incidence of injury in outdoor soccer. *American Journal of Sports Medicine* 22, 364–371.

Lund-Hassen, H., Gannon, J., Engebretsen, L. *et al.* (1994) Intercondylar notch width and risk of ACL rupture in female varsity team handball players. A case control study. *Acta Orthopaedica Scandinavica* 65(5), 529–532.

Lysens, R., Steverlynck, A., van de Auweele, Y. *et al.* (1984) The predictability of sports injuries. *Sports Medicine* 1, 6–10.

McConnell, J. (1986) The management of chondromalacia patellae: a long term solution. *Australian Journal of Physiotherapy* 33, 215.

McCue, F.C., Dinsmore, H. & Kowalk, D. (1998) Athletic injuries to the hand and wrist. In R.J. Johnson & J. Lombardo (eds) *Current Review of Sports Medicine*, 2nd edn, pp. 43–53. Current Medicine, Philadelphia.

Macera, C.A., Jackson, K.L., Hagenmaier, G.W., Kronenfeld, J.J., Kohl, H.W. & Blair, S.N. (1989a) Age, physical activity, physical fitness, body composition, and incidence of orthopaedic problems. *Research Quarterly for Exercise and Sport* 60, 225–233.

Macera, C.A., Pate, R.R. & Powell, F.P. (1989b) Predicting lower extremity injuries among habitual runners. *Archives of Internal Medicine* 149, 2565–2568.

Markolf, K.L., Gorek, J.F., Kabo, J.M. & Shapiro, J.S. (1990) Direct measurement of resultant forces in the anterior cruciate ligament. *Journal of Bone and Joint Surgery* 72A, 557–567.

Matsen, F.A., Fu, F.H. & Hawkins, R.J. (eds) (1993) *The Shoulder: a Balance of Mobility and Stability.* Proceedings of a workshop, Vail, Colorado, September 1992. American Academy of Orthopedic Surgeons, Rosemont, Illinois.

Mattov, A., Arendt, E. & Riehl, R. (1996) The female athlete. In J. Zachazewski, D. Magee & W. Quillen (eds) *Athletic Injuries and Rehabilitation*, pp. 841–851. W.B. Saunders, Philadelphia.

Micheli, L. (1985) Sports following spinal surgery in the young athlete. *Clinical Orthopaedics and Related Research* 196, 152–157.

Micheli, L., Hall, J. & Miller, M. (1980) Use of the modified Boston brace for back injuries in athletes. *American Journal of Sports Medicine* 8, 351–356.

Milgrom, C., Shlamkovitch, N., Finestone, A. *et al.* (1991) Risk factors for lateral ankle sprain: a prospective study among military recruits. *Foot and Ankle* 12, 26–30.

Molnar, T.J. (1993) Patellofemoral rehabilitation. In J.M. Fox & W. Del Pizzo (eds) *The Patellofemoral Joint*, pp. 291–304. McGraw-Hill, New York.

Moore, J.R. & Wade, G. (1989) Prevention of ACL injuries. *National Strength Conditioning Society* 6, 35–40.

Moretz, J.A., Walters, R. & Smith, L. (1982) Flexibility as a predictor of knee injuries in college football players. *Physician and Sportsmedicine* 10, 93–97.

Muneta, T., Takakuda, K. & Yamamoto, H. (1997) Intercondylar notch width and its relation to the configuration and cross-sectional area of the anterior cruciate ligament. *American Journal of Sports Medicine* 25, 69–72.

Myklebust, G., Maehlum, S., Engebretsen, L., Strand, T. & Solheim E. (1997) Registration of cruciate ligament injuries in Norwegian top level team handball. A prospective study covering two sessions. *Scandianvian Journal of Medicine and Science in Sports* 7(5), 289–292.

Nicholas, J.A. (1970) Injuries to knee ligaments: relationship to looseness and tightness in football players. *Journal of the American Medical Association* 212, 2236–2239.

Noyes, F.R., Mooar, P.A., Matthews, D.S. & Grood, E.S. (1983) The symptomatic ACL deficient knee. Part II: the results of rehabilitation activity modification and counseling on functional disability. *Journal of Bone and Joint Surgery* 65A, 154–174.

O'Neill, D.B., Micheli, L.J. & Warner, J.P. (1992) Patellofemoral stress: a prospective analysis of exercise treatment in adolescents and adults. *American Journal of Sports Medicine* 20, 151–156.

Ott, J., Clancy, W. & Wilk, K. (1994) Soft tissue injuries of the shoulder. In J. Andrew & K. Wilk (eds) *The Athlete's Shoulder*, pp. 241–259. Churchill Livingstone, New York.

Ozaki, J., Nakagawa, Y., Sakurai, G. & Tanai, F. (1989) Recalcitrant chronic adhesive capsulitis of the shoulder. *Journal of Bone and Joint Surgery* 71A, 1511–1522.

Parker, R., Froimson, A., Winsberg, D. & Arsham, N. (1989) Frozen shoulder. Part I: chronology, pathogenesis and clinical picture and treatment. *Orthopedics* 12, 869–873.

Pink, M. & Jobe, F. (1991) Shoulder injuries in the athlete. *Clinical Management* 11, 39–47.

Podesta, L. & Sherman, M.F. (1988) Knee bracing. *Orthopedic Clinics of North America* 19, 737–745.

Protzman, R. (1979) Physiologic performance of women compared to men. *American Journal of Sports Medicine* 7, 191–194.

Rettig, A. & Patel, D. (1995) Epidemiology of the elbow, forearm, and wrist injuries in the athlete. *Clinics in Sports Medicine* 14, 289–297.

Roub, L.W., Gumerman, L.W. & Hanley, E.N. (1979) Bone stress: a radionuclide imaging prospective. *Radiology* **132**, 431–438.

Roy, S., Caine, D. & Singer, K. (1985) Stress changes of the distal radial epiphysis in young gymnasts. *American Journal of Sports Medicine* **13**, 301–308.

Ryan, J. & Pearl, A. (1994) Pathophysiology and healing of musculoskeletal tissues. In L. Griffin (ed.) *Orthopedic Knowledge Update: Sports Medicine*, p. 21. American Academy of Orthopedic Surgeons, Rosemont, Illinois.

Sailer, S. & Lewis, S. (1995) Rehabilitation and splinting of common upper extremity injuries in athletes. *Clinics in Sports Medicine* **14**, 411–446.

Savola, C.J. (1971) Stress fracture: a classification of earliest radiographic signs. *Radiology* **100**, 519–524.

Schickdatz, M.S. & Weiker, G.G. (1993) The predictive value of radiographs in the evaluation of unilateral and bilateral anterior cruciate ligament injuries. *American Journal of Sports Medicine* **21**(1), 110–113.

Sciore, P., Smith, S., Frank, C.B. & Hart, D.A. (1997) Detection of receptors for estrogen and progesterone in human ligaments and rabbit ligaments and tendons by RT-PCR. *Transactions of the Orthopaedic Research Society* **22**, 51.

Shangold, M., Rebor, R.W. & Wentz, A.C. (1990) Evaluation and management of menstrual dysfunction in athletes. *Journal of the American Medical Association* **263**, 1665–1669.

Shelbourne, K.D., Davis, T.J. & Klootwyk, T.E. (1998) The relationship between intercondylar notch width of the femur and the incidence of anterior cruciate ligament tears. A prospective study. *American Journal of Sports Medicine* **26**(3), 402–408.

Shively, R.A., Grana, W.A. & Ellis, D. (1981) High school sports injuries. *Physician and Sportsmedicine* **8**, 46–50.

Silliman, J. & Hawkins, R. (1994) Clinical examination of the shoulder complex. In J. Andrews & K. Wilk (eds) *The Athlete's Shoulder*, pp. 45–58. Churchill Livingstone, New York.

Skinner, H.B., Wyatt, M.P., Stone, M.L., Hogdon, J.A. & Barrack, R.L. (1986) Exercise related knee joint laxity. *American Journal of Sports Medicine* **14**, 30–34.

Slaughterbeck, J.R., Narayan, R.S., Clevenger, C. *et al.* (1997) Effects of estrogen level on the tensile properties of the rabbit anterior cruciate ligament (ACL). *Transactions of the Orthopaedic Research Society* **22**, 76.

Souryal, T.O. & Freeman, T.R. (1993) Intercondylar notch size and anterior cruciate ligament injuries in athletes. A prospective study. *American Journal of Sports Medicine* **21**, 535–539.

Souryal, T.O., Moore, H.A. & Evans, J.P. (1998) Bilaterality in anterior cruciate ligament injuries: associated intercondylar notch stenosis. *American Journal of Sports Medicine* **16**, 449–454.

Staheli, L.T. (1987) Rotational problems of the lower extremities. *Orthopedic Clinics of North America* **18**, 503–512.

Staheli, L.T. (1993) Rotational problems in children. *Journal of Bone and Joint Surgery* **75A**, 939–948.

Steiner, M.E., Grana, W.A., Chillag, K. & Schelberg-Karnes, E. (1986) The effect of exercise on anterior–posterior knee laxity. *American Journal of Sports Medicine* **14**, 24–29.

Steinkamp, L.A., Dillingham, M.F., Markel, M.D., Hill, J.A. & Kaufman, K.R. (1993) Biomechanical considerations in patellofemoral joint rehabilitation. *American Journal of Sports Medicine* **21**, 438–444.

Steyers, C. & Schelkun, P. (1995) Practical management of carpal tunnel syndrome. *Physician and Sportsmedicine* **23**, 83–87.

Strand, T., Wisnes, A.R. & Tvedte, R. (1990) ACL injuries in team handball. *Journal of the Norwegian Medical Association* **110**, 45–48.

Tanner, J.M. (ed.) (1962) *Growth at Adolescence, with a General Consideration of the Effects of Hereditary and Environmental Factors upon Growth and Maturation from Birth to Maturity*, 2nd edn. Blackwell Scientific Publications, Oxford.

Tomasi, L.F., Peterson, J.A. & Pettit, G.P. (1977) Women's response to army training. *Physician and Sportsmedicine* **5**, 32–37.

Tria, A.J. Jr, Palumbo, R.C. & Alicea, J.A. (1992) Conservative care for patellofemoral pain. *Orthopedic Clinics of North America* **23**, 545–554.

Vainiopaa, S., Laasonen, E., Silvennoinen, T., Vasenius, J. & Rokkanen, P. (1990) Acute dislocation of the patella: a prospective review of operative treatment. *Journal of Bone and Joint Surgery* **72B**, 365–369.

Warren, M.P., Brooks-Gunn, J. & Hamilton, L.H. (1986) Scoliosis and fractures in young ballet dancers. *New England Journal of Medicine* **314**, 1348–1353.

Weesner, C.L., Albohm, M.J. & Ritter, M.A. (1986) A comparison of anterior and posterior cruciate ligament laxity between female and male basketball players. *Physician and Sportsmedicine* **14**, 149–154.

Weinstein, S. & Buckwalter, J. (1994) *Turek's Orthopaedics*, 5th edn, pp. 447–485. J.B. Lippincott, Philadelphia.

Whiteside, P. (1980) Men's & women's injuries in comparable sports. *Physician and Sportsmedicine* **8**, 130–140.

Wiesler, E.R., Hunter, D.M., Martin, D.F., Curl, W.W. & Hoen, H. (1996) Ankle flexibility and injury patterns in dancers. *American Journal of Sports Medicine* **24**, 754–757.

Wilk, K., Arrigo, C. & Andrews, J. (1994) Current concepts in the rehabilitation of the athlete's shoulder. *Journal of the Southern Orthopedic Association* **3**, 205–215.

Wilson, F., Andrews, J., Balckburn, T. & McCaulskey, G. (1983) Valgus extension overload in the pitching elbow. *American Journal of Sports Medicine* **11**, 83–87.

Winter, E.M. & Brookes, F.B. (1991) Electromechanical response times and muscle elasticity in men and women. *European Journal of Applied Physiology* **63**, 124–128.

Wojtys, E.M. & Huston, L.J. (1994) Neuromuscular performance in normal and anterior cruciate ligament-deficient lower extremities. *American Journal of Sports Medicine* **22**, 89–104.

Yu, C. & Garfin, S. (1994) Recognizing and managing lumbar spondylolisthesis. *Journal of Musculoskeletal Medicine* **11**, 55–64.

Zelisko, J.A., Noble, H.B. & Porter, M. (1982) A comparison of men's and women's professional basketball injuries. *American Journal of Sports Medicine* **10**, 297–299.

Zillmer, D.A., Powell, J.W. & Albright, J.P. (1991) Gender-specific injury patterns in high school varsity basketball. *Journal of Women's Health* **1**, 69–76.

Chapter 16

Cardiovascular Issues

PATRICIA SANGENIS

Introduction

For many years young girls and women in general were discouraged from participating in sports, exhaustive training and competition. The underlying idea was that physical activity could harm the reproductive system, diminishing fertility; another interesting concept was that a woman had a weaker heart. However, time passed and the evolution of female performance in sports, some amazing records and mothers who became world champions persuaded sports scientists to question these concepts.

Do the differences in performance between female and male reflect biological differences or are they the result of education and social and cultural restrictions placed on young girls? Do a smaller heart and smaller blood volume play an important role in performance? In the past, very few of the large epidemiological studies examined the female cardiovascular system, coronary heart disease not being considered a major issue. Today we know that cardiovascular disease is the leading cause of death in women, in many countries claiming more lives than all forms of cancer, accidents and diabetes combined. Exercise is one of the most effective tools for maintaining a healthy heart via modification of such risk factors as hypertension, elevated lipids and lipoproteins, obesity and diabetes. Exercise is also considered an independent factor in the prevention of coronary heart disease.

Cardiovascular system

The cardiovascular system comprises the heart, blood vessels and blood. The heart serves as a muscular pump that circulates the blood, oxygen and nutrients to all the tissues and organs of the body through the blood vessels. The heart has two atria that act as receiving chambers and two ventricles that serve as pumping chambers. The heart is a muscular pump and its walls are composed of three layers: the inner layer, the endocardium; the middle layer of muscle, the myocardium; and the outer layer, the epicardium. The heart is encased in a protective membrane, the pericardium.

The heart is a double-system pump, the right and left sides being completely separated by a thick muscle wall called the septum. The systemic circuit is the left side of the heart and the pulmonary circuit the right side of the heart. The left atrium receives the oxygenated blood from the lungs through the pulmonary veins. From the left atrium the blood passes through the mitral valve into the left ventricle, which pumps blood through the aortic semilunar valve into the aorta. This blood supplies every cell with oxygen and nutrients and also transports carbon dioxide and other waste products. The deoxygenated blood returns via the superior and inferior venae cavae to the right atrium and then passes through the tricuspid valve into the right ventricle. This chamber pumps the blood through the pulmonary semilunar valve into the pulmonary artery, which carries the deoxygenated blood to the lungs for reoxygenation.

Cardiac muscle has the ability to generate its own electrical signal, the conduction system allowing the heart muscle to contract rhythmically. The intrinsic heart rate averages 60–80 beats·min^{-1}. Disturbances of heart rhythm are called dysrhythmias, the degree of seriousness varying widely: bradycardia is a resting heart rate < 60 beats·min^{-1}; tachycardia is a resting heart rate > 100 beats·min^{-1}. Complex dysrhythmias may cause symptoms such as dizziness, fatigue, lightheadedness and fainting.

Preparticipation cardiovascular physical examination

Although exercise is the best way to maintain a healthy heart, it is important to identify the presence of heart disease in an athlete before participation in sport. The traditional established goals of the preparticipation physical examination are to prepare the athlete for safe participation in sports, to uncover any life-threatening conditions the athlete may have and to satisfy legal requirements set forth by various governing bodies.

Medical history

• A history of sudden cardiac death or cardiac problems in family members < 50 years of age might need further evaluation.
• Has the athlete been told that she has an extra heart beat, high blood pressure, a heart murmur, a click or any other heart abnormality?
• Has she ever stopped exercising because of dizziness, chest pain or palpitations?
• Has she ever passed out during exercise?

Medical examination

The medical examination should be mainly screening in nature. Any chest wall or other skeletal abnormality seen with Marfan's syndrome should be noted, including pectus excavatum, long arms, arachnodactyly and abnormal vision. The cardiac evaluation should emphasize pulse, auscultation and blood pressure.

• Radial and femoral pulses should be palpated.
• Resting heart rate indicates cardiovascular fitness and may be abnormal in anaemia, cardiac disorders and anorexia nervosa.
• To confirm elevated blood pressure, abnormal measurements should be found on at least three occasions. The upper limits of normal for athletes aged 11 years or younger are 130/75 mmHg (17.3/10 kPa) and for those aged 12 years or older 140/85 mmHg (18.6/11.3 kPa).
• Heart murmurs are the most common abnormality found during the examination. Most murmurs in young, healthy athletes fall into the II/VI systolic ejection group that usually suggests 'flow' murmurs or well-conditioned athletic hearts. Any murmurs with a grade greater than II/VI, any diastolic murmur or any murmur that increases during the Valsalva manoeuvre or other methods that increase intra-abdominal pressure deserves special consideration before the athlete is allowed to participate in sport activity. An abnormal sound can indicate the turbulent flow of blood through a narrowed or leaky valve. It could also indicate errant blood flow through a hole in the septum that separates the right and left sides of the heart (septal defect). Most murmurs in athletes are benign, although they can indicate diseased valves or septal defects.

Evaluation techniques

The examiner should be ready to refer the athlete for further testing or to order more tests if any of the above findings are noted. The following is a list of evaluation techniques that may be helpful:
• 12-lead ECG;
• chest X-ray;
• blood lipid profile;
• stress test;
• echocardiography;
• Holter monitoring;
• angiography.
If the athlete is over 40 or is a high-risk individual, a very thorough cardiac examination should

be given before athletic clearance is granted. A high-risk individual may be defined as one with two or more major risk factors for coronary heart disease and symptoms suggestive of cardiac, pulmonary or metabolic disease. Major risk factors include cigarette smoking, hypertension [> 160/90 mmHg (21.3/12 kPa)], serum cholesterol > 240 mg·dl⁻¹, diabetes or a family history of cardiac disease prior to age 65. The American College of Sports Medicine (1994) suggests that graded exercise testing of all such individuals be included in any preparticipation screening process. If congenital or other anatomical defects are present, echocardiographic evaluation of the anatomy should be done, perhaps supplemented by angiography.

Clinical manifestations of the athlete's heart

Many athletes, particularly those who have undergone endurance training, will have various manifestations of exercise training that are occasionally misinterpreted as organic cardiac disease. Most of these findings are related to the physiological adaptations that occur as a result of exercise training and do not represent true organic heart disease.

Cardiac enlargement in athletes may be detected during palpation of the chest as a displaced apical impulse or a right ventricular lift. Third and fourth heart sounds are frequently heard in athletes. The third heart sound is related to a prominent rapid filling phase of the left ventricle during early diastole and has no clinical significance. The mechanism of production of the fourth heart sound is related to heart rate, PR interval or changes in the intrinsic diastolic properties of the left ventricle. The combination of a long PR interval and a thin chest wall may result in an audible fourth heart sound. The large stroke volumes seen in well-trained athletes may result in mid-systolic murmurs. These murmurs are due to a large stroke volume being ejected through normal semilunar valves. The murmurs related to large volumes decrease in intensity or disappear in the upright position as a result of decreased ventricular filling and stroke volume.

Common physical findings in athletes

- Carotid upstroke: normal or hyperdynamic, reflecting increased stroke volume.
- Jugular venous pulse: normal unless pattern associated with conduction abnormalities.
- Enlarged heart on percussion.
- Prominent apical impulse and right ventricular lift.
- S1 and S2 normal.
- Third heart sound.
- Fourth heart sound.
- Mid-systolic flow murmur.
- Diastolic flow murmur: rare.
- Peripheral pulses: normal or hyperdynamic, reflecting increased stroke volume.

Electrocardiogram

The ECG alterations found in well-trained athletes may mimic those observed in patients with organic heart disease. Alterations may be noted in all the waves of the ECG. These alterations are generally thought to represent manifestations of the physiological adaptations that occur within the heart and cardiovascular system as a result of exercise training. Changes in the waveforms are due to cardiomegaly and an increased myocardial mass. The disturbances of rhythm are largely related to alterations in the autonomic nervous system, specifically increased parasympathetic activity. The ECG findings in athletes are summarized below.

1 Rhythm:
    (a) sinus bradycardia;
    (b) first-degree atrioventricular (AV) block;
    (c) second-degree AV block, Wenckebach type;
    (d) high-grade AV block.
2 Axis: normal or slightly rightward.
3 P wave:
    (a) notched;
    (b) left atrial enlargement;
    (c) right atrial enlargement.
4 QRS complex:

(a) left ventricular hypertrophy voltage;

(b) right ventricular hypertrophy voltage;

(c) intraventricular conduction defects;

(d) incomplete right bundle branch block;

(e) pseudoanteroseptal myocardial infarction with QS in leads V1–V3.

5 ST segment:

(a) early repolarization;

(b) ST segment elevation.

6 T wave:

(a) increased amplitude;

(b) biphasic or inverted T waves in anterior precordial leads.

7 QT interval: normal or variable.

8 U wave: normal or increased amplitude.

Sinus bradycardia at rest is a well-recognized hallmark of a cardiovascular training effect. The resting heart rate tends to be lower in endurance-trained athletes. In general the heart rate at rest varies inversely with $\dot{V}O_{2max}$ or exercise capacity. Heart rates of < 40 beats·min^{-1} may be seen frequently in well-trained athletes, with even lower rates during sleep. Differentiating athlete's heart from an underlying true organic heart disease can be difficult, although lack of symptoms, a history of exercise training and participation in athletic events without symptoms are helpful signs. Nevertheless, if the physical examination reveals evidence suggestive of valvular or myocardial disease, other evaluation techniques might be useful.

Cardiovascular diseases in women

Mitral valve prolapse

This condition occurs with greater frequency in women than men (Levy & Savage, 1987). It is characterized by a variety of cardiac symptoms, some patients reporting chest pain and ventricular dysrhythmias but most not having any symptoms. Signs are those associated with auscultatory features (mid-systolic non-ejection click and late systolic murmur). Echocardiographic or cineangiographic evidence of systolic billowing of the mitral valve leaflets in the left atrium and a thickened mitral valve may

also be present. Other symptoms include chest pain, palpitations, dizziness, abnormal ECG, atrial or ventricular dysrhythmia, systemic emboli, mitral regurgitation, syncope and even sudden death.

Mitral valve prolapse is generally a benign syndrome and most patients can exercise without restrictions. The American College of Cardiology (Maron et al., 1985) recommends limiting competitive participation in those patients whose chest pain is worsened by exercise and in those with a history of syncope, supraventricular tachycardia, ventricular dysrhythmias, moderate or severe mitral regurgitation, or a family history of sudden death due to mitral valve prolapse. Exercise should be restricted, especially if the dysrhythmias are worsened during physical activity. Mitral valve prolapse may also be associated with Marfan's syndrome. Other valvular heart diseases affect male and female athletes equally.

Recommendations regarding eligibility for competition and limitations for physical activity and sports have been published by the American College of Cardiology and the American College of Sports Medicine.

Hypertrophic cardiomyopathy

This syndrome, characterized by a thickened left ventricle, is idiopathic, genetically transmitted and the most common cause of sudden death in young people during exercise. Any athlete with a history of dizziness or exercise-related syncope must be suspected of having hypertrophic cardiomyopathy and should be evaluated by an experienced cardiologist.

This cardiomyopathy may or may not have an outflow tract gradient. Some of the findings include ECG abnormalities, a family history of sudden death or cardiomyopathy, systolic anterior motion of the mitral valve in the echocardiogram, asymmetric septal hypertrophy and diastolic filling abnormalities. Those women with significant left ventricular outflow tract obstruction, a personal history of syncope, or complex dysrhythmias should not participate in any form of athletic competition. Regardless of disease severity, no participation in high-intensity competitive sports is recommended by the American College of Cardiology (Maron *et al.*, 1985).

Coronary heart disease

While there is still a general misconception among the lay public that coronary heart disease is a man's disease, there is increasing awareness of the problem in women. Although it has a later onset in life among women, it has a worse prognosis. Even the rate of early death after myocardial infarction is higher for women (Lerner & Kannel, 1986). The frequency of silent or unrecognized myocardial infarction is higher in women than in men, and women are referred for revascularization at a later stage of illness (Gardner *et al.*, 1985) and have higher operative mortality rates and periprocedural complications with coronary bypass surgery (Loop *et al.*, 1983). Since women participate in competitive sports well past their sixties, it is important to realize that they are not immune to heart disease.

Atherosclerosis begins in infancy, with lipid being deposited in the endothelium of the artery. Atherosclerotic plaques develop in coronary arteries when the amount of low-density lipoprotein cholesterol (LDL-C) entering the subintimal space exceeds removal, resulting in the accumulation of LDL-C in the form of cholesterol esters. The trigger may be an injury to, or disruption of, the endothelial cells lining the intima. The injury to the endothelium increases its permeability and exposes the subintimal and medial layers of the artery wall to infiltration by monocytes, platelets, LDL-C and other vasoactive substances. Another hypothesis about the development of the plaque assumes that lipid filtration occurs through the endothelium when the concentration of LDL-C in the blood is elevated. LDL-C is filtered into the subintimal space and followed by monocytes that assimilate the extracellular lipid and become macrophages. The progressive accumulation of lipid by macrophages leads to their conversion to foam cells, which are the principal constituent of the early lipid-filled plaque. Macrophages and platelets release a variety of growth factors and chemoattractants that result in the proliferation of smooth muscle cells.

The rate at which coronary atherosclerosis progresses will be mainly determined by genetics and lifestyle factors such as diet, smoking, physical activity and stress. Although the prevalence of coronary heart disease is lower among the active population, the risk factors and symptoms such as chest pain are equally important for both women and men (Hubbard *et al.*, 1992) (Table 16.1). Misperception of angina pectoris in women may delay the evaluation, increasing the risk. Exercise ECG testing is recommended for women who have a history typical of angina pectoris even if the resting ECG is normal (Hlatky *et al.*, 1984). Among young and middle-aged women, coronary heart disease has a low prevalence (Wenger *et al.*, 1993), so a normal exercise ECG has high specificity for excluding the illness (Weiner *et al.*, 1979). When indicated, perfusion imaging with thallium improves the specificity of exercise testing in women (Friedman *et al.*, 1982).

Hypertension

The pathophysiology of hypertension is not well understood. Of hypertensive adults, 90% are classified as having idiopathic hypertension. Idiopathic hypertension is also referred to as essential hypertension and its origin is unknown. Some of the factors that may contribute to or cause essential hypertension include obesity, insulin resistance, physical inactivity, high sodium intake, stress and genetic factors.

Role of exercise in the prevention of cardiovascular heart disease

The representation of women in prospective studies relating exercise to cardiovascular disease has been inadequate. Therefore it is difficult to determine possible gender differences in the effect of exercise on the risk of heart disease.

Table 16.1 Risk of developing coronary artery disease on the basis of specific values for the various risk factors. (From Wilmore & Costill, 1994 with permission)

Risk factor	Relative level of risk				
	Very low	Low	Moderate	High	Very high
Blood pressure (mmHg)					
Systolic	< 110	120	130–140	150–160	> 170
Diastolic	< 70	76	82–88	94–100	> 106
Cigarettes (per day)	Never or none in 1 year	5	10–20	30–40	> 50
Cholesterol (mg·dl^{-1})	< 180	< 200	220–240	260–280	> 300
Cholesterol : HDL*	< 3.0	< 4.0	< 4.5	> 5.2	> 7.0
Triglycerides (mg·dl^{-1})	< 50	< 100	130	200	> 300
Glucose (mg·dl^{-1})	< 80	90	100–110	120–130	> 140
Body fat (%)					
Men	12	16	25	30	> 35
Women	16	20	30	35	> 40
Body mass index†	< 25	25–30	30–40	> 40	
Stress tension	Never	Almost never	Occasional	Frequent	Nearly constant
Physical activity (min·week^{-1}) > 25 kJ·min^{-1} (5 MET)‡	240	180–120	100	80–60	< 30
> 60% Maximal heart rate reserve	120	90	30	0	0
ECG abnormality (ST depression in mV)§	0	0	0.05	0.10	0.20
Family history of premature heart attack (blood relative)¶	0	0	1	2	+ 3
Age (years)	< 30	40	50	60	> 70

*HDL, high-density lipoprotein.
†Body mass index = weight (kg)/height (m²).
‡1 MET is equal to the oxygen cost at rest.
§Other ECG abnormalities are also potentially dangerous and are not listed here.
¶Premature heart attack refers to persons younger than 60 years of age.

Most risk factors are shared equally by women and men. However, there are two factors under study that may uniquely affect the female cardiovascular system: the use of oral contraceptives and postmenopausal hormone replacement.

Physical activity might play an important role in preventing or delaying the onset of coronary artery disease in women. Possible mechanisms involve a reduction in risk factors as a result of physical activity and/or physiological adaptations with training. Some studies do show lower all-cause and cardiovascular mortality rates for more physically active women (Magnus et al., 1979; Salonen et al., 1982) and for fit older and younger women (Ekelund et al., 1988; Blair et al., 1989). Studies also support an inverse relation between blood pressure and fitness or physical activity status (Gibbons et al., 1983; Reaven et al., 1991). Exercise has little or no effect in severe hypertension. Powell et al. (1987), in an extensive review of epidemiological studies on physical inactivity and coronary artery disease, found that the relative risk from physical inactivity is similar to the risk associated with the three other major risk factors. In 1992 the American Heart Association declared that physical inactivity is a primary risk factor for coronary artery disease.

Physical activity, especially endurance training, exerts a beneficial effect on blood lipid levels: there is an increase in high-density lipoprotein cholesterol (HDL-C), a decrease in triglycerides, a decrease in LDL-C and total cholesterol, and almost all studies show benefits in the LDL-C: HDL-C and total cholesterol:HDL-C ratios (Haskell, 1984; Goldberg & Elliot, 1985). Exercise has also been reported to be effective in weight reduction, in the control of diabetes and for reducing anxiety (Kirkcaldy, 1989). No evidence is yet available to indicate that exercise leads to cessation of smoking.

Sudden death

Sudden cardiovascular deaths in athletes during training or competitive events are rare but have attracted a great deal of attention. The instantaneous nature of the deaths suggests that cardiac arrhythmias are probably the immediate cause of death in most instances. In children and adults under the age of 30, atherosclerotic heart disease is an unusual cause of exercise-related deaths. Hypertrophic cardiomyopathy is well recognized as a high risk factor for exercise-induced sudden death (McManus *et al.*, 1982). It is unknown which of several factors present in this disease is the initiating cause of sudden death. These athletes present with marked septal hypertrophy, disarray of ventricular myocardial fibres, and predisposition to ventricular arrhythmias and sudden death. The resting ECG is usually abnormal. A massive screening effort to identify competitive athletes at high risk for sudden death appears impractical.

Congenital anomalies of the coronary arteries are also reported as a cause of sudden death. When the left coronary artery has its origin from the right sinus of Valsalva and passes between the aorta and pulmonary artery, the blood flow through the artery is compromised during exercise as a result of its anatomical position (Levin *et al.*, 1978).

The causes of sudden death in athletes are summarized below.
1 Myocardial:
  (a) hypertrophic cardiomyopathy (asymmetric septal hypertrophy);
  (b) idiopathic cardiomyopathy;
  (c) myocarditis;
  (d) myocardial infarction.
2 Conduction system disorders:
  (a) primary conduction system disease;
  (b) accessory bypass tracts (Wolff–Parkinson–White syndrome);
  (c) congenital long QT interval syndrome.
3 Coronary artery disorders:
  (a) coronary atherosclerosis;
  (b) coronary artery anomalies;
  (c) coronary artery hypoplasia;
  (d) myocardial bridging, intramural coronary artery.
4 Valvular:
  (a) aortic stenosis;
  (b) mitral valve prolapse.
5 Vascular:
  (a) aortic dissection (Marfan's syndrome or atherosclerosis);
  (b) subarachnoid haemorrhage.

Conclusion and recommendations for future research

Research should be directed towards understanding the basic mechanisms of the cardiovascular system and should focus on aspects unique to women, especially in areas in which comparisons between women and men are inadequate or data are unavailable. The aspects of cardiovascular disease that need to be clarified are summarized below.
• Investigations need to address why there is a later onset of coronary heart disease in women compared with men, as well as a later onset of other cardiovascular disorders such as aortic stenosis, hypertension, stroke, heart failure and peripheral vascular disease (Wenger *et al.*, 1993).
• Research should determine why women undergo intensive or invasive evaluations less frequently or later than men who have symp-

toms of similar or lesser severity, particularly in the evaluation of chest pain.

• Educational messages focusing on cardiovascular disease in women should be increased to promote the objective of enhancing cardiovascular health.

• A vigorous antismoking campaign is needed to enhance awareness about the relation between cigarette smoking and cardiovascular disease. The prevalence of smoking among adolescent girls has exceeded that among boys for the past decade (Gilchrist *et al.*, 1989).

• **More women should be encouraged to adopt** an active lifestyle. Also, as more female athletes challenge the limits of endurance and resistance performance, scientists will have more opportunities to collect information on the respiratory and cardiovascular responses to exercise.

• A gender-specific pattern of cardiovascular regulation during exercise may exist. It is important to understand the health and performance implications of these gender-related differences.

References

American College of Sports Medicine (1994) Recommendations for determining eligibility for competition in athletes with cardiovascular abnormalities. *Medicine and Science in Sports and Exercise* **26**, S223–283.

Blair, S.N., Khol, H.W., Paffenbarger, R.S., Clark, D.G., Cooper, K.H. & Gibbons, L.W. (1989) Physical fitness and all-cause mortality: a prospective study of healthy men and women. *Journal of the American Medical Association* **262**, 2395–2401.

Ekelund, L., Haskell, W.L., Troung, Y.L., Gordon, E.H. & Shepps, D.S. (1988). Physical fitness as predictor of cardiovascular (CVD) mortality in asymptomatic females. *Circulation* **78** (Suppl. 11), Abstract 110.

Friedman, T.D., Greene, A.C., Iskandrian, A.S., Hakki, A.H., Kane, S.A. & Segal, B.L. (1982) Exercise thallium-201 myocardial scintigraphy in women: correlation with coronary arteriography. *American Journal of Cardiology* **49**, 1632–1637.

Gardner, T.J., Horneffer, P.J., Gott, V.L. *et al.* (1985) Coronary artery bypass grafting in women: a ten-year perspective. *Annals of Surgery* **201**, 780–784.

Gibbons, L.W., Blair, S.N., Cooper, K.H. & Smith, M. (1983) Association between coronary heart disease risk factors and physical fitness in healthy adult women. *Circulation* **67**, 977–983.

Gilchrist, L.D., Schinke, S.P. & Nurius, P. (1989) Reducing onset of habitual smoking among women. *Prevention Medicine* **18**, 235–248.

Goldberg, L. & Elliot, D.L. (1985) The effect of physical activity on lipid and lipoprotein levels. *Medical Clinics of North America* **69**, 41–55.

Haskell, W.L. (1984) The influence of exercise on the concentrations of triglyceride and cholesterol in human plasma. *Exercise and Sport Sciences Reviews* **12**, 205–244.

Hlatky, M.A., Pryor, D.B., Harrell, F.E. Jr, Califf, R.M., Mark, D.B. & Rosati, R.A. (1984) Factors affecting sensitivity and specificity of exercise electrocardiography: multivariable analysis. *American Journal of Medicine* **77**, 64–71.

Hubbard, B.L., Gibbons, R.J., Lapeyre, A.C. III, Zinsmeister, A.R. & Clements, I.P. (1992) Identification of severe coronary artery disease using simple clinical parameters. *Archives of Internal Medicine* **152**, 309–312.

Kirkcaldy, B. (1989) Exercise as a therapeutic modality. *Medicine and Sports Science* **29**, 166–187.

Lerner, D.J. & Kannel, W.B. (1986) Patterns of coronary heart disease morbidity and mortality in the sexes: a 26-year follow-up of the Framingham population. *American Heart Journal* **111**, 383–390.

Levin, D.C., Fellows, K.E. & Abrams, H.L. (1978) Hemodynamically significant primary abnormalities of the coronary arteries: angiographic aspects. *Circulation* **58**, 25–34.

Levy, D. & Savage, D. (1987) Prevalence and clinical features of mitral valve prolapse. *American Heart Journal* **113**, 1281–1290.

Loop, F.D., Golding, L.R., MacMillan, J.P., Cosgrove, D.M., Lytle, B.W. & Sheldon, W.C. (1983) Coronary artery surgery in women compared with men: analyses of risk and long-term results. *Journal of the American College of Cardiology* **1**, 383–390.

McManus, B.M., Waller, B.F., Graboys, T.B. *et al.* (1982) Exercise and sudden death. Part 1. *Current Problems in Cardiology* **6**, 1–89.

Magnus, K., Matroos, A. & Strackee, J. (1979) Walking, cycling, or gardening, with or without seasonal interruptions, in relation to acute coronary events. *American Journal of Epidemiology* **110**, 724–733.

Maron, B.J., Gaffney, F.A., Jeresaty, R.M., McKenna, W.J. & Miller, W.W. (1985) Cardiovascular abnormalities in the athlete: recommendations regarding eligibility for competition. Task force III: Hypertrophic cardiomyopathy, other myopericardial diseases and mitral valve prolapse. *Journal of the American College of Cardiology* **6**, 1215–1217.

Powell, K.E., Thompson, P.D. & Caspersen, C.J. (1987) Physical activity and the incidence of coronary heart disease. *Annual Reviews in Public Health* **8**, 253–287.

Reaven, P.D., Barrett-Connor, E. & Edelstein, S. (1991). Relation between leisure-time physical activity and blood pressure in older women. *Circulation* **83**, 559–565.

Salonen, J., Puska, P. & Tuomilehto, J. (1982) Physical activity and risk of myocardial infarction, cerebral stroke and death. *American Journal of Epidemiology* **115**, 526–537.

Weiner, D.A., Ryan, T.J., McCabe, C.H. *et al.* (1979) Exercise stress testing: correlations among history of angina, ST-segment response and prevalence of coronary-artery disease in the Coronary Artery Surgery Study (CASS). *New England Journal of Medicine* **301**, 230–235.

Wenger, N.K., Speroff, L. & Packard, B. (1993) Cardiovascular health and disease in women. *New England Journal of Medicine* **329**, 247–256.

Wilmore, J.H. & Costill, D.L. (1994) *Physiology of Sports and Exercise*. Human Kinetics Publishers, Champaign, Illinois.

Chapter 17

Physical Activity and Risk for Breast Cancer

PATTY S. FREEDSON, CHUCK E. MATTHEWS AND
PHILIP C. NASCA

Introduction

Interest in the relationship between physical
activity and breast cancer began with an observational study of former college athletes (Frisch *et
al.*, 1985). This study was the first to suggest that
physical activity confers a protective effect
against the development of breast cancer.
'Athlete' was defined as a woman who had been
on one varsity, house or intramural team for at
least 1 year and/or who had been recognized for
athletic distinction. Training had to be regular
and occur at least two times per week during the
season. The relative risk for breast cancer among
non-athletes was 1.86 [95% confidence interval
(CI) 1.0–3.47] compared with former athletes
after controlling for age, family history of breast
cancer, age at menarche, number of pregnancies,
oral contraceptive use, oestrogen use during
menopause, smoking and body composition.
Since 1985, a number of epidemiological studies
have examined this issue using several different
approaches and experimental designs. The
notion that physical activity may provide protection from breast cancer is appealing, as this
disease is a major public health concern for
women.

Breast cancer is the most common cancer
among women in the USA. In 1994, it was estimated that there were 182 000 new cases and
46 000 deaths from the disease. Nearly one-third
of all new cancer cases among women were
cancers of the breast (Gloeckler *et al.*, 1994). In
1991, the age-adjusted breast cancer mortality

rates for white and black women were 26.8 and
31.9 per 100 000 respectively. Although the mortality rate has remained relatively constant since
1950, the incidence of breast cancer has been
increasing in the USA, particularly since 1980
(Fig. 17.1). A significant portion of this increase
can be attributed to changes in the diagnostic
criteria for the disease and increased detection
by screening programmes since the early 1980s
(Kelsey & Horn-Ross, 1993). However, some
studies have reported that the incidence of the
disease is increasing independent of enhanced
screening and diagnostic changes (White *et al.*,
1990; Kelsey & Horn-Ross, 1993; Hankey *et al.*,
1994). Given the relatively stable mortality rates
and increased incidence rates for breast cancer,
primary prevention of the disease is an important public health concern. This chapter reviews
the existing epidemiological literature, evaluating the association between regular physical
activity and breast cancer and potential biological mechanisms through which physical activity
may mediate the relationship.

Physical activity and breast
cancer risk

Since 1994, several epidemiological studies have
examined the association between physical
activity and risk of breast cancer (Bernstein *et al.*,
1994; Dorgan *et al.*, 1994; Friedenreich & Rohan,
1995; Mittendorf *et al.*, 1995; Taioli *et al.*, 1995;
D'Avanzo *et al.*, 1996; McTiernan *et al.*, 1996; Tretli
& Gaard, 1996; Chen *et al.*, 1997; Coogan *et al.*,

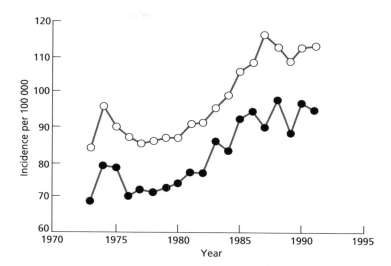

Fig. 17.1 Age-adjusted breast cancer incidence rates per 100 000 white (○) and black (●) women in the USA, 1973–91.

1997; Hu *et al.*, 1997; Thune *et al.*, 1997). These reports have provided conflicting results, with Bernstein *et al.* (1994), Mittendorf *et al.* (1995) and Thune *et al.* (1997) providing the most compelling evidence of a protective effect. Bernstein *et al.* (1994) reported that lifelong participation in physical activity was associated with a protective effect, while Mittendorf *et al.* (1995) concluded that activity every day of the year between the ages of 14 and 22 years was related to a reduced risk of breast cancer. In the study by Thune *et al.* (1997), adult physical activity conferred the protective effect. In contrast, Dorgan *et al.* (1994) reported a small increased risk of breast cancer among physically active women and Chen *et al.* (1997) reported a minimal protective effect of either lifelong or adult leisure-time physical activity.

Tables 17.1 and 17.2 summarize study design, subject characteristics, outcome measures, physical activity assessment techniques and results from all epidemiological studies conducted since 1985. It should be noted that even though the association between regular physical activity and breast cancer risk remains equivocal, several lines of evidence point to potential mechanisms through which physical activity may possibly modify the risk of developing the disease.

Influence of physical activity assessment methods

A common observation emerges from the group of published retrospective studies that found a reduced risk of breast cancer in more active women, i.e. quantifying lifelong participation in physical activity, rather than at a single point in time, may be important in observing a reduced risk for the disease. Among the five retrospective cohort studies that reported a protective effect, each either directly quantified or had a reasonable proxy measure of lifetime activity levels, e.g. usual occupational activity or reported exercise habits throughout life (Frisch *et al.*, 1985; Vena *et al.*, 1987; Vihko *et al.*, 1992; Zheng *et al.*, 1993; Bernstein *et al.*, 1994).

A single measure of physical activity in retrospective cohort studies may not reflect the lifelong participation of women in physical activity. Indeed, Dorgan *et al.* (1994) present evidence that activity scores on the physical activity index in 1954–56 were only weakly correlated ($r = 0.18$ and 0.25) to the physical activity index scores measured 14 and 16 years later. In the investigations of Albanes *et al.* (1989) and Paffenbarger *et al.* (1992), no data were presented on the changes in physical activity in the interval between baseline and follow-up.

There are no longitudinal data on the trends for physical activity behaviour in the USA that date back to the baseline of these investigations; however, survey data have been available for the USA and Canada since the early and mid 1980s. In both countries there has been a trend towards increasing participation in physical activities, predominantly in moderate intensity activities (e.g. walking, gardening, social dancing) (Stephens & Casperson, 1994). Trend data from the Minnesota Heart Survey between 1980–82 and 1985–87 suggest that women increased their total activity [+55 kJ·day^{-1} (+13 kcal·day^{-1})] in leisure time over this time period (Jacobs et al. 1991). Therefore, it is likely that a single assessment of physical activity is a poor indicator of lifelong activity behaviour, particularly when trends for activity appear to be changing.

Summary of observational studies

Of the 18 published studies presented in Tables 17.1 and 17.2, only three suggest a moderate to strong protective effect of physical activity where the 95% relative risk CI does not include 1.0 (Bernstein et al., 1994; Mittendorf et al., 1995; Thune et al., 1997). Investigations that have observed a protective effect for high levels of activity on the risk of breast cancer appear to have better information for physical activity over much of the individual's lifetime or to have a proxy lifetime measure (e.g. occupational physical activity). Based on these findings, physical activity accumulated over a lifetime appears to attenuate breast cancer risk in women. The remainder of this review examines the experimental evidence supporting the notion that

Table 17.1 Selected features of studies examining the association between physical activity and breast cancer

Reference	Design	Sample	Breast cancer cases	Physical activity assessment
Frisch et al. (1985)	Retrospective cohort	5398 US college alumnae graduating between 1925 and 1981; aged 21–81 years in 1981	Self-reported breast cancer in 1981; 69 cases	Classified as athletes or non-athletes based on college participation in sport or physical training
Vena et al. (1987)	Retrospective cohort	25 000 residents of Washington dying between 1974 and 1979	Death certificate diagnosis of breast cancer; 791 cases	Occupational job classification
Albanes et al. (1989)	Prospective cohort	7407 from NHANES I and NHEFS	Review of hospital admission, death records and self-report; histologically confirmed in all but one case; 122 cases	Recreational and non-recreational activity self-classified into one of three categories: low, moderate or high
Paffenbarger et al. (1992)	Prospective cohort	4706 University of Pennsylvania alumnae graduating between 1916 and 1950	Incident cases of breast cancer; 46 cases	College sport participation: ≤ 5 h·week^{-1} or > 5 h·week^{-1}

Continued

Table 17.1 (*Continued*)

Reference	Design	Sample	Breast cancer cases	Physical activity assessment
Vihko *et al.* (1992)	Retrospective cohort	8619 language teachers and 1499 physical education teachers	Incident cases of breast cancer verified by Finnish Cancer Registry; 128 cases	Job classification
Dosemeci *et al.* (1993)	Hospital-based case control	Hospital patients from Turkey; 244 controls	Histologically confirmed cases of breast cancer; 241 cases	Occupation titles and years in occupation used to estimate energy expenditure and sitting time at work
Zheng *et al.* (1993)	Record linkage	3783 incident cancer cases in Shanghai, China diagnosed between 1980 and 1984	2736 verified by Chinese Cancer Registry	Occupational physical activity, sitting time and energy expenditure; three levels of activity
Bernstein *et al.* (1994)	Population case-control	University of Southern California Cancer Surveillance Program, 1983–89; < 40 years of age; 545 controls	545 cases matched on birth date, race parity, neighbourhood residence	Lifetime (since menarche) physical activity ($\geq 2\,h\cdot week^{-1}$); interviewer administered
Dorgan *et al.* (1994)	Prospective cohort	2298 from Framingham Heart Study	Incident cases based on hospital admission, death records and self-report; all but one case histologically confirmed; 117 cases	Usual $h\cdot day^{-1}$ in sedentary, light, moderate and heavy activities; index weighted for energy expenditure; low vs. high quartile
Friedenreich & Rohan (1995)	Population case-control	Cancer registry in Adelaide and controls from electoral roll	444 cases	Recreational physical activity converted to $kcal\cdot week^{-1}$; low vs. high quartile
Mittendorf *et al.* (1995)	Population case-control	Cancer registries in Massachusetts, Maine, New Hampshire, Wisconsin and controls from drivers' licenses or Medicare lists	6888 cases	Strenuous recreational physical activity at 14–18 and 18–22 years of age

Continued p. 254

Table 17.1 (*Continued*)

Reference	Design	Sample	Breast cancer cases	Physical activity assessment
Taioli *et al.* (1995)	Hospital case-control	One hospital source for cases and controls	617 cases	Strenuous recreational physical activity at ages 15–21, 22–44 and 45 +; < 3 vs. ≥ 3 h·week^{-1}
Tretli & Gaard (1996)	Ecological	Norwegian Cancer Registry	20 111 cases	Increased physical activity during the Second World War
D'Avanzo *et al.* (1996)	Multicentre population case-control	Hospitals in Italy were sources for cases and 2588 controls	2569 cases	Occupational and leisure-time physical activity at ages 15–19, 30–39 and 50–59 years; lowest vs. highest quartile
McTiernan *et al.* (1996)	Population case-control	Washington State Cancer Registry and RDD controls	537 cases	Recreational activity at ages 12–21 years and 2 years before interview
Hu *et al.* (1997)	Hospital case-control	Hospital in Japan for cases and breast cancer screening programme for 369 controls	157 cases	Recreational activity in adolescence and in twenties
Thune *et al.* (1997)	Prospective cohort	25 624 from three counties in Norway in 1974–78 and 1977–83 health survey	351 cases	Occupational and recreational activity in years preceding survey; sedentary vs. regularly active
Chen *et al.* (1997)	Population case-control	Seattle–Puget Sound SEER Registry and 961 RDD controls	747 cases	Recreational activity 2 years before survey and from 12 to 21 years; no activity vs. ≥ 4 h·week^{-1}

NHANES, National Health and Nutrition Examination Survey; NHEFS, NHANES I Epidemiologic Follow-up Study; RDD, random digit telephone dialling; SEER, surveillance, epidemiology and end results.

Table 17.2 Results of studies examining the association between physical activity and breast cancer

Reference	Variables controlled in analyses	Contrasts	Results
Frisch *et al.* (1985)	Age	Non-athletes vs. athletes	54% increased risk for non-athletes
	Age, number of pregnancies, family history of cancer, body composition, age at menarche, smoking, oral contraceptive or oestrogen use	Non-athletes vs. athletes	86% increased risk for non-athletes
Vena *et al.* (1987)	Age	Job activity level: 1 (low active) 2 3, 4 and 5	15% increased mortality 17% reduced mortality 15% reduced mortality
Albanes *et al.* (1989)	Age at menarche and menopause, parity, age at first birth, family history of breast cancer, body mass index, dietary fat intake	*Premenopausal* Recreational (low vs. high) Non-recreational (low vs. high) *Postmenopausal* Recreational (low vs. high) Non-recreational (low vs. high)	40% reduced risk for low 60% reduced risk for low 50% reduced risk for low 70% increased risk for low All, $P > 0.05$
Paffenbarger *et al.* (1992)	Age	≤ 5 vs. > 5 h·week^{-1} in college sports	No association
	Age, BMI, maternal history of cancer	≥ 4600 vs. < 4600 kJ·week^{-1} (1095 kcal·week^{-1})	12% reduced risk for more active ($P > 0.05$)
Vihko *et al.* (1992)	Age	Language vs. physical education teachers	20% increased risk for language teachers (NS)
	Age, observation period, age at first birth, number of children	Language vs. physical education teachers	30% increased risk for language teachers (NS)
Dosemeci *et al.* (1993)	Age, smoking, socioeconomic status	Energy expenditure [< 8 vs. > 12 kJ·min^{-1} (<1.9 vs. > 2.8 kcal·min^{-1})]	30% increased risk for low energy expenditure ($P > 0.05$)
Zheng *et al.* (1993)	Age	Sitting time Long (> 80% of work) Moderate (20–80% of work Short (< 20% of work) Energy expenditure Low [< 8 kJ·min^{-1} (1.9 kcal·min^{-1})] Moderate [8–12 kJ·min^{-1} (1.9–2.8 kcal·min^{-1})] High [> 12 kJ·min^{-1} (>2.8 kcal·min^{-1})]	 27% increased incidence 10% increased incidence 7% lower incidence 31% increased incidence 5% increased incidence ($P > 0.05$) 21% reduced incidence

Continued p. 256

Table 17.2 (*Continued*)

Reference	Variables controlled in analyses	Contrasts	Results
Bernstein *et al.* (1994)	Age at menarche, first full-term pregnancy, number of full-term pregnancies, lactation, family history of breast cancer, Quetelet's index, oral contraceptive use	Lowest vs. highest weekly activity quintile	58% reduced risk for high (95% relative risk CI 0.27–0.64)
Dorgan *et al.* (1994)	Age at first pregnancy, education, occupation, alcohol consumption	Lowest vs. highest physical activity quartile	60% greater risk for high (95% relative risk CI 0.9–2.9)
Friedenreich & Rohan (1995)	Quetelet's index, energy intake	Lowest vs. highest quartile	27% greater risk for low (95% relative risk CI 0.50–1.05)
Mittendorf *et al.* (1995)	Age, age at menarche, age at menopause, menopausal status, first full-term pregnancy, parity, family history of breast cancer, history of benign breast disease, type of menopause, alcohol consumption, BMI, BMI/ menopausal status	No strenuous activity vs. activity every day of the year	50% reduced risk for active (95% relative risk CI 0.4–0.7
Taioli *et al.* (1995)	Age, education, BMI, age at menarche, parity	< 3 vs. ≥ 3 h·week⁻¹ of exercise	1.0 relative risk (95% relative risk CI 0.6–1.8)
Tretli & Gaard (1996)	None	Increased physical activity during Second World War	Decreased incidence of breast cancer among women in puberty during Second World War
D'Avanzo *et al.* (1996)	Age, centre, menarche age, first full-term pregnancy, parity, menopausal status, age at menopause, caloric intake, previous BBD, breast cancer family history	Lowest vs. highest quartile	15–19 years: 6% decreased risk for low (95% relative risk CI 0.77–1.16) 30–39 years: 27% decreased risk for low (95% relative risk CI 0.56–1.06) 50–59 years: 32% decreased risk for low (95% relative risk CI 0.4–1.09)

Continued

Table 17.2 (*Continued*)

Reference	Variables controlled in analyses	Contrasts	Results
McTiernan *et al.* (1996)	Age, education	No exercise vs. ≥ 3 h·week⁻¹ of high-intensity exercise	40% reduced risk (95% relative risk CI 0.4–1.0)
Hu *et al.* (1997)	None	No exercise vs. highest tertile of energy expenditure	*Premenopausal breast cancer* Activity in adolescence: 28% reduced risk (95% relative risk CI 0.38–1.38) Activity during twenties: 1.01 (95% relative risk CI 0.54–1.87) *Postmenopausal breast cancer* Activity in adolescence: 1.39 (95% relative risk CI 0.61–3.13) Activity in twenties: 0.53 (95% relative risk CI 0.19–1.52)
Thune *et al.* (1997)	Age at study entry, BMI, height, residence, number of children	Sedentary vs. consistently active	33% reduced risk (95% relative risk CI 0.40–1.1)
Chen *et al.* (1997)	Age	No activity vs. ≥ 4 h·week⁻¹	8% reduced risk (95% relative risk CI 0.71–1.22)

BMI, body mass index; CI, confidence interval; NS, not significant.

regular participation in physical activity reduces the risk of breast cancer before and after menopause.

Biological mechanisms: hormonal effects

Although the aetiology of breast cancer is not completely understood, several factors have been clearly associated with increased risk of the disease. The most striking observation is that many of the risk factors are related to exposure to endogenous or exogenous hormones (Kelsey, 1993; Pike *et al.*, 1993). Pike *et al.* (1993) have pro-

posed a model which suggests that combined exposure to oestrogens and progesterone is important to an increased risk for breast cancer. Reviewing several studies that examined the proliferative activity of breast tissue during the menstrual cycle, these authors provide evidence suggesting that higher rates of breast cell proliferative activity are associated with increased levels of both oestradiol and progesterone during the luteal phase of the cycle. This mechanism appears to be the direct link between circulating hormones and risk of breast cancer (Preston-Martin *et al.*, 1990). An increased level of cell proliferation in breast tissue may lead to a greater number of genetic errors, which in turn increases the risk of cell mutations and the development of cancer.

Pike *et al.* (1993) suggest that their model provides a mechanism to explain the following epidemiological findings: (i) lower risk for women after the menopause (naturally occurring or following ovarian removal); (ii) increased risk among women exposed to oestrogen replacement therapy or oral contraceptives; and (iii) lower risk for obese women before, but not after, the menopause. The latter paradoxical finding of a reduced risk for premenopausal obesity and increased risk for postmenopausal obesity may be explained by this model. Pike *et al.* (1993) present evidence which suggests that premenopausal obesity is associated with a greater number of anovulatory cycles and lower levels of circulating progesterone levels; thus this group of women have a favourable hormonal profile (Hartz *et al.*, 1979). Postmenopausal obese women have increased levels of circulating oestrogen, thus elevating their breast cancer risk (Simpson & Mendelson, 1987; Barbosa *et al.*, 1990). The recent Women Nurses Study findings by Huang *et al.* (1997) support this hypothesis. They reported that a higher body mass index and weight gain after 18 years of age was unrelated to breast cancer risk before menopause, but was associated with breast cancer risk after menopause. Finally, the model of Pike *et al.* (1993) fits several other epidemiological findings related to reduced exposure to ovarian hormones and lower breast cancer risk, including later menarche, a greater number of pregnancies and more years of breast-feeding (Kelsey, 1993). The epidemiological findings which suggest that high levels of regular physical activity confer a protective effect on breast cancer risk may also be explained in terms of the model suggested by Pike *et al.* (1993).

Impact of physical activity on endogenous hormones

Regular vigorous exercise has been associated with an alteration of normal menstrual function,

resulting in primary amenorrhoea (menarche at >16 years), secondary amenorrhoea (lack of menstruation for three to four consecutive months) or 'unobtrusive' but hormonally important alterations in menstrual function (Bullen *et al.*, 1985; Bernstein *et al.*, 1987; Bonen, 1994). In the two latter situations, circulating levels of oestrogen and/or progesterone are reduced from those observed in a regular menstrual cycle and this could be a mechanism whereby exposure to these hormones is reduced. In each of these instances, the cessation of exercise results in return to normal menstrual functioning (Bonen, 1994). The fluctuations of oestradiol and progesterone over the course of a typical menstrual cycle are presented in Fig. 17.2. This illustration clearly shows the sharp peak of oestradiol at the end of the follicular phase and the abrupt rise in progesterone accompanied by a mild elevation of oestradiol during the luteal phase of the cycle.

Female athletes training at very high volumes have often reported secondary amenorrhoea (Bonen, 1994). In experimental studies, female athletes have low levels of oestradiol and progesterone and have greatly reduced peak hormone concentrations over the course of a menstrual cycle (Loucks *et al.*, 1989; Bonen, 1994). Similar hormonal changes have been observed in groups of inactive women following the initiation of vigorous high-volume (>20 h·week^{-1}) exercise programmes (Bullen *et al.*, 1985). In experimental studies of lower exercise volume (1–2 h·week^{-1}), unobtrusive changes, lower progesterone levels or a shortened luteal phase have been observed in some but not all investigations (Bernstein *et al.*, 1987; Bonen, 1992).

Data from Loucks *et al.* (1989) provide a vivid example of secondary amenorrhoea and the 'unobtrusive' alterations in hormonal profile associated with high levels of athletic training. These investigators examined urinary markers for oestrogen and progesterone, oestrone glucuronide (E_1G) and pregnanediol glucuronide (PdG), over 30 days in three groups of women who differed in their menstrual and exercise status. The athletic women were competitive runners, cyclists, swimmers or triathletes

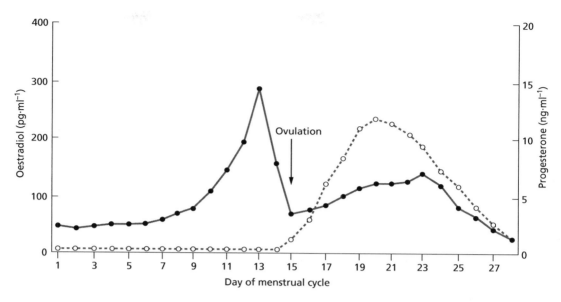

Fig. 17.2 Serum concentrations of oestradiol (●) and progesterone (○) by day of the menstrual cycle. Day 1 is the first day of menses and a 28-day cycle is assumed, with ovulation occurring on day 14. (From Pike *et al.*, 1993 with permission.)

who had been training for more than 8 years. Comparisons of urinary excretion of E_1G and PdG were made between regularly cycling sedentary, regularly cycling athletic and amenorrhoeic athletic groups (Fig. 17.3). Amenorrhoeic athletes appeared to have very low levels of oestradiol and progesterone, with little fluctuation over the cycle. Among the regularly cycling athletes, although a normal oestrogen profile was observed, luteal-phase progesterone levels were significantly reduced ($P < 0.05$) and the length of the luteal phase was significantly shortened (by 2 days, $P < 0.05$) compared with sedentary women (Fig. 17.3). Thus, it appears that the hormonal profile associated with lower risk of breast cancer may be achieved via physical activity. However, the exercise volume needed to attain this profile is quite large. Moderate levels of exercise may not always provide the hypothesized hormonal profile.

Alterations in hormonal function among women who undertake regular vigorous exercise appear to be related to an energy conservation adaptation within the human organism (Warren,

1980; Bonen, 1994). Under conditions of low caloric availability or deficit the body limits energy expenditure to systems within the body that are of lesser importance. For instance, the luteal phase of the menstrual cycle is marked by an increase in resting metabolic rate of 10–15%. Therefore, shortening its length during times of moderate caloric deficit will conserve energy (Bonen, 1994; Heymsfield *et al.*, 1994). A consequence of this adaptation may be to lower a woman's exposure to endogenous progesterone.

Warren (1980) hypothesized that the 'energy drain' associated with exercise may be related to many of the observed reproductive disorders among exercising women. This hypothesis is consistent with observations that energy availability is directly related to reproductive function in many species of mammals (Bronson, 1988). Loucks and Callister (1993) have also speculated that energy availability is an important factor in human reproductive function and have presented evidence that the low-T_3 (triiodothyronine) syndrome, which is associated with secondary amenorrhoea, can be prevented in

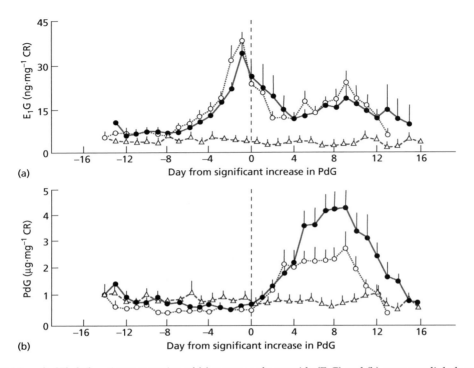

Fig. 17.3 Mean (± SE) daily urinary excretion of (a) oestrone glucuronide (E_1G) and (b) pregnanediol glucuronide (PdG) in different groups of women. Days are orientated from a significant increase in urinary PdG excretion, with day 1 being the day of first significant increase. ●, cycling sedentary; ○, cycling athletic; △, amenorrhoeic athletic. CR, creatinine. (From Loucks *et al.*, 1989 with permission.)

exercising women who balance their energy expenditure with intake. To our knowledge no studies have directly examined the influence of energy availability on progesterone levels during the luteal phase or on the length of the luteal phase. Interestingly, Bonen (1992) provide indirect evidence that length of the luteal phase and progesterone levels are not altered in exercising women who maintain their energy balance (e.g. maintain body mass and percentage body fat). Their results provide indirect evidence that length of the luteal phase and progesterone levels may be influenced by energy availability in the physiological system rather than by physical activity only.

If energy availability rather than physical activity is the key to a 'low-risk' hormonal profile for breast cancer, the variability of the epidemiological studies may be more under-standable. Since physical activity and caloric intake can each be independently manipulated to achieve a reduced energy availability and the attendant protective hormonal profile, the classification of exposure to breast cancer risk by evaluating only one side of the energy balance equation (e.g. physical activity) may be limited. It is possible that the inconsistencies in the existing literature on physical activity and breast cancer are related to the inability to classify this 'low-risk' hormonal profile accurately by examining only one side of the energy balance equation. No studies of the association between physical activity and breast cancer have examined the interaction of energy expenditure and energy intake on breast cancer risk. The greater protective effect of physical activity in lean women observed by Thune *et al.* (1997) indirectly supports this energy balance theory.

Alternative biological mechanisms: obesity attenuation and enhanced immunosurveillance

In addition to the potential impact of physical activity on endogenous hormones, high levels of activity may influence the risk of breast cancer beneficially via an influence on the development of obesity and on immunosurveillance of early tumour growth. Obesity has been associated with increased risk of breast cancer in post-menopausal women and decreased risk in pre-menopausal women (Kelsey, 1993; Pike et al., 1993; Huang et al., 1997). The protective effect of obesity before the menopause is transient because an increase in body mass after the menopause has been associated with an approximately 2.5-fold increased risk of the disease (Lubin et al., 1985; Ballard-Barbash et al., 1990).

The recent study by Huang et al. (1997) reported that weight gain after age 18 was strongly associated with an increased risk of postmenopausal breast cancer in women who had never used hormone replacement therapy. The relative risk was 1.99 (95% CI 1.43–2.76) for a ≥20-kg weight gain compared with women who were weight stable. Thus it appears that weight gain is a potent stimulus for the development of breast cancer after the menopause for women who have not used hormone replacement therapy.

Accumulation of fat mass in central locations on the body appears to be a particularly strong risk factor for the disease. Schapira et al. (1990) found that higher levels of centrally located fat conferred a five- to six-fold increased risk for developing breast cancer. These findings are consistent with the hypothesis that after menopause obesity creates a high-risk hormonal environment. In postmenopausal women, the predominant circulating oestrogen is oestrone, which is produced in an aromatization reaction from circulating androgens within adipose tissue (Simpson & Mendelson, 1987). Increased levels of adiposity have been associated with increased serum concentrations of oestrone and greater concentrations of free oestrone (Siiteri, 1987; Barbosa et al., 1990).

It is generally understood that higher levels of physical activity aid in the maintenance of fat-free mass and attenuate gains in fat mass over the lifespan. Studies of the age-related changes in body composition suggest that following the menopause there is an acceleration in both accumulation of fat mass and loss of fat-free mass. Moreover, the accumulation of fat mass tends to increase on the trunk and intra-abdominally (Heymsfield et al., 1994). Regular participation in physical activity appears to attenuate these changes. Interestingly, a recent study observed that abdominal fat was lost preferentially in response to exercise training and that loss of overall fat mass was highly correlated with loss of visceral fat ($r = 0.70$) in obese women (Despres et al., 1991). These findings strongly support the role of regular physical activity in blunting the age-related gain in fat mass and in reducing fat mass after it has been accumulated.

Our understanding of the interrelations between the immune system and physical activity is only beginning to emerge. The published data provide some support for the hypothesis that moderate levels of activity can improve host defence against tumour growth by enhancing macrophage and monocyte function (Hoffman-Goetz, 1994; Woods & Davis, 1994). Additionally, it has been hypothesized that physical activity may buffer the neuroendocrine stress response, which is known negatively to affect immune function, and therefore exercise may enhance immune function indirectly (LaPierre et al., 1994). Unfortunately, our current understanding of the relationship of physical activity to the immune system is in its infancy. The field is only beginning to derive preliminary findings, which are exceedingly complex and often interrelated to many systems in the body.

Conclusion

The mechanisms presented to explain some of the epidemiological findings of a reduced risk of breast cancer in more physically active women are plausible. The concept that high levels of physical activity reduce exposure to oestrogen and progesterone before the menopause and influence oestrone levels indirectly by attenuating fat-mass gains after the menopause are generally supported in the literature. Presently, the data supporting the proposed mechanisms are stronger than the current epidemiological findings. Studies that report a protective effect of physical activity on breast cancer have shown that lifelong exposure to activity is important. Studies that did not demonstrate consistent patterns of activity over the lifespan did not generally report this effect. There is no clear explanation why some studies have observed an adverse effect of higher levels of physical activity on risk of breast cancer, although these findings may be related to: (i) the assessment of activity at only a single point in time; (ii) the lack of control for factors that increased breast cancer risk in more active women; or (iii) incomplete assessment of energy availability.

If the findings of Bernstein et al. (1994) and Thune et al. (1997) are reproduced, showing that very high levels of physical activity reduce breast cancer risk by appoximately 50% and that the proposed hormonal changes are responsible, then consideration would have to be given to public health recommendations for physical activity in this group of women. Such high levels of physical activity may lead to reduced risk of breast cancer. However, if the hypothesized hormonal changes do take place, they may lead to adverse outcomes for bone health. Secondary amenorrhoea has been associated with lower bone density (lower peak bone mass and/or enhanced bone resorption) in young women consequent to reduced exposure to endogenous oestrogens (Constantini, 1994).

If public health recommendations are to be made specifically for women, then these recommendations should be formulated so that the risk of breast cancer and cardiovascular disease is reduced optimally and the risk of osteoporosis is not increased. Since most cases of breast cancer in the USA are detected in postmenopausal women (88% after age 50 years) and there is a clear increased risk for obese women in this group, recommendations for physical activity aimed at attenuating excessive weight gain in adulthood could be made (Hankey et al., 1994). Such recommendations should focus on reducing the gain in adult body mass often seen with ageing rather than promoting high levels of exercise training, which may produce secondary amenorrhoea.

Currently in the USA, participation rates of women in regular vigorous or moderate-intensity physical activity are relatively low for both the adolescent and adult populations. Among 9th to 12th grade girls, participation in vigorous activity three or more times weekly was only 27.5% for whites, 17.4% for blacks and 20.9% for Hispanics. During high school, participation rates dropped in each successive grade: 30.6, 27.1, 23.4 and 17.3% for 9th through 12th grades, respectively (Centers for Disease Control and Prevention, 1991). By middle age, only about 10% of women in the USA report participation in regular vigorous activity and only 40% participate in regular activity of any kind (Stephens & Casperson, 1994). If the association between regular physical activity and breast cancer is eventually confirmed, significant population-wide effects on the development of breast cancer may be possible by increasing activity levels in a large proportion of the population.

References

Albanes, D., Blair, A. & Taylor, P.R. (1989) Physical activity and risk of cancer in the NHANES I population. *American Journal of Public Health* **79**, 744–750.

Ballard-Barbash, R., Schatzkin, A., Taylor, P. & Kahle, L. (1990) Association of change in body mass with breast cancer. *Cancer Research* **50**, 2152–2155.

Barbosa, J.C., Schulz, T.D., Filley, S.J. & Nieman, D.C. (1990) The relationship among adiposity, diet, and hormone concentrations in vegetarian and non-vegetarian post menopausal women. *American Journal of Clinical Nutrition* **51**, 798–803.

Bernstein, L., Ross, R.K., Lobo, R.A., Hanisch, R., Krailo, M.D. & Henderson, B.E. (1987) The effects of moderate physical activity on menstrual cycle patterns in adolescence: implications for breast cancer prevention. *British Journal of Cancer* **55**, 681–698.

Bernstein, L., Henderson, B.E., Hanisch, R., Sullivan-Halley, J. & Ross, R.K. (1994) Physical exercise and reduced risk of breast cancer in young women. *Journal of the National Cancer Institute* **86**, 1403–1408.

Bonen, A. (1992) Recreational exercise does not impair menstrual cycles: a prospective study. *International Journal of Sports Medicine* **13**, 110–120.

Bonen, A. (1994) Exercise induced menstrual cycle changes: a functional temporary adaptation to metabolic stress. *Sports Medicine* **17**, 373–392.

Bronson, F.H. (1988) Seasonal regulation of reproduction in mammals. In E. Knobil & J.D. Neill (eds) *The Physiology of Reproduction*, Vol. 2, pp. 1831–1871. Raven Press, New York.

Bullen, B.A., Skrinar, G.S., Beitins, I.Z., von Mering, G., Turnbull, B.A. & McArthur, J.W. (1985) Induction of menstrual disorders by strenuous exercise in untrained women. *New England Journal of Medicine* **312**, 1349–1353.

Centers for Disease Control and Prevention. (1991) Chronic disease and health promotion. Reprints from *Morbidity and Mortality Weekly Reports: 1990–1991*. Youth Risk Behavior Surveillance System, US Department of Health and Human Services, Atlanta.

Chen, C.-L., White, E., Malone, K.E. & Daling, J.R. (1997) Leisure-time physical activity in relation to breast cancer among young women (Washington, United States). *Cancer Causes and Control* **8**, 77–84.

Constantini, N.W. (1994) Clinical consequences of athletic amenorrhea. *Sports Medicine* **17**, 213–223.

Coogan, P.F., Newcomb, P.A., Clapp, R.W., Trentham-Dietz, A., Baron, J.A. & Longnecker, M.P. (1997) Physical activity in usual occupation and risk of breast cancer (United States). *Cancer Causes and Control* **8**, 626–631.

D'Avanzo, B., Nanni, O., La Vecchia, C. *et al.* (1996) Physical activity and breast cancer risk. *Cancer Epidemiology* **5**, 155–160.

Despres, J.P., Pouliot, M.C., Mooranji, S. *et al.* (1991) Loss of abdominal fat and metabolic response to exercise training in obese women. *American Journal of Physiology* **261**, E159–E167.

Dorgan, J.F., Brown, C., Barrett, M. *et al.* (1994) Physical activity and risk of breast cancer in the Framingham Heart Study. *American Journal of Epidemiology* **139**, 622–669.

Dosemeci, M., Hayes, R.B., Vetter, R. *et al.* (1993) Occupational physical activity, socioeconomic status and risks of 15 cancer sites in Turkey. *Cancer Causes and Control* **4**, 313–321.

Friedenreich, C.M. & Rohan, T.E. (1995) Physical activity and risk of breast cancer. *European Journal of Cancer Prevention* **4**, 145–151.

Frisch, R.E., Wyshak, G., Albright, N.L. *et al.* (1985) Lower prevalence of breast cancer and cancers of the reproductive system among former college athletes compared to non-athletes. *British Journal of Cancer* **52**, 885–891.

Gloeckler, L.A., Miller, B.A., Hankey, B.F., Kosary, C.L., Harras, A. & Edwards, B.K. (eds) (1994) *Cancer Statistics Review, 1973–1991*. NIH pub. no. 94-2789. National Cancer Institute, Bethesda, Maryland.

Hankey, B.F., Miller, B., Curtis, R. & Kosary, C. (1994) Trends in breast cancer in younger women in contrast to older women. *Monographs of the National Cancer Institute* **16**, 7–16.

Hartz, A.J., Barboriak, P.N., Wong, A., Katayama, K.P. & Rimm, A.A. (1979) The association of obesity with infertility and related menstrual abnormalities in women. *International Journal of Obesity* **3**, 57–73.

Heymsfield, S.B., Gallagher, D., Poehlman, E.T. *et al.* (1994) Menopausal changes in body composition and energy expenditure. *Experimental Gerontology* **29**, 377–389.

Hoffman-Goetz, L. (1994) Exercise, natural immunity, and tumor metastasis. *Medicine and Science in Sports and Exercise* **26**, 157–164.

Hu, Y.-H., Nagata, C., Shimizu, H., Kaneda, N. & Kashiki, Y. (1997) Association of body mass index, physical activity, and reproductive histories with breast cancer: a case-control study in Gifu, Japan. *Breast Cancer Research and Treatment* **43**, 65–72.

Huang, Z., Hankinson, S.E., Colditz, G.A. *et al.* (1997) Dual effects of weight and weight gain on breast cancer risk. *Journal of the American Medical Association* **278**, 1407–1411.

Jacobs, D.R., Hahn, L.P., Folsom, A.R., Hannan, P.J., Sparfka, J.M. & Burke, G.L. (1991) Time trends in leisure-time physical activity in the upper midwest 1957–1987: University of Minnesota studies. *Epidemiology* **2**, 8–15.

Kelsey, J.L. (1993) Breast cancer epidemiology: summary and future directions. *Epidemiologic Reviews* **15**, 1256–1263.

Kelsey, J.L. & Horn-Ross, P.L. (1993) Breast cancer: Magnitude of the problem and descriptive epidemiology. *Epidemiologic Reviews* **15**, 7–16.

LaPierre, A., Ironson, G., Antoni, M.H., Schneideman, N., Klimas, N. & Fletcher, M.A. (1994) Exercise and psychoneuroimmunology. *Medicine and Science in Sports and Exercise* **26**, 182–191.

Loucks, A.B. & Callister, R. (1993) Induction and prevention of low-T3 syndrome in exercising women. *American Journal of Physiology* **264**, R924–R930.

Loucks, A.B., Mortola, J.F., Girton, L. & Yen, S.C. (1989) Alterations in the hypothalamic–pituitary–ovarian and hypothalamic–pituitary–adrenal axes in athletic women. *Journal of Clinical Endocrinology and Metabolism* **68**, 402–411.

Lubin, F., Ruder, A.M., Wax, Y. & Modan, B. (1985) Overweight and changes in weight throughout adult life in breast cancer etiology. *American Journal of Epidemiology* **122**, 579–588.

McTiernan, A., Stanford, J.L., Weiss, N.S., Daling, J.R. & Voigt, L.F. (1996) Occurrence of breast cancer in relation to recreational exercise in women age 50–64. *Epidemiology* **7**, 598–604.

Mittendorf, R., Longnecker, M.P., Newcomb, P.A. *et al.* (1995) Strenuous physical activity in young adulthood and risk of breast cancer (United States). *Cancer Causes and Control* **6**, 347–353.

Paffenbarger, R.S., Lee, I.M. & Wing, A.L. (1992) The influence of physical activity on the influence of site-specific cancers in college alumni. In M.M. Jacobs (ed.) *Exercise, Calories, Fat, and Cancer*, pp. 7–15. **Plenum** Press, New York.

Pike, M.C., Spicer, D.V., Dahmoush, L. & Press, M.F. (1993) Estrogens, progestogens, normal breast cell proliferation, and breast cancer risk. *Epidemiologic Reviews* **15**, 17–35.

Preston-Martin, S., Pike, M.C. & Ross, R.K. (1990) Increased cell division as a cause of human cancer. *Cancer Research* **50**, 7415–7421.

Schapira, D.V., Kumar, N.B., Lyman, G.H. & Cox, C.E. (1990) Abdominal obesity and breast cancer risk. *Annals of Internal Medicine* **112**, 182–186.

Siiteri, P.K. (1987) Adipose tissue as a source of hormones. *American Journal of Clinical Nutrition* **45**, 277–282.

Simpson, E.R. & Mendelson, C.R. (1987) Effect of aging and obesity on aromatase activity of human adipose cells. *American Journal of Clinical Nutrition* **45**, 290–295.

Stephens, T. & Casperson, C.J. (1994) The demography of physical activity. In C. Bouchard, R.J. Shepard & T. Stephens (eds) *Physical Activity, Fitness, and Health*, pp. 204–213. Human Kinetics Publishers, Champaign, Illinois.

Taioli, E., Barone, J. & Wynder, E.L. (1995) A case-control study on breast cancer and body mass. *European Journal of Cancer* **31A**, 723–728.

Thune, I., Brenn, T., Lund, E. & Gaard, M. (1997) Physical activity and the risk of breast cancer. *New England Journal of Medicine* **336**, 1269–1275.

Tretli, S. & Gaard, M. (1996) Lifestyle changes during adolescence and risk of breast cancer: an ecological study of the effect of World War II in Norway. *Cancer Causes and Control* **7**, 507–512.

Vena, J.E., Graham, S. & Zielezny, M. (1987) Occupational exercise and risk of cancer. *American Journal of Clinical Nutrition* **45**, 18–27.

Vihko, V.J., Apter, D.L. & Pukkala, E.A. (1992) Risk of breast cancer among female teachers of physical education and languages. *Acta Oncologica* **31**, 201–204.

Warren, M.P. (1980) The effects of exercise on pubertal progression and reproductive function in girls. *Journal of Clinical Endocrinology and Metabolism* **51**, 1150–1157.

White, E., Lee, C.Y. & Kristal, A.R. (1990) Evaluation of the increase in breast cancer incidence in relation to mammography use. *Journal of the National Cancer Institute* **82**, 1546–1552.

Woods, J.A. & Davis, J.M. (1994) Exercise, monocyte/macrophage function, and cancer. *Medicine and Science in Sports and Exercise* **26**, 147–157.

Zheng, W., Shu, X.O., McLaughlin, J.K., Chow, W., Gao, Y.T. & Blott, W.J. (1993) Occupational physical activity and the incidence of cancer of the breast, corpus uteri, and ovary in Shanghai. *Cancer* **71**, 3620–3624.

Chapter 18

Diabetes and Sport

BARBARA N. CAMPAIGNE

Introduction

Exercise is well known as an adjunct therapy in the management of diabetes. One of the earliest indications that exercise was effective in diminishing the sweetness of urine was made in 600 BC by the Indian physician Shushruta (1938). After the discovery of insulin in the early 1920s, the three cornerstones of diabetes care became insulin, diet and exercise. Exercise has been shown to be beneficial in controlling blood glucose in non-insulin-dependent diabetes mellitus (NIDDM) (Horton, 1991a) and gestational diabetes mellitus (GDM) (Bung *et al.*, 1991) for reasons that are discussed in the specific sections below. Exercise can be safe and effective in maintaining cardiovascular health in individuals with insulin-dependent diabetes mellitus (IDDM) (Campaigne & Gunnarsson, 1988; Campaigne & Lampman, 1994). This chapter covers exercise in women with diabetes, focusing on athletes. Issues that are specific to women throughout the lifespan are discussed. Because very little research has been conducted on women only, studies on men with diabetes have been included. Since athletes affected by diabetes are primarily those with IDDM, this is the focus of the chapter and not NIDDM.

Overview of diabetes

Diabetes mellitus is a chronic illness that is recognized as two major diseases with several other minor or less prevalent types. Most cases of diabetes are diagnosed as either type I (IDDM) or type II (NIDDM). NIDDM is the most common form and frequently is undiagnosed until the later stages of the disease. NIDDM is an inherited disorder revealed by environmental factors, particularly obesity. NIDDM is evident as hyperinsulinaemia and diminished insulin sensitivity. IDDM has a strong hereditary component, which may be triggered by an environmental factor such as a viral infection. IDDM, previously known as juvenile diabetes, primarily occurs in children or young adults. At the onset of IDDM, unusual weight loss may occur in conjunction with excessive thirst, urination and tiredness. Another form of diabetes specific to women is GDM, which manifests itself during pregnancy. The origin of GDM may be multifactorial and is probably related to ineffective glucose clearance. The primary clinical manifestation of GDM is hyperinsulinaemia (Summary and Recommendations of the Second International Workshop-Conference on Gestational Diabetes Mellitus, 1991). The effects of exercise on each of these types of diabetes are discussed. Because NIDDM occurs primarily in overweight individuals, most athletes with diabetes will have IDDM. Therefore, managing the athlete or physically active individual with IDDM is covered in depth in the following section.

Exercise and managing the athlete with IDDM

Acute exercise

Acute exercise brings about an increase in glucose utilization; thus an increase in glucose production is necessary in order to maintain near-normal glucose levels. Depending on its duration and intensity, exercise is characterized by individual endocrine and neural responses. The control of the availability and utilization of metabolic fuel is influenced principally by a balance of insulin, glucagon and the catecholamines adrenaline and noradrenaline. Other factors that may have a significant influence on metabolic fuel during exercise in type I diabetes include the central nervous system (Kjaer *et al.*, 1987), state of glucose control (Jenkins *et al.*, 1986) and the overall metabolic profile (Wasserman & Vranic, 1985; Cooper *et al.*, 1986; Katz *et al.*, 1986). Diabetes may alter all or some of these factors and thus the individual with IDDM may be unable to respond properly to the increased glucose usage brought about by exercise.

Figure 18.1 illustrates the importance of insulin in influencing blood glucose levels in physically active individuals with type I diabetes. Three possible consequences need to be considered.

1 If treatment with intravenous insulin infusion generates normal portal insulin levels, glucose production will equal glucose utilization and circulating glucose homeostasis will be maintained.

2 If circulating insulin levels are low (insulin deficiency), glucose utilization may not be adequately stimulated by exercise. This, in conjunction with an increase in hepatic glucose production produced by exercise, may result in hyperglycaemia.

3 If insulin absorption is enhanced by insulin being administered subcutaneously prior to exercise (overadministration of insulin), inhibition of glucose production may result. This, along with the increased glucose utilization induced by exercise, may lead to hypoglycaemia.

Hormonal changes that affect glucose utilization take place during the menstrual cycle, possibly making the response to exercise variable. Hormones play a role in insulin sensitivity and thus glucose utilization; changes in insulin sensitivity that occur during the menstrual cycle possibly influence circulating glucose levels. Because of the many considerations indicated, careful glucose monitoring and appropriate adjustments including diet and\or insulin are necessary to make exercise safe and prevent hypoglycaemia or hyperglycaemia in women with IDDM. The following points have been shown to be helpful when considering insulin treatment in relation to exercise.

• Consider timing of insulin action in relation to exercise (e.g. rapid acting vs. long acting).
• Inject insulin away from exercising muscle.
• Decrease insulin dose, especially for those receiving insulin subcutaneously (see Table 18.2).
• Individualize insulin treatment.
• Consider dietary intake.

Other possible ways to prevent exercise-induced hypoglycaemia, though less effective than altering insulin treatment and dietary carbohydrate intake, include the following.

Status of plasma insulin	Hepatic glucose production	Muscle glucose utilization	Blood glucose
Normal or slightly diminished	⬆	⬆	→
Markedly diminished	⬆	↑	↑
Increased	↑	↑	↓

Fig. 18.1 The influence of plasma insulin on blood glucose levels of individuals with type I diabetes. The size of arrow pointing up or down indicates a varying rate of increase or decrease; horizontal arrow shows no change. (From Campaigne & Lampman, 1994 with permission.)

• Inject insulin in non-exercising muscle group.
• Prevent intramuscular injection by avoiding perpendicular injection, injecting into the skin-fold and using needles < 8 mm long for thigh injection.

Physical training

Physical training is defined as the effects of repeated bouts of exercise performed on a regular basis over a period of weeks. The effects of physical training in IDDM are well documented (Horton, 1991a; Campaigne & Lampman, 1994; Ruderman & Devlin, 1995). Exercise has been shown to have beneficial effects on insulin sensitivity, glucose transport, blood lipids and lipoproteins, and skeletal muscle enzymes in individuals with IDDM. Regular exercise can be beneficial when conscientious screening and close monitoring of the individual's progress are applied. Table 18.1 lists the benefits of regular exercise for individuals with IDDM. Very little information is available specifically on women; however, several of the studies cited in these findings included groups of men and women.

Glucose control

Most studies in adults with IDDM have not shown improvements in haemoglobin (Hb)A_{1c} with training (Wallberg-Henriksson et al., 1982, 1984; Yki-Jarvinen et al., 1984; Zinman et al.,

Table 18.1 Benefits of exercise on insulin-dependent diabetes mellitus

---

Improved insulin sensitivity
Improved blood lipids and lipoproteins
Increased caloric expenditure, resulting in reduction or
   maintenance of body weight, reduction in body fat
   and preservation of lean body mass
Improved physical fitness
Improved flexibility and strength
Decreased blood pressure in hypertension
Reduced risk of cardiovascular disease
Improved psychological well-being, including
   enhanced quality of life, improved self-esteem

1984). Wallberg-Henriksson et al. (1982, 1984) found no change in blood glucose control, as determined by home-monitored blood glucose levels, HbA_{1c} or urinary glucose, in men after 8–16 weeks of physical training. Zinman et al. (1984) studied adult men and women over 12 weeks of training compared with a non-diabetic control group. Maximal oxygen uptake ($\dot{V}O_{2max}$) increased significantly and similarly in the two groups. In those with diabetes, exercise sessions resulted in a significant decrease in blood glucose, while HbA_1 was unchanged after the 12 weeks. There was no change in insulin dose or in the number of reported hypoglycaemic episodes during the study period. According to self-report, caloric intake increased on exercise days. In well-controlled patients on insulin-pump treatment, Yki-Jarvinen et al. (1984) were unable to demonstrate any further improvement in blood glucose by exercise, beyond the improvements noted at the start of pump treatment.

Insulin sensitivity

It has been suggested that people with diabetes become more sensitive to insulin after physical training. Some studies cite no decrease in insulin need or a slight fall during physical training, although Costill et al. (1979) noted a significant decrease in insulin dose during training and Bak et al. (1989) found a 12% decrease in insulin dose after 6 weeks of physical training.

Whole-body insulin sensitivity as assessed by the glucose clamp technique is accepted as a measure of skeletal muscle insulin sensitivity (DeFronzo et al., 1979). Wallberg-Henriksson et al. (1982), Yki-Jarvinen et al. (1984) and Landt et al. (1985) have all documented significant increases in insulin sensitivity in adults and adolescents with IDDM. These studies reported about a 20% increase in insulin sensitivity with physical training. Because well-trained, non-diabetic individuals have been found to have a higher insulin sensitivity compared with their sedentary counterparts, the increase in insulin sensitivity brought about by physical training appears to be a normal physiological adaptation that is due, in part, to an increase in insulin action.

The precise mechanism behind increases in insulin sensitivity with physical training is currently unknown. The nature of this change in insulin sensitivity is probably related to glucose transport, which has been indicated by recent findings. Clarification of the mechanism responsible for increased insulin sensitivity with exercise in diabetes is an important area of research.

Blood lipids

Most studies have been done in men or in gender-diverse groups. In a cross-sectional study, Gunnarson et al. (1987) examined the relationship between serum lipoprotein levels, glycaemic control and physical fitness in female type I diabetic patients. Subjects were divided into three groups based on glycaemic control: good (HbA$_1$, 9.5%), acceptable (HbA$_1$, 9.6–10.9%) and poor (HbA$_1$, 11.0%). Those in good control were found to have the lowest triglyceride concentrations, mainly attributable to lower levels of very low-density lipoprotein (VLDL) triglyceride. The patients in good control also had higher concentrations of high-density lipoprotein (HDL) cholesterol and HDL-2 cholesterol, while HDL-3 cholesterol was similar in all groups. When patients were grouped by a measure of aerobic capacity ($\dot{V}_{O_{2max}}$), triglycerides were also lower in those with higher aerobic capacity, consistent with a lower low-density lipoprotein (LDL) fraction. HDL-2 cholesterol and the HDL-2 : HDL-3 ratio were found to be significantly elevated in subjects with high aerobic capacity. Adding HbA$_1$ to the multiple regression analysis with $\dot{V}_{O_{2max}}$ and the lipid and lipoprotein parameters did not further explain the variability of the lipid fraction under study. These authors concluded that both good glycaemic control and high aerobic capacity may be important for favourable lipid status in patients with type I diabetes. These findings support the use of physical training for women with type I diabetes.

Favourable but limited information is cur-rently available regarding the long-term effects of exercise in patients with IDDM. Moy et al. (1993) followed 548 patients with IDDM over 7 years. Baseline physical activity was inversely related to risk of mortality during the 7-year period. Males expending < 4200 kJ·week^{-1} (1000 kcal·week^{-1}) had a threefold greater risk of death than those expending > 8400 kJ·week^{-1} (2000 kcal·week^{-1}). In females, the findings were similar but not as apparent. Data from the Joslin Clinic on 48 patients at 25-year follow-up indicate that men who developed complications associated with diabetes reported a lower frequency of physical activity throughout life compared with those who had no complications (Chazan et al., 1970). A lower incidence of macrovascular disease has been observed in individuals with IDDM who engaged in team sports in high school and college compared with their sedentary counterparts (LaPorte et al., 1986). These investigators also reported a lower incidence of mortality after 25 years in the physically active group. These results agree with findings in non-diabetic individuals (Paffenbarger et al., 1978). These findings further support evidence that even moderate levels of activity performed regularly are beneficial in improving longevity in individuals with diabetes.

The above findings show that in individuals who begin an exercise programme in good glucose control, regular exercise may have little or no effect on long-term blood glucose control. There are known atherogenic effects of insulin and some individuals can decrease their insulin dose after beginning a regular exercise programme. Exercise does improve insulin sensitivity and may be beneficial in improving blood lipids in patients with IDDM. These findings indicate that regular physical activity may decrease the overall risk of the development of coronary heart disease in those with diabetes. Though clinical correlates of glucose control may not be improved by regular exercise, research on subcellular increases in glucose transport and glucose metabolism may be beneficial. In addition, there is some epidemiological evidence to suggest that individuals with IDDM who exercise regularly throughout life may develop fewer complications and live longer than those who have not exercised.

Dietary intake

Diabetes can be effectively controlled by diet, exercise and insulin, with consistency of management and lifestyle being key to good control. Dietary intake is an essential component of any athlete's training programme; in the case of the athlete with diabetes it may be a life-saving factor. The athlete should be monitored carefully to maintain ideal body weight, blood glucose levels and normal growth (Peterson & Peterson, 1988). Regular dietary histories may be required if problems arise in maintaining normal weight, growth and glucose levels. Clinical screening on a regular basis (every 3–6 months) should include a blood lipid profile, electrolyte values, HbA_{1c} (a measure of long-term glucose control) and dietary factors. The athlete should receive careful instruction by a trained nutritionist on the use of dietary exchange lists and on maintaining a dietary history. Nutritional counselling should be a part of the initial screening and management of individuals with diabetes. In the case of those beginning an exercise programme, it may be necessary to design meal plans for exercise days and non-exercise days as a part of the training programme. In planning the diet of the athlete with diabetes, the type of insulin needs to be considered as does the means of insulin administration and the type, intensity and duration of exercise. Regular meals and snacks should be emphasized, as should the importance of emergency feeds and self-care. In general, the well-balanced diet and sound nutrition advocated for the individual with diabetes is recommended for everyone.

During intense exercise (heavy training or competition) it may be necessary to replace glucose through supplemental carbohydrate feeding. Athletes performing sustained exercise (e.g. tennis players, swimmers and distance runners) need to receive snacks during training. All individuals with diabetes need to monitor their blood glucose levels on a regular basis (several times each day), including before and after exercise. A readily absorbable form of carbohydrate should be available at all times (something small, convenient and concentrated), such as glucose tablets, hard candy, fruit juice or some sports nutrition bars. In order to achieve stable glucose levels a balance between insulin dose and dietary intake is essential. As with non-diabetic athletes, the focus on extra carbohydrate consumed before activity should be shifted to extra carbohydrate during activity.

Coaches, professional staff and individuals training with athletes who have diabetes need to be aware of the signs of hypoglycaemia, such as confusion, weakness, tiredness and unusual irritability. If these symptoms are not recognized and treated, hypoglycaemia could potentially lead to unconsciousness or convulsions. In most cases, activities done alone (e.g. scuba diving, sky diving and independent mountain climbing or hiking) should be avoided.

An area of extreme importance to the athlete with diabetes is the long-lasting effect of prolonged exercise. Insulin adjustments are necessary and specific dietary changes need to be made. Low blood glucose reactions often occur nocturnally with little warning, are inconsistent and are difficult to prevent or correct. Several new products exist that are specifically designed to prevent hypoglycaemia over a prolonged time period or during the night (e.g. Z-bar, Nite-bite). These 'bars' are a slow-release carbohydrate source that are designed to have a 'timed-release' effect and prevent hypoglycaemia hours after they are consumed. Athletes may need to keep careful records and report any adverse blood glucose reactions to the healthcare team so that a specific programme can be designed to alter the timing and amount of exercise, diet and insulin to achieve optimal blood glucose levels.

Timing and mode of insulin treatment

The majority of individuals with IDDM are treated with multiple subcutaneous insulin injections throughout the day. Most insulin treatment plans consist of a mixed split dose of insulin. This includes a combination of short-acting and longer-acting (sustained-release) insulin administered in the morning and afternoon in order to optimize blood glucose control. Carbohydrate and total caloric intake need to be matched with the amount and timing of insulin given. There are several times of day that are optimal for exercise in relation to glucose control. General recommendations include not exercising at the time of peak insulin action. If an individual is required to exercise at a specific time, insulin dose can be reduced to prevent its peak effect during exercise. This strategy would include decreasing long-acting insulin in order to prevent hypoglycaemia during exercise occurring in the late afternoon. Exercise should be recommended when the effects of insulin are lowest and blood glucose is rising. When exercise is unplanned, a quickly absorbed carbohydrate snack can be consumed before exercise to prevent hypoglycaemia. Exercising before insulin administration and breakfast may decrease the need for short- or rapid-acting insulin. It is best to develop an exercise routine so that caloric intake and insulin dose can be adjusted to optimize blood glucose control. Table 18.2 lists effective ways to prevent hypoglycaemia in relation to exercise in IDDM. Table 18.3 provides information on the action of various insulin preparations to be considered in relation to exercise timing. It is important to note that the optimal level of blood glucose before beginning exercise or an athletic event should be individualized based on the length and intensity of the activity and the individual's metabolic profile in relation to exercise. A *general* guideline is that blood glucose should be > 120 but < 220 $mg \cdot dl^{-1}$ immediately prior to exercise.

Specific sports

Because of their unique requirements, which may affect the individual with diabetes, certain sports have specific guidelines and recommendations (e.g. scuba diving, mountain climbing). The American Diabetes Association provides

Table 18.2 General guidelines for preventing hypoglycaemia in relation to exercise

Blood glucose monitoring
Monitor blood glucose immediately before, during (approximately every 30 min) and after exercise
Delay exercise if blood glucose is ≥ 250 $mg \cdot dl^{-1}$ or ketosis is present, or if blood glucose level is ≥ 300 $mg \cdot dl^{-1}$
　　whether or not ketosis is present
Consume carbohydrates if blood glucose is ≤ 100 $mg \cdot dl^{-1}$
Learn individual glucose response to different types of exercise
Avoid exercising late at night

Diet
When exercise is unplanned extra carbohydrate should be consumed (e.g. 20–30 g for every 30 min of exercise)
During exercise consume easily absorbable carbohydrate when necessary
After exercise a carbohydrate snack may be required

Insulin
Indications for reductions in insulin dose may occur before and after exercise, depending on the intensity and
　　duration of exercise and the individual's experience
Suggestions for altering insulin dose:
　　(a) Intermediate-acting insulin: decrease by 30–35% on the day of exercise
　　(b) Intermediate- and short-acting insulin: omit dose of short-acting insulin that precedes exercise
　　(c) Multiple doses of short-acting insulin: reduce the dose prior to exercise by 30–35% and supplement
　　　　carbohydrates
　　(d) Continuous subcutaneous infusion: eliminate meal-time bolus or increment that precedes or
　　　　immediately follows exercise
Do not exercise at the time of peak insulin action

Table 18.3 Activity characteristics of insulin. (From Roitman, 1998 with permission.)

	Onset (hours)	Peak (hours)	Duration (hours)
Rapid-acting: regular	0.5–1	2–4	6–8
Intermediate-acting: lente or NPH	1–3	6–12	18–26
Long-acting: ultralente or human	4–8	12–18	24–28

Onset, peak and duration of action vary considerably and may depend upon the individual patient, injection site, vascularity and temperature.

Table 18.4 Benefits of exercise on non-insulin-dependent diabetes mellitus

Reduced blood glucose and glycosylated haemoglobin levels
Improved glucose tolerance
Improved insulin response to oral glucose stimulus
Improved peripheral and hepatic insulin sensitivity
Improved blood lipid and lipoprotein levels
Decreased blood pressure in hypertension
Reduced risk of cardiovascular disease
Improved physical fitness
Increased caloric expenditure, resulting in reduction or maintenance of body weight, reduction in body fat and preservation of lean body mass
Improved flexibility and strength
Improved psychological well-being, including enhanced quality of life, increased self-esteem

guidelines on these sports in relation to diabetes management (Ruderman & Devlin, 1995). A few of the key points that need attention with regard to these activities are listed below.

SCUBA DIVING

• The diabetic diver should perform frequent self-monitoring of blood glucose, particularly before exercise.
• Before exercise, determine the expected physical exertion.
• Fast-acting glucose gel should be carried by the diving partner.
• Divers affected by hypoglycaemia should leave the water.
• Diving is a high-risk activity for those with cardiovascular disease or cardiac autonomic neuropathy.

MOUNTAIN CLIMBING

• The individual with diabetes should hike or climb with a partner.
• Blood glucose levels should be self-monitored frequently.
• Insulin should be stored so that it does not freeze and is not exposed to direct sunlight and extremes in temperature.
• The diabetic climber should be screened for

complications that may be particularly hazardous (i.e. retinopathy, peripheral and autonomic neuropathy).

Exercise, NIDDM and the recreational athlete

The benefits of regular exercise for individuals with NIDDM have been clearly documented (Horton, 1991b; Campaigne & Lampman, 1994) (Table 18.4). Regular physical activity as part of the treatment plan for NIDDM is a current recommendation of the American Diabetes Association (1990). Regular exercise results in improved blood glucose control on a daily basis and a decrease in HbA_{1c} levels as a result of improved long-term blood glucose control (Schneider *et al.*, 1984). The mechanism of improved glucose control during regular exercise in NIDDM has been studied. Individuals with NIDDM have improved insulin sensitivity with physical training (Bjorntorp *et al.*, 1972, 1983). Regular exercise lowers the risk of cardiovascular disease by reducing blood pressure in individuals with hypertension and improving blood lipid profiles (Huttunen *et al.*, 1979; Haskell, 1986). Specific lipid and lipoprotein changes include decreased triglycerides and VLDLs and increased HDLs. Decreases in both systolic and diastolic blood pressure have been shown to occur in mild to moderate hypertension (Boyer & Kasch, 1970; Choquette & Ferguson, 1973) and may be associated with the effects of lowering insulin levels on renal sodium retention (Horton, 1991b). An important effect of regular exercise for NIDDM can be weight reduction in conjunction with dietary intervention, with the combination resulting in the preservation of lean tissue (Pavlou et al., 1985; Hill et al., 1987; Lampman et al., 1987; Lucas et al., 1987).

Data comparing rural and urban cultures provide evidence of a lower prevalence of NIDDM among active rural populations (Zimmet et al., 1981, 1990). Some data from cross-sectional studies show that glucose tolerance and diabetes occur more frequently in sedentary individuals compared with individuals who are more active (King et al., 1984; Taylor et al., 1984; Dowse et al., 1991), independent of body mass and age. Physical activity has been indicated as a significant approach to preventing NIDDM in men (Helmrich et al., 1991) and women (Manson et al., 1991). In a prospective cohort study of 87 253 women aged 34–59 years, Manson et al. (1991) found that women who exercised vigorously at least once per week had a significantly lower risk of NIDDM compared with women who did not exercise weekly. Of importance is that the beneficial effect of exercise was not modified by a family history of diabetes. Statistical adjustment for age, family history of diabetes, body mass index and other variables did not alter the beneficial effects of exercise on diabetes risk. Table 18.5 provides guidelines for screening the individual with IDDM or NIDDM prior to designing and beginning an exercise programme.

Foot care

Of particular importance for anyone with diabetes is the need to care for the feet. Individuals who have developed peripheral neuropathy need special attention in this area, as insensitivity in the feet may cause a callus or blister to go unnoticed. Infections can develop quickly and

Table 18.5 Recommended screening procedures for diabetes

History and physical examination (for newly diagnosed patients or without current records)
Review all systems
Identification of medical conditions (e.g. asthma, arthritis)

Diabetes evaluation
Glycosylated haemoglobin
Ophthalmoscopic examination (retinopathy)
Neurological examination (neuropathy)
Nephrological evaluation (micro-albumin or protein in urine)
Nutritional status evaluation (underweight/overweight, eating disorders)

Cardiovascular evaluation
Blood pressure with orthostatic measurements
Peripheral pulses
Bruits
12-lead electrocardiogram
Serum lipid profile (total cholesterol, triglycerides, HDL and LDL cholesterol)
Graded exercise test (those > 30 years of age with IDDM, those > 35 years of age with NIDDM, those with suspected history of or documented cardiovascular disease, those with multiple cardiovascular disease risk factors present, or those with diabetes of > 10 years)

HDL, high-density lipoprotein; IDDM, insulin-dependent diabetes mellitus; LDL, low-density lipoprotein; NIDDM, non-insulin-dependent diabetes mellitus.

therefore the feet should be examined regularly by the individual and the physician. Helpful tips for those who are physically active include: (i) wear proper fitting, well-cushioned shoes (e.g. gel or air soles); (ii) have clean dry socks available after activity; (iii) check for blisters regularly; and (iv) wear special water footwear when walking on rough surfaces near the water (pool or ocean).

Complications of diabetes

Detailed information on determining the appropriate types and levels of physical activity for individuals with complications of diabetes is available (Campaigne & Lampman, 1994; Ruderman & Devlin, 1995). After an initial screening is completed, the existence of complications can be established and recommendations for exercise or physical activity can be made.

Absolute contraindications for *strenuous* exercise include:

- poor glycaemic control;
- proliferative retinopathy;
- microangiopathy;
- neuropathy;
- nephropathy;
- evidence of cardiovascular disease.

Exercise and diabetic pregnancy

Very little research has been done on the effects of exercise during pregnancy in women with IDDM. Artal *et al.* (1985) found low-level exercise to be safe for women with IDDM and not to affect plasma glucose or glucagon concentrations. Others have found no improvement in postprandial glucose levels following the evening meal in pregnant women with IDDM (Hollingsworth & Moore, 1987). During diabetic pregnancy, a blood glucose level greater than four standard deviations from the mean increases the risk of spontaneous abortion, with the risk rising markedly as hyperglycaemia increases (Mills *et al.*, 1988). If complications of diabetes are present (retinopathy, neuropathy, etc.) precautions should be taken, including the restriction of certain types of exercise (Graham & Lasko-McCarthey, 1990). Any conditions that require bed rest during pregnancy would be clear contraindications to exercise.

Certain types of exercise have been shown to be safe during normal pregnancy. The American College of Obstetricians and Gynecologists (1994) has established guidelines for exercise during pregnancy. The safest form of exercise during pregnancy should not bring about: (i) uterine contraction; (ii) low birth weight infants; or (iii) fetal distress (Ruderman & Devlin, 1995). Exercises that primarily use the upper body and avoid mechanical stress to the trunk have been shown to be the safest during pregnancy (Durak

et al., 1990). These types of exercise result in less chance of fetal distress than activities utilizing the lower body, while still achieving a cardiovascular workout. Pregnant women with IDDM need to adhere to strict glucose control in order to ensure the optimal health of the fetus. The danger of exercise for the woman with diabetes is a possible deleterious effect on blood glucose control. Therefore, very careful counselling and close monitoring of glucose control and insulin dose need to be emphasized for the pregnant woman with IDDM. Since the primary goal is to achieve near-normal blood glucose levels (Jovanovic *et al.*, 1981), beginning a *vigorous* exercise programme before or during gestation is not recommended for women with diabetes.

Exercise and gestational diabetes

There are three significant factors that influence the development of GDM: genetic predisposition, decrease in insulin action and impaired pancreatic β-cell function (Horton, 1991b). During pregnancy the development of insulin resistance depends on a host of factors, including the hormonal environment, hereditary predisposition, age, excess body weight and the level of physical activity (Horton, 1991b). It is documented that glucose tolerance deteriorates during the course of gestation (Ruderman & Devlin, 1995). Because of the effects of exercise on insulin secretion, insulin sensitivity and glucose metabolism, it seems reasonable to infer that regular exercise may be effective in preventing or treating GDM. However, very few data are available that illustrate this possibility (Jovanovic-Peterson *et al.*, 1989). Improvements in glucose tolerance with exercise training in women with GDM have been demonstrated (Jovanovic-Peterson & Peterson, 1990). These authors found that the hyperglycaemia occurring with GDM can be managed by arm ergometry. In the sixth week of training, women achieved near-normal glucose levels, HbA_{1c} and response to glucose challenge. In contrast, women who had been managed by diet alone showed no significant improvement in glucose control. These results indicate that insulin administration may be avoided in some women with GDM by the safe application of regular exercise (Jovanovic-Peterson & Peterson, 1991). The use of exercise in the healthcare management of GDM has great potential. Further study needs to be done in this area.

Special considerations

Women have specific health needs that change during the lifespan. These need to be considered when working with the athlete with diabetes. Women with diabetes have special health needs and physiological conditions that predispose them to certain health problems, such as delayed pubertal development, osteoporosis, coronary heart disease and obesity. The sections below describe specific areas of concern that need to be considered in women with diabetes.

Adolescence

The adolescent girl with diabetes has certain physiological and psychological considerations specific to her disease. Fluctuations in blood glucose are frequently seen in relation to emotional swings, hormonal changes and specific dietary patterns that occur during the adolescent years. It becomes increasingly necessary to consider these factors when making participation in sports safe for the diabetic adolescent. In most circumstances, undertaking regular physical activity and sports can be recommended for children and adolescents with diabetes, as it may be effective in preventing complications later in life, promote optimal bone density, increase socialization and improve self-esteem. Before participation in regular exercise, careful clinical evaluation should be carried out by the diabetes management team to ensure optimal health and safety of the individual.

Amenorrhoea

Long-term hyperglycaemia is associated with short stature and delayed puberty (Jovanovic-Peterson, 1995). When blood glucose is normal-ized, the growth spurt is initiated and menarche follows (Drash et al., 1980). In adolescents with diabetes, if blood glucose is normalized rapidly there is a risk of diabetic retinopathy in some pre-disposed individuals (Drash et al., 1980). Thus during adolescence blood glucose levels need to be carefully monitored in order to ensure optimal growth and normal development as well as to prevent the long-term complications of diabetes. Menarche has been found to occur later in athletes (non-diabetic) compared with non-athletes (Marcus et al., 1985; Ding et al., 1988; Loucks et al., 1989). However, there is no evidence documenting delayed menarche in athletes. Certain types of athletes appear to have the highest occurrence of amenorrhoea, such as long-distance runners and gymnasts (Brownell et al., 1992). Exercise combined with other conditions, such as a calorie-deficient diet and low body weight, increases the risk of amenorrhoea, particularly among competitive athletes (Tanner & Davies, 1985; Loucks et al., 1992). In light of the previously mentioned concerns that chronic hyperglycaemia is associated with delayed menarche, adolescent girls with diabetes who exercise regularly need careful dietary monitoring in order to prevent or reverse exercise-associated amenorrhoea and maintain near-normal blood glucose levels (Jovanovic-Peterson, 1995). All girls, diabetic and non-diabetic, who exercise regularly need careful evaluation and regular monitoring for the occurrence of amenorrhoea. If amenorrhoea is present, the athlete should be evaluated for other associated factors such as possible osteoporosis and eating disorders (Yeager et al., 1993). Disordered eating behaviour among young women with IDDM is common (Rydall et al., 1997) and is associated with non-compliance with the diabetes treatment plan and poor blood glucose control. Anyone exhibiting the signs of eating disorders should be evaluated and managed appropriately in a timely fashion (see Chapter 25).

Menopause

The onset of the menopause brings about several health implications, including an increased risk of developing osteoporosis and cardiovascular disease. Both these health risks are associated with decreasing oestrogen levels at menopause. The postmenopausal loss of endogenous oestrogen influences the woman with diabetes in several ways. Oestrogen alters glucose metabolism by affecting gluconeogenesis and glycogenolysis; oestrogen also has a beneficial influence on lipid metabolism (van der Mooren et al., 1994). Menopause changes the diabetes management plan in women with NIDDM because of the associated decrease in metabolism and associated weight gain. Caloric intake needs to be reduced by 20% in order to prevent weight gain; thus the insulin dose needs to be decreased equally (Reilly et al., 1993). If exercise is added to the management programme, caloric intake may not need marked alteration, insulin sensitivity may be improved along with the prevention of weight gain and menopause-associated hyperglycaemia may be diminished.

Osteoporosis

Osteoporosis and risk of fracture are major health problems, especially for postmenopausal women. The relationship between regular weight-bearing exercise and bone density has been documented (Smith & Gilligan, 1991; Marcus et al., 1992; Suominen, 1993; Alekel et al., 1995; Drinkwater et al., 1995). Regular exercise increases peak bone mass in adolescents, slows the decline in bone mass in middle age and may increase bone density in women with osteoporosis (Marcus et al., 1992). A greater muscle mass appears to enhance bone mass by imposing a greater mechanical stress on bone (Sandler, 1988; Marcus et al., 1992). Active individuals are stronger and have a greater muscle mass than their inactive counterparts, which reduces the risk of falls in the former (Pocock et al., 1989). When counselling individuals with diabetes it should be emphasized that women with poor glycaemic control are at increased risk of osteoporosis (Jovanovic-Peterson, 1995). Bone demineralization and fractures are complications of diabetes, as are osteoarthritis and Charcot's joints. In addition, there is a higher risk of falls in

individuals with these problems, brought on by muscle disuse and the resulting muscle atrophy. Good glucose control decreases the prevalence of these problems (Jovanovic-Peterson, 1995). Glucose control, calcium intake, oestrogen status and physical activity should be assessed, as each contributes to the promotion of optimal bone health and prevention of osteoporosis in women with diabetes. Regular exercise should be recommended for adolescent girls and may be particularly beneficial for those with an increased risk of osteoporosis later in life.

Cardiovascular disease

Women with diabetes have a markedly increased risk of developing cardiovascular disease compared with non-diabetic women (Solomon, 1996). This risk has been documented to be as much as five to seven times higher in diabetic women compared with non-diabetic women (Manson et al., 1991). In fact, the risk of developing cardiovascular disease in diabetic women is equal to that in non-diabetic men. Insulin is an indirect risk factor for cardiovascular disease, possibly because of its secondary effects on physiological parameters such as blood pressure and lipid metabolism. The protective effects of oestrogen are lost after the menopause, unless hormone replacement therapy is used (Freedman, 1996). As in women without diabetes, the risk of cardiovascular disease increases at menopause possibly because of the loss of the protective effects of oestrogen. Exercise is important in the prevention of cardiovascular disease and in the management of the risk factors for cardiovascular disease both before and after the menopause (Blair, 1996). Active, physically fit women without diabetes have been shown to receive comparable benefits from regular physical activity as men (Blair, 1996). In addition, individuals with diabetes appear to reap similar benefits from physical activity as those without diabetes (Berlin & Colditz, 1990; Ford & DeStefano, 1991). It has been noted that women with diabetes who engage in regular vigorous physical activity have reduced rates of coronary heart disease compared with those who are not as physically active (Solomon, 1996). As indicated in previous sections, regular exercise can decrease the risk of cardiovascular disease via several beneficial effects, such as decreasing blood pressure in those with elevated blood pressure, increasing insulin sensitivity, decreasing insulin need, increasing the HDL : total cholesterol ratio and decreasing LDL and triglyceride levels, as well as improving cardiovascular fitness. It should be noted that women are likely to have non-specific electrocardiographic changes in response to exercise; thus alternative methods, such as radionuclide stress testing, may be required for those considered at risk of cardiovascular disease.

Conclusion and recommendations for future research

Regular physical activity can be an important part of the management plan for the woman with diabetes and particularly for those with NIDDM. Girls and women with IDDM can exercise and participate in sports with careful management specific to their needs. Regular physical activity reduces the risk of many diseases to which women with diabetes are predisposed, including hypertension, coronary heart disease, obesity and osteoporosis. The woman with diabetes needs comprehensive healthcare management, taking into account diet, insulin dose, hormone replacement therapy and exercise, in order to ensure optimal blood glucose and lipid levels, to assist in weight management and to prevent accelerated bone loss. Because very little research has been undertaken on women, areas for future research include: (i) the effects of exercise on the risk of osteoporosis in women with IDDM; (ii) exercise, glucose control and menarche in girls with diabetes; (iii) evaluation of strength training in women with diabetes; and (iv) further investigations on exercise and diabetic pregnancy.

References

Alekel, L., Clasey, J.L., Fehling, P.C. et al. (1995) Contributions of exercise, body composition, and age to bone mineral density in premenopausal women. Medicine and Science in Sports and Exercise 27, 1477–1485.

American College of Obstetricians and Gynecologists (1994) Exercise During Pregnancy and the Postpartum Period. ACOG, Washington, DC.

American Diabetes Association (1990) Diabetes mellitus and exercise. Diabetes Care 13, 804–805.

Artal, R., Wiswell, R. & Romem, Y. (1985) Hormonal responses to exercise in diabetic and nondiabetic pregnant patients. Diabetes 34 (Suppl. 2), 78–80.

Bak, J.F., Jacobsen, U.K., Jorgensen, F.S. & Pedersen, O. (1989) Insulin receptor function and glycogen synthase activity in skeletal muscle biopsies from patients with insulin dependent diabetes mellitus: effects of physical training. Journal of Clinical Endocrinology and Metabolism 69, 158–164.

Berlin, J.A. & Colditz, G.A. (1990) A meta-analysis of physical activity in the prevention of coronary heart disease. American Journal of Epidemiology 132, 612–628.

Bjorntorp, P., Fahlen, M., Grimby, G. et al. (1972) Carbohydrate and lipid metabolism in middle-aged physically well-trained men. Metabolism 21, 1037–1044.

Bjorntorp, P., de Jounge, D., Sjostrom, L. & Sullivan, L. (1983) The effect of physical training on insulin production in obesity. Metabolism 19, 631–637.

Blair, S.N. (1996) Physical inactivity and cardiovascular disease risk in women. Medicine and Science in Sports and Exercise 28, 9–10.

Boyer, J. & Kasch, F. (1970) Exercise therapy in hypertensive men. Journal of the American Medical Association 211(10), 1668–1671.

Brownell, K.D., Rodin, J. & Wilmore, J.H. (1992) Eating, Body Weight and Performance in Athletes. Lea and Febiger, Philadelphia.

Bung, P., Atral, R., Khodiguian, N. & Kjos, S. (1991) Exercise in gestational diabetes: an optional therapeutic approach? Diabetes 40 (Suppl. 2), 182–185.

Campaigne, B.N. & Gunnarsson, R. (1988) The effects of physical training in people with insulin-dependent diabetes. Diabetic Medicine 5, 429–433.

Campaigne, B.N. & Lampman, R.L. (1994) Exercise in the Clinical Management of Diabetes Mellitus. Human Kinetics Publishers, Champaign, Illinois.

Chazan, B.I., Balodimos, M.C., Ryan, J.R. & Marble, A. (1970) Twenty-five to forty-five years of diabetes with and without vascular complications. Diabetologia 6, 565–569.

Choquette, G. & Ferguson, R. (1973) Blood pressure reduction in borderline hypertensives following physical training. Canadian Medical Association Journal 108, 699–703.

Cooper, D.M., Wasserman, D.H., Vranic, M. & Wasserman, K. (1986) Glucose turnover in response to exercise during high- and low-flow breathing in humans. American Journal of Physiology 14, E209–E214.

Costill, D.L., Cleary, P., Find, W., Foster, C., Ivy, J.L. & Witzmann, F. (1979) Training adaptations in skeletal muscles of juvenile diabetics. *Diabetes* **28**, 818–822.

DeFronzo, A., Tobin, J.D. & Andres, R. (1979) Glucose clamp technique: a method for quantifying insulin secretion and resistance. *American Journal of Physiology* **237**, E214–E223.

Ding, J.H., Sheckter, C.B., Drinkwater, B.L. *et al.* (1988) High cortisol levels in exercise-associated amenorrhea. *Annals of Internal Medicine* **108**, 530–534.

Dowse, G.K., Zimmet, P.Z., Gareeboo, H. *et al.* (1991) Abdominal obesity and physical inactivity as risk factors for NIDDM and impaired glucose tolerance in Indians, Creole, and Chinese Mauritians. *Diabetes Care* **14**, 271–282.

Drash, A.L., Daneman, D. & Travis, L. (1980) Progressive retinopathy with improved metabolic control in diabetic dwarfism (Mauriac's syndrome). *Diabetes* **29** (Suppl. 2), 1A.

Drinkwater, B.D., Grimston, S.K., Raab-Cullen, D.M. & Snow-Harter, C.M. (1995) Osteoporosis and exercise. *Medicine and Science in Sports and Exercise* **27**, i–vii.

Durak, E.P., Jovanovic-Peterson, L. & Peterson, C.M. (1990) Comparative evaluation of uterine response to exercise on five aerobic machines. *American Journal of Obstetrics and Gynecology* **162**, 754–756.

Ford, E.S. & DeStafano, F. (1991) Risk factors for mortality from all causes and from coronary heart disease among persons with diabetes. Findings from the National Health and Nutrition Examination Survey I Epidemiologic Follow-up Study. *American Journal of Epidemiology* **133**, 1220–1230.

Freedman, M. (1996) Postmenopausal hormone replacement therapy and cardiovascular disease risk. *Medicine and Science in Sports and Exercise* **28**, 17–18.

Graham, C. & Lasko-McCarthey, P. (1990) Exercise options for persons with diabetic complications. *Diabetes Educator* **16**, 212–220.

Gunnarsson, R., Wallberg-Henriksson, H., Rossner, S. & Wahren, J. (1987) Serum lipid and lipoprotein levels in female Type I diabetics: relationships to aerobic capacity and glycaemic control. *Diabetes and Metabolism* **13**, 417–421.

Haskell, W.L. (1986) The influence of exercise training on plasma lipids and lipoproteins in health and disease. *Acta Medica Scandinavica* Suppl. 711, 25–37.

Helmrich, S.P., Raglund, D.R., Leung, R.W. & Paffenbarger, R.S. (1991) Physical activity and reduced occurrence of non-insulin dependent diabetes mellitus. *New England Journal of Medicine* **325**, 147–152.

Hill, J.O., Sparling, P.B., Shields, T.W. & Heller, P.A. (1987) Effects of exercise and food restriction on body composition and metabolic rate in obese women. *American Journal of Clinical Nutrition* **46**, 622–630.

Hollingsworth, D.R. & Moore, T.R. (1987) Postprandial walking exercise in pregnant insulin-dependent (type I) diabetic women: reduction of plasma lipid levels but absence of a significant effect on glycemic control. *American Journal of Obstetrics and Gynecology* **157**, 1359–1363.

Horton, E.S. (1991a) Exercise. In H.E. Leovitz (ed.) *Therapy for Diabetes Mellitus and Related Disorders*, pp. 103–111. American Diabetes Association, Alexandria, Virginia.

Horton, E.S. (1991b) Exercise in the treatment of NIDDM: applications for GDM? *Diabetes* **40** (Suppl. 2), 175–178.

Huttunen, J.K., Lansimies, E., Voutilainen, E. *et al.* (1979) Effect of moderate physical exercise on serum lipoproteins. *Circulation* **60**, 1220–1229.

Jenkins, A.B., Furler, S.M., Chisholm, D.J. & Kraegen, E.W. (1986) Regulation of hepatic glucose output during exercise by circulating glucose and insulin in humans. *American Journal of Physiology* **250**, R411–R417.

Jovanovic, L., Druzin, M. & Peterson, C.M. (1981) The effect of euglycemia on the outcome of pregnancy in insulin-dependent diabetics as compared to normal controls. *American Journal of Medicine* **71**, 92–97.

Jovanovic-Peterson, L. (1995) Women and exercise: In N. Ruderman & J.T. Devlin (eds) *The Health Professionals Guide to Diabetes and Exercise*, p. 211. American Diabetes Association, Alexandria, Virginia.

Jovanovic-Peterson, L. & Peterson, C.M. (1990) Dietary manipulation as a primary treatment strategy for pregnancies complicated by diabetes. *Journal of the American College of Nutrition* **9**, 320–325.

Jovanovic-Peterson, L. & Peterson, C.M. (1991) Is exercise safe or useful for gestational diabetic women? *Diabetes* **40** (Suppl. 2), 179–181.

Jovanovic-Peterson, L., Durak, E.P. & Peterson, C.M. (1989) Randomized trial of diet vs. diet plus cardiovascular conditioning on glucose levels in gestational diabetes. *American Journal of Obstetrics and Gynecology* **161**, 415–419.

Katz, A., Broberg, S., Sahlin, K. & Wahren, J. (1986) Leg glucose uptake during maximal dynamic exercise in humans. *American Journal of Physiology* **251**, E65–E70.

King, H., Zimmet, P., Raper, L.R. & Balkau, B. (1984) Risk factors for diabetes in three Pacific populations. *American Journal of Epidemiology* **119**, 396–409.

Kjaer, M., Secher, N.H., Bach, F.W. & Galbo, H. (1987) Role of motor center activity for hormonal changes and substrate mobilization in humans. *American Journal of Physiology* **253**, R687–R695.

Lampman, R.M., Schteingart, D.E., Santinga, J.T. *et al.* (1987) The influence of physical training on glucose tolerance, insulin sensitivity, and lipid and lipoprotein concentrations in middle aged hypertriglyceridemic and carbohydrate intolerant men. *Diabetologia* **30**, 380–385.

Landt, K.W., Campaigne, B.N., James, F.W. & Sperling, M.A. (1985) Effects of exercise training on insulin sensitivity in adolescents with type 1 diabetes. *Diabetes Care* **8**, 461–465.

LaPorte, R.E., Dorman, J.S. & Taiima, N. (1986) Pittsburgh insulin-dependent diabetes mellitus morbidity and mortality study: physical activity and diabetic complications. *Pediatrics* **78**, 1027–1033.

Loucks, A.B., Mortola, J.F., Girton, L. & Yen, S.C.C. (1989) Alterations in hypothalamic–pituitary–ovarian and the hypothalamic–pituitary–adrenal axes in athletic women. *Journal of Clinical Endocrinology and Metabolism* **68**, 402–411.

Loucks, A.B., Vaitukaitis, J., Cameron, J.L. *et al.* (1992) The reproductive system and exrcise in women. *Medicine and Science in Sports and Exercise* **24**, S288–S293.

Lucas, C.P., Patton, S., Stepke, T. *et al.* (1987) Achieving therapeutic goals in insulin-using diabetic patients with non-insulin-dependent diabetes mellitus. A weight reduction–exercise–oral agent approach. *American Journal of Medicine* **83**(3A), 3–9.

Manson, J.E., Rimm, E.B., Stampfer, M.J. *et al.* (1991) Physical activity and incidence of non-insulin-dependent diabetes mellitus in women. *Lancet* **338**, 774–778.

Marcus, R., Cann, C. & Madvig, P. (1985) Menstrual function and bone mass in elite women distance runners: endocrine and metabolic features. *Annals of Internal Medicine* **102**, 158–163.

Marcus, R., Drinkwater, B., Dalsky, G. *et al.* (1992) Osteoporosis and exercise in women. *Medicine and Science in Sports and Exercise* **24**, S301–S307.

Mills, J.L., Simpson, J.L., Driscoll, S.G. *et al.* (1988) The National Institutes of Childhealth and Family Development Diabetes in Early Pregnancy Study: incidence of spontaneous abortion among normal women and insulin-dependent diabetic women whose pregnancies were identified within 21 days of conception. *New England Journal of Medicine* **319**, 1617–1623.

Moy, C.S., Songer, T.J., LaPorte, R.E. *et al.* (1993) Insulin-dependent diabetes mellitus, physical activity, and death. *American Journal of Epidemiology* **137**, 74–81.

Paffenbarger, R.S. Jr, Wing, A.L. & Hyde, R.T. (1978) Physical activity as an index of heart attack risk in college alumni. *American Journal of Epidemiology* **108**, 161–175.

Pavlou, K.N., Steffee, W.P., Lerman, R.H. & Burrows, B.S. (1985) Effects of dieting and exercise on lean body mass, oxygen uptake and strength. *Medicine and Science in Sports and Exercise* **17**, 466–471.

Peterson, M.S. & Peterson, K. (1988) *Eat to Compete: A Guide to Sports Nutrition*. Medical Year Book Publishers, Chicago.

Pocock, N.J., Eisman, J. & Gwinn, T. (1989) Muscle

strength, physical fitness and weight but not age predict fermoral neck bone mass. *Journal of Bone and Mineral Research* **4**, 441–447.

Reilly, J.J., Lord, A., Bunker, V.W. *et al.* (1993) Energy balance in healthy elderly women. *British Journal of Nutrition* **69**, 21–27.

Roitman, J.L. (ed.) (1998) *American College of Sports Medicine Resource Manual for Guidelines for Exercise Testing and Prescription*, 3rd edn. Baltimore, Williams and Wilkins.

Ruderman, N. & Devlin, J.T. (eds) (1995) *The Health Professionals Guide to Diabetes and Exercise*. American Diabetes Association, Alexandria, Virginia.

Rydall, A.C., Rodin, G.M., Olmsted, M.P., Devenyi, R.G. & Daneman, D. (1997) Disordered eating behavior and microvascular complications in young women with insulin-dependent diabetes mellitus. *New England Journal of Medicine* **336**, 1849–1854.

Sandler, R.B. (1988) Muscle strength and skeletal competence: implications for early prophylaxis. *Calcified Tissue International* **42**, 281–283.

Schneider, S.H., Amorosa, L.F., Khachadurian, A.K. & Ruderman, N.B. (1984) Studies on the mechanism of improved glucose control during regular exercise in type 2 (non-insulin dependent) diabetes. *Diabetologia* **26**(5), 355–360.

Shushruta, S.C.S. (1938) *Vaidya Jayayaii Trikamji Acharia*. Nimyar Sagar Press, Bombay.

Smith, E.L. & Gilligan, C. (1991) Physical activity effects on bone metabolism. *Calcified Tissue International* **49** (Suppl.), S50–S54.

Solomon, C.G. (1996) Diabetes mellitus and risk of cardiovascular disease in women. *Medicine and Science in Sports and Exercise* **28**, 15–16.

Summary and Recommendations of the Second International Workshop-Conference on Gestational Diabetes Mellitus (1991) *Diabetes* **34** (Suppl. 2), 179–181.

Suominen, H. (1993) Bone mineral density and long term exercise. *Sports Medicine* **16**, 316–330.

Tanner, J.M. & Davies, S.W.D. (1985) Clinical longitudinal standards for height and height velocity for North American children. *Journal of Paediatrics* **107**, 317–329.

Taylor, R., Ram, P., Zimmet, P., Raper, L.R. & Ringrose, H. (1984) Physical activity and prevalence of diabetes in Melanesian and Indian men in Fiji. *Diabetologia* **27**, 578–582.

Van der Mooren, M.J., de Graaf, J., Demacker, P.N., de Haan, A.F. & Rolland, R. (1994) Changes in low-density lipoprotein profile during 17 beta-estradiol-hydrogesterone therapy in post-menopausal women. *Metabolism: Clinical and Experimental* **43**, 799–802.

Wallberg-Henriksson, H., Gunnarsson, R. & Henriksson, J. (1982) Increased peripheral insulin sensitivity and muscle mitochondrial enzymes but unchanged blood glucose control in type I diabetics after physical training. *Diabetes* **31**(12), 1044–1050.

Wallberg-Henriksson, H., Gunnarsson, R., Henriksson, J., Ostman, J. & Wahren, J. (1984) Influence of physical training on formation of muscle capillaries in type I diabetes. *Diabetes* **33**, 851–857.

Wasserman, D.R. & Vranic, M. (1985) Interaction between insulin, glucagon, and catecholamines in the regulation of glucose production and uptake during exercise: physiology and diabetes. In B. Saltin (ed.) *Biochemistry of Exercise*, Vol. VI, pp. 167–179. International Series on Sports Sciences, Copenhagen.

Yeager, K.K., Agostini, R., Nattiv, A. & Drinkwater, B. (1993) The female athlete triad: disordered eating, amenorrhea, osteoporosis. *Medicine and Science in Sports and Exercise* **25**, 775–777.

Yki-Jarvinen, H., DeFronzo, P. & Koivisto, V.A. (1984) Normalization of insulin sensitivity in Type I diabetic subjects by physical training during insulin pump therapy. *Diabetes Care* **7**, 520–527.

Zimmet, P., Faaiuso, S., Ainuu, S., Whitehouse, S., Milne, B. & DeBoer, W. (1981) The prevalence of diabetes in the rural and urban Polynesian population of Western Samoa. *Diabetes* **30**, 45–51.

Zimmet, P., Dowse, G., Finch, C., Serjeantson, S. & King, H. (1990) The epidemiology and natural history of NIDDM: lessons from the South Pacific. *Diabetes Metabolism Reviews* **6**, 91–124.

Zinman, B., Zuniga-Guajardo, S. & Kelly, D. (1984) Comparison of the acute and longterm effects of exercise on glucose control in Type I diabetes. *Diabetes Care* **7**, 515–519.

Chapter 19

Sport and Bone

ILKKA VUORI AND ARI HEINONEN

Introduction

Bone is a metabolically active tissue that is continuously formed and lost during one's lifetime. The basic form and development of the bones comprising the skeleton are genetically determined, but their mass and architecture are influenced by several factors. The most important of these are mechanical, nutritional and hormonal factors. The significance of mechanical factors, i.e. physical loading, was recognized over 100 years ago, when Wolff (1892) suggested that bone accommodates the habitual stress imposed upon it. Based on a great number of experimental, epidemiological and interventional studies, Frost (1987) has proposed a 'mechanostat' theory to explain the adaptation of bone architecture and mass to its typical mechanical environment. This theory maintains that physical loading causes locally microscopical structural deformations called strains in the bone. The strains induce various biophysical and chemical events that influence the metabolism and thus the structure of bone. Under habitual loading conditions the 'mechanostat' is in balance, resulting in maintenance of bone mass and architecture. When loading exceeds the customary loading of the bone, the strain-induced events result in increased bone formation. Therefore athletes in some disciplines have unusually strong bones. If the loading is less than what the bone is adapted to, the lack of stimuli caused by the strain leads to diminished local bone formation and loss of

bone. This happens typically as a consequence of immobilization.

Different sports load the skeleton at various sites in different ways. The induced strains vary in localization, magnitude, number or cycles, rate of development, and distribution at the bone site. All these variables have been shown to be associated with the regulation of bone mass (Lanyon, 1996). However, the type, intensity, frequency and duration of exercise that best enhances bone mineral accumulation are still largely unknown. The extent to which a bone can alter its form due to exercise and the extent to which growing and mature bones have similar adaptive capacities also remain unclear (Biewener & Bertram, 1993).

Thorough investigation and analysis of bone characteristics of athletes practising various sports is important because sports offer a large variety of 'natural experiments' that would be difficult or impossible to conduct in any other way. The knowledge gained may be valuable not only in a descriptive sense but also in testing ideas and hypotheses related to bone metabolism and physical characteristics, examining dose–response issues and evaluating potential benefits and risks to bone health of various sports at different ages.

Bone turnover

Physical loading influences bone mass, geometry and internal architecture through bone turnover. Three tissue-level mechanisms, growth, modelling and remodelling, are involved in bone turnover. Each of them has a specific purpose and mechanical loading can influence all of them.

Growth determines the bone size. Growth can only add, not remove, bone (Parfitt, 1994). The growth of bone stops at around 16–18 years of age. Consequently, the highest or peak bone mass and areal density are achieved around age 20 (Matkovic *et al.*, 1994; Haapasalo *et al.*, 1996a). Growth is under strong genetic influence, especially the maternal influence on daughters (Jouanny *et al.*, 1995). However, mechanical loading, nutrition and hormonal factors also influence growth.

Modelling is simultaneous removal and formation of bone at different sites by two mediator mechanisms, called resorption and formation drifts. It continues throughout life. Modelling determines the shape of bones and increases bone strength by improving geometric properties and adding mass (Kimmel, 1993).

Bone remodelling is a process by which bone is removed and formed at the same site but at different times. It maintains the functional competence of bone by replacing aged bone with new bone and repairing microcracks at scattered locations on bone surfaces through a biologically coupled activation–resorption–formation sequence (Jee, 1988; Frost, 1990, 1992; Turner, 1991). In a normal adult, activation and resorption last 1 month and formation another 3 months; thus the time scale for one complete remodelling cycle, called sigma, is about 4 months (Jee, 1988; Frost, 1989). Mineralization is completed in another 3–4 months (Jee, 1988). Bone remodelling is a complex process that is regulated by the balance between physiological signals due to mechanical factors and those due to systemic non-mechanical factors (polypeptide, steroid and thyroid hormones) as well as local factors (growth factors and prostaglandins) (Lanyon, 1987, 1990, 1996; Canalis, 1993).

Mechanical adaptation of bone

The magnitude of the force and the rate of force application affecting the human skeleton are mainly determined by movement conditions (velocity of body segments, number of repetitions, the muscular activity) and boundary conditions (anthropometric factors, fitness level, type of shoes, surface and weather) (Nigg, 1985). Thus changes in movement conditions affect the kinematics and kinetics of the movement and probably also the stress on, and strain of, bone. Therefore, the differences in the movement and boundary conditions of different sports may induce various strain distributions and different strain rates on bones. The rate of force application rather than the magnitude of force may be more important for the degree of strain. In tennis, for instance, the forces and the influence of the friction of the playing surface produce high torques on the bones of the lower extremity (Nigg, 1985). Furthermore, the relationship between force and acceleration–deceleration ($F = ma$) implies that sports involving impact loading (e.g. highly accelerating and decelerating movements) may produce high stresses and thus effective strains on bones.

Each bone can be regarded as a mechanical unit whose characteristics are adjusted to the demands of the loading environment. Bone adapts to changes in the effective stresses by adjusting its characteristics in a direction that tends to keep the internal strain within a physiologically reasonable range. If mechanical loading or disuse causes the strain level to shift outside the 'customary mechanical range', the bone is either overloaded or underloaded, which leads to bone adaptation and imbalance between bone formation and resorption. An example of adaptation of bone to altered loading conditions is illustrated in Fig. 19.1. The capability of bone to respond to mechanical loading is probably determined by a genetically controlled set-point that has been further modified by past site-specific loading and several biochemical factors related to age and disease. Biochemical agents can influence bone mass independently or they can influence bone structure by changing the set-point of the mechanical feedback system (Frost, 1987, 1993; Lanyon, 1987, 1996; Turner, 1991).

All the strain-related variables, namely magni-

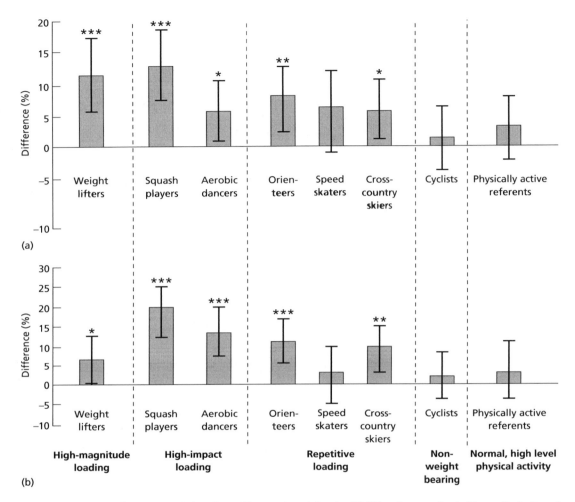

Fig. 19.1 Relative difference in weight-adjusted bone mineral density (BMD) at the most loaded lower limb sites of different female athlete groups ($n = 18–30$) and a physically active reference group ($n = 25$) compared with that of the sedentary reference group ($n = 25$). (a) Proximal tibia BMD and (b) calcaneus BMD. The grouping of the athletes was based on the specific bone-loading characteristics of the respective sports. The bars indicate the 95% confidence intervals. *, $P < 0.05$; **, $P < 0.01$; ***, $P < 0.001$. (From Heinonen, 1997 with permission.)

tude, cycles, rate and pattern of distribution, are integrated into dynamic loading conditions. However, the exact characteristics of an optimal stimulus for mechanically induced bone formation are not known. According to current knowledge, an effective exercise programme should involve high strains and/or high strain rates and unusual strain distributions. In practical terms, effective exercise regimens should consist of high mechanical forces and/or high rates of force application produced in versatile movements.

Other factors modifying bone adaptation to mechanical loading

Frost (1983, 1987) has proposed a hypothesis for a feedback control system that describes the interaction between mechanical and other factors, such as nutrition, age, hormonal stimuli and body composition. Bone mass is also determined by several interacting genetic, metabolic and environmental factors (Brandi *et al.*, 1994; Bronner, 1994). Genetic influences account for 60–80% of the interindividual variation of bone mass as assessed in the adult years (Pocock *et al.*, 1987; Slemenda *et al.*, 1991; Seeman *et al.*, 1996). In addition, adequate calcium intake is considered essential in order to attain and maintain optimal bone mineral mass and size (Dawson-Hughes *et al.*, 1990; Johnston *et al.*, 1992; Bronner, 1994; Parfitt, 1994; Nieves *et al.*, 1995; Specker, 1996).

Decreased oestrogen influence as reflected in menstrual irregularities and amenorrhoea is associated with low lumbar spine bone mineral density (BMD) (Drinkwater *et al.*, 1984; Marcus *et al.*, 1985; Prior *et al.*, 1990; Myburgh *et al.*, 1993), but other bone sites may also be affected (Drinkwater *et al.*, 1990). Therefore, in female athletes a significant risk factor for stress fractures is low bone density (Bennell *et al.*, 1996).

Complex associations exist between various parameters of body composition and bone density. A positive association may be explained, at least in part, by skeletal responses to mechanical forces induced by greater body weight and a weight-related beneficial effect of higher oestrogen concentrations (Slemenda, 1995; Albala *et al.*, 1996). Lean mass seems to be a stronger predictor of bone density or mass than fat mass (Nichols *et al.*, 1995; Young *et al.*, 1995; Chen *et al.*, 1997), although Reid *et al.* (1992) found that total body fat mass was the most significant predictor of total body BMD in premenopausal and postmenopausal women. In addition, muscle mass is positively related to bone density in older men and women (Doyle *et al.*, 1970; Snow-Harter *et al.*, 1990; Hughes *et al.*, 1995). The weight of muscle reflects the forces exerted on the bone to which it is attached, and muscle weight is an important determinant of bone mass (Doyle *et al.*, 1970).

Methodological considerations

The most commonly assessed bone parameters have been BMD and bone mineral content (BMC), while other important parameters related to bone strength, such as bone size and diameter, cortex–cavity ratio in long bones, geometric shape and trabecular architecture, have been assessed in only a few studies (Genant *et al.*, 1996; Sievänen *et al.*, 1996). Dual energy X-ray absorptiometry is the method of choice for measuring BMC and areal BMD. Most studies report the results as BMD. However, BMD does not represent true material density or apparent density and depends strongly on bone size and maturation of subjects (Bailey *et al.*, 1996; Genant *et al.*, 1996; Sievänen *et al.*, 1996). In many studies on athletes the subjects have been children or adolescents and since body size and phase of sexual maturity have great influence on bones, these variables need to be controlled. Quantitative computed tomography and peripheral quantitative computed tomography offer new possibilities for assessing bone geometry and mass distribution and for estimating bone strength (Genant *et al.*, 1996; Sievänen *et al.*, 1997). Broadband ultrasound attenuation has also been used to study bone mineral mass and other characteristics of bone strength that are potentially independent of density (Genant *et al.*, 1996).

The vast majority of studies have been cross-sectional and only a few have included follow-up or have investigated the effects of training programmes. An inherent problem in cross-sectional studies is the possible self-selection of subjects. Studies on athletes practising unilateral sports, such as racquet sports, offer possibilities for escaping this bias. Studies of tennis and squash players show large side-to-side differences in BMD and BMC in the players' arms but no significant differences in BMD or BMC in the non-dominant arm of the players and control subjects (Haapasalo *et al.*, 1994; Kannus *et al.*, 1995), indicating that local mechanical loading can greatly increase bone mass, at least in growing subjects. Consequently, carefully designed cross-sectional studies on female athletes could offer valuable insights into the effects of various long-standing exercise habits.

It has been shown convincingly that mechanical loading influences bone only at the sites where it causes strains, i.e. the effects are site specific. Therefore the effects of various sports on bones should be sought and expected at loaded sites. If the exercise mainly involves the lower limb, it may improve femoral neck bone density with no effect on the radius. Thus, if exercise training is intended to be osteogenic, it should provide loading targeted to specific sites, e.g. the femoral neck or lumbar vertebrae.

Bone mineral density and content in female athletes

BMD or BMC has been assessed in female athletes representing at least 20 sports. Most of the studies have been cross-sectional. In order to reveal true associations between bone characteristics and sports, the studies have to be analysed in a theoretically sound way. Thus, the characteristics of both the athletes, e.g. age, and of the sport, especially the loading characteristics, have to be taken into account.

Bones of child and adolescent athletes

The response of the skeleton to sport may vary at different stages of growth and maturation due to factors such as hormonal influences. It is known

that the adolescent growth spurt is the only time in life when bone is added substantially to both the inside and outside of the cortices (Parfitt, 1994). Furthermore, trabecular bone is more sensitive than cortical bone to changes in hormonal concentrations, which are especially large at puberty. These features may partially explain why the ability of bone to adapt to mechanical loading is greater during growth than during maturity (Slemenda *et al.*, 1994; Gunnes & Lehmann, 1996). In a cross-sectional study of female tennis and squash players, Kannus *et al.* (1995) showed that the influence of mechanical loading on the BMC of the playing arm is about two times greater if playing is begun before compared with after menarche (Fig. 19.2). This finding suggests that in order to attain the highest possible peak bone mass the bones should be loaded effectively at a rather young age, during the few years before and at puberty.

Bones of female athletes representing various sports

Table 19.1 is an attempt to assess the loading and consequently strain characteristics of sports in which bone mineral measurements of female athletes have been determined. Tables 19.2–19.4

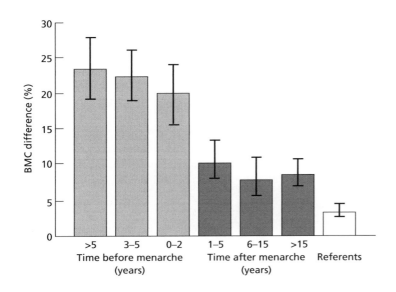

Fig. 19.2 Benefit of mechanical loading with respect to bone mineral content (BMC). The BMC of the playing arm (humeral shaft) of the subjects was about two times greater if the girls started playing at or before, rather than after, menarche. The bars represent the 95% confidence intervals. (From Kannus *et al.*, 1995 with permission.)

Table 19.1 Assessment of the loading characteristics of the different sports in which bone measurements of female athletes have been made

| Sport | Loading characteristics | | | | |
	Weight-bearing	High magnitude	High impact	Repetitive	Varied
Strength sports					
Body-building	xxx	xxx	x	x	x
Power-lifting	xxx	xxx	x	x	x
Weight-lifting	xxx	xxx	xx	x	xx
Endurance sports					
Running	xx	x	xx	xxx	xx
Orienteering	xx	x	xx	xxx	xx
Speed skating	xx	x	xx	xxx	xx
Cross-country skiing	xx	x	x	xxx	x
Rowing	x	x	x	xxx	x
Cycling	x	x	x	xxx	x
Swimming	0	x	x	xxx	x
Speed and power					
Aerobic dancing	xxx	xx	xxx	xxx	xxx
Ballet dancing	xxx	xx	xxx	xx	xxx
Gymnastics	xxx	xx	xxx	xx	xxx
Figure skating	xxx	xx	xxx	xx	xxx
Basketball	xxx	xx	xxx	xx(x)	xxx
Soccer	xxx	xx	xxx	xx(x)	xxx
Volleyball	xxx	xx	xxx	xx	xxx
Squash	xxx	xx	xxx	xx	xxx
Tennis	xxx	xx	xxx	xx	xxx

Assumption: duration of exposure is sufficient.
xxx, high, broad; xx, medium; x, low, limited; 0, none.

summarize the main features and findings of valid studies carried out on female athletes representing various sports, classified on the basis of their loading characteristics. Figure 19.1 has been constructed on the same basis and shows the summary of results of studies that have used the same design and methodology in the same laboratory, thus allowing good comparability between various types of sports.

BONE MINERAL MASS OF ATHLETES IN HIGH-MAGNITUDE LOADING SPORTS

Table 19.1 shows that strength sports produce high-magnitude loading of bones. Table 19.2 summarizes the findings of three cross-sectional studies on mature female athletes representing strength sports. In all studies, the BMD of the athletes at the loaded sites is substantially greater than that in the control subjects.

The results of the study of Heinonen *et al.* (1993) are also shown in Fig. 19.1. Although the possiblity of self-selection to competition in strength sports by subjects with stronger or better-adapting bones cannot be excluded, there is no evidence that this has occurred. Studies on female tennis and squash players showing no difference in BMD or BMC of the non-playing arm between athletes and controls (Haapasalo *et al.*, 1994; Kannus *et al.*, 1995) do not suggest any substantial selection bias. However, prospective weight-training studies on women have

Table 19.2 Bone mineral mass in female athletes taking part in high-magnitude loading sports (results selected from cross-sectional studies)

Reference	Athlete group	No.	Age (years)	Bone site	Bone mineral mass — Difference between athletes and controls (%)	Technique
Davee et al. (1990)	Muscle-building	9	20–30	L2–L4	+ 10*	DPA
	Controls	9				
Heinonen et al. (1993)	Weight-lifters	18	25 ± 5	L2–L4	+ 15*	DXA
				Femoral neck	+ 10*	
				Distal femur	+ 19*	
				Patella	+ 22*	
				Proximal tibia	+ 12*	
				Calcaneus	+ 4*	
				Distal radius	+ 29*	
	Controls	25	23 ± 3			
Heinrich et al. (1990)	Body-builders	11	26 ± 5	L2–L4	+ 12*	DPA
				Femoral neck	+ 15*	
				Ward triangle	+ 23*	
				Greater trochanter	+ 12*	
				Proximal radius	+ 9	SPA
				Distal radius	+ 16*	
	Controls	18	25 ± 4			

*$P < 0.05$.
DPA, dual photon absorptiometry; DXA, dual-energy X-ray absorptiometry; SPA, single photon absorptiometry.

demonstrated only small to moderate (0.8–3.8%) gain in regional bone mineral mass (Gleeson et al., 1990; Peterson et al., 1991; Pruitt et al., 1992; Snow-Harter et al., 1992; Nelson et al., 1994; Vuori et al., 1994; Friedlander et al., 1995; Lohman et al., 1995) or no effect (McCartney et al., 1995; Pruitt et al., 1995; Heinonen et al., 1996b; Sinaki et al., 1996). The likely explanations for the differences between cross-sectional and prospective training studies include more intensive, strenuous and longer training started in childhood or adolescence in the athletes compared with the subjects in the training studies. Furthermore, in many of the prospective studies, training consisted of slow, smooth, similar repetitions of movements produced by the use of various types of training machine (Peterson et al., 1991; Pruitt et al., 1992; Snow-Harter et al., 1992; Nelson et al., 1994; Vuori

et al., 1994; Friedlander et al., 1995). Bone-loading effects are likely to be substantially less in these exercises compared with those used by weight-lifters, whose training consists of a number of different exercises using free weights. This type of training not only produces high-magnitude strains but also a favourable rate and distribution of the strains in terms of osteogenesis.

BONE MINERAL MASS OF
ATHLETES IN REPETITIVE LOADING
WEIGHT-BEARING SPORTS

The most commonly practised sport that involves a large number of repetitive loadings is running (Table 19.1). Several studies have shown that mineral mass of the loaded bones, e.g. several sites in the lower legs and lumbar spine, of female athletes in running sports is greater than in control subjects (Table 19.3, Fig. 19.1). However, the difference is not as great as between athletes in strength sports and control subjects. In cross-country skiers and speed skaters there is, or tends to be, greater regional bone mineral mass at the loaded sites compared with control subjects (Table 19.3, Fig. 19.1). In these sports the movements are gliding, resulting in very small, or no, impact with the ground; also they are likely to produce less stress on various sites in the lower legs than running. The reaction forces acting on the lower limb during running can be two to five times body weight (Subotnick, 1985) and those on the vertebrae can be 1.75 times body weight (Capozzo, 1983). Thus, the greater regional bone mineral mass at loaded sites of athletes in running sports is probably due to both the great number of loading cycles and the moderate impact in running. The regional bone mineral mass of rowers and cyclists (Table 19.3, Fig. 19.1) as well as of swimmers (Orwoll et al., 1989; Risser et al., 1990; Fehling et al., 1995; Lee et al., 1995; Taaffe et al., 1995, 1997) has not been found to be greater in the athletes compared with controls. The reason is very likely the partial or complete lack of weight-bearing activity in these sports.

There are no published data on regional bone mineral mass of competitive walkers. In addition, the data regarding the influence of occupational or recreational walking are contradictory. In premenopausal women there were no differences in weight-adjusted regional bone mineral mass between mail and newspaper carriers walking 6 km daily and more sedentary office workers (average walking distance about 2 km daily) of the same age and from the same work sites (Uusi-Rasi et al., 1994). In postmenopausal women both habitual walking (>12 km·week⁻¹) (Krall & Dawson-Hughes 1994) and walking plus callisthenics (Dalsky et al., 1988; Hatori et al., 1993; Krall & Dawson-Hughes, 1994; Kohrt et al., 1995; Prince et al., 1995) have been found to have positive influence on the loaded sites. It may be that only fast walking causes sufficient strain in the bone tissue (Rubin & Lanyon, 1982). During

fast walking, the direction and rate of loading on the lower limb are altered by the short heel strike and high ground reaction forces (Subotnick, 1985; Grove & Londeree, 1992) and hip reaction forces (Bergman et al., 1993) compared with ordinary walking. This mechanism might also explain why there seems to be an intensity threshold (70–90% of maximal oxygen consumption), corresponding to sufficient speed of walking or running for aerobic training to influence regional bone mineral mass (Dalsky et al., 1988; Hatori et al., 1993; Martin & Notelovitz, 1993; Heinonen et al., 1998).

BONE MINERAL MASS OF ATHLETES IN HIGH-IMPACT SPORTS

Speed and power sports are characterized by fast, forceful, acceleratory and deceleratory, impact-producing movements, often in multiple directions. These sports produce strains in bones at a high rate and in multiple directions (Table 19.1). On the basis of animal experiments (Lanyon, 1992, 1996; Rubin & McLeod, 1996), the osteogenic effect of the loading profile produced by speed and power sports should be greater than that caused by strength or endurance sports. This notion is supported by the results of both cross-sectional and prospective studies on female athletes (Table 19.4), as well as by controlled training studies. The differences in areal bone mineral mass at loaded sites between speed and power athletes and referents (Table 19.4, Fig. 19.1) are generally larger than those in strength and endurance athletes (Tables 19.2 & 19.3, Fig. 19.1).

Direct comparisons of groups of athletes corroborate this picture. One of our previous studies showed that, compared with regularly exercising controls, squash players had the highest weight-adjusted BMD values (7–19%) at all measured sites of any sport group (Heinonen et al., 1995). Robinson et al. (1995) investigated bone mineral mass in two groups of competitive young female athletes, gymnasts and runners, with different skeletal loading patterns. The gymnasts exhibited higher bone mineral mass in the femoral

Table 19.3 Bone mineral mass in female athletes taking part in repetitive loading (weight-bearing) sports (results selected from cross-sectional studies)

Reference	Athlete group	No.	Age (years)	Bone site	Bone mineral mass — Difference between athletes and controls (%)	Technique
Dook et al. (1997)	Running and field hockey	20	46 ± 3	Whole body	+ 7*	DXA
				Regional leg	+ 7*	
				Regional arm	+ 3	
	Sedentary controls	20	46 ± 2			
Harber et al. (1991)	Eumenorrhoeic runners	17	27 ± 5	Calcaneus	− 2	CST
	Amenorrhoeic runners	11	26 ± 6	Calcaneus	0	
	Normoactive controls	14	27 ± 7			
Heinonen et al. (1993)	Orienteers	30	23 ± 3	L2–L4	0	DXA
				Femoral neck	+ 2	
				Distal femur	+ 5*	
				Patella	+ 3	
				Proximal tibia	+ 4*	
				Calcaneus	+ 4	
				Distal radius	+ 1	
	Cross-country skiers	28	21 ± 3	L2–L4	0	
				Femoral neck	+ 5	
				Distal femur	+ 5	
				Patella	+ 2	
				Proximal tibia	+ 3	
				Calcaneus	+ 3	
				Distal radius	− 1	
	Active controls	25	23 ± 3			
Heinonen et al. (1995)	Orienteers	30	23 ± 3	L2–L4	+ 8	DXA
				Femoral neck	+ 3	
				Distal femur	+ 6*	
				Patella	+ 4	
				Proximal tibia	+ 7*	
				Calcaneus	+ 11*	
				Distal radius	− 4	
	Speed skaters	14	21 ± 9	L2–L4	+ 6	
				Femoral neck	+ 4	
				Distal femur	+ 7*	
				Patella	+ 5	
				Proximal tibia	+ 6	
				Calcaneus	+ 3	
				Distal radius	− 6	

Continued

Table 19.3 (*Continued*)

Reference	Athlete group	No.	Age (years)	Bone site	Bone mineral mass — Difference between athletes and controls (%)	Technique
	Cross-country skiers	28	21 ± 3	L2–L4	+ 3	
				Femoral neck	+ 5	
				Distal femur	+ 5	
				Patella	+ 2	
				Proximal tibia	+ 5*	
				Calcaneus	+ 9*	
				Distal radius	− 7*	
	Sedentary controls	25	24 ± 5			
Kirk *et al.* (1989)	Long-distance runners	10	25–35	T12–L3	+ 1	QCT
				Mid-radius	+ 12	SPA
	Sedentary controls	10				
	Long-distance runners	9	55–65	T12–L3	− 7	
				Mid-radius	+ 1	
	Sedentary controls	9				
Lane *et al.* (1986)	Long-distance runners	6	56	L1	+ 35*	QCT
	Matched controls	6	56			
Myerson *et al.* (1992)	Eumenorrhoeic runners	13	30 ± 1	Total body	+ 10*	DPA
	Amenorrhoeic runners	13	30 ± 1	Total body	− 7	
	Controls	12	27 ± 1			
Suominen *et al.* (1992)	Long-distance runners, skiers	18	66–85	Calcaneus	+ 12 and + 6	SPA
	Population sample	42	70–81			
Wolman *et al.* (1991)	Runners	21	25–28	Femoral shaft	+ 8*	DPA
	Rowers	36	24–26	Femoral shaft	+ 2	
	Sedentary controls	13	27–30			

* $P < 0.05$.
CST, compton scattering technique; DPA, dual photon absorptiometry; DXA, dual-energy X-ray absorptiometry; QCT, quantitative computed tomography; SPA, single photon absorptiometry.

Table 19.4 Bone mineral mass in female athletes taking part in sports producing strains on bones at a high rate (e.g. impacts) and usually from many directions (results selected from cross-sectional studies)

Reference	Athlete group	No.	Age (years)	Bone site	Bone mineral mass — Difference between athletes and controls (%)	Technique
Dook et al. (1997)	Basketball and netball	20	46 ± 3	Whole body	+ 8*	DXA
				Regional leg	+ 8*	
				Regional arm	+ 4	
	Sedentary controls	20	46 ± 2			
Düppe et al. (1996)	Active football players	96	18 ± 4	Total body	+ 4*	DXA
				Lumbar spine	+ 5	
				Femoral neck	+ 11*	
				Trochanter	+ 11*	
				Ward's triangle	+ 11*	
	Controls	90	20 ± 5			
	Former football players	25	40 ± 5	Total body	+ 4*	
				Lumbar spine	− 2	
				Femoral neck	+ 7*	
				Trochanter	+ 11*	
				Ward's triangle	+ 9*	
	Controls	57	37 ± 4			
Fehling et al. (1995)	Volleyball players	8	20 ± 1	L2–L4	+ 11*	DXA
				Femoral neck	+ 15*	
				Ward's triangle	+ 17*	
				Total body	+ 13*	
				left arm	+ 5*	
				right arm	+ 7*	
				left leg	+ 15*	
				right leg	+ 12*	
				right pelvis	+ 19*	
	Gymnasts	7	20 ± 1	L2–L4	+ 14*	
				Femoral neck	+ 15*	
				Ward's triangle	+ 17*	
				Total body	+ 11*	
				left arm	+ 15*	
				right arm	+ 16*	
				left leg	+ 10*	
				right leg	+ 10*	
				right pelvis	+ 15	
	Controls	13	20 ± 1			
Fogelholm et al. (unpublished observations)	Gymnasts	12	17 ± 1	L2–L4	+ 7*	DXA
				Femoral neck	+ 17*	
				Distal radius	0	
	Soccer players	12	19 ± 2	L2–L4	+ 14*	
				Femoral neck	+ 16*	
				Distal radius	+ 10*	
	Controls	12	17 ± 1			

Continued

Table 19.4 (*Continued*)

Reference	Athlete group	No.	Age (years)	Bone site	Bone mineral mass Difference between athletes and controls (%)	Technique
Haapasalo *et al.* (1994)	Squash players	19	18–32	Proximal humerus	+ 9*	DXA
				Humeral shaft	+ 10*	
				Radial shaft	+ 1*	
				Ulnar shaft	− 1*	
				Distal radius	+ 10*	
				Distal ulna	+ 24*	
				Calcaneus	+ 12*	
	Controls	19	19–33			
Heinonen *et al.* (unpublished observations)	Triple jumpers	4	23 ± 4	L2–L4	+ 38*	DXA
				Femoral neck	+ 26*	
				Distal femur	+ 34*	
				Patella	+ 25*	
				Proximal tibia	+ 35*	
				Calcaneus	+ 35*	
				Distal radius	+ 11	
	Controls	25	24 ± 5			
Heinonen *et al.* (1995)	Squash players	18	25 ± 4	L2–L4	+ 14*	DXA
				Femoral neck	+ 17*	
				Distal femur	+ 11*	
				Patella	+ 7*	
				Proximal tibia	+ 13*	
				Calcaneus	+ 19*	
				Distal radius	+ 11*	
	Aerobic dancers	27	28 ± 4	L2–L4	+ 3	
				Femoral neck	+ 9*	
				Distal femur	+ 3	
				Patella	+ 2	
				Proximal tibia	+ 6*	
				Calcaneus	+ 14*	
				Distal radius	− 8*	
	Controls	25	24 ± 5			
Jacobson *et al.* (1984)	Tennis players	11	18–22	Spine	+ 11*	DPA
				Distal radius	+ 17*	SPA
				Mid-radius	+ 12*	
				Metatarsal	+ 23*	
	Age-matched controls	11				
Kannus *et al.* (1995)	Tennis and squash players	105	16–50	Proximal humerus	+ 10*	DXA
				Humeral shaft	+ 10*	
				Radial shaft	+ 3	
				Distal radius	+ 8*	

Continued p. 292

Table 19.4 (*Continued*)

Reference	Athlete group	No.	Age (years)	Bone site	Bone mineral mass — Difference between athletes and controls (%)	Technique
				Calcaneus	+ 11*	
	Controls	50	16–48			
Kirchner *et al.* (1995)	Gymnasts	26	20 ± 0.2	Lumbar spine	+ 18*	DXA
				Total proximal femur	+ 21*	
				Femoral neck	+ 22*	
				Ward's triangle	+ 25*	
				Whole body	+ 10*	
	Controls	26	20 ± 0.2			
Kirchner *et al.* (1996)	Former gymnasts	18	36 ± 1	Lumbar spine	+ 16*	DXA
				Femoral neck	+ 18*	
				Ward's triangle	+ 22*	
				Whole body	+ 9*	
	Controls	15	37 ± 1			
Lee *et al.* (1995)	Volleyball players	11	19 ± 1	Total body	+ 17	DXA
				Lumbar spine	+ 18	
				Femoral neck	+ 11	
				Trochanter	+ 17	
				Ward's triangle	+ 4	
				Spine	+ 6*	
				Pelvis	+ 10*	
				Left arm	+ 12*	
				Right arm	+ 13*	
				Left leg	+ 17*	
				Right leg	+ 15*	
	Basketball players	7	20 ± 2	Total body	+ 9*	
				Lumbar spine	+ 14*	
				Femoral neck	+ 20*	
				Trochanter	+ 24*	
				Ward's triangle	+ 18*	
				Spine	+ 5*	
				Pelvis	+ 11*	
				Left arm	+ 12*	
				Right arm	+ 17*	
				Left leg	+ 15*	
				Right leg	+ 17*	
	Soccer players	9	19 ± 1	Total body	+ 4	
				Lumbar spine	+ 6*	
				Femoral neck	+ 10*	
				Trochanter	+ 16*	
				Ward's triangle	+ 12	

Continued

Table 19.4 (*Continued*)

Reference	Athlete group	No.	Age (years)	Bone site	Bone mineral mass — Difference between athletes and controls (%)	Technique
				Spine	+ 5	
				Pelvis	+ 7*	
				Left arm	+ 1	
				Right arm	+ 3	
				Left leg	+ 11*	
				Right leg	+ 11*	
	Sedentary controls	11	22 ± 1			
Nichols *et al.* (1994)	Gymnasts	11	19 ± 1	Preseason: lumbar spine	+ 8*	DXA
				femoral neck	+ 11*	
	Controls	11	21 ± 2			
Nichols *et al.* (1995)	Basketball players	14	19 ± 1	L2–L4	+ 10*	DXA
				Femoral neck	+ 14*	
				Total body	+ 10*	
				Leg	+ 15*	
				Arm	+ 8*	
	Gymnasts	15	19 ± 1	L2–L4	+ 9*	
				Femoral neck	+ 11*	
				Total body	+ 5*	
				Leg	+ 7*	
				Arm	+ 12*	
	Tennis players	6	23 ± 4	L2–L4	+ 4	
				Femoral neck	+ 3*	
				Total body	+ 6*	
				Leg	+ 9*	
				Arm	+ 6*	
	Volleyball players	13	19 ± 1	L2–L4	+ 13*	
				Femoral neck	+ 14*	
				Total body	+ 10*	
				Leg	+ 15*	
				Arm	+ 8	
	Non-athletes	12	21 ± 2			
Pearce *et al.* (1996)	Ballet dancers: < 40 months oligomenorrhoea	17	14 ± 0.2	Lumbar spine	− 2	DXA
				Femoral neck	+ 9*	
				Ward's triangle	+ 10*	
				Trochanter	+ 9*	
				Arms	− 4	
	> 40 months oligomenorrhoea	24	18 ± 0.2	Lumbar spine	− 4	
				Femoral neck	+ 4	
				Ward's triangle	+ 4	
				Trochanter	+ 2	

Continued p. 294

Table 19.4 (*Continued*)

Reference	Athlete group	No.	Age (years)	Bone site	Bone mineral mass: Difference between athletes and controls (%)	Technique
				Arms	− 8	
	Controls	46	18 ± 0.2			
Risser *et al.* (1990)	Volleyball players	12	20 ± 2	Lumbar spine	+ 15*	DPA
				Calcaneus	+ 26*	SPA
	Basketball players	9	20 ± 1	Lumbar spine	+ 12	
				Calcaneus	+ 36*	
	Non-athletes	13	20 ± 1			
Robinson *et al.* (1995)	Gymnasts	21	22 ± 3	Whole body	+ 2	DXA
				Lumbar spine	+ 6	
				Femoral neck	+ 12*	
	Controls	19	19 ± 2			
Slemenda & Johnston (1993)	Figure skaters	22	10–23	Total body	+ 7*	DXA
				Spine	+ 6	
				Trunk	+ 8*	
				Legs	+ 10*	
				Pelvis	+ 14*	
				Arm	+ 4	
	Controls	22	10–23			
Taaffe *et al.* (1995)	Gymnasts	13	19 ± 1	Whole body	+ 3	DXA
				Lumbar spine	+ 8	
				Femoral neck	+ 15*	
				Trochanter	+ 15*	
	Controls	19	19 ± 2			
Taaffe *et al.* (1997)	Gymnasts, 8-month cohort	26	20 ± 1	Whole body	+ 1	DXA
				Lumbar spine	+ 6	
				Femoral neck	+ 14	
	Controls	14	19 ± 2			
	Gymnasts, 12-month cohort	8	19 ± 1	Whole body	+ 4	
				Lumbar spine	+ 4	
				Femoral neck	+ 20*	
	Controls	11	20 ± 2			

*$P < 0.05$.
DPA, dual photon absorptiometry; DXA, dual-energy X-ray absorptiometry; SPA, single photon absorptiometry.

neck and lumbar spine (6–12%) compared with runners and controls. Taaffe *et al.* (1995) found similar results: young female gymnasts had greater bone mineral mass at both appendicular and axial sites compared with swimmers and controls. Fehling *et al.* (1995) and Kirchner *et al.* (1995) also showed that when height and weight were controlled, the impact-loading group (gymnasts and volleyball players) had higher bone mineral mass than swimmers and controls. The very substantial differences between the playing and non-playing arm sites in squash and tennis players (Jacobson *et al.*, 1984; Haapasalo *et al.*, 1994; Kannus *et al.*, 1995; Nichols *et al.*, 1995) also speak for the effectiveness of high-impact loading as an osteogenic stimulus. The strongest evidence for this view is provided by recent prospective studies and clinical trials. Young female gymnasts had a higher bone mineral mass in the lumbar spine compared with controls, and the bone mass increased even further after 27 weeks of gymnastic training (Nichols *et al.*, 1994). Taaffe *et al.* (1997) demonstrated that BMD of the lumbar spine and femoral neck responded dramatically to 8 and 18 months of gymnastic training in young women.

Clinical trials also support the aforementioned concept. In our recent study (Heinonen *et al.*, 1996a), in which an exercise regimen with a rapidly rising force profile (jumping) was applied for 18 months, we showed significant increases in BMD (1.4–3.7%) at the loaded sites (lumbar spine, femoral neck, distal femur, patella, proximal tibia and calcaneus) in pre-menopausal women. The training consisted of aerobic jumping and step exercises, in which the magnitude of the ground reaction forces was gradually increased by increasing the height of the foam fences and the number of step-benches (Heinonen *et al.*, 1996a). Bassey and Ramsdale (1994, 1995) and Grove and Londeree (1992) also used an impact training regimen and have shown an increase or maintenance of bone mineral mass in premenopausal and post-menopausal women.

Conclusion

Studies on athletes provide a wealth of 'natural experiments' with which to gain information and insight about the influence and significance of physical loading on human bones. Cross-sectional studies strongly support the adaptation hypothesis expressed by Wolff (1892) more than 100 years ago and also the 'mechanostat' theory of Frost (1987). Thus, a substantial increase in physical loading produced by sports activity leads to a local increase in bone mineral mass, while unloading below the habitual level, beneath the 'physiological window' (Turner, 1991), produces a local decrease in bone mass.

However, preliminary evidence suggests that if an athlete decreases the intensity and volume of her training but still remains physically active, at least part of the training-induced bone mass is retained (Kirchner *et al.*, 1996).

Studies on weight-lifters and athletes involved in unilateral sports, such as tennis and squash, have probably explored the upper limits of adaptive capacity attainable for human bones through natural exercise. This is because the amount, intensity, duration and even versatility of the training of these athletes is hard to surpass and also because they started their systematic training during the optimal phase of growth and maturation. This optimal phase has also been identified by cross-sectional studies on athletes; prospective training studies on this issue are in progress. Studies on athletes in unilateral sports have also provided strong evidence that the unusually high bone mass at the loaded sites is the result of training and not self-selection and genetic factors. Furthermore, studies on athletes have revealed the risks of excessive training volume and intensity, i.e. fatigue fractures, hormonal imbalance and osteopenia.

Experimental studies on animals have shown that the magnitude and rate of development of strains are more powerful osteogenic characteristics of physical loading than the number of strain cycles. Cross-sectional studies on athletes reveal similar findings. These have been further corroborated by training studies showing that the strongest osteogenic effect in non-athletic women has been induced by exercises producing a high rate of strain (as impact) at high magnitude and from many directions.

Cumulative evidence shows that bones are no different from other tissues and organs of the body. Training strengthens them to tolerate the stress caused by training, but they get weaker and lighter when stress decreases. Consequently, the bones of athletes training sensibly tolerate even temporary excess stresses without damage if the internal milieu determined by hormonal and nutritional factors is also in balance. On the other hand, errors in training such as an unduly rapid increase in volume or intensity, inappropriate training during recovery from injuries or strengthening muscles excessively by using drugs may lead to serious bone damage.

Recommendations for future research

There are still many opportunities for acquiring new knowledge on how bone responds to physical loading by studying athletes. Assessment techniques such as quantitative computed tomography can be used to study the geometric properties and adaptations of bones and estimate their strength more accurately than bone mass measurement. These techniques are important because training may result in an improvement in bone strength due to changes in bone geometry and material quality without a notable increase in bone mineral mass. In addition, the role of the entire biomechanical environment should be taken into consideration in future studies. The knowledge that will be acquired from these studies will be especially valuable for the development of 'bone-training' methods for the prevention of osteoporosis as well as for the treatment and rehabilitation of patients with injuries and bone diseases. The applications may include training machines comparable to those used for strength and aerobic training; in fact, the first versions of these machines have been developed.

References

Albala, C., Yýñez, M., Devoto, E., Sostin, C., Zeballos, L. & Santos, J.L. (1996) Obesity as a protective factor for postmenopausal osteoporosis. *International Journal of Obesity* **20**, 1027–1032.

Bailey, D.A., Faulkner, R.A. & McKay, H.A. (1996) Growth, physical activity, and bone mineral acquisition. *Exercise and Sports Sciences Reviews* **24**, 233–266.

Bassey, E.J. & Ramsdale, S.J. (1994) Increase in femoral bone density in young women following high-impact exercise. *Osteoporosis International* **4**, 72–75.

Bassey, E.J. & Ramsdale, S.J. (1995) Weight-bearing exercise and ground reaction forces: a 12-month randomized controlled trial of effects on bone mineral density in healthy postmenopausal women. *Bone* **16**, 469–476.

Bennell, K.L., Malcom, S.A., Thomas, S.A. *et al.* (1996) Risk factors for stress fractures in track and field athletes. A twelve-month prospective study. *American Journal of Sports Medicine* **24**, 810–818.

Bergman, G., Graichen, F. & Rohlman, A. (1993) Hip joint loading during walking and running, measured in two patients. *Journal of Biomechanics* **26**, 969–990.

Biewener, A.A. & Bertram, J.E.A. (1993) Skeletal strain patterns in relation to exercise training during growth. *Journal of Experimental Biology* **185**, 51–69.

Brandi, M.L., Bianchi, M.L., Eisman, J.A. *et al.* (1994) Genetics of osteoporosis. *Calcified Tissue International* **55**, 161–163.

Bronner, F. (1994) Calcium and osteoporosis. *American Journal of Clinical Nutrition* **60**, 831–836.

Canalis, E. (1993) Regulation of bone remodelling. In M.J. Favus (ed.) *Primer on the Metabolic Bone Disease and Disorders of Mineral Metabolism*, 2nd edn, pp. 33–37. Raven Press, New York.

Capozzo, A. (1983) Force actions in the human trunk during running. *Journal of Sports Medicine* **23**, 14–22.

Chen, Z., Lohman, T.G., Stini, W.A., Ritenbaugh, C. & Aickin, M. (1997) Fat or lean tissue mass: which one is the major determinant of bone mineral mass in healthy postmenopausal women? *Journal of Bone and Mineral Research* **12**, 144–151.

Dalsky, G.P., Stocke, K.S., Ehsani, A.A., Slatopolsky, E., Lee, W.C. & Birge, J.S. (1988) Weight-bearing exercise training and lumbar bone mineral content in postmenopausal women. *Annals of Internal Medicine* **108**, 824–828.

Davee, A.M., Rosen, C.J. & Adler, R.A. (1990) Exercise patterns and trabecular bone density in college women. *Journal of Bone and Mineral Research* **5**, 245–250.

Dawson-Hughes, B., Dallal, G.E., Krall, E.A., Sadowski, L., Sahyoun, N. & Tannenbaum, S. (1990) A controlled trial of the effect of calcium supplementation on bone density in postmenopausal women. *New England Journal of Medicine* **322**, 878–883.

Dook, J.E., James, C., Henderson, N.K. & Price, R.I. (1997) Exercise and bone mineral density in mature female athletes. *Medicine and Science in Sports and Exercise* **29**, 291–296.

Doyle, F., Brown, J. & Lachance, C. (1970) Relation between bone mass and muscle weight. *Lancet* **i**, 391–393.

Drinkwater, B.L., Nilson, K., Chesnut, C. III, Bremner, W.J., Shainholtz, S. & Southworth, M.B. (1984) Bone mineral content of amenorrheic and eumenorrheic athletes. *New England Journal of Medicine* **311**, 277–286.

Drinkwater, B.L., Bruemner, B. & Chesnut, C.H. (1990) Menstrual history as determinant of current bone density in young athletes. *Journal of the American Medical Association* **263**, 545–548.

Düppe, H., Gärdsell, P., Johnell, O. & Ornstein, E. (1996) Bone mineral density in female junior, senior and former football players. *Osteoporosis International* **6**, 437–441.

Fehling, P.C., Alekel, L., Clasey, J. & Rector, A. (1995) A comparison of bone mineral densities among female athletes in impact loading and active loading sports. *Bone* **17**, 205–210.

Friedlander, A.L., Genant, H.K., Sadowsky, S., Byl, N.N. & Gluer, C.C. (1995) A two-year program of aerobics and weight training enhances bone mineral density of young women. *Journal of Bone and Mineral Research* **10**, 574–585.

Frost, H.M. (1983) The skeletal intermediary organization. *Metabolic Bone Disease and Related Research* **4**, 281–290.

Frost, H.M. (1987) Bone 'mass' and the 'mechanostat': a proposal. *Anatomical Record* **219**, 1–9.

Frost, H.M. (1989) Some effects of basic multicellular unit-based remodeling on photon absorptiometry of trabecular bone. *Bone and Mineral* **7**, 47–65.

Frost, H.M. (1990) Skeletal structural adaptations to mechanical usage (SATMU). 2. Redefining Wolff's law: the remodeling problem. *Anatomical Record* **226**, 414–422.

Frost, H.M. (1992) The role of changes in mechanical usage set points in the pathogenesis of osteoporosis. *Journal of Bone and Mineral Research* **7**, 253–261.

Frost, H.M. (1993) Suggested fundamental concepts in skeletal physiology. *Calcified Tissue International* **52**, 1–4.

Genant, H.K., Engele, K., Fuerst, T. *et al.* (1996) Noninvasive assessment of bone mineral and structure: state of the art. *Journal of Bone and Mineral Research* **11**, 707–730.

Gleeson, P.B., Protas, E.J., LeBlanc, A.D., Schneider, V.S. & Evans, H.J. (1990) Effects of weight lifting on bone mineral density in premenopausal women. *Journal of Bone and Mineral Research* **5**, 153–158.

Grove, K.A. & Londeree, B.R. (1992) Bone density in postmenopausal women: high impact vs. low impact exercise. *Medicine and Science in Sports and Exercise* **24**, 1190–1194.

Gunnes, M. & Lehmann, E.H. (1996) Physical activity and dietary constituents as predictors of forearm cortical and trabecular bone gain in healthy children and adolescents: a prospective study. *Acta Paediatrica Scandinavica* **85**, 19–25.

Haapasalo, H., Kannus, P., Sievänen, H., Heinonen, A., Oja, P. & Vuori, I. (1994) Long-term unilateral loading and bone mineral density and content in female squash players. *Calcified Tissue International* **54**, 249–255.

Haapasalo, H., Kannus, P., Sievänen, H. *et al.* (1996a) Development of mass, density, and estimated mechanical characteristics of bones in caucasian females. *Journal of Bone and Mineral Research* **11**, 1751–1760.

Haapasalo, H., Sievänen, H., Kannus, P., Heinonen, A., Oja, P. & Vuori, I. (1996b) Dimensions and estimated mechanical characteristics of the humerus after long-term tennis loading. *Journal of Bone and Mineral Research* **11**, 864–872.

Harber, V.I., Webber, L.E., Sutton, J.R. & MacDougall, J.D. (1991) The effect of amenorrhea on calcaneal bone density and total bone turnover in runners. *International Journal of Sports Medicine* **12**, 505–508.

Hatori, M., Hasegawa, A., Adachi, H. *et al.* (1993) The effects of walking at anaerobic threshold level on vertebral bone loss in postmenopausal women. *Calcified Tissue International* **52**, 411–414.

Heinonen, A. (1997) *Exercise as an osteogenic stimulus*. Studies in Sport, Physical Education and Health No. 49. Academic dissertation, University of Jyväskylä.

Heinonen, A., Oja, P., Kannus, P., Sievänen, H., Mänttäri, A. & Vuori, I. (1993) Bone mineral density in female athletes of different sports. *Bone and Mineral* **23**, 1–14.

Heinonen, A., Oja, P., Kannus, P. *et al.* (1995) Bone mineral density in female athletes representing sports with different loading characteristics of the skeleton. *Bone* **17**, 197–203.

Heinonen, A., Kannus, P., Sievänen, H. *et al.* (1996a) Randomised controlled trial of effect of high-impact exercise on selected risk factors for osteoporotic fractures. *Lancet* **348**, 1343–1347.

Heinonen, A., Sievänen, H., Kannus, P., Oja, P. & Vuori, I. (1996b) Effects of unilateral strength training and detraining on bone mineral mass and estimated mechanical characteristics of upper limb bones in young women. *Journal of Bone and Mineral Research* **11**, 490–501.

Heinonen, A., Oja, P., Sievänen, H., Pasanen, M. & Vuori, I. (1998) Effect of two training regimens on bone mineral density in healthy perimenopausal women: a randomized controlled trial. *Journal of Bone and Mineral Research* **13**, 483–490.

Heinrich, C.H., Going, S.B., Pamenter, R.W., Perry, C.D., Boyden, T.W. & Lohman, T.G. (1990) Bone mineral content of cyclically menstruating female resistance and endurance trained athletes. *Medicine and Science in Sports and Exercise* **22**, 558–563.

Hughes, V.A., Frontera, W.R., Dallal, G.E., Lutz, K.J., Fisher, E.C. & Evans, W.J. (1995) Muscle strength and body composition: associations with bone density in older subjects. *Medicine and Science in Sports and Exercise* **27**, 967–974.

Jacobson, P.C., Beaver, W., Grubbs, S.A., Taft, T.N. & Talmage, R.V. (1984) Bone density in women: college athletes and older athletic women. *Journal of Orthopaedic Research* **2**, 328–332.

Jee, W.S.S. (1988) The skeletal tissues. In L. Weiss (ed.) *Cell and Tissue Biology. A Textbook of Histology*, 6th edn, pp. 213–254. Urban & Schwerzenberg, Baltimore.

Johnston, C.C., Miller, J.Z., Slemenda, C.W. *et al.* (1992) Calcium supplementation and increases in bone mineral density in children. *New England Journal of Medicine* **327**, 82–87.

Jouanny, P., Guillemin, F., Kuntz, C., Jeandel, C. & Pourel, J. (1995) Environmental and genetic factors affecting bone mass: similarity of bone density among members of healthy families. *Arthritis and Rheumatism* **38**, 61–67.

Kannus, P., Haapasalo, H., Sankelo, M. *et al.* (1995) Effects of starting age of physical activity on bone mass in dominant arm of tennis and squash players. *Annals of Internal Medicine* **123**, 27–31.

Kimmel, D.B. (1993) A paradigm for skeletal strength homeostasis. *Journal of Bone and Mineral Research* **8**, S515–S522.

Kirchner, E.M., Lewis, R.D. & O'Connor, P.J. (1995) Bone mineral density and dietary intake of female college gymnasts. *Medicine and Science in Sports and Exercise* **27**, 543–549.

Kirchner, E.M., Lewis, R.D. & O'Connor, P.J. (1996) Effect of past gymnastics participation on adult bone mass. *Journal of Applied Physiology* **80**, 226–232.

Kirk, S., Sharp, C.F., Elbaum, N. *et al.* (1989) Effect of long-distance running on bone mass in women. *Journal of Bone and Mineral Research* **4**, 515–522.

Kohrt, W.M., Snead, D.B., Slatopolsky, E. & Birge, S.J. (1995) Additive effects of weight-bearing exercise and estrogen on bone mineral density in older women. *Journal of Bone and Mineral Research* **10**, 1303–1311.

Krall, E.A. & Dawson-Hughes, B. (1994) Walking is related to bone density and rates of bone loss. *American Journal of Medicine* **96**, 20–26.

Lane, N.E., Bloch, D.A., Jones, H.H., Marshall, W.H., Wood, P.D. & Fries, J.F. (1986) Long-distance running, bone density and osteoarthritis. *Journal of the American Medical Association* **255**, 1147–1151.

Lanyon, L.E. (1987) Functional strain in bone tissue as an objective and controlling stimulus for adaptive bone remodeling. *Journal of Biomechanics* **20**, 1083–1093.

Lanyon, L.E. (1990) Bone loading: the functional determinant of bone architecture and a physiological contributor to the prevention of osteoporosis. In R. Smith (ed.) *Osteoporosis*, pp. 63–78. Royal College of Physicians, London.

Lanyon, L.E. (1992) Control of bone architecture by functional load bearing. *Journal of Bone and Mineral Research* **7**, S369–S375.

Lanyon, L.E. (1996) Using functional loading to influence bone mass and architecture: objectives, mecha-

nisms, and relationship with estrogen of the mechanically adaptive process in bone. *Bone* **18**, S37–S43.

Lee, E.J., Long, K.A., Risser, W.L., Poindexter, H.B.W., Gibbons, W.E. & Goldzierh, J. (1995) Variations in bone status of contralateral and regional sites in young athletic women. *Medicine and Science in Sports and Exercise* **27**, 1354–1361.

Lohman, T., Going, S., Pamenter, R. *et al.* (1995) Effects of resistance training on regional and total bone mineral density in premenopausal women: a randomized prospective study. *Journal of Bone and Mineral Research* **10**, 1015–1024.

McCartney, N., Hicks, A.L., Martin, J. & Webber, C.E. (1995) Long-term resistance training in the elderly: effects on dynamic strength, exercise capacity, muscle, and bone. *Journal of Gerontology* **50A**, B97–B104.

Marcus, R., Cann, C., Madvig, P. *et al.* (1985) Menstrual function and bone mass in elite women distance runners. *Annals of Internal Medicine* **102**, 158–163.

Martin, D. & Notelovitz, M. (1993) Effects of aerobic training on bone mineral density of postmenopausal women. *Journal of Bone and Mineral Research* **8**, 931–936.

Matkovic, V., Jelic, T., Wardlaw, G.M. *et al.* (1994) Timing of peak bone mass in caucasian females and its implication for the prevention of osteoporosis: inference from a cross-sectional model. *Journal of Clinical Investigation* **93**, 799–808.

Myburgh, K.H., Bachrach, L.K., Lewis, B., Kent, K. & Marcus, R. (1993) Low bone mineral density at axial and appendicular sites in amenorrheic athletes. *Medicine and Science in Sports and Exercise* **25**, 1197–1202.

Myerson, M., Gutin, B., Warren, M.P. *et al.* (1992) Total body bone density in amenorrheic runners. *Obstetrics and Gynecology* **79**, 973–978.

Nelson, M.E., Fiatarone, M.A., Morganti, C.M., Trice, I., Greenberg, R.A. & Evans, W.J. (1994) Effects of high-intensity strength training on multiple risk factors for osteoporotic fractures. A randomized controlled trial. *Journal of the American Medical Association* **272**, 1909–1914.

Nichols, D.L., Sanborn, C.F., Bonnick, S.L., Benezra, V., Gench, B. & Dimarco, N.M. (1994) The effects of gymnastics training on bone mineral density. *Medicine and Science in Sports and Exercise* **26**, 1220–1225.

Nichols, D.L., Sanborn, C.F., Bonnick, S.L., Gench, B. & Dimarco, N. (1995) Relationship of regional body composition to bone mineral density in college females. *Medicine and Science in Sports and Exercise* **27**, 178–182.

Nieves, J.W., Golden, A.L., Siris, E., Kelsey, J.L. & Lindsay, R. (1995) Teenage and current calcium intake are related to bone mineral density of hip and forearm in women aged 30–39 years. *American Journal of Epidemiology* **141**, 342–351.

Nigg, B.M. (1985) Biomechanics, load analysis and sports injuries in the lower extremities. *Sports Medicine* **2**, 367–379.

Orwoll, E.S., Ferar, J., Oviatt, S.K., McClung, R.M. & Huntington, K. (1989) The relationship of swimming exercise to bone mass in men and women. *Archives of Internal Medicine* **149**, 2197–2200.

Parfitt, A.M. (1994) The two faces of growth: benefits and risks to bone integrity. *Osteoporosis International* **4**, 382–398.

Pearce, G., Bass, S., Young, N., Formica, C. & Seeman, E. (1996) Does weight-bearing exercise protect against the effect of exercise induced oligomenorrhea on bone density? *Osteoporosis International* **6**, 448–452.

Peterson, S.E., Peterson, M.D., Raymond, G., Gilligan, C., Checovich, M.M. & Smith, E.L. (1991) Muscular strength and bone density with weight training in middle-aged women. *Medicine and Science in Sports and Exercise* **23**, 499–504.

Pocock, N.A., Eisman, J.A., Hopper, J.L., Yeates, M.G., Sambrook, P.N. & Eben, S. (1987) Genetic determinants of bone mass in adults: a twin study. *Journal of Clinical Investigation* **80**, 706–710.

Prince, R., Devine, A., Dick, I. *et al.* (1995) The effects of calcium supplementation (milk powder or tablets) and exercise on bone density in postmenopausal women. *Journal of Bone and Mineral Research* **10**, 1068–1075.

Prior, J.C., Vigna, M.Y., Schecter, M.T. & Burgess, A.E. (1990) Spinal bone loss and ovulatory disturbances. *New England Journal of Medicine* **323**, 1221–1227.

Pruitt, L.A., Jackson, R.D., Bartels, R.L. & Lehnhard, H.J. (1992) Weight training effects on bone mineral density in early postmenopausal women. *Journal of Bone and Mineral Research* **7**, 179–185.

Pruitt, L.A., Taaffe, D.R. & Marcus, R. (1995) Effects of a one-year high-intensity vs. low-intensity resistance training program on bone mineral density in older women. *Journal of Bone and Mineral Research* **10**, 1788–1795.

Reid, I.R., Plank, L.D. & Evans, M.C. (1992) Fat mass is an important determinant of whole body bone density in premenopausal women but not in men. *Journal of Clinical Endocrinology and Metabolism* **75**, 779–782.

Risser, W.L., Lee, E.J., Leblanc, A., Poindexter, H.B.W., Risser, J.M.H. & Schneider, V. (1990) Bone density in eumenorrheic female college athletes. *Medicine and Science in Sports and Exercise* **22**, 570–574.

Robinson, T.L., Snow-Harter, C., Taaffe, D.R., Gillis, D., Shaw, J. & Marcus, R. (1995) Gymnasts exhibit higher bone mass than runners despite similar prevalence

of amenorrhea and oligomenorrhea. *Journal of Bone and Mineral Research* **10**, 26–35.

Rubin, C.T. & Lanyon, L.E. (1982) Limb mechanics as a function of speed and gait: a study of functional strain in the radius and tibia of horse and dog. *Journal of Experimental Biology* **101**, 187–211.

Rubin, C.T. & Mcleod, K.J. (1996) Inhibition of osteopenia by biophysical intervention. In R. Marcus, D. Feldman & J. Kelsey (eds) *Osteoporosis*, pp. 351–371. Academic Press, San Diego.

Seeman, E., Hopper, J.L., Young, N.R., Formica, C., Goss, P. & Tsalamandris, C. (1996) Do genetic factors explain associations between muscle strength, lean mass, and bone density? A twin study. *American Journal of Physiology* **270**, E320–E327.

Sievänen, H., Heinonen, A. & Kannus, P. (1996) Adaptation of bone to altered loading environment: a biomechanical approach using x-ray absorptiometric data from the patella of a young woman. *Bone* **19**, 55–59.

Sievänen, H., Koskue, V., Rauhio, A., Kannus, P., Heinonen, A. & Vuori, I. (1998) Peripheral quantitative computed tomography in human long bones: evaluation of *in vitro* and *in vivo* precision. *Journal of Bone and Mineral Research* **13**, 871–882.

Sinaki, M., Wahner, H.W., Bergstrahl, E.J. *et al.* (1996) Three-year controlled, randomized trial of the effect of dose-specific loading and strengthening exercise on bone mineral density of spine and femur in nonathletic, physically active women. *Bone* **19**, 233–244.

Slemenda, C.W. (1995) Body composition and skeletal density: mechanical loading or something more. *Journal of Clinical Endocrinology and Metabolism* **80**, 1761–1763.

Slemenda, C.W. & Johnston, C.C. (1993) High intensity activities in young women: site specific bone mass effects among male figure skaters. *Bone and Mineral* **20**, 125–132.

Slemenda, C.W., Miller, J.Z., Hui, S.L., Reister, T.K. & Johnston, C.C. Jr (1991) Role of physical activity in the development of skeletal mass in children. *Journal of Bone and Mineral Research* **6**, 1227–1233.

Slemenda, C.W., Reister, T.K., Hui, S.L., Miller, J.Z., Christian, J.C. & Johnston, C.C. (1994) Influences on skeletal mineralization in children and adolescents: evidence for varying effects of sexual maturation and physical activity. *Journal of Pediatrics* **125**, 201–207.

Snow-Harter, C.M., Bouxsein, M.L., Lewis, B.T., Charette, S., Weinstein, P. & Marcus, R. (1990) Muscle strength as a predictor of bone mineral density in young women. *Journal of Bone and Mineral Research* **5**, 589–595.

Snow-Harter, C., Bouxsein, M.L., Lewis, B.T., Carter,

D.R. & Marcus, R. (1992) Effects of resistance and endurance exercise on bone mineral status of young women: a randomized exercise intervention trial. *Journal of Bone and Mineral Research* **7**, 761–769.

Specker, B.L. (1996) Evidence for an interaction between calcium intake and physical activity. *Journal of Bone and Mineral Research* **11**, 1539–1544.

Subotnick, S.I. (1985) The biomechanics of running: implications for prevention of foot injuries. *Sports Medicine* **2**, 144–153.

Suominen, H., Cheng, S. & Rahkila, P. (1992) Physical training and bone in elderly male and female athletes. In *Abstracts of the 3rd International Conference of Physical Activity, Aging and Sports*, pp. 90–91. University of Jyväskylä, Jyväskylä.

Taaffe, D.R., Snow-Harter, C., Connolly, D.A., Robinson, T.L., Brown, M.D. & Marcus, R. (1995) Differential effects of swimming vs. weight-bearing activity on bone mineral status of eumenorrheic athletes. *Journal of Bone and Mineral Research* **10**, 586–593.

Taaffe, D.R., Robinson, T.L., Snow, C.M. & Marcus, R. (1997) High-impact exercise promotes bone gain in well-trained female athletes. *Journal of Bone and Mineral Research* **12**, 255–260.

Turner, C.H. (1991) Homeostatic control of bone structure: an application of feedback theory. *Bone* **12**, 203–217.

Uusi-Rasi, K., Nygård, C.-H., Oja, P., Pasanen, M., Sievänen, H. & Vuori, I. (1994) Walking at work and bone mineral density of premenopausal women. *Osteoporosis International* **4**, 336–340.

Vuori, I., Heinonen, A., Sievänen, H., Kannus, P. & Oja, P. (1994) Effects of unilateral strength training and detraining on bone mineral density and content in young women: a study of mechanical loading on humans bones. *Calcified Tissue International* **55**, 59–67.

Wolff, J. (1892) *Das Gesetz der Transformation der Knochen*. Berlin, Germany. Cited in A. Hirschwald.

Wolman, R.L., Faulman, L., Clark, P., Hesp, R. & Harries, M.G. (1991) Different training patterns and bone mineral density of the femoral shaft in elite, female athletes. *Annals of the Rheumatic Diseases* **50**, 487–489.

Young, D., Hopper, J.L., Nowson, C.A. *et al.* (1995) Determinants of bone mass in 10- to 26-year-old females: a twin study. *Journal of Bone and Mineral Research* **10**, 558–567.

Chapter 20

Women with Disabilities

KAREN P. DEPAUW

Introduction

Individuals with disabilities have participated in sport, including competitive sport, for much of the 20th century. Despite this, athletes with disabilities are only now gaining recognition as athletes. They are experiencing increased visibility, greater inclusion and 'true' acceptance in sport. As this century comes to a close, disability sport is finally coming into its own.

Disability sport refers to sport 'that has been designed for or specifically practiced by athletes with disabilities' (DePauw & Gavron, 1995). As an umbrella term, 'disability sport' is understood throughout the world to encompass sport for individuals with disabilities and includes numerous international competitive events, primarily the Paralympic Games, World Games for the Deaf and the International Special Olympics (for a thorough discussion of disability sport, see DePauw & Gavron, 1995).

The experience of athletes with disabilities in sport is complicated by the intersection of gender and disability, as well as by the type of impairment (e.g. spinal cord injury or cerebral palsy), the severity of impairment (e.g. paraplegia or quadriplegia, visual impairment or blindness) and the sport. In the fight for rights as athletes, much of the struggle in disability sport has been focused on disability rather than on gender or race/ethnicity (see DePauw & Gavron, 1995). Female athletes with disabilities, fewer in number than their male counterparts, have been present in disability sport since the early 1920s but have yet to gain the visibility afforded male athletes with disabilities (Sherrill, 1997).

Historical perspectives

Similar to many able-bodied women who have participated in sport and sought competitive opportunities throughout history, females with disabilities have also sought physical activity and sport. Although history primarily records the experiences of men, women with disabilities have participated in a variety of sport events spanning the 20th century.

Women with disabilities have competed in the Olympic Games. For example, Liz Hartel (post polio, Denmark) won a silver medal in dressage at the 1952 Helsinki Olympics. More recently, Ms Neroli Fairhall, representing New Zealand, competed in archery during the 1984 Olympic Games in Los Angeles. As a fully acknowledged Olympian, she competed from her wheelchair. In addition to these women who participated in full Olympic events, male and female athletes with disabilities competed in their first exhibition events at the 1984 Winter Olympics in Sarajevo and the 1984 Summer Olympics in Los Angeles. Exhibition events for the Winter Games (selected alpine and Nordic events for physically impaired and blind athletes) and the Summer Games (1500 m wheelchair for men, 800 m wheelchair for women) have continued since then. In 1997, after a concerted effort to integrate athletes with disabilities into the Olympic Games, the President of the International Olympic Committee (IOC), Juan Antonio Samaranch, agreed to bring a proposal to the IOC to incorporate these two events as part of the Olympic Games. Although these efforts have not yet been successful, there is increasing acknowledgement of disability sport by the IOC and the general public.

Women with disabilities have also participated in élite national and international competitions beyond the Olympic Games. The Paralympic Games represent the largest single event in which female athletes with disabilities are found. The Summer Paralympic Games were founded by Sir Ludwig Guttman 50 years ago at Stoke Mandeville Hospital in Aylesbury, England. The first Paralympic Games, held in 1960 in Rome, marked the deliberate attempt by Guttman to link these games to the Olympic Games (Tiessen, 1996). Since then, the Summer Paralympic Games and the Olympic Games have shared the same country (Germany 1972, Canada 1976, USA 1984) and, more recently, the same city for the Summer and Winter Games (Seoul 1988, Albertville 1992, Barcelona 1992, Lillehammer 1994, Atlanta 1996). Bidding for the Olympic Games now includes consideration for the Paralympic Games as well (e.g. Nagano 1998, Sydney 2000, Salt Lake City 2002). Although competitors, females have been underrepresented in the Paralympic Games (DePauw, 1994; Sherrill, 1997). According to Sherrill (1997), the male–female ratio for the Barcelona Paralympic Games was 3 : 1 and decreased to 4 : 1 at the 1996 Atlanta Paralympic Games. In Atlanta, of the 104 participating countries 49 (47%) brought no female athletes and most countries brought fewer than nine female athletes (Sherrill, 1997). Given this trend and growing concern, the International Paralympic Committee (IPC) Sports Council established a Women's Initiative to address the issue of female representation and participation in future Paralympic Games.

In addition to the Paralympic Games, a large contingent of women participates in the World Games for the Deaf. Women were among the first competitors in the 1924 World Games for the Deaf (Paris) and continue to participate in the

summer and winter competitions every 4 years in the year following the Olympic Games. The International Special Olympics also includes girls and women with mental retardation among the competitors.

The Boston Marathon stands as an additional example of competitive opportunities for athletes with disabilities. Wheelchair athletes were among its entrants as early as 1974. The first female wheelchair competitor, Sharon Rahn (Hedrick), won the 1977 Women's Wheelchair Division with a time of 3 hours 48 min 51 s. Since then, not only have the times decreased dramatically but the gap between the winning times for women and for men has narrowed as well (Fig. 20.1). Currently, wheelchair men regularly finish under 1 hour 30 min and wheelchair women under 1 hour 45 min. Although the performances have improved, the number of wheelchair women competitors remains relatively few (three to four per year).

The Boston Marathon is but one example of marathons and other road races that regularly offer competitive divisions for athletes with disabilities. These have resulted in increased opportunities for male and female athletes with disabilities to compete professionally in wheelchair road racing and marathons. Competitive sport opportunities at the collegiate and even the interscholastic level exist as well. Individuals with physical impairments in selected universities, such as the University of Illinois and Wright State University, and deaf athletes at Gallaudet University have been provided with collegiate sport experiences, including athletic scholarships in some cases. Although these sport opportunities have been available to female as well as male athletes with disabilities, the numbers have favoured men (DePauw & Gavron, 1995).

In an attempt to provide a historical perspective of sport for women with disabilities, a selection of 'firsts' and other significant milestones are highlighted in the Appendix. Selected world records held by female athletes with disabilities appear in Table 20.1.

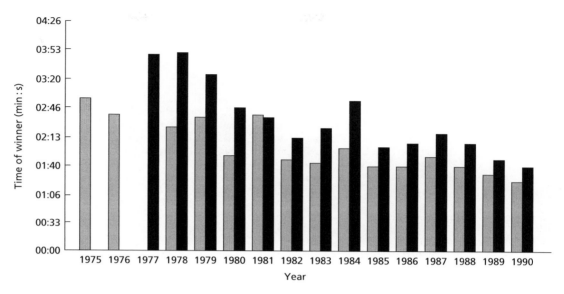

Fig. 20.1 Winning times for the wheelchair divisions of the first 15 years of the Boston Marathon. ☐, men; ■, women.

Disability, sport and society

Disability rights movement

Throughout history, individuals with disabilities have resided in the margins of society. The historical roots of disability can be traced back to the medical model that described those with disabilities as having a limiting condition that adversely affected one's performance (World Health Organization, 1980). This definition places the 'problem in the person' and thereby avoids any consideration of the role of society in the 'creation' of disabling conditions. The traditional medical approach to disability tends to emphasize categorization and disability-specific programmes. Thus, it follows that individuals with disabilities continue to be marginalized in society and removed from its various social institutions (e.g. education, employment) including sport.

The disability rights movement, the most recent of the civil rights movements, has challenged us to revisit the traditional definition of disability (Shapiro, 1993). That is, the disability

rights movement forced society to view disability in the context of social relationships (Hanks & Poplin, 1981; Brown & Smith, 1989; Chappell, 1992; Shapiro, 1993) and therefore as socially constructed (constituted for, and by, those with power). Viewing disability as a social construct forces us to reconceptualize sport as well.

Sport as contested terrain

Historically, sport has been viewed as the domain of the élite. Furthermore, sport has been dominated by males and masculinity and has played a significant role in the preservation of a patriarchal social order (Theberge, 1985). The sporting ideals of physicality and masculinity have served as the basis for certain groups to be excluded from, or marginalized within, sport. Among the marginalized groups are women and individuals with disabilities and some interesting parallels can be drawn among the groups.

Although female athletes and athletes with disabilities are participants in sport and have made great strides towards acceptance as athletes, this is far from complete. Inclusion is

Table 20.1 Selected world records held by female athletes with disabilities

Event*	Record	Name
Athletics		
100 m (T12)	12.43 s	R. Takbulatova (former USSR)
200 m (T11)	26.32 s	B. Mendoza (Spain)
200 m (T32)	35.30 s	L. Mastandrea (USA)
400 m (T10)	57.79 s	P. Santamarta (Spain)
1500 m (T11)	4 min 37.02 s	R. Batalova (former USSR)
1500 m (wheelchair)	3 min 30.45 s	L. Sauvage (Australia)
Discus (F42, 43, 44)	38.92 m	J. Barrett (USA)
Long jump (F11)	5.31 m	R. Lazaro (Spain)
Shot put (F12)	12.54 m	T. Sivakova (former USSR)
Swimming		
100 m backstroke (S7)	1 min 26.41 s	K. Hakonard (Iceland)
200 m breaststroke (B3)	3 min 3.24 s	G. Tjernberg (Sweden)
50 m butterfly (S7)	42.65 s	E. Nesheim (Norway)
100 m butterfly (S10)	1 min 9.76 s	G. Dashwood (Australia)
100 m butterfly (B3)	1 min 7.07 s	E. Scott (USA)
100 m freestyle (B2)	1 min 4.33 s	T. Zorn (USA)
100 m freestyle (S10)	1 min 4.01 s	C. Hengst (Germany)
400 m freestyle (S10)	4 min 43.79 s	G. Dashwood (Australia)

* Classification of disability is given in brackets. B, blind swimming; F, field; S, swimming; T, track. T10, visually impaired, no light perception; T11/F11/B2, visually impaired, 2/60 vision; T12/F12/B3, visually impaired, 2/60 to 6/60 vision; T32, cerebral palsy, full upper body strength, independent wheelchair propulsion; F42, 43, 44, amputations (single above knee, double below knee, single below knee); S7, good hand and arm propulsion, good trunk control, hips level, stand or sit dive start (includes individuals with amputations, cerebral palsy and other physical impairments); S10, full hand and arm propulsion, full trunk control, strong leg kick, dive start and propulsion in turns.

related to conformity to the ideals of physicality within the limits of masculinity. As the ideals of physicality and masculinity are questioned and redefined we will see more inclusion and acceptance in sport of women and female athletes with disabilities (Fig. 20.2). Beyond the experience of able-bodied female athletes, female athletes with disabilities face a double jeopardy in sport, that of being female and of having an impairment. It follows that conformity to the ideals of sport assumes even greater significance.

Given that disability is socially constructed, disability sport has been, and will continue to be, influenced and constructed by and through society. For example, the history of disability sport has been written through the eyes of white males with spinal cord injuries who use a wheelchair for sport competitions. Specifically, the first competitive events for athletes with disabilities in premier competitions (e.g. Olympic Games, marathon races) were wheelchair events. Male and female athletes who use a wheelchair exemplify the ideals of physicality (e.g. athletic beautiful body, strength, endurance, grace) and athletic performance (e.g. upper body physicality with lower spinal cord lesions or lower limb amputations), but are still required to conform to stereotypically masculine and feminine images.

Sport has been viewed as a reflection of society.

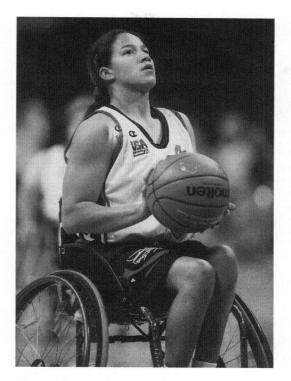

Fig. 20.2 Since 1974, wheelchair basketball has been considered a premier sport for female athletes with disabilities. (© Disability Today Publishing Group / Dan Galbraith.)

Recently, sport has been examined for its role in the production and reproduction of social inequality (Donnelly, 1996). That is, sport has served to produce and reinforce dominant societal values that are often rooted in power and oppression. On the other hand, sport can also be a site for resistance to those same dominant cultural values and for the production of social equality. Much of current disability sport, including female athletes with disabilities, reflects the able-bodied model of sport and has therefore contributed to the reproduction of dominant cultural values. On the other hand, the mere presence of athletes with disabilities in sport is an act of resistance and can contribute to the transformative power of sport and effect change in sport and society.

Research perspectives

Background

Beginning in the1970s, research on sport for individuals with disabilities was focused in two areas: (i) physiological aspects of sport performance (i.e. fitness, response to exercise); and (ii) biomechanical aspects (i.e. wheelchair propulsion) of sport performance (DePauw, 1988). Males with spinal cord injury or recovering from polio were utilized as subjects for these early research studies. Although limited, the findings of these studies provided the basis for the following three general statements.

1 Individuals with disabilities demonstrate physiological responses to exercise similar to those of athletes without disabilities. Any differences are identified with alterations in functional muscle mass, due to factors such as paralysis, amputation, osteoporosis in paralysed limbs or severity of the physical impairment, or are observed because of difficulties in comprehension, motivation or mechanical inefficiency related to specific types of impairment (e.g. mental retardation, cerebral palsy) (Shephard, 1990). In some cases, it remains unclear whether the differences in physiological responses are due to differences in physiological function or in assessment techniques.

2 Although a specific disability may affect the degree of intensity, duration and frequency of exercise, evidence suggests that physiological training effects can be achieved with individuals with disabilities. For example, the type of activity (endurance vs. strength) influences maximum oxygen consumption, e.g. wheelchair athletes who compete in track and swimming events have larger maximum oxygen uptake than those who compete in strength events.

3 Movement efficiency of wheelchair propulsion has been studied in terms of rim diameter, stroke frequency, seat height, technique, speed, level of impairment and sporting event (sprint vs. distance). With the decrease in mass of the chair, in addition to individual adaptations to seat height and inclination, wheel camber and handrim

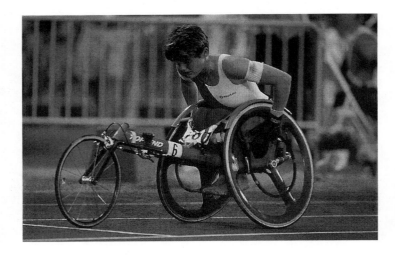

Fig. 20.3 Improved technology and training have enhanced wheelchair racing for women with disabilities into a highly visible and competitive sport. (© Disability Today Publishing Group / Dan Galbraith.)

sizes, athletic performance (movement efficiency) has increased substantially (Fig. 20.3) (DePauw, 1996).

These statements emphasize the complexity of research about athletes with disabilities. Yet only two aspects of sport performance (physiology and biomechanics) have been highlighted and research studies have used a highly selective subject pool (e.g. white males with spinal cord injuries or post polio who use wheelchairs). Since the 1970s, disability sport research has become more sport specific, disability specific, performance related and subdiscipline related (e.g. sport sociology, sport physiology, sport medicine) (DePauw, 1988). However, given the complexity of disability sport, it is not surprising that a significant body of scientific literature is still lacking.

Under the auspices of the Committee on Sport for the Disabled of the United States Olympic Committee, the following seven research areas have been identified for disability sport (DePauw, 1986): (i) effects of training and/or competition, including fitness, sport performance and sport classification; (ii) selection and training of coaches, volunteers and officials; (iii) technological advances, including prostheses and wheelchair design; (iv) sociological/psychological aspects of sport, including motivation, impact of society on sport and influence of age,

gender, ethnicity and disability; (v) differences and similarities among athletes with and without disabilities, especially from physiological, biomechanical, sport injury and nutritional perspectives; (vi) demographics of disability sport, including youth sport; and (vii) legal, philosophical and historical bases of sport. These have served as a framework for much of the disability sport research conducted to date.

Recently, Reid (1998) performed a documentary analysis of the disability sport research conducted over a 10-year period using the seven research areas outlined above. He identified a total of 344 articles on disability sport published between 1986 and 1996; only 149 of these were data-based publications. He concluded that the number of data-based publications was not sufficient to contribute significantly to the body of knowledge about disability sport and to advance the field. It is clear that a concerted research effort is needed to increase the body of knowledge. Efforts to revise and re-establish research priorities are currently underway through the Sport Science Committee of the International Paralympic Committee.

Female athletes with disabilities

In a recent literature review, Turk (1996) found the number of studies limited although there was 'growing interest in exercise for persons with disabilities'. She reported that while women were represented in a number of these studies, women were found more frequently in studies on arthritis, were less well represented in studies of spinal cord injuries and were missing altogether from other studies.

Women with disabilities were likewise found to be underrepresented in a literature review reported by DePauw (1996). Up to 1993 the literature produced only a few studies on selected physiological parameters of individuals with disabilities (i.e. body composition, pulmonary function, cardiovascular response, handgrip, forearm cranking and training regimens). The subjects for these investigations were primarily active males with spinal cord injuries who used wheelchairs for physical activity. None of the studies were conducted with females only. Among the findings of these studies were the following (adapted from Shephard, 1990).

1 Normal wheelchair propulsion does not provide a sufficient stimulus to maintain physical condition.

2 Amputation and muscle atrophy due to impairment may restrict lean body mass and adversely influence accurate measures of body composition and prediction of ideal body mass.

3 Resting oxygen consumption and cardiac output may be lessened because of physical impairment (e.g. limb paralysis).

4 Increase in heart rate with exercise in spinally injured tetraplegics is less than that found in able-bodied individuals.

5 Regular participation in wheelchair sport increases cardiac stroke volume.

6 Shoulder and elbow strength in wheelchair users is greater than that in able-bodied individuals.

7 Maximum oxygen uptake is more limited in spinally injured tetraplegics compared with paraplegics; wheelchair athletes have the advantage of peak oxygen uptake and peak power output relative to their inactive peers.

8 Higher values for isometric and isokinetic muscle force data are found in wheelchair athletes; males with disabilities have been found to be stronger than females with disabilities.

These findings can be used as the foundation for further studies designed to investigate the impact of sex and/or type and severity of impairment (disability) on physiological performance. Because females have not been studied systematically, the studies to date 'fall short of speaking to the experience of women with spinal cord injury or the experience of other women with physical disabilities such as cerebral palsy' (DePauw, 1996).

Although females with disabilities do participate in physical activity and sport (Fig. 20.4), very little is known about the physical activity patterns of girls and women with disabilities. A comprehensive study conducted by Fitness

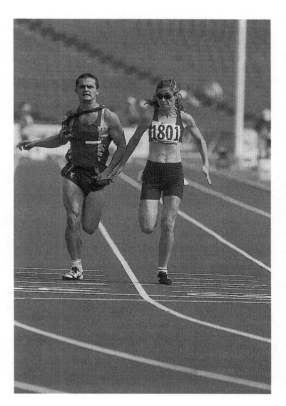

Fig. 20.4 Blind runner and sighted guide finish a middle-distance race in stride. (© Disability Today Publishing Group / Dan Galbraith.)

Canada provides the clearest data about these patterns. The results of this study indicate that only 31% of the females were physically active but that these females sought higher levels of participation.

Gender-specific or gender-neutral phenomena have not been systematically studied in disability sport (DePauw, 1994; DePauw & Gavron, 1995). Although some sport studies have included females and some have used female subjects only, definitive findings about the female experience and the performances of female athletes with disabilities are lacking in the scientific literature. Although female athletes with disabilities are being sought as subjects in sport studies, the results of these studies are not yet available.

Recommendations for future research

It is apparent that more research is needed that specifically addresses female athletes with disabilities. In order to study physical activity/exercise among females with disabilities, DePauw (1996) argued for research on the biological or mechanical responses to exercise among women via a model of interaction between gender and disability (impairment). When this model is extended to disability sport, it implies that there are: (i) biological and mechanical responses that are gender and disability independent (i.e. responses that occur regardless of one's sex or physical impairment, such as an increase in heart rate and improved performance after training); and (ii) biological and mechanical responses to exercise that are gender or disability specific or dependent (i.e. responses that vary with sex, with impairment or with the interaction of sex and impairment, such as thermal regulation, maximum oxygen uptake or gait efficiency).

For those responses that do not vary with sex or impairment, it follows that the physiological and mechanical principles that exist for able-bodied athletes can be applied to athletes with disabilities, including females; this information can be drawn from the existing research literature. On the other hand, when the responses vary with sex or with disability, or both, research

should be undertaken to identify and understand those biological and mechanical responses and adaptations to exercise that are gender and disability dependent and to investigate their relationship to sport performance (DePauw, 1996). This approach could be helpful in determining research foci and in providing meaningful results for athletes with disabilities.

Research on females athletes with disabilities should draw on the literature about sport performance in general, as well as specific research on female athletes. In addition to research about sport performance, disability sport research can also examine the experience of female athletes with disabilities, including the influence of the social context of sport and the sociopsychological perspectives of gender, race, disability, class and sexual orientation in disability sport. Morris (1992) has advocated emancipatory research, through which traditional notions of disability are challenged. In order to conduct emancipatory research, it is necessary to design studies in collaboration with female athletes with disabilities so that the results are applicable and meaningful to them.

Conclusion

Many argue that sport is a microcosm of society. As a social institution, it is certain that sport cannot remain unaffected by the political, social and cultural changes occurring throughout the world. A number of social changes have taken place during the 20th century: virtually all social institutions, from the religious to the military, have been profoundly influenced by challenges from women, members of racial and ethnic minority groups, lesbians and gays, and individuals with disabilities. The target of these protests are those who control most major social institutions in society; those who hold power over others and those with privilege.

Disability sport has come a long way in its relatively short history. Female athletes with disabilities are beginning to gain visibility and acceptance as athletes alongside their male counterparts. Though the disability sport movement came together around disability, concerns about equity within disability sport are increasing and gender is but the first of these issues to face disability sport.

References

Brown, H. & Smith, H. (1989) Whose 'ordinary life' is it anyway? *Disability, Handicap and Society* **4**, 105–119.

Chappell, A.L. (1992) Towards a sociological critique of the normalization principle. *Disability, Handicap and Society* **7**, 35–50.

DePauw, K.P. (1988) Sport for individuals with disabilities: research opportunities. *Adapted Physical Activity Quarterly* **5**, 80–89.

DePauw, K.P. (1994) A feminist perspective on sport and sports organizations for persons with disabilities. In R.D. Steadward, E.R. Nelson & G.D. Wheeler (eds) *VISTA '93: The Outlook*, pp. 467–477. Rick Hansen Centre, Edmonton, Alberta.

DePauw, K.P. (1996) Adapted physical activity and sport. In D.M. Krostoski, M.A. Nosek & M.A. Turk (eds) *Women with Physical Disabilities: Achieving and Maintaining Health and Well-being*, pp. 419–430. Paul H. Brookes Publishing Co., Baltimore.

DePauw, K.P. & Gavron, S.J. (1995) *Disability and Sport*. Human Kinetics Publishers, Champaign, Illinois.

Donnelly, P. (1996) Approaches to social inequality in the sociology of sport. *Quest* **48**, 221–242.

Fitness Canada. *Physical Activity and Women with Disabilities: A National Survey*. Fitness Canada Women's Program, Ottawa.

Hanks, M. & Poplin, D.E. (1981) The sociology of physical disability: a review of literature and some conceptual perspectives. *Deviant Behavior: An Interdisciplinary Journal* **2**, 309–328.

Morris, J. (1992) Personal and political: a feminist perspective on researching physical disability. *Disability, Handicap and Society* **7**, 157–166.

Reid, G. (1998) A documentary analysis of research priorities in disability sport. *Adapted Physical Activity Quarterly* **2**, 168–178.

Shapiro, J. (1993) *No Pity: People with Disabilities Forging a New Civil Rights Movement*. Times Books, New York.

Shephard, R.J. (1990) *Fitness in Special Populations*. Human Kinetics Publishers, Champaign, Illinois.

Sherrill, C. (1997) Paralympic Games 1996: feminist and other concerns. What's your excuse? *Palaestra* **13**, 32–38.

Theberge, N. (1985) Toward a feminist alternative to sport as a male preserve. *Quest* **37**, 193–202.

Tiessen, K. (1996) Paralympic history. In *Xth Paralympic Games: The Official Commemorative Program*, p. 24. Disability Today Publishing Group.

Turk, M.A. (1996) The impact of disability on fitness in women: musculoskeletal issues. In D.M. Krostoski,

M.A. Nosek & M.A. Turk (eds) *Women with Physical Disabilities: Achieving and Maintaining Health and Well-Being*, pp. 391–406. Paul H. Brookes Publishing Co., Baltimore.

World Health Organization (1980) *International Classification of Impairments, Disabilities, and Handicaps: A Manual of Classification Relating to the Consequence of Disease*. WHO, Geneva.

Appendix: selected 'firsts' and significant milestones for women with disabilities

1924   First International Silent Games (Paris, France); women among the competitors.

1952   Liz Hartel (post polio, Denmark) wins silver medal in dressage at Summer Olympic Games.

1957   First US National Wheelchair Games (New York) includes women.

1960   First International Games for Disabled (Paralympics) in Rome, Italy; women among the competitors.

1968   International Special Olympics founded by Eunice Kennedy Shriver; first competition held in Chicago; girls and women among competitors.

1974   UNESCO conference establishes right of individuals with disabilities to participate in physical education and sport; rights secured for females as well as males.

1977   Sharon Rahn (Hedrick) becomes the first athlete to win the women's wheelchair division of the Boston Marathon with a winning time of 3 hours 48 min 51 s.

1982   Karen Farmer (a single-leg amputee) becomes one of the first to earn an athletic scholarship and to compete in the track team for Eastern Washington University. Karen also the first winner of the Women's Sports Foundation Up and Coming Award in the physically challenged division.

Blind women compete for the first time in the World Goal Ball Championships at Butler University.

1983   First international women's wheelchair basketball tounament held in France separately from the Paralympics.

1984 Neroli Fairhall (New Zealand) becomes first wheelchair athlete to be eligible for and compete in Summer Olympic Games; competes in women's archery.

First wheelchair races as exhibition events for 1984 Olympic Games: 1500 m won by Paul Van Winkle (Belgium) in 3 min 58.5 s; 800 m won by Sharon Rahn Hedrick (USA) in 2 min 15.5 s.

October issue of *Runner's World* is the first commercial magazine to run a full-length article on a disabled athlete, Linda Down, a Class 5 cerebral palsied athlete who completed the 1982 New York Marathon in 11 hours 15 min.

1988 Candace Cable-Brooks wins the women's wheelchair division of the Boston Marathon for the sixth time in 2 hours 10 min 44 s.

After her gold medal performance in the disabled skiing exhibition event during the Winter Olympics in Calgary, Daina Golden becomes an official spokesperson for the ChapStick Challenge for Disabled Skiing and signs a corporate sponsorship agreement with Subaru, who supply the official car for the US Disabled Ski Team.

Winter Olympics in Calgary include exhibition events (three alpine, blind Nordic) for males and females.

Summer Olympics (South Korea) include wheelchair races as exhibition events (1500 m for men, 800 m for women); Sharon Hedrick wins second gold medal in 800 m wheelchair event in a time of 2 min 11.49 s.

1989 Seven women (and seven men) become first winners of the US Disabled Athletes of the Year Award.

1990 Dr Donalda Ammons is appointed the first deaf female director of the US team for the World Games for the Deaf.

1991 Jean Driscoll (USA) becomes the first athlete with a disability to win the Sudafed Female Athlete of the Year.

Sue Moucha (USA) is the first athlete with a disability to attend the International Olympic Academy in Greece.

Jan Wilson is named the first Coordinator, Disabled Sport Programs, US Olympic Committee.

1992 Connie Hansen (Denmark) and Candace Cable (USA) become the only two women to compete in all Summer Olympic exhibition events.

Tanni Grey (UK) is named the *Sunday Times* Sportswoman of the Year by Her Majesty the Queen.

Tricia Zorn (USA) wins 12 medals (10 gold, 2 silver) at the Paralympic Games in Barcelona (also won 12 at 1988 Paralympic Games in Seoul, South Korea).

1994 Monique Kalkman (The Netherlands) earns the title of Amsterdam's Sportswoman of the Year.

1996 Jean Driscoll (USA) becomes the first athlete to win the Boston Marathon for the seventh time.

(Adapted from DePauw & Gavron, 1995.).

Chapter 21

Exercise-related Anaemia

SALLY S. HARRIS

Introduction

Anaemia is one of the most common medical conditions encountered among adolescent and adult women, and may be more common in female athletes than non-athletes for a variety of reasons. When unrecognized and untreated, anaemia can impair athletic performance and general well-being. Anaemia is easily diagnosed and treated and is usually preventable, and therefore is particularly amenable to screening. Iron-deficiency anaemia is the most common type of anaemia seen among female athletes. Although frank anaemia is easy to diagnose, mild iron-deficiency anaemia can be difficult to distinguish from non-anaemic iron deficiency and other types of exercise-related anaemias. Two types of anaemia are unique to athletes: dilutional pseudoanaemia and exercise-induced haemolysis. These conditions must be differentiated from iron-deficiency anaemia when evaluating and treating anaemia in female athletes.

Criteria for anaemia: interpretation of haemoglobin and haematocrit values

By strict criteria, anaemia is present if haemoglobin (Hb) or haematocrit (Hct) values fall below the normal range. In adolescent and adult females, the normal range for Hb is between 12 and 16 g·dl^{-1} and for Hct is between 36% and 46%. Normal ranges represent two standard deviations from the mean (i.e. 95% of the population will fall into this range). Hb is typically

0.5 g·dl^{-1} lower in Blacks, while Hct is 4% higher for each 1000 m (3280 feet) increase in altitude. On an individual basis, significant overlap exists between normal and abnormal values, so the diagnosis of anaemia must be made *relative* to an individual's baseline normal range. For example, an Hb value of 13 g·dl^{-1}, although within the normal range, may represent anaemia for a woman whose normal baseline Hb level is 13.5 g·dl^{-1}. Alternatively, an Hb value of 11.5 g·dl^{-1}, although below the normal range, may not represent anaemia for a woman in whom this is the normal baseline level.

Dilutional pseudoanaemia: 'sports anaemia'

In active women, low Hb and Hct values may not represent disease if they are due to dilutional psuedoanaemia, also referred to as 'sports anaemia'. In this condition a natural dilution of Hb occurs as a result of the increased plasma volume associated with endurance exercise training, resulting in artificially low values of Hb and Hct. The acute effect of exercise is to reduce plasma volume by 10–20%, resulting in haemoconcentration. Three mechanisms are thought to cause this change: (i) increased capillary hydrostatic pressure due to increased mean arterial pressure and muscular compression on venules; (ii) increased tissue osmotic pressure due to production of lactic acid and other metabolites; and (iii) filtered plasma lost as perspiration. A compensatory rise in baseline plasma volume then occurs due to exercise-induced release of aldosterone, renin and vasopressin. This increase in plasma volume is proportional to the amount and intensity of endurance exercise. For example, a 5% increase in plasma volume can result from a moderate jogging programme, while the training of an élite distance runner can induce a 20% increase (Brown *et al.*, 1985). The increase in plasma volume appears and disappears within a few days of initiation or cessation of training.

The compensatory increase in plasma volume artificially lowers Hb and Hct values. Although Hb concentration decreases due to this dilutional effect, red blood cell mass remains normal or is often increased; therefore, the oxygen-carrying capacity of the blood is not impaired (hence the term 'pseudoanaemia'). In fact, the phenomenon may represent a favourable adaptive response to training whereby increased plasma volume and less viscous blood allows increased oxygen delivery to tissues during exercise.

This condition is most commonly observed in élite endurance athletes, in previously sedentary individuals initiating an exercise programme and among athletes who are increasing their training intensity. This type of anaemia can be distinguished from iron-deficiency anaemia because it is not hypochromic or microcytic, iron indices are normal, it does not respond to iron supplementation and it is unlikely to result in severe anaemia.

Exercise-induced haemolytic anaemia

Exercise-induced haemolytic anaemia results from intravascular haemolysis during exercise and can result in iron depletion. Intravascular haemolysis can occur in both high- and low-impact sports. In high-impact sports such as running, it is thought that the physical trauma of repetitive hard foot strikes leads to the destruction of red blood cells (RBCs). For this reason the terms 'runner's macrocytosis' and 'foot strike haemolysis' have been used to describe this condition. However, intravascular haemolysis has also been documented among competitive swimmers and other athletes not participating in

running activities and seems to be associated with duration of activity (Selby & Eichner, 1986). In these circumstances, RBCs may be damaged by injury caused by muscular contraction, acidosis or increased body temperature.

This form of anaemia can be distinguished from other forms by the diagnostic triad of macrocytosis, reticulocytosis and low haptoglobinaemia with or without haemoglobinuria. Macrocytosis occurs because older, smaller RBCs are preferentially destroyed. Reticulocytosis occurs in response to haemolysis; however, it is often absent if haemolysis is mild. Low haptoglobin occurs because destroyed RBCs release Hb that is then bound by haptoglobin and removed by the liver. If the haptoglobin supply in the bloodstream is depleted, free Hb is excreted into the urine producing haemoglobinuria.

The condition is most commonly observed in middle-aged distance runners, particularly those who are overweight, run on hard surfaces, wear poorly cushioned shoes and run with a stomping gait. Prevention and treatment therefore focuses on encouraging runners to have lean body composition, run on soft surfaces, run light on their feet and wear well-cushioned shoes and insoles. For most athletes, exercise-induced haemolysis is of little consequence, since it is rarely severe enough to cause appreciable iron loss. However, the potential for haemolysis to limit RBC mass can cause fractional physiological differences that may result in a competitive disadvantage for world-class athletes.

Iron-deficiency anaemia

Pathophysiology: the three stages of iron deficiency

There are three stages of iron deficiency. Iron stores are depleted before clinically recognized anaemia occurs. In stages I and II, which represent non-anaemic iron deficiency, Hb and Hct levels are normal. Low Hb and Hct values are only present in stage III, which represents clinically recognized anaemia. The characteristics of each stage are shown in Table 21.1.

Table 21.1 Stages of iron deficiency

Stage I: iron depletion
Characterized by ferritin $< 12\,\mu g \cdot l^{-1}$ indicating
    depletion of iron stores in the bone marrow
Other indices of iron status remain normal
    (haemoglobin, haematocrit, free erythrocyte
    protoporphyrin (FEP), serum iron, total iron-
    binding capacity (TIBC), transferrin saturation)
Duration of several months

Stage II: iron-deficient erythropoiesis
Characterized by decreased iron transport, marked by
    low serum iron, increased TIBC, decreased
    transferrin saturation, increased FEP
Haemoglobin and haematocrit remain normal
Duration of several weeks

Stage III: iron-deficiency anaemia
This is the stage that is clinically recognized as
    anaemia
Characterized by diminished haemoglobin production
    Low haemoglobin and haematocrit
    Decreased mean corpuscular volume
    Hypochromic microcytic red blood cells

Differential diagnosis of iron deficiency

When frank anaemia is present, the diagnosis of iron-deficiency anaemia can be made on the basis of RBC indices alone. These will indicate the classic findings of hypochromic (low mean corpuscular volume) microcytic (low mean corpuscular Hb concentration) anaemia. Medical history is usually sufficient to distinguish iron-deficiency anaemia from the other causes of hypochromic microcytic anaemia, such as lead toxicity (rare outside of childhood), thalassaemia (associated family history and ethnicity) and chronic disease. Since Hb and Hct values below the normal range, as well as hypochromic and microcytic changes, are very late indicators of anaemia, it is often necessary to look beyond Hb and Hct when screening for the earlier stages of iron-deficiency anaemia. There are numerous haematological indicators of iron status (Table 21.2) whose values are affected during different stages of iron deficiency (see Table 21.1) and which can be helpful in differentiating iron-

deficiency anaemia from other exercise-related anaemias (Table 21.3). In most cases, however, a ferritin level will be sufficient to make the diagnosis.

FERRITIN

Ferritin is the most useful indicator of iron deficiency because it most closely reflects the status of iron stores in the body. A serum ferritin concentration of $< 12\,\mu g \cdot l^{-1}$ represents complete depletion of iron stores in the bone marrow; $12–20\,\mu g \cdot l^{-1}$ represents minimal iron stores; $>20\,\mu g \cdot l^{-1}$ represents adequate iron stores. An average ferritin value for young women is 30 $\mu g \cdot l^{-1}$. Ferritin values are elevated by acute inflammation, infection and liver disease. Training intensity can also affect ferritin values, as well as other haematological indicators of iron status. During high-intensity training, ferritin decreases while serum iron and transferrin saturation increase. When training is reduced, these changes reverse and ferritin increases while transferrin saturation decreases (Banister & Hamilton, 1985). While ferritin and Hb values usually suffice to make the diagnosis of iron deficiency and distinguish it from other exercise-related anaemias (Table 21.3), occasionally other iron indices are needed to sort out the effects that inflammation, infection and training can have on iron status.

Prevalence of iron deficiency in female athletes

Iron deficiency is a prevalent condition among women due to iron loss in menstrual blood. For this reason, the prevalence is higher in females than males after puberty. Adolescent girls may be particularly susceptible because of increased iron needs to meet the demands of growth and to counteract the onset of menses; their suboptimal dietary practices may play a role as well. Similarly, pregnant women need additional iron to support red cell volume expansion and the growth of the fetus and placenta. Postmenopausal women and amenorrhoeic women have

Table 21.2 Diagnostic tests for iron deficiency

Test	Normal range (women)
Haemoglobin	$12–16\,g\cdot dl^{-1}$ ($1.86–2.48\,mmol\cdot l^{-1}$)
Haematocrit	36–46%
Serum ferritin concentration	$12–150\,\mu g\cdot l^{-1}$ in females
	$15–200\,\mu g\cdot l^{-1}$ in males
Transferrin saturation	20–55%
Serum iron	$40–150\,\mu g\cdot dl^{-1}$ in females
	($7.16–26.85\,\mu mol\cdot l^{-1}$)
	$50–160\,\mu g\cdot dl^{-1}$ in males
	($8.95–28.64\,\mu mol\cdot l^{-1}$)
Total iron-binding capacity	$250–400\,\mu g\cdot dl^{-1}$
	($44.75–71.60\,\mu mol\cdot l^{-1}$)
Serum erythroprotoporphyrin concentration	$< 1.24\,\mu mol\cdot l^{-1}$
Mean corpuscular volume	80–100 fl
Mean corpuscular haemoglobin concentration	$4.81–5.74\,mmol\cdot l^{-1}$
Reticulocyte count	0.5–1.5%
Haptoglobin	$30–175\,mg\cdot dl^{-1}$ ($6.20–27.90\,\mu mol\cdot l^{-1}$)

Table 21.3 Laboratory test profile of exercise-related anaemias

	Haemoglobin/ haematocrit	Red blood cell size	Serum ferritin	Reticulocyte count
Non-anaemic iron deficiency	–	–	↓	–
Iron-deficiency anaemia	↓	↓	↓	–
Dilutional pseudoanaemia	↓	–	–	–
Exercise-induced anaemia	↓	↑	–	↑ or –

↑, increase; ↓, decrease; –, no change.

reduced iron needs due to lack of menstruation. In the USA, the prevalence of non-anaemic iron deficiency in the general population is estimated to be approximately 30% for adult women and 39% for adolescent girls; the prevalence of iron-deficiency anaemia is just under 6% for both adolescent and adult females (Expert Scientific Working Group, 1985).

It is unclear whether the prevalence is higher among female athletes than non-athletes because prevalence estimates vary according to the population studied. Most studies have shown the iron status of female athletes to be similar or somewhat worse than non-athletes (Parr *et al.*, 1984; Brown *et al.*, 1985; Risser *et al.*, 1988). However, studies of some female athletes have shown a substantially higher prevalence, particularly in high-school runners (Plowman & McSwegin, 1981; Brown *et al.*, 1985) and swimmers (Rowland & Kelleher, 1989). In general, studies in high-school and college female athletes report prevalences of 0–19% for iron-deficiency anaemia and 20-62% for non-anaemic iron deficiency (Plowman & McSwegin, 1981; Nickerson

& Tripp, 1983; Clement & Asmundson, 1984; Parr *et al.*, 1984; Brown *et al.*, 1985; Nickeson *et al.*, 1985; Haymes *et al.*, 1986; Risser *et al.*, 1988; Haymes & Spillman, 1989; Nickerson *et al.*, 1989; Rowland & Kelleher, 1989).

Effects of training on iron status

A higher than normal prevalence of iron deficiency among some female athletes suggests that training may contribute to negative iron balance. A study in female field hockey players found a progressive decline in ferritin values over each of three consecutive seasons (30–37% reduction of ferritin per season), normalizing between seasons (Deihl *et al.*, 1986). Studies following the iron status of female high-school and college athletes over a competitive season found that 16% of males and 20% of females with initially normal iron status developed non-anaemic iron deficiency but none developed anaemia (Frederickson *et al.*, 1983; Nickerson *et al.*, 1985, 1989; Haymes *et al.*, 1986; Rowland *et al.*, 1987; Risser *et al.*, 1988). Most athletes who developed non-anaemic iron deficiency were treated with iron supplementation; therefore it is unknown what proportion would have developed anaemia in the absence of intervention. In most studies, the development of non-anaemic iron deficiency during training was found to be preventable by iron supplementation. Poor response in some studies may have been due to inadequate iron dosage, poor compliance or ongoing gastrointestinal blood loss.

Mechanisms of iron deficiency in athletes

Besides exercise-induced haemolysis, a number of other mechanisms may contribute to negative iron balance during training. These mechanisms include loss of iron through the gastrointestinal tract, sweat, urine or menses; impaired gastrointestinal absorption of iron; and inadequate iron intake. However, the predominant cause of iron deficiency is inadequate iron intake to compensate for menstrual loss of iron.

GASTROINTESTINAL LOSSES

Occult gastrointestinal blood loss is common in runners. An estimated 8–85% of runners test positive for faecal occult blood following their runs (McMahon *et al.*, 1984; Stewart *et al.*, 1984; McCabe *et al.*, 1986; Robertson *et al.*, 1987; Baska *et al.*, 1990) and 2% of marathon runners and triathletes have visible blood in stools after races (Eichner, 1989). Average gastrointestinal loss of iron for a sedentary woman is 0.45 mg daily (Dubach *et al.*, 1955). A recent study showed that physically active women expending >2520 kJ (600 kcal) daily during exercise lost 1 mg of iron through faecal blood loss daily, which was twice as much as that lost by sedentary women expending <420 kJ (100 kcal) daily during exercise (Lampe *et al.*, 1991). Although the exact cause is unclear, gastrointestinal blood loss probably occurs as a result of bowel ischaemia. Some evidence suggests that individuals who experience gastrointestinal symptoms during exercise, such as diarrhoea or cramping, have higher gastrointestinal blood loss. Use of aspirin or non-steroidal anti-inflammatory drugs may also increase gastrointestinal blood loss.

IMPAIRED GASTROINTESTINAL ABSORPTION OF IRON

Iron absorption from the gastrointestinal tract usually increases in response to iron deficiency. However, evidence suggests that this compensatory response is blunted in athletes. For example, one study found that iron-deficient runners absorb 16% of iron from the gastrointestinal tract compared with 30% in iron-deficient non-athletes (Ehn *et al.*, 1980).

SWEAT LOSSES

Iron lost in sweat by female runners during exercise averages 0.28 mg·h^{-1} (Lamanca *et al.*, 1988). Unless exercise is prolonged, iron loss through sweat is usually negligible.

URINARY LOSSES

Urinary loss of iron can occur due to haematuria resulting from urinary tract microtrauma or haemoglobinuria secondary to marked intravascular haemolysis. Under usual circumstances, urinary loss of iron is minimal.

MENSTRUAL LOSSES

Menstrual blood loss is the primary source of iron loss in female athletes and non-athletes. Average menstrual blood loss during a period is approximately 34 ml (Hallberg et al., 1966), which translates to an additional iron requirement of 0.55 mg daily (Haymes, 1993). However, menstrual blood loss during a period can range from 1.6 to 200 ml and therefore iron loss can vary significantly (Hallberg et al., 1966). Women who lose more than 60 ml during a period are more susceptible to iron deficiency (Hallberg et al., 1966). The method of contraception may also affect the amount of blood lost per menses; use of oral contraceptives can decrease blood loss by 50%, while use of an intrauterine device can double the amount of blood loss (Hallberg & Rossander-Hulten, 1991). While one would expect amenorrhoeic athletes to have a lower prevalence of iron deficiency because they do not menstruate, a study of élite marathon runners found that the prevalence was higher in amenorrhoeic than eumenorrhoeic runners (Deuster et al., 1986). Presumably a lower dietary intake of iron counteracts the protective effect of lack of menstruation in these amenorrhoeic runners.

INADEQUATE DIETARY INTAKE OF IRON

Inadequate dietary intake of iron is the preeminent cause of iron deficiency in female athletes. In the USA, the recommended daily allowance (RDA) for iron to meet basal requirements is 15 mg of females and 10 mg for males. The iron needs of some women may be appreciably greater. The average diet in the USA contains 5–7 mg of iron per 4200 kJ (1000 kcal). Therefore, women need 12.6 MJ (3000 kcal) daily to obtain the RDA of iron. However, many female athletes consume <8400 kJ (2000 kcal) daily, particularly female athletes participating in sports emphasizing lean body physique. In addition, many female athletes eat a modified vegetarian diet, which poses increased risk due to lower bioavailability and quantities of iron in non-meat foods.

Effects on performance

Anaemia clearly impairs physical performance and correlates with diminished maximum oxygen consumption, decreased physical work capacity, lower endurance, increased lactic acidosis and increased fatigue (Nickerson & Tripp, 1983; Risser et al., 1988; Rowland et al., 1988). The correlation between Hb levels and exercise capacity and diminished performance by athletes participating in endurance events is well known. The unresolved question is whether iron deficiency in the absence of anaemia (non-anaemic iron deficiency) impairs performance. In the absence of a reduction in Hb levels, iron deficiency is unlikely to reduce oxygen delivery to the tissues, as is the case when anaemia is present. However, non-anaemic iron deficiency may diminish performance by other mechanisms, for example impairment of iron-dependent metabolic processes at the cellular level such as energy production by mitochondrial cytochromes.

Studies in rats suggest that iron deficiency in the absence of anaemia can impair physical performance and endurance capacity (Finch et al., 1976; McLane et al., 1981). However, these findings have not been replicated in humans. Celsing et al. (1986) induced anaemia in men by repeated phlebotomies and then reinfused RBCs in order to restore RBC volume, creating a non-anaemic iron-deficient state. Although maximal oxygen consumption and endurance were clearly diminished when the men were tested while anaemic, both measures returned to normal when RBC volume was restored (although the men were still iron deficient), suggesting that anaemia impairs performance as a consequence of reduced oxygen-carrying capacity.

Studies of the effects of iron supplementation on the performance of non-anaemic iron-deficient athletes have produced conflicting results. No studies have shown improvements in maximal oxygen consumption, although studies in female runners following iron supplementation have shown improvements in measures of endurance, such as treadmill times (Rowland *et al.*, 1988), run times (Yoshida *et al.*, 1990), lower blood lactate levels during submaximal exercise (Schoene *et al.*, 1983; Lamanca & Haymes, 1989) and appreciable improvements in treadmill times that did not reach statistical significance (Lamanca & Haymes, 1989). In many instances, iron supplementation also led to improvements in Hb levels, suggesting that the beneficial effects were seen because of correction of a mild anaemia. These studies illustrate two important points: (i) it is clinically difficult to distinguish mild anaemia from non-anaemic iron deficiency; and (ii) although an Hb value may technically fall in the normal range, it may nevertheless represent mild anaemia that will respond to iron supplementation. However, other studies have failed to show beneficial effects on performance of the iron supplementation of non-anaemic iron-deficient athletes (Matter *et al.*, 1987; Newhouse *et al.*, 1989; Fogelholm *et al.*, 1992), suggesting that when Hb levels are not improved iron supplementation does not improve performance, despite an increase in ferritin levels.

Should non-anaemic iron deficiency be treated?

Iron should not be administered solely to improve athletic performance, as it is unclear whether non-anaemic iron deficiency impairs performance. Iron therapy may be indicated for non-anaemic iron-deficient athletes in order to prevent development of anaemia and reduce the non-haematological manifestations of iron deficiency. From a practical standpoint, it is often difficult to distinguish non-anaemic iron deficiency from mild anaemia. Many women with pre-sumed non-anaemic iron deficiency do respond to iron supplementation and will show increases in Hb values that can lead to improvements in performance. Therefore, these women are actually mildly anaemic, although their Hb falls within the normal range, and will benefit from iron supplementation. One must weigh the potential benefits of supplementation against the potential risks, such as cost of supplementation, gastrointestinal distress and haemochromatosis associated with overdosage.

Screening for iron deficiency

The clinical manifestations of iron deficiency are rare unless anaemia is severe. Potential signs and symptoms of iron deficiency include exercise fatigue, muscle burning, nausea, dyspnoea, pagophagia, pica, pallor, koilonychia, cheilosis and glossitis. Non-haematological manifestations of iron deficiency include susceptibility to infection, impaired attention span and altered mental function (Oski, 1979; Dallman, 1982; Bruner *et al.*, 1996). However, in most cases the condition will be asymptomatic and will not be recognized unless screening blood work is done. While it would be ideal to screen all female athletes for iron deficiency on a yearly basis, in many settings this is not feasible and the cost may be prohibitive. Therefore screening should be directed towards those athletes at highest risk. Table 21.4 lists risk factors for anaemia that can be addressed during a medical history to identify

Table 21.4 Risk factors for anaemia in female athletes

Disadvantaged socioeconomic background
Dietary restriction: vegetarian diet, weight-loss diets
  or fad diets
Intense or prolonged endurance training
Personal or family history of anaemia, bleeding
  disorders or chronic disease
Excessive menstrual flow: increased duration,
  frequency or volume
Use of anti-inflammatory medications
Volunteer blood donor
Childbirth

Table 21.5 Prevention of iron deficiency: strategies to increase dietary intake of iron

Ingest iron-rich foods
    Meat sources: lean red meat, dark meat of poultry, fish
    Non-meat sources: cereals, pasta and bread enriched with iron, dried fruits, beans, tofu, spinach
Meat sources of iron are absorbed better than non-meat sources of iron
Enhance iron absorption from foods by concurrently ingesting foods containing vitamin C, such as fruit juices
Avoid inhibitors of iron absorption: tannic acid (tea), **phytic acid (wheat bran), calcium salts (milk)**, antacids
Cook in iron skillets
If unable to meet daily iron needs through diet, a supplement containing the RDA for iron (15 mg), such as a multivitamin with iron, is recommended

RDA, recommended daily allowance.

Prevention of iron deficiency

Preventive efforts should focus on ensuring adequate dietary intake of iron. This depends on not only the amount of iron ingested but also the bioavailability of iron sources. Strategies to increase dietary intake of iron are presented in Table 21.5. The bioavailability of iron is greater in food sources than in iron supplements so it is preferable to meet daily iron needs through food sources. However, if unable to meet daily iron needs through diet alone, iron supplements containing the RDA for iron (15 mg) are recommended.

Treatment of iron deficiency

Iron supplementation is the mainstay of treatment of iron deficiency, as it is usually not feasible to increase dietary intake of iron sufficiently to reverse iron deficiency. Dosage and practical tips for iron supplementation are provided in Table 21.6.

Table 21.6 Treatment of iron deficiency: iron supplementation

Dosage
For iron-deficiency anaemia (ferritin < 12 μg·l^{-1}, low haemoglobin)
    50–100 mg elemental iron three times daily (6 mg·kg^{-1} daily), e.g. 325 mg ferrous sulphate three times daily
    Confirm response to supplementation by rise of 1 g·dl^{-1} in haemoglobin after 4–6 weeks
    Serum haemoglobin concentration is usually completely corrected within 2 months
    Reticulocytosis is seen in 5–10 days
    Continue **treatment for 6–8 months to replenish iron** stores and restore normal ferritin level
For non-anaemic iron deficiency (ferritin 12–20 μg·l^{-1}, normal haemoglobin)
    50–100 mg elemental iron once daily*, e.g. 325 mg ferrous sulphate daily
    Continue supplementation until ferritin > 20 μg·l^{-1} (several months)*

Practical tips
Iron salts contain varying amounts of elemental iron: sulphate, 20%; fumarate, 11%; gluconate, 33%
Ferrous salts are better absorbed than ferric salts
There is little difference in rate of absorption among various ferrous salt forms
Ferrous sulphate is cheapest
Avoid sustained-release or enteric-coated products
Enhance absorption by taking supplements with vitamin C, without other competing supplements, on an empty stomach
Side-effects of gastrointestinal symptoms are lessened by gradual progression of the dosage from once daily to three times daily as tolerance develops

*Risser & Risser (1990).

References

Banister, E.W. & Hamilton, C.L. (1985) Variations in iron status with fatigue modelled from training in female distance runners. *European Journal of Applied Physiology* **54**, 16–23.

Baska, R.S., Moses, F.M., Graeber, G. & Kearny, G. (1990) Gastrointestinal bleeding during an ultramarathon. *Digestive Diseases and Science* **35**, 276–279.

Brown, R.I., McIntosh, S.M. & Seaboth, V.R. (1985) Iron status of adolescent female athletes. *Journal of Adolescent Health Care* **6**, 349–352.

Bruner, A.B., Joffe, A., Duggan, A.K., Casella, J.F. & Bandt, J. (1996) Randomised study of cognitive effects of iron supplementation in non-anemic iron-deficient adolescent girls. *Lancet* **348**, 992–996.

Celsing, F., Blomstrand, E., Werner, B., Pihlstedt, P. & Ekblom, B. (1986) Effects of iron deficiency on endurance and muscle enzyme activity in man. *Medicine and Science in Sports and Exercise* **18**, 156–161.

Clement, D.B. & Asmundson, R.C. (1984) Iron status and sports performance. *Sports Medicine* **1**, 65–74.

Dallman, P.R. (1982) Manifestations of iron deficiency. *Seminars in Hematology* **19**, 19–30.

Deihl, D.M., Lohman, T.G., Smith, S.C. & Kertzer, R. (1986) The effects of physical training on iron status of female field hockey players. *International Journal of Sports Medicine* **7**, 264–270.

Deuster, P.A., Kyler, S.B., Moser, P.B., Vigersky, R.A., Singh, A. & Schoomaker, E.B. (1986) Nutritional intakes and status of highly trained amenorrheic and eumenorrheic women runners. *Fertility and Sterility* **46**, 636–643.

Dubach, R., Moore, C.V. & Callender, S. (1955) Studies in iron transportation and metabolism. IX. The excretion of iron as measured by the isotope technique. *Journal of Laboratory and Clinical Medicine* **45**, 599–615.

Ehn, L., Carmark, B. & Hoglund, S. (1980) Iron status in athletes involved in intense physical activity. *Medicine and Science in Sports and Exercise* **12**, 61–64.

Eichner, E.R. (1989) Gastrointestinal bleeding in athletes. *Physician and Sportsmedicine* **17**, 128–140.

Expert Scientific Working Group (1985) Summary of a report on assessment of the iron nutritional status of the United States population. *American Journal of Clinical Nutrition* **42**, 1318–1330.

Finch, C.A., Miller, L.R., Inamdar, A.R., Person, R., Seiler, K. & Mackler, B. (1976) Iron deficiency in the rat. *Journal of Clinical Investigation* **58**, 447–453.

Fogelholm, M., Jaakkola, L. & Lampisjavi, T. (1992) Effects of iron supplementation in female athletes with low serum ferritin concentration. *International Journal of Sports Medicine* **13**, 158–162.

Frederickson, L.A., Puhl, J.L. & Runyan, W.S. (1983) Effects of training on indices of iron status of young female crosscountry runners. *Medicine and Science in Sports and Exercise* **15**, 271–276.

Hallberg, L. & Rossander-Hulten, L. (1991) Iron requirements in menstruating women. *American Journal of Clinical Nutrition* **54**, 1047–1058.

Hallberg, L., Hogdahl, A.M., Nilsson, L. & Rybo, G. (1966) Menstrual blood loss: a population study. *Acta Obstetricia et Gynecologica Scandinavica* **45**, 320–351.

Haymes, E.M. (1993) Dietary iron needs in exercising women: a rational plan to follow in evaluating iron status. *Medicine, Exercise, Nutrition and Health* **2**, 203–212.

Haymes, E.M. & Spillman, D.M. (1989) Iron status of women distance runners, sprinters, and control

women. *International Journal of Sports Medicine* **10**, 430–433.

Haymes, E.M., Puhl, J.L. & Temples, T.E. (1986) Training for crosscountry skiing and iron status. *Medicine and Science in Sports and Exercise* **18**, 162–167.

Lamanca, J. & Haymes, E. (1989) Effects of dietary iron supplementation on endurance. *Medicine and Science in Sports and Exercise* **21**, S77.

Lamanca, J.J., Haymes, E.M., Daly, J.A., Moffatt, R.J. & Waller, M.F. (1988) Sweat iron loss of male and female runners during exercise. *International Journal of Sports Medicine* **9**, 52–55.

Lampe, J.W., Slavin, J.L. & Apple, F.S. (1991) Iron status of active women and the effect of running a marathon on bowel function and gastrointestinal blood loss. *International Journal of Sports Medicine* **12**, 173–179.

McCabe, M.E., Peura, D.A., Kadakia, S.C., Bocek, Z. & Johnson, L.F. (1986) Gastrointestinal blood loss associated with running a marathon. *Digestive Diseases and Science* **31**, 1229–1232.

McLane, J.A., Fell, R.D., McKay, R.H., Winder, W.W., Brown, E.B. & Hollosszy, J.O. (1981) Physiological and biochemical effects of iron deficiency on rat skeletal muscle. *American Journal of Physiology* **241**, C47–C54.

McMahon, L.F., Ryan, M.J. & Larson, D.L. (1984) Occult gastrointestinal blood loss in marathon runners. *Annals of Internal Medicine* **100**, 846–847.

Matter, M., Stittfall, I., Graves, J. *et al.* (1987) The effect of iron and folate therapy on maximal exercise performance in female marathon runners with iron and folate deficiency. *Clinical Science* **72**, 415–422.

Newhouse, I.J., Clement, D.B., Taunton, J.E. & McKenzie, D.C. (1989) The effect of prelatent/latent iron deficiency on physical work capacity. *Medicine and Science in Sports and Exercise* **21**, 263–268.

Nickerson, H.J. & Tripp, A.D. (1983) Iron deficiency in adolescent cross-country runners. *Physician and Sportsmedicine* **11**, 60–66.

Nickerson, H.J., Holubets, M., Tripp, A.D. & Pierce, W.E. (1985) Decreased iron stores in high school female runners. *American Journal of Diseases of Children* **139**, 1115–1119.

Nickerson, H.J., Holubets, M. & Weiler, B.R. (1989) Causes of iron deficiency in adolescent athletes. *Journal of Pediatrics* **114**, 657–659.

Oski, F.A. (1979) The nonhematologic manifestations of iron deficiency. *American Journal of Diseases of Children* **133**, 315–322.

Parr, R.B., Bachman, L.A. & Moss, R.A. (1984) Iron deficiency in female athletes. *Physician and Sportsmedicine* **12**, 81–86.

Plowman, S.A. & McSwegin, P.C. (1981) The effects of iron supplementation on female cross country runners. *Journal of Sports Medicine and Physical Fitness* **21**, 407–416.

Risser, W.L. & Risser, J.M. (1990) Iron deficiency in adolescents and young adults. *Physician and Sportsmedicine* **18**, 87–101.

Risser, W.L., Lee, E.J., Poindexter, H.B. *et al.* (1988) Iron deficiency in female athletes: its prevalence and impact on performance. *Medicine and Science in Sports and Exercise* **20**, 116–121.

Robertson, J.D., Maughan, R.J. & Davidson, R.J.L. (1987) Faecal blood loss in response to exercise. *British Medical Journal* **295**, 303–305.

Rowland, T.W. & Kelleher, J.F. (1989) Iron deficiency in athletes: insights from high school swimmers. *American Journal of Diseases of Children* **143**, 197–200.

Rowland, T.W., Black, S.A. & Kelleher, J.F. (1987) Iron deficiency in adolescent endurance athletes. *Journal of Adolescent Health Care* **8**, 322–326.

Rowland, T.W., Deisroth, M.B., Green, G.M. & Kelleher, J.F. (1988) The effect of iron therapy on the exercise capacity of nonanemic iron-deficient adolescent runners. *American Journal of Diseases of Children* **142**, 165–169.

Schoene, R.B., Escourrou, P., Robertson, H.T., Nilson, K.L., Parsons, J.R. & Smith, N.J. (1983) Iron repletion decreases maximal exercise lactate concentration in female athletes with minimal iron deficiency anaemia. *Journal of Laboratory and Clinical Medicine* **102**, 306–312.

Selby, G.B. & Eichner, E.R. (1986) Endurance swimming, intravascular hemolysis, anemia, and iron depletion: new perspective on athlete's anemia. *American Journal of Medicine* **81**, 791–794.

Stewart, J.G., Ahlquist, D.A., McGill, D.B., Ilstrup, D.M., Schwartz, S. & Owen, R.A. (1984) Gastrointestinal blood loss and anemia in runners. *Annals of Internal Medicine* **100**, 843–845.

Yoshida, T., Udo, M. & Chida, M. (1990) Dietary iron supplement during severe physical training in competitive female distance runners. *Sports Training and Medical Rehabilitation* **1**, 279–285.

Chapter 22

Nutritional and Pharmacological Ergogenic Aids

PRISCILLA M. CLARKSON AND MELINDA M. MANORE

Introduction

Use of dietary supplements to improve performance dates back as far as 400 BC. However, in the 20th century, many new supplements have been developed, and their use has grown precipitously. This increased interest in supplements has been largely due to a better understanding of how muscles function and what fuels are used to provide energy (Grivetti *et al.*, 1996). Nutritional supplements to enhance performance are popular with athletes, and sales of these products abound. However, when dietary interventions are not sufficient to gain a competitive edge, many athletes turn to pharmaceutical interventions.

Today a wealth of studies exist on the effects of various nutrients as ergogenic aids. However, the science of sport is no different from the science of medicine, and most studies have been undertaken using males as subjects. Likewise, studies of the effects of drugs on performance have predominantly used male subjects. Thus, we do not have a full understanding of the effective-ness of ergogenic aids in female athletes. This chapter reviews nutritional and pharmaceutical ergogenic aids and emphasizes the state of knowledge of these interventions in female subjects.

Nutritional ergogenic aids

Nutritional ergogenic aids are substances that if added to the diet may directly enhance sports performance. They are usually divided into three general categories: macronutrients, micronutrients and metabolic intermediates. In general, macronutrients, such as supplemental carbohydrate, amino acids and medium-chain triglycerides (MCTs), contribute to improved athletic performance by providing additional energy or essential substrates required for fuelling the body before and during exercise and refuelling or repairing the body after exercise. Micronutrients (vitamins and minerals) act to improve overall health and thus may improve performance indirectly. It is difficult to document improved athletic performance by supplementing with a single vitamin and/or mineral unless there is a deficiency initially. Consequently, this chapter does not address vitamin and mineral use in active females as a means of improving athletic performance directly. However, some of the metabolic intermediates that are frequently marketed as ergogenic aids are discussed.

Macronutrients

CARBOHYDRATE

Carbohydrate is one of the most extensively researched and reviewed nutritional ergogenic aids for the enhancement of exercise performance (Coggan & Coyle, 1991; Sherman, 1991, 1995; Sherman & Wimer, 1991; Costill & Hargreaves, 1992; Coyle, 1992, 1995). It is well established that providing adequate carbohydrate before, during and after exercise improves exercise performance (Coyle, 1992, 1995). This ergogenic effect may be due to a number of mechanisms (Coyle, 1992, 1995; Walberg-Rankin, 1995). The muscles require carbohydrate to fuel exercise and to replenish the body's glycogen stores after exercise. Thus, carbohydrate fed before or after exercise increases glycogen stores, while carbohydrate fed during exercise provides the body with additional fuel and helps maintain blood glucose. This additional energy, whether stored or provided exogenously during exercise, improves performance (Coyle, 1992, 1995; Tsintzas et al., 1993). The amount of carbohydrate required both during and after exercise depends on the intensity and duration of the exercise, the level of physical training and the nutritional state of the individual. However, it is generally recommended that athletes consume a high-carbohydrate diet (6–10 g·kg⁻¹) during periods of intense exercise training (Walberg-Rankin, 1995). The amount of energy provided by carbohydrate (percentage of energy intake) will depend on the total energy intake; for most female athletes consuming 10.5–14.7 MJ (2500–3500 kcal) daily, this means that about 50–70% of energy will come from carbohydrate.

There is very limited research that has specifically examined the carbohydrate needs of active females and the gender differences in carbohydrate metabolism during exercise. However, recent research indicates that trained females oxidize more lipids and less carbohydrate and protein during exercise compared with males matched for training (Tarnopolsky et al., 1990, 1995; Phillips et al., 1993). In addition, females appear to store muscle glycogen differently in response to a high-carbohydrate diet. Tarnopolsky et al. (1995) examined the ability of matched endurance-trained males and females to increase muscle glycogen content in response to a high-carbohydrate diet (75% of energy from carbohydrate vs. 55–60% in a typical diet). Differences in exercise performance and substrate metabolism during 60 min of cycling at 75% $\dot{V}_{O_{2max}}$ were also examined. Females did not increase glycogen content nor did exercise performance time increase in

response to a 4-day high-carbohydrate diet. Conversely, the males increased glycogen content by 41% and exercise performance by 5%. The females also oxidized more lipid and less carbohydrate and protein during exercise than the men.

A couple of factors may contribute to the gender differences observed in the study by Tarnopolsky et al. (1995). First, the absolute amount of carbohydrate consumed daily was different: the females on the typical and high-carbohydrate diets consumed 5.9 and 7.7 g·kg⁻¹ respectively, while the males consumed 7.9 and 9.6 g·kg⁻¹ respectively. Fallowfield and Williams (1993) report that a carbohydrate supplement of 5.8 g·kg⁻¹ did not replenish glycogen levels after exhaustive exercise in male runners, while a supplement of 8.8 g·kg⁻¹ was adequate. Carbohydrate loading studies typically provide a carbohydrate intake >8.5 g·kg⁻¹; however, this level of carbohydrate is not attainable for active females consuming <11.76 MJ (2800 kcal) daily. Thus, for the females in the study by Tarnopolsky et al. (1995) to achieve the same relative level of glycogen storage as observed in the men, more carbohydrate may be required. Second, this study was conducted in the follicular phase of the menstrual cycle. Nicklas et al. (1989) have reported greater glycogen repletion during the luteal phase vs. the follicular phase.

In summary, the studies cited above indicate that trained females utilize fuel substrates differently from males and that the ergogenic effect of a high-carbohydrate diet may not be as readily apparent in females. However, females still require carbohydrate to replace muscle glycogen used during exercise. Based on these studies and others (Keith et al., 1991; Walberg-Rankin, 1995), active women appear to need a minimum carbohydrate requirement of 5–6 g·kg⁻¹ during periods of exercise training. In order to obtain the same ergogenic effect as frequently observed in men, this carbohydrate intake might need to be higher. However, the ergogenic effect of carbohydrate feeding (30–70 g·h⁻¹) during exercise appears to be similar in males and females (Tsintzas et al., 1993).

PROTEIN SUPPLEMENTS AND AMINO ACIDS

Athletes frequently supplement their diet with protein powders and/or single amino acids (i.e. branched-chain amino acids (BCAA), lysine, arginine and ornithine). The popularity of these supplements is evidenced by the numerous products available for sale at health food stores, in sports magazines and local drug stores. Protein powders are marketed to athletes as a way of increasing their total protein intake and, in turn, increasing muscle mass and repairing muscle tissue damage associated with exercise. Competitive athletes, regardless of gender, have greater protein requirements than their sedentary counterparts (Phillips et al., 1993; Lemon, 1995). However, there is no research supporting the hypothesis that protein powders and/or amino acids are better sources of this protein than food or that they offer an ergogenic edge.

During exercise, blood levels of BCAA decrease as the exercising muscles use these amino acids as a source of energy (Ahlborg et al., 1974; Lehmann et al., 1995; Blomstrand et al., 1997). Researchers have hypothesized that providing supplemental BCAA during exercise would help maintain blood BCAA and decrease endogenous protein oxidation. This in turn has been hypothesized to improve muscular performance. Studies of both acute (Maresh et al., 1994; Varnier et al., 1994; Blomstrand et al., 1995) and chronic (Bigard et al., 1996) exercise report no strong evidence to support this hypothesis.

Another mechanism whereby BCAA may influence exercise performance is by preventing central fatigue (Davis, 1995; Meeusen & De Meirleir, 1995). The central fatigue hypothesis states that the decline in blood BCAA observed with exercise causes an increase in brain serotonin levels, which in turn cause a deterioration in sport and exercise performance. As blood BCAA levels decrease, the competitive inhibition of tryptophan across the blood–brain barrier is removed. This allows more tryptophan to enter the brain, resulting in greater serotonin production. Although this mechanism is well documented, there is little evidence that supplemental BCAA improves exercise performance (van Hall et al., 1995; Blomstrand et al., 1997) or prevents exercise-related fatigue. However, other studies report decreased perceived exertion (7% decrease) and mental fatigue (15% decrease) during moderate-intensity exercise (70% $\dot{V}_{O_{2max}}$ for 60 min) but not during maximum exercise (Blomstrand et al., 1997).

Single amino acids or combinations of amino acids (i.e. ornithine and arginine) are marketed as a dietary means of stimulating muscle growth and/or facilitating fat loss through the endogenous production and release of human growth hormone (HGH) (Macintyre, 1987) and/or insulin (Bucci et al., 1992). These hormones are anabolic in nature and therefore athletes believe that increasing endogenous secretion will improve muscle mass and strength. There is no evidence to suggest that either arginine or ornithine, or any mixture of amino acids, increases strength, power or the endogenous production of either HGH (Bucci, 1994) or insulin (Bucci et al., 1992).

All the studies that have examined the use of supplemental amino acids as a way of increasing endogenous anabolic hormone production have used male subjects, except for the study by Bucci et al. (1992). These authors included three female and nine male body-builders in their study, in which supplemental ornithine was given and insulin production measured; however, all data were presented in aggregate form. Similarly, all human studies that have examined the mechanism of the central fatigue hypothesis have used male subjects or did not classify results by gender.

MEDIUM-CHAIN TRIGLYCERIDES

MCTs are composed of medium-chain fatty acids (MCFAs) that are 6–12 carbons in length. These fats are found naturally in coconut and palm kernel oils or are prepared synthetically by the hydrolysis of coconut oil (Bach & Babayan, 1982). MCTs are metabolized differently from regular fats and oils: (i) most MCFAs are quickly absorbed from the gut directly into the portal system and transported to the liver rather than passing through the lymphatic system (Swift *et al.*, 1990); (ii) they do not require carnitine for transport into the mitochondria of heart, liver or kidney of adults; and (iii) they are quickly oxidized and used for energy with little opportunity for storage as fat (Bach & Babyan, 1982; Johnson *et al.*, 1990). MCTs are becoming more popular with athletes because they are energy dense [34.9 kJ·g^{-1} (8.3 kcal·g^{-1})], providing twice the energy per gram of carbohydrate. In addition, they are easily absorbed (Beckers *et al.*, 1992) and preferentially used for energy before carbohydrate (Jeukendrup *et al.*, 1995). If MCTs are consumed as part of a high-carbohydrate isocaloric diet, ketone production is minimal (Bach & Babayan, 1982). Thus, these fats may be added to the athlete's diet in order to increase daily energy intake (i.e. when an athlete needs to gain weight) or to boost energy intake during an exercise event when immediate energy is needed (i.e. added to sports beverages or foods).

Because MCTs are absorbed rapidly into the bloodstream as MCFAs and metabolized as quickly as glucose, it has been hypothesized that they may enhance performance by sparing glycogen utilization during exercise (Berning, 1996). Endurance studies using trained males exercising for 60–120 min at 60–70% $\dot{V}O_{2max}$ show no carbohydrate-sparing effect of supplemental MCTs (Décombaz *et al.*, 1983; Massicotte *et al.*, 1992; Borghouts *et al.*, 1995). Studies using either a combination of moderate- and high-intensity exercise or only high-intensity exercise show mixed results. Some report a carbohydrate-sparing effect (Van Zyl *et al.*, 1996), while others do not (Horowitz *et al.*, 1995). All the above studies used male subjects or did not give the gender of their subjects. No study has specifically examined the use of MCTs as an ergogenic aid in female athletes.

Although the research does not support a clear ergogenic effect for MCTs, they can be used to increase total daily energy intake during periods of intense training, when energy intake fre-

quently decreases. They also can be used during endurance exercise events (i.e. triathlons, marathons, etc.) to increase energy intake above that provided by carbohydrate drinks or sports bars. We have successfully used MCTs with female triathletes to increase energy intake during exercise (M. Manore, personal communication). However, athletes should experiment with this fat prior to competitions in order to avoid any unexpected gastrointestinal disturbances.

Metabolic intermediates

CARNITINE

Carnitine is a vitamin-like substance produced in the body from the amino acids methionine and lysine. The enzymes involved in carnitine synthesis also require vitamin C, vitamin B$_6$, niacin and iron as cofactors (Broquist, 1994). Carnitine is obtained in the diet from red meats and dairy products, while vegetables, cereals and fruits have negligible amounts. Thus, vegans have low dietary intakes of carnitine. Supplemental carnitine can be found in either the L or D form; L-carnitine is the active form, while D-carnitine causes depletion of L-carnitine within the body and can have potentially toxic effects (Wagenmaker, 1991).

The majority of the body's carnitine is found in muscle (98%) where it has a number of physiological functions that could possibly affect exercise performance, thus making it a potential ergogenic aid (Wagenmaker, 1991; Heinonen, 1996). However, the most common reason given for supplementation with carnitine is the role it plays in fatty acid metabolism. Carnitine is a component in several enzymes involved in transporting long-chain fatty acids across the inner mitochondrial membrane for β-oxidation. Thus, it has been hypothesized that supplemental carnitine increases the transfer of lipids across the mitochondrial membrane during prolonged exercise, increasing fat oxidation and sparing muscle glycogen. This alteration in substrate metabolism should improve performance and delay fatigue. One fundamental premise of this hypothesis is that supplemental carnitine will increase muscle concentrations of carnitine, thus altering cellular metabolism. However, research now indicates that while supplemental carnitine (2–5 g daily for >14 days) increases both blood and urinary carnitine concentrations, it does not change total muscle carnitine levels significantly (Décombaz *et al.*, 1992; Barnett *et al.*, 1994; Vukovich *et al.*, 1994; Constantin-Teodosiu *et al.*, 1996). Numerous reviews of the literature have concluded that supplemental carnitine does not increase fat oxidation or decrease carbohydrate oxidized in healthy active individuals during exercise (Wagenmaker, 1991; Clarkson, 1992; Brass & Hiatt, 1994; Kanter & Williams, 1995; Heinonen, 1996). This is true even when muscle glycogen is depleted, making less carbohydrate available for oxidation (Décombaz *et al.*, 1993). Thus, there is no convincing evidence to suggest that supplemental carnitine alters substrate oxidation during endurance exercise or improves performance in healthy adults. However, supplemental carnitine is used in clinical settings where the ability to synthesize carnitine endogenously is compromised. In these situations, supplemental carnitine does improve lipid oxidation (Broquist, 1994).

Carnitine is also frequently added to products advertised as 'fat burners' or dieting agents. These products supposedly increase the body's oxidation of fat at rest and thus alter body composition (i.e. decrease body fat). There is no theoretical basis for this assumption and no research data supporting this hypothesis. Yet these products are popular with athletes and the general public who want to decrease body fat.

Most research studies that have examined the ergogenic effects of carnitine have used male subjects. Those studies that have included females usually do not report results based on gender; thus, specific information on how females differ from males with regard to carnitine supplementation and exercise performance is not available. Females do have a smaller total body carnitine pool than males due to their smaller muscle mass (Heinonen, 1996). However,

there is no evidence that females, including vegans, are at risk for carnitine deficiency (Lombard *et al.*, 1989).

COENZYME Q_{10}

Coenzyme Q_{10} (ubiquinone) is a naturally occurring lipid-soluble substance that is synthesized endogenously. It functions primarily as an electron carrier in mitochondria but may have a secondary role as an antioxidant in muscle. It has been hypothesized that supplemental coenzyme Q_{10} could increase the rate of flux through the electron-transport chain and thus enhance ATP production. In addition, coenzyme Q_{10} might help to scavenge free radicals and regenerate the antioxidant form of vitamin E, thus acting as an antioxidant (Jenkins, 1993; Beyer, 1994).

Studies that have examined the performance-enhancing effects of coenzyme Q_{10} have produced inconclusive results. Numerous studies have found no ergogenic effect of supplementation on exercise performance in healthy young trained or sedentary males (Braun *et al.*, 1991; Snider *et al.*, 1992; Laaksone *et al.*, 1995) or middle-aged untrained males (Porter *et al.*, 1995). Conversely, Karlsson *et al.* (1996) report a positive relationship between muscle ubiquinone levels and maximal exercise performance and the onset of blood lactate accumulation. Karlsson *et al.* (1992) also report lower plasma concentrations of ubiquinone in trained male athletes compared with sedentary controls.

Studies that have examined the antioxidant effect of coenzyme Q_{10} have also produced mixed results. Some report positive effects of supplementation (Karlsson *et al.*, 1996; Karlsson, 1997), while others report no effect (Braun *et al.*, 1991) or increased cell damage (Malm *et al.*, 1996) with supplementation. Currently, there appears to be no strong evidence that coenzyme Q_{10} improves exercise performance. However, its role as an antioxidant is still equivocal.

None of the studies examining the ergogenic effect of coenzyme Q_{10} on exercise performance have included female athletes. Hence, specific information on how females differ from males with regard to coenzyme Q_{10} supplementation and exercise performance is not available.

CREATINE PHOSPHATE

Creatine supplementation is one of the newest ergogenic aids to hit the sports market (Greenhaff, 1995; Maughan, 1995). The popularity of creatine soared after the 1992 Olympic Games, when British athletes, including a gold medallist, reported using the supplement (Anderson, 1993). Besides being present in the diet (flesh foods), creatine is synthesized in the liver from the amino acids lysine and arginine. Creatine is then transported to the muscle where 95% of the body's creatine is found. Within the resting muscle, 60% of this creatine is found as creatine phosphate (CP). Oral supplementation of creatine decreases endogenous synthesis, but this is reversible when supplementation stops. The creatine pool is relatively stable with approximately 1.7% (2 g) of the pool turning over daily. However, the size of this pool depends on a number of factors, such as dietary intake, gender, age and amount of muscle mass. Ingestion of 20 g of exogenous creatine (4 g daily for 5 days) increases muscle creatine levels by about 20% (Hultman et al., 1996).

Individuals with the lowest muscle creatine levels appear to respond the most to creatine supplementation (Harris et al., 1992). Thus, some individuals may benefit more than others. In addition, creatine taken with high levels of carbohydrate appears to augment creatine retention in the muscle (Green et al., 1996). However, the muscle does have an upper limit for creatine uptake that cannot be exceeded. Once the muscle is saturated, the concentration of creatine will not increase even though high doses of supplemental creatine are still being used (Greenhaff, 1995).

Within the muscle, CP is used to regenerate ATP from ADP. Since the availability of CP is one of the limiting factors in muscle performance during short-term high-intensity exercise (Greenhaff, 1995), it follows that supplemental creatine could boost muscle CP levels. If CP increases, it could increase the ability to regenerate ATP both during and after repeated bouts of high-intensity exercise. One confounding factor

in testing this assumption is that the washout period from the muscle after creatine supplementation is 4–6 weeks, which makes crossover designs impractical. Greenhaff et al. (1993) examined the effect of creatine supplementation on repeated bouts of maximal isokinetic contractions interspersed with a 1-min rest period. They found that supplementation significantly increased muscle peak torque by 5–7%. All subjects in the creatine treatment group (six males) improved with supplementation; three females were included in the study but all were in the placebo group.

Subsequent studies using high-intensity exercise, such as sprint swimming, running and cycling, have shown mixed results. Some researchers report no effect (Burke et al., 1996; Mujika et al., 1996; Redondo et al., 1996; Odland et al., 1997), while others report positive results (Balsom et al., 1993; Birch et al., 1994). These discrepancies may be due to a number of factors: (i) no increase in muscle creatine in response to supplementation due to high initial muscle creatine levels; (ii) muscle creatine is not the limiting factor in some of the exercise protocols used, such as sprint swimming; and (iii) the length of active recovery between exercise bouts varies greatly among studies. Consequently, the ergogenic effect of creatine is still debatable, and may depend on the type of exercise, the initial muscle creatine level and other factors associated with performance.

Many of the studies that have examined the ergogenic effect of creatine included females in their subject pool; however, no study has specifically examined whether females respond differently to creatine supplementation compared with men. Because many female athletes limit their intake of flesh foods or practise a vegetarian lifestyle, their intake of dietary creatine may be low. These individuals may benefit from creatine supplementation if they participate in high-intensity exercise.

Pharmacological interventions

The use of drugs to enhance athletic performance has had a long and varied history. The popularity of certain drugs waxes and wanes. In the late 1940s and 1950s, amphetamines were popular because they were purported to be used by German soldiers as stimulants to ward off fatigue and enhance performance in battle. Most recently, ephedrine has been the stimulant of choice. Anabolic steroids became popular in the 1950s after Russian athletes were suspected of taking them. The ease of testing for anabolic steroids has prompted athletes to seek drugs, such as growth hormone, that cannot be detected by urinalysis. Recent attention has also focused on clenbuterol as a drug to increase muscle mass because it is believed to have less side-effects. Athletes who want to lose weight fast or cut weight for competition have long been known to use diuretics. For more lasting weight loss, many athletes, especially female athletes, have turned to new drugs that have been developed to treat obese individuals. The following sections briefly review research on drugs used to enhance performance or alter body composition.

Drugs used as stimulants

AMPHETAMINES

Amphetamines have been used to enhance performance because they stimulate the central nervous system and also mimic sympathetic neural activity. Prior to 1950, the effects of amphetamines on performance were examined because of their potential usefulness as ergogenic aids for soldiers (Wagner, 1989). Most studies used males as subjects and found improvement in some motor tasks, although there was a large interindividual variability in the responses (Alles & Feigen, 1942; Cuthbertson & Knox, 1947). In one study of three subjects (one female), the effect of 20 mg of benzedrine on several psychomotor tasks, including reaction time, handgrip, speed of movement and steadiness, was examined in a double-blind design (Thornton et al., 1939). Although the female responded similarly to the males in several tests, she showed a more marked increase in maintained handgrip (holding time) performance (121%) compared with the two males (9% and 58%).

Karpovich (1959) investigated the effects of 10–20 mg amphetamine on treadmill run to exhaustion and performance of other track and swim tests in male college students and noted only minimal performance enhancement with the drug. Other studies also reported no performance changes when male subjects were given amphetamines (Haldi & Wynn, 1946; Blyth et al., 1960; Golding & Barnard, 1963; Blum et al., 1964; Williams & Thompson, 1973). Blum et al. (1964) did include some female subjects but their data were pooled with the males. Although there was considerable interindividual variability in the responses, some subjects showed performance benefits in most of the studies.

Smith and Beecher (1959, 1960) performed six experiments on male athletes who were given 0.2 mg·kg^{-1} amphetamine sulphate before several types of exercise. Over 67% of the athletes performed better with the amphetamines compared with the placebo group, with improvements ranging from 0.6% to 4.0%. With the drug, the athletes felt bold, elated and 'revved up' before the performance and perceived that they had improved coordination, strength and endurance.

The action of amphetamines in altering pain perception was highlighted in a field study by Cuthbertson and Knox (1947), in which 55 male soldiers were kept without sleep for 24 hours. The soldiers were then placed into three marching groups, one group receiving 15 mg methedrine, another group receiving placebo and the third group receiving either methedrine or placebo. There appeared to be no effect of the amphetamine on marching performance. However, there were more complaints of severe foot trouble in the placebo group, even though the severity of blisters was greater in the group who took the amphetamines. The number of soldiers who fell out of the march was greater in the placebo group compared with the drug group. Although performance was not enhanced by the drug, subjects felt better.

Studies that found performance benefits reported that amphetamines may mask fatigue, enhance ability to tolerate discomfort and allow subjects to exercise longer (Wyndham et al., 1971;

Chandler & Blair, 1980). However, amphetamines could also diminish performance because of a failure to detect warning signs for serious health complications, for example ignoring the early signs of heat stroke (Wyndham *et al.*, 1971). Athletes may ignore pain from injuries while taking amphetamines, which could exacerbate the injury (Laties & Weiss, 1981). We know little about the effects of amphetamines on female athletes, although there is no reason to suspect that they would be any more or less effective than in males or result in less interindividual variability in response.

The use of amphetamines in college athletes has dropped in the past 10 years for both males and females. A survey performed by the National Collegiate Athletic Association (NCAA) examined the responses of 13 914 athletes from 637 institutions; 34% of the respondents were females. It was found that 4.7% of female softball players and swimmers took amphetamines, while ≤3% of male athletes in various sports took the drug. Also, the reason athletes use amphetamines has changed. In 1993, most athletes reported that they took amphetamines in order to improve performance and provide more energy. In 1997, there was an increase in the number of respondents who reported that they used amphetamines as an appetite suppressant, while there was a significant drop in those indicating they used amphetamines to improve performance (NCAA, 1997). Amphetamines are effective appetite suppressants. However, because of their side-effects, other drugs are more commonly used for this purpose. These are described in the section on drugs used to alter body weight.

EPHEDRINE

Ephedrine is structurally related to the amphetamines and also functions as a central nervous system stimulant but is not as potent as the amphetamines (Wagner, 1991). Examples of the 'ephedrines' are ephedrine, pseudoephedrine and phenylpropanolamine (Cowan, 1994). Phenylpropanolamine is commonly found as the

active ingredient, i.e. appetite suppressant, in commercially available diet pills (Greenway, 1992).

Limited data exist concerning the effects of ephedrine on performance. Bright *et al.* (1981) studied six male subjects who were given 60 and 120 mg ephedrine (or placebo) before submaximal treadmill exercise. No significant difference was found in the time to reach 85% of predicted maximum heart rate, blood pressure or recovery heart rate. Two subjects showed sinus arrhythmias during recovery on the 120-mg dose. In a study of male cyclists, Gillies *et al.* (1996) found that 120 mg pseudoephedrine taken 120 min prior to a 40-km cycling time trial and 90 min prior to isometric strength tests did not affect cycling performance time or isometric strength of the quadriceps muscle. The authors concluded that a single therapeutic dose did not enhance performance in well-trained cyclists.

Two studies have assessed the effects of ephedrine in females. Clemons and Crosby (1993) gave 60 mg pseudoephedrine or placebo to 10 female subjects 70 min before performing a graded exercise test. There was no difference in total exercise time or several other physiological changes, except that heart rate during and after exercise was higher in the ephedrine group. Sidney and Lefcoe (1978) administered 24 mg ephedrine and 130 mg theophylline to six male and six female track athletes. These drugs did not affect simple reaction time, handgrip strength or isometric holding time but resulted in a 4% increase in the number of sit-ups that could be performed. There was no difference between the drug and placebo on time to exhaustion for a high- or low-intensity treadmill run or on psychomotor performance. Data for the females and males were not presented separately so it is not clear whether the changes were similar for males and females.

One study reported that females and males differ in their subjective response to ephedrine (Chait, 1994). Capsules containing the drug or placebo, which were distinguishable only by colour, were offered to the subjects; then on a subsequent occasion subjects were able to choose one or none. Subjects were told that capsules of the same colour always contained the same substance. Males chose ephedrine more frequently (33.3%) than females (9.3%). Males also showed a very positive mood response to the drug. This study highlights the fact that males and females may respond differently to drugs, and this may influence whether they take the drug and/or whether the drug is effective. In fact, the NCAA survey found that the use of ephedrine was quite low for female athletes (<1.9%) compared with male athletes (1.5–5.3%). About half the respondents claimed that the main reason for using ephedrine was to improve athletic performance.

Ephedrine has also been used as an agent for causing weight loss, but it is not known to what extent female athletes use the drug for this purpose. There are no studies to show that ephedrine acts as a 'fat burner' in order to promote leanness in athletes, although it is rumoured that athletes who want to maintain low body weight and who want to increase muscle definition are using ephedrine (see section Thermogenic and anorectic agents).

COCAINE

Cocaine functions as a stimulant of the central nervous system and sympathetic nervous system. It stimulates the release of noradrenaline from neurones and also blocks the reuptake of noradrenaline and dopamine, thereby potentiating the effects of these transmitters. Athletes who use cocaine do so mainly as a social drug rather than as a performance enhancer. However, the sense of euphoria that cocaine produces could allow an athlete to perceive that they are faster and stronger than they actually are (Tennant, 1984; Lombardo, 1986; Haupt, 1989).

Studies on the effects of cocaine have all been performed using only male subjects. A few early reports suggested that cocaine could increase work time, improve performance or enhance recovery (see Conlee, 1991). However, Asmussen and Bøje (1948) gave 129 mg cocaine to three male athletes 15 min before two cycling ergometer tests and found no improvement in performance.

No recent studies of the effects of cocaine ingestion on performance exist other than the effects of coca leaf chewing in Peruvian males. The leaves of the coca plant (*Erythroxylon coca*) naturally contain cocaine. These studies, which were not well controlled, reported only small benefits from chewing coca leaves (Hanna, 1970, 1971). It was concluded that coca exerted an effect by altering the perception of effort so that the effects of fatigue were reduced (Hanna, 1971). Two other studies examined the physiological response to coca chewing before exercise and found that chewers had increased fatty acid levels in the blood before the exercise and these remained elevated during exercise (Favier *et al.*, 1996; Spielvogel *et al.*, 1996). The authors suggested that the increased free fatty acid levels in the blood may benefit endurance performance, although the mechanism to explain this is not clear.

Although few studies have examined the effect of cocaine on performance, there does not seem to be any significant performance benefits from using cocaine. In fact, the euphoria that cocaine produces may cause athletes to perform poorly but think they are performing well. According to the NCAA survey, cocaine use by both males and females has declined dramatically since 1985. It appears that the reason for use is more social than any direct ergogenic benefits. The percentage of female athletes using cocaine ranges from 0.2% for track and field athletes to 1.8% for softball athletes; the range for males is 0.6–2.1%.

CAFFEINE

Several excellent reviews on caffeine and performance have been published (Dodd *et al.*, 1993; Tarnopolsky, 1994; Spriet, 1995). Caffeine may exert an ergogenic effect by acting on the central nervous system, increasing free fatty acids in the blood and/or acting directly on skeletal muscle (Spriet, 1997). In some individuals, especially those who are sensitive to caffeine, ingestion could impair performance of motor skills by exacerbating tremor (Wagner, 1991). Review of the many studies on the effects of caffeine shows that moderate doses (5–7 mg·kg^{-1}) taken about 1 hour before exercise benefits performance, with the exception of sprint exercises lasting <90 s, high-intensity exercise (>90% $\dot{V}_{O_{2max}}$) and incremental exercise tests (Tarnopolsky, 1994; Spriet, 1995). Beneficial effects of ingestion of caffeine have been found in both recreationally active and trained individuals. The mechanisms to explain the ergogenic effect that occurs across a wide variety of exercise types remain to be determined (Spriet, 1997).

Most studies of the ergogenic effect of caffeine have used males as subjects or included a small number of females; however, the female data were pooled with the male data. There may be reasons to suspect that females could respond differently to caffeine. Oestrogen and caffeine are metabolized similarly, such that oestrogen can affect the half-life of caffeine and possibly affect the response to caffeine. Urinary clearance of caffeine is reduced in females using oral contraceptive (Schwenk, 1997). Further studies of the effects of caffeine on exercise performance in females is warranted. Also, studies should control the menstrual status because of the interaction between oestrogen and caffeine (Spriet, 1997).

Females given an acute dose of caffeine exhibited increased excretion of minerals in the urine similar to that in males (Massey & Wise, 1992). Differences in body size and composition between males and females were accounted for by calculating mineral–creatinine ratios. However, because females have lower body stores of minerals, they lost proportionally more of their body stores (Massey & Wise, 1992). Considering that calcium is lost in this manner, chronic caffeine consumption could negatively affect bone mineral density. Chronic use of excessive caffeine as an ergogenic aid, in addition to normal dietary use (coffee, soda, etc.), could jeopardize mineral status in female athletes who do not ingest sufficient quantities of minerals in their diet.

Caffeine has also been used to promote weight loss but, by itself, has not been proved effective (Astrup *et al.*, 1992a). However, Donelly and McNaughton (1992) have reported that caffeine increased metabolic rate above normal levels in untrained females during, and for a short period of time after, exercise. The effectiveness of caffeine combined with exercise to enhance weight loss has not been fully investigated.

Drugs used to reduce heart rate and tremor

β-BLOCKERS

The β-adrenergic blockers prevent binding of the neurotransmitter noradrenaline to its receptors, which reduces the stimulatory effects of the sympathetic nervous system. Hence, β-blockers can reduce heart rate and tremor, a valuable effect for sporting activities like shooting where steadiness is important (Tesch, 1985; Williams, 1991). The β-blockers have proved useful in treating stage-fright in musicians, although most studies have used males as subjects (James *et al.*, 1977; Brantigan *et al.*, 1982). Those participating in sports like pistol shooting and ski jumping can benefit from the reduced anxiety provided by β-blockers (Imhof *et al.*, 1969; Siitonen *et al.*, 1997; Videman *et al.*, 1979; Antal & Good, 1980; Kruse *et al.*, 1986).

Previous studies have shown that there is a large interindividual variability in response to β-blockers; while many athletes improve performance, some show impaired performance. Very few females were included in these studies and their data were pooled with the male data, so it is not clear whether females exhibit, or benefit from, reduced heart rate and tremor after taking β-blockers. In a recent study, Eston and Thompson (1997) examined perceived exertion during exercise in a control group and in patients taking the cardioselective β-blocker atenolol. Females taking the drug had the lowest predicted maximal work rate, which suggests that the drug may affect females differently. Because β-blockers reduce heart rate, decrease cardiac output and reduce $\dot{V}_{O_{2max}}$, they probably impair performance that is metabolically stressful (Tesch, 1985; Wilmore, 1988).

Drugs used to alter body weight

ANABOLIC–ANDROGENIC STEROIDS AND GROWTH HORMONE

Anabolic steroids are synthetic derivatives of testosterone. Although they have been synthesized to maximize anabolic effects, some androgenic effects are still produced. Several reviews of anabolic–androgenic steroids and performance have been published (Haupt & Rovere, 1984; Lamb, 1984; Hough, 1990; Lombardo et al., 1991; Bahrke & Yesalis, 1994; Bahrke et al., 1996). Published studies have primarily used males as subjects. Many studies lack controls for diet and exercise and used doses lower than those used by athletes. Bhasin et al. (1996), in a well-controlled study, examined the effects of 600 mg testosterone (a supraphysiological dose) weekly for 10 weeks in four groups of males who had weight-training experience: (i) placebo with no exercise; (ii) testosterone with no exercise; (iii) placebo with resistance training; and (iv) testosterone with resistance training. Dietary intake and exercise level were controlled. The non-exercising subjects taking testosterone were found to have a larger increase in muscle size and strength than the non-exercising controls. However, the males who exercised and injected testosterone demonstrated the greatest increase in both muscle size and strength. For example, the increases in fat-free mass for the non-exercise plus placebo group, non-exercise plus testosterone group, exercise plus placebo group and exercise plus testosterone group were 0.01%, 4.6%, 2.8% and 9.3%, respectively. Also, the corresponding increases in bench-press forces were 2.9%, 12.6%, 19.8% and 37.3%.

We uncovered no studies that have assessed the effects of anabolic steroids in female athletes, although studies of therapeutic doses do show that body weight is increased (American College of Sports Medicine, 1987). In the NCAA survey, <1% of female athletes used anabolic steroids; softball players showed the highest use (0.9%). This value is consistent with the results of some studies, while others suggest that the rate of use

is higher (Strauss et al., 1985; Strauss & Yesalis, 1991; Cordova, 1996). Terney and McLain (1990) found that 3.9% of female high-school athletes and 6.6% of male high-school athletes reported taking steroids. Korkia (1996) reported that of 349 females who attended gyms in England, Scotland and Wales, eight (2.3%) responded that they had taken anabolic steroids.

Strauss and Yesalis (1991) reported that female athletes were taking steroids in order to increase strength and muscle mass, the same reasons that males take steroids. Strauss et al. (1985) reported that 10 weight-trained females who took anabolic steroids used stacking and cycling techniques and took up to nine times the manufacturer's recommended doses. Females who took steroids had abnormalities of the menstrual cycle and depressed levels of high-density lipoprotein cholesterol (Cordova, 1996). The secondary male sex characteristics caused by the androgenic effects of anabolic steroids have perhaps reduced the likelihood of female athletes taking these drugs.

HGH is a peptide hormone secreted by the anterior pituitary that regulates growth and metabolism. There are a few studies of the effects of HGH on muscle mass, and these have used young and older males as subjects (Christ et al., 1988; Rudman et al., 1990; Yarasheski et al., 1992, 1993, 1995; Deyssig et al., 1993; Taafe et al., 1994; Welle et al., 1996). Findings were fairly consistent in that HGH increased fat-free mass but did not increase protein synthesis in the muscle. Thus, HGH may increase lean body mass and decrease fat mass. However, the increase in lean tissue is probably not skeletal muscle but may reflect increases in fluid retention or increases in connective tissue or organ mass (Wirth & Gieck, 1996).

For both anabolic–androgenic steroids and HGH there is a paucity of well-controlled studies in females. It is unlikely that HGH will be any more effective at increasing muscle mass in females than it is in males. However, because females are taking anabolic–androgenic steroids, it is important to understand the effects in females. A well-controlled study, such as that of

Bhasin *et al.* (1996), using females as subjects is needed.

β_2-AGONISTS

Clenbuterol has received recent attention as a drug for enhancing muscle mass. Clenbuterol and its relatives, salbutamol (albuterol) and orciprenaline (metaproterenol), are classified as sympathomimetic amines (Cowan, 1994) and act at β_2-adrenergic receptors. When used in aerosol form, their action is relatively selective for the receptors in bronchial muscle. Aerosol forms of β_2-agonists are used in the treatment of asthma (Morton & Fitch, 1992). Clenbuterol has a long half-life of about 35 hours compared with 5 hours for salbutamol; the long half-life may allow clenbuterol to have anabolic effects (Schwenk, 1997).

In studies on animals, clenbuterol has been shown to result in muscle hypertrophy, decreases in fat deposition and conversion of slow-twitch fibres to fast-twitch fibres (Spann & Winter, 1995; Dodd *et al.*, 1996). However, there are no studies that have examined the effects of clenbuterol on muscle mass gains in humans. Two studies have assessed the effects of clenbuterol or orciprenaline on the recovery of strength and muscle mass after injury in male patients. These studies generally showed a faster recovery of strength (Maltin *et al.*, 1993; Signorile *et al.*, 1995), but only the latter study reported an improvement in muscle size. Martineau *et al.* (1992) found that salbutamol improved strength but did not affect lean body mass in healthy males. Another study examined the effect of salbutamol during a resistance training programme for 9 weeks in subjects whose gender was not specified (presumably male) and also found that the drug improved strength but not muscle mass (Caruso *et al.*, 1995). Although β_2-agonists can enhance strength, the mechanisms responsible are not clear. No change in muscle mass was found in most of these studies, although this is the primary reason athletes use these drugs. However, the amount of the drug taken by athletes is probably much greater. Whether these drugs increase strength or muscle mass in females has yet to be determined.

While recent attention has focused on the role of β_2-agonists in increasing muscle mass, earlier concern was that these drugs may exert stimulatory effects and thereby enhance performance. Because β_2-agonists are used in the treatment of asthma, it was important to identify their possible ergogenic effects in order to determine whether asthmatic athletes had an advantage when taking β_2-agonists. In the treatment of asthma these drugs are inhaled, which limits the amount administered. Three studies of males found that therapeutic aerosol doses of salbutamol or salmeterol (structurally related to salbutamol) did not produce ergogenic effects in trained athletes (Meeuwisse *et al.*, 1992; Lemmer *et al.*, 1995; Morton *et al.*, 1996). McKenzie *et al.* (1983) examined the effects of aerosol salbutamol on treadmill performance in 10 highly trained female and 9 highly trained male athletes and reported no benefit of the drug on performance. Data were analysed by gender and neither group showed an ergogenic effect. In contrast, two studies reported that inhaled salbutamol exerted an ergogenic effect on power output (Bedi *et al.*, 1988; Signorile *et al.*, 1992). One of these studies (Signorile *et al.*, 1992) tested eight males and seven females, but whether gender influenced the results is not known as the data were not analysed by gender. The differences among the studies are probably due to the fact that the latter study used recreational athletes rather than the trained athletes used in the other studies (Spann & Winter, 1995). However, Bedi *et al.* (1988) reported performance benefits of salbutamol in trained cyclists (14 males and 1 female). Thus, the data are equivocal on whether aerosol β_2-agonists improve performance. Also, whether these drugs have different effects in males and females has not been comprehensively examined, but it seems unlikely.

THERMOGENIC AND ANORECTIC AGENTS

Many female athletes try to achieve a low body weight because they believe it is associated with improved performance. When dieting fails, some athletes have turned to pharmacological interventions. Drugs have been identified that act as agonists to receptors in the sympathetic nervous system, which is a primary regulator of dietary thermogenesis (Landsberg & Young, 1993). Ephedrine has both thermogenic (energy expending) and anorectic (appetite suppressant) effects. Other drugs function primarily as anorectic agents and suppress appetite by increasing catecholamine or serotonin levels. Unlike most of the studies examined in this chapter, studies of this group of drugs have predominantly used females as subjects.

Several studies have reported that ephedrine is more effective than placebo in reducing weight in obese subjects (Dulloo & Miller, 1986; Astrup *et al.*, 1992b; Pasquali & Casimirri, 1993) and reducing nitrogen loss, thereby sparing protein (Pasquali *et al.*, 1987; Dulloo, 1993). Ephedrine also prevents the decrease in resting metabolic rate associated with low-calorie diets (Pasquali *et al.*, 1992). To enhance its effectiveness in producing weight loss, ephedrine has been coupled to caffeine and aspirin, which potentiate the sympathetic effects of ephedrine. A combination of ephedrine and caffeine increases energy expenditure and enhances weight loss in obese subjects (Astrup *et al.*, 1991, 1992c; Astrup & Toubro, 1993; Breum *et al.*, 1994). Astrup and Toubro (1993) estimated that about 80% of the weight loss was due to an anorectic effect and 20% to a thermogenic effect. The combination of ephedrine, caffeine and aspirin is also effective in producing weight loss in obese subjects (Daly *et al.*, 1993).

The effectiveness of these drugs for those who are already relatively lean (such as athletes) has not been determined. The reason the drugs may be effective for obese subjects is that these individuals have a lower thermogenesis and the drugs increase thermogenesis (Geissler, 1993). In fact, ephedrine, aspirin and caffeine were more effective in increasing the thermic response in obese compared with lean subjects (Horton & Geissler, 1991). Another reason why athletes should be discouraged from using these drugs is that they have side-effects that could hinder athletic performance.

Amphetamines and the newer adrenergic drugs (diethylpropion, phentermine and mazindol) have been used as anorectic drugs and act as catecholaminergic agents (Atkinson & Hubbard, 1994). Recently, the drugs fenfluramine (dexfenfluramine) and fluoxetine, which act as serotoninergic agents, have also proved successful as anorectic agents (Silverstone & Goodall, 1992). Several studies reported that fenfluramine (Guy-Grand *et al.*, 1989; Guy-Grand, 1992; Breum *et al.*, 1994; O'Connor *et al.*, 1995) and fluoxetine (currently approved for the treatment of depression) result in weight loss in obese subjects (Wise, 1992; Stinson *et al.*, 1992). Due to heart valve problems and cardiac disturbances in patients taking fenfluramine, this drug was withdrawn from the maket in 1997 at the Food and Drug Administration's request.

Pharmacological agents like ephedrine that increase energy expenditure may impair performance because they act on the sympathetic nervous system and can increase tremor and nervousness and exert effects on the cardiovascular system. Anorectic drugs may also result in adverse symptoms that can impair ability to accomplish optimal training and performance. Thus, pharmacological agents are more likely to impair performance than they are to benefit performance by inducing weight loss. It is still unclear how effective these drugs are in nonobese subjects. Moreover, weight loss caused by these drugs is regained when the diet pills are discontinued (Munro *et al.*, 1992) and many weight-loss drugs have serious side-effects.

DIURETICS

Diuretics are used by athletes to induce rapid weight loss. Many diuretics act by blocking the reabsorption of electrolytes in the kidneys, thus facilitating water loss from the body. Wrestlers, light-weight crew, body-builders and jockeys who must make a particular weight classification or who want to reduce body weight for competition have used diuretics. Diuretics can produce a weight loss of about 3–4% within a 24-hour period (Claremont *et al.*, 1976; Caldwell *et al.*, 1984; Wagner, 1991). Laboratory studies have found that use of diuretics can impair performance (Steen, 1991; Horswill, 1994), although whether diuretics adversely affect performance during competition has not been determined. However, diuretics probably do not impair performance that is not metabolically stressful.

The extent of diuretic use by female athletes is not known, but diuretics represent about 6% of the drugs abused by athletes (Al-Zaki & Talbot-Stern, 1996). Female athletes may be taking diuretics in order to reduce the effect of premenstrual bloating. Also, diuretic use often becomes part of the behaviour of those with eating disorders. Chronic use of diuretics can lead to electrolyte imbalance, which can produce symptoms of muscle cramps, spasms and paralysis, as well as disturbances in cardiac function that can be life-threatening.

Conclusion

Adequate carbohydrate before, during and after exercise is important in ensuring optimal performance. However, there are some data to suggest that a high-carbohydrate diet may not be as effective in females as it is in males, but this warrants further study. Amino acid supplements, MCTs, carnitine and coenzyme Q_{10} have not proved beneficial for males, and there is no reason to suspect that they would be any more effective for females. The most popular nutritional supplement today is probably creatine. Several studies have found that creatine supplementation enhances performance of short-term high-intensity exercise. Because many females limit their intake of meat or are vegetarians, they may have lower creatine stores. Further research is needed to determine whether creatine may be an even more effective performance enhancer in females than males.

It appears that fewer females compared with males are taking drugs in order to improve performance. However, a small percentage of females are using drugs so it is important to determine whether these drugs are effective. Because of the large interindividual variability in response to drugs, it is uncertain whether a given individual will experience an enhancement of performance. Furthermore, most drugs are probably contraindicated as ergogenic aids because of the side-effects. For example, ephedrine, which is often considered harmless by athletes, results in augmentation of myocardial contraction and cardiac output, elevated systolic blood pressure and can produce dizziness, headache, irritability and anxiety. There is now a strong movement in the USA to increase the regulation of ephedrine. Female athletes are using drugs to induce weight loss, but these drugs are also contraindicated because of side-effects that could impair performance. There is a lack of information to show that these drugs are effective in relatively lean individuals as studies have used obese subjects. Moreover, the discontinuation of drugs that induce weight loss results in regain of the weight.

There is a paucity of research on female athletes with regard to both nutritional and pharmacological ergogenic aids. To improve performance in female athletes as well as to safeguard their health, it is important that future research identifies possible ergogenic and ergolytic effects of these supplements specifically for female subjects.

References

Ahlborg, G., Felig, P., Hagenfeldt, L., Hendler, R. & Wahren, J. (1974) Substrate turnover during prolonged exercise in man. *Journal of Clinical Investigation* **53**, 1080–1090.

Alles, G.A. & Feigen, G.A. (1942) The influence of benzedrine on work-decrement and patellar reflex. *American Journal of Physiology* **136**, 392–400.

Al-Zaki, T. & Talbot-Stern, J. (1996) A bodybuilder with diuretic abuse presenting with symptomatic hypotension and hyperkalemia. *American Journal of Emergency Medicine* **14**, 96–98.

American College of Sports Medicine (1987) Position stand on the use of anabolic–androgenic steroids in sports. *Medicine and Science in Sports and Exercise* **19**, 534–539.

Anderson, O. (1993) Creatine propels British athletes to Olympic gold medals: is creatine the one true ergogenic aid? *Running Research News* **9**, 1–5.

Antal, L.C. & Good, C.S. (1980) Effects of oxprenolol on pistol shooting under stress. *Practitioner* **224**, 755–760.

Asmussen, E. & Bøje, O. (1948) The effect of alcohol and some drugs on the capacity for work. *Acta Physiologica Scandinavica* **15**, 109–118.

Astrup, A. & Toubro, S. (1993) Thermogenic, metabolic,

and cardiovascular responses to ephedrine and caffeine in man. *International Journal of Obesity* **17** (Suppl. 1), S41–S43.

Astrup, A., Toubro, S., Cannon, S., Hein, P. & Madsen, J. (1991) Thermogenic synergism between ephedrine and caffeine in healthy volunteers: a double-blind, placebo-controlled study. *Metabolism* **40**, 323–329.

Astrup, A., Toubro, S., Christensen, N.J. & Quaade, F. (1992a) Pharmacology of thermogenic drugs. *American Journal of Clinical Nutrition* **55**, 246S–248S.

Astrup, A., Breum, L., Toubro, S., Hein, P. & Quaade, F. (1992b) The effect and safety of an ephedrine/caffeine compound compared to ephedrine, caffeine and placebo in obese subjects on an energy restricted diet. A double blind trial. *International Journal of Obesity* **16**, 269–277.

Astrup, A., Buemann, B., Christensen, N.J. *et al.* (1992c) The effect of ephedrine/caffeine mixture on energy expenditure and body composition in obese women. *Metabolism* **41**, 686–688.

Atkinson, R.L. & Hubbard, V.S. (1994) Report on the NIH workshop on pharmacologic treatment of obesity. *American Journal of Clinical Nutrition* **60**, 153–156.

Bach, A.C. & Babayan, V.K. (1982) Medium-chain triglycerides: an update. *American Journal of Clinical Nutrition* **36**, 950–962.

Bahrke, M.S. & Yesalis, C.E. III (1994) Weight training: a potential confounding factor in examining the psychological and behavioral effects of anabolic–androgenic steroids. *Sports Medicine* **18**, 309–318.

Bahrke, M.S., Yesalis, C.E. III & Wright, J.E. (1996) Psychological and behavioural effects of endogenous testosterone and anabolic–androgenic steroids: an update. *Sports Medicine* **22**, 367–390.

Balsom, P.D., Ekblom, B., Soderlund, K., Sjodin, B. & Hultman, E. (1993) Creatine supplementation and dynamic high-intensity intermittent exercise. *Scandinavian Journal of Medicine and Science in Sports* **3**, 143–149.

Barnett, C., Costill, D.L., Vukovich, M.D. *et al.* (1994) Effect of L-carnitine supplementation on muscle and blood carnitine content and lactate accumulation during high-intensity sprint cycling. *International Journal of Sports Nutrition* **4**, 280–288.

Beckers, E.J., Jeukendrup, A.E., Brouns, F., Wagenmakers, A.J.M. & Saris, W.H.M. (1992) Gastric emptying of carbohydrate–medium chain triglyceride suspensions at rest. *International Journal of Sports Medicine* **13**, 581–584.

Bedi, J.F., Gong, H. Jr & Horvath, S.M. (1988) Enhancement of exercise performance with inhaled albuterol. *Canadian Journal of Sport Sciences* **13**, 144–148.

Berning, J. (1996) The role of medium-chain triglycerides in exercise. *International Journal of Sports Nutrition* **6**, 121–133.

Beyer, R.E. (1994) The role of ascorbate in antioxidant protection of biomembranes: interaction with vitamin E and coenzyme Q. *Journal of Bioenergetics and Biomembranes* **26**, 349–358.

Bhasin, S., Storer, T.W., Berman, N. *et al.* (1996) The effects of supraphysiologic doses of testosterone on muscle size and strength in normal men. *New England Journal of Medicine* **335**, 1–7.

Bigard, A.X., Lavier, P., Ullmann, L., Legrand, H., Douce, P. & Guezennec, C.Y. (1996) Branched-chain amino acid supplementation during repeated prolonged skiing exercises at altitude. *International Journal of Sports Nutrition* **6**, 295–306.

Birch, R., Noble, D. & Greenhaff, P.L. (1994) The influence of dietary creatine supplementation on performance during repeated bouts of maximal isokinetic cycling in man. *European Journal of Applied Physiology* **69**, 268–270.

Blomstrand, E., Andersson, S., Hassmen, P., Ekblom, B. & Newsholme, E.A. (1995) Effect of branched-chain amino acid and carbohydrate supplementation on the exercise-induced change in plasma and muscle concentration of amino acids in human subjects. *Acta Physiologica Scandinavica* **153**, 87–96.

Blomstrand, E., Hassmen, P., Ek, S., Ekblom, B. & Newsholme, E.A. (1997) Influence of ingesting a solution of branched-chain amino acids on perceived exertion during exercise. *Acta Physiologica Scandinavica* **159**, 41–49.

Blum, B., Stern, M.H. & Melville, K.I. (1964) A comparative evaluation of the action of depressant and stimulant drugs on human performance. *Psychopharmacologia* **6**, 173–177.

Blyth, C.S., Allen, E.M. & Lovingood, B.W. (1960) Effects of amphetamines (Dexedrine) and caffeine on subjects exposed to heat and exercise stress. *Research Quarterly* **31**, 553–559.

Borghouts, L., Juekendrup, A.E., Saris, W.H.M., Brouns, F. & Wagenmakers, A.J.M. (1995) No effect of medium chain triglyceride (MCT) ingestion during prolonged exercise on muscle glycogen utilization. *Medicine and Science in Sports and Exercise* **27** (Suppl. 5), S101.

Brantigan, C.O., Brantigan, T.A. & Joseph, N. (1982) Effect of beta blockade and beta stimulation on stage fright. *American Journal of Medicine* **72**, 88–94.

Brass, E.P. & Hiatt, W.R. (1994) Minireview: carnitine metabolism during exercise. *Life Sciences* **54**, 1383–1393.

Braun, B., Clarkson, P.M., Freedson, P.S. & Kohl, R.L. (1991) Effects of coenzyme Q_{10} supplementation on exercise performance, $\dot{V}O_{2max}$, and lipid peroxidation in trained cyclists. *International Journal of Sports Nutrition* **1**, 353–365.

Breum, L., Pedersen, J.K., Ahlstrøm, F. & Frimodt-Møller, J. (1994) Comparison of an ephedrine/caffeine combination and dexfenfluramine in the treatment of obesity. A double-blind multi-centre trial in general practice. *International Journal of Obesity* **18**, 99–103.

Bright, T.P., Sandage, B.W. & Fletcher, H.P. (1981) Selected cardiac and metabolic responses to pseudoephedrine with exercise. *Journal of Clinical Pharmacology* **21**, 488–492.

Broquist, H.P. (1994) Carnitine. In M.E. Shils, J.A. Olson & M. Shike (eds) *Modern Nutrition in Health and Disease*, 8th edn, pp. 459–465. Lea & Febiger, Philadelphia.

Bucci, L.R. (1994) Nutritional ergogenic aids. In I.Wolinsky & J.F. Hickson (eds) *Nutrition in Exercise and Sport*, 2nd edn, pp. 295–346. CRC Press, Boca Raton, Florida.

Bucci, L.R., Hickson, J.F., Wolinsky, I. & Pivarnik, J.M. (1992) Ornithine supplementation and insulin release in bodybuilders. *International Journal of Sports Nutrition* **2**, 287–291.

Burke, L.M., Pyne, D.B. & Telford, R.D. (1996) Effect of oral creatine supplementation on single-effort sprint performance in elite swimmers. *International Journal of Sports Nutrition* **6**, 222–233.

Caldwell, J.E., Ahonen, E. & Nousiainen, U. (1984) Differential effects of sauna-, diuretic-, and exercise-induced hypohydration. *Journal of Applied Physiology* **57**, 1018–1023.

Caruso, J.F., Signorile, J.F., Perry, A.C. *et al.* (1995) The effects of albuterol and isokinetic exercise on the quadriceps muscle group. *Medicine and Science in Sports and Exercise* **27**, 1471–1476.

Chait, L.D. (1994) Factors influencing the reinforcing and subjective effects of ephedrine in humans. *Psychopharmacology* **113**, 381–387.

Chandler, J.V. & Blair, S.N. (1980) The effect of amphetamines on selected physiological components related to athletic success. *Medicine and Science in Sports and Exercise* **12**, 65–69.

Christ, D.M., Peake, G.T., Egan, P.A. & Waters, D.L. (1988) Body composition response to exogenous GH during training in highly conditioned adults. *Journal of Applied Physiology* **65**, 579–584.

Claremont, A.D., Costill, D.L., Fink, W. & Van Handel, P. (1976) Heat tolerance following diuretic induced dehydration. *Medicine and Science in Sports and Exercise* **8**, 239–243.

Clarkson, P.M. (1992) Nutritional ergogenic aids: carnitine. *International Journal of Sports Nutrition* **2**, 185–190.

Clemons, J.M. & Crosby, S.L. (1993) Cardiopulmonary and subjective effects of a 60 mg dose of pseudoephedrine on graded treadmill exercise. *Journal of Sports Medicine and Physical Fitness* **33**, 405–412.

Coggan, A.R. & Coyle, E.F. (1991) Carbohydrate ingestion during prolonged exercise: effects on metabolism and performance. *Exercise and Sport Sciences Reviews* **19**, 1–40.

Conlee, R.K. (1991) Amphetamine, caffeine, and cocaine. In D.R. Lamb & M.H.Williams (eds) *Perspectives in Exercise Science and Sports Medicine, Vol. 4. Ergogenics: Enhancement of Performance in Exercise and Sport*, pp. 285–329. Brown and Benchmark, Carmel, Indiana.

Constantin-Teodosiu, D., Howell, S. & Greenhaff, P.L. (1996) Carnitine metabolism in human muscle fiber types during submaximal dynamic exercise. *Journal of Applied Physiology* **80**, 1061–1064.

Cordova, M.L. (1996) Steroid use and the female athlete. *Strength and Conditioning* **18**, 17–19

Costill, D.L. & Hargreaves, M. (1992) **Carbohydrate** nutrition and fatigue. *Sports Medicine* **13**, 86–92.

Cowan, D.A. (1994) Drug abuse. In M. Harries, C. Williams, W.D. Stanish & L.J. Micheli (eds) *Oxford Textbook of Sports Medicine*, pp. 314–329. Oxford University Press, New York.

Coyle, E.F. (1992) Carbohydrate supplementation during exercise. *Journal of Nutrition* **122**, 788–795.

Coyle, E.F. (1995) Substrate utilization during exercise in active people. *American Journal of Clinical Nutrition* **61** (Suppl.), 968S–979S.

Cuthbertson, D.P. & Knox, J.A.C. (1947) The effects of analeptics on the fatigued subject. *Journal of Physiology* **106**, 42–58.

Daly, P.R., Krieger, D.R., Dulloo, A.G., Young, J.B. & Landsberg, L. (1993) Ephedrine, caffeine and aspirin: safety and efficacy for treatment of human obesity. *International Journal of Obesity* **17** (Suppl. 1), S73–S78.

Davis, J.M. (1995) Carbohydrate, branched-chain amino acids, and endurance: the central fatigue hypothesis. *International Journal of Sports Nutrition* **5**, S29–S38.

Décombaz, J., Arnaud, M.J., Milon, H. *et al.* (1983) Energy metabolism of medium-chain triglycerides vs. carbohydrates during exercise. *European Journal of Applied Physiology* **52**, 9–14.

Décombaz, J., Gmuender, B., Sierro, G. & Cerretelli, P. (1992) Muscle carnitine after strenuous endurance exercise. *Journal of Applied Physiology* **72**, 423–427.

Décombaz, J., Deriza, O., Acheson, K., Gmuender, B. & Jequier, E. (1993) Effect of L-carnitine on submaximal exercise metabolism after depletion of muscle glycogen. *Medicine and Science in Sports and Exercise* **25**, 733–740.

Deyssig, R., Frisch, H., Blum, W.F. & Waldhör, T. (1993) Effect of growth hormone treatment on hormonal parameters, body composition and strength in athletes. *Acta Endocrinologica* **128**, 313–318.

Dodd, S.L., Herb, R.A. & Powers, S.K. (1993) Caffeine and exercise performance: an update. *Sports Medicine* **15**, 14–23.

Dodd, S.L., Powers, S.K., Vrabas, I.S., Criswell, D.,

Stetson, S. & Hussain, R. (1996) Effects of clenbuterol on contractile and biochemical properties of skeletal muscle. *Medicine and Science in Sports and Exercise* **28**, 669–676.

Donelly, K. & McNaughton, L. (1992) The effects of two levels of caffeine ingestion on excess postexercise oxygen consumption in untrained women. *European Journal of Applied Physiology* **65**, 459–463.

Dulloo, A.G. (1993) Ephedrine, xanthines and prostaglandin-inhibitors: actions and interactions in the stimulation of thermogenesis. *International Journal of Obesity* **17** (Suppl. 1), S35–S40.

Dulloo, A.G. & Miller, D.S. (1986) The thermic properties of ephedrine/methylxanthine mixtures: human studies. *International Journal of Obesity* **10**, 467–481.

Eston, R.G. & Thompson, M. (1997) Use of ratings of perceived exertion for predicting maximal work rate and prescribing exercise intensity in patients taking atenolol. *British Journal of Sports Medicine* **31**, 114–119.

Fallowfield, J.L. & Williams, C. (1993) Carbohydrate intake and recovery from prolonged exercise. *International Journal of Sports Nutrition* **3**, 150–164.

Favier, R., Caceres, E., Koubi, H., Sempore, B., Sauvain, M. & Spielvogel, H. (1996) Effects of coca chewing on hormonal and metabolic responses during prolonged submaximal exercise. *Journal of Applied Physiology* **80**, 650–655.

Geissler, C.A. (1993) Effects of weight loss, ephedrine and aspirin on energy expenditure in obese women. *International Journal of Obesity* **17** (Suppl. 1), S45–S48.

Gillies, H., Derman, W.E., Noakes, T.D., Smith, P., Evans, A. & Gabriels, G. (1996) Pseudoephedrine is without ergogenic effects during prolonged exercise. *Journal of Applied Physiology* **81**, 2611–2617.

Golding, L.A. & Barnard, J.R. (1963) The effect of *d*-amphetamine sulfate on physical performance. *Journal of Sports Medicine and Physical Fitness* **3**, 221–224.

Green, A.L., Simpson, E.J., Littlewood, J.J., Macdonald, I.A. & Greenhaff, P.L. (1996) Carbohydrate ingestion augments creatine retention during creatine feeding in humans. *Acta Physiologica Scandinavica* **158**, 195–202.

Greenhaff, P.L. (1995) Creatine and its application as an ergogenic aid. *International Journal of Sports Nutrition* **5**, S100–S110.

Greenhaff, P.L., Casey, A., Short, A.H., Harris, R., Soderlund, K. & Hultman, E. (1993) Influence of oral creatine supplementation on muscle torque during repeated bouts of maximal voluntary exercise in man. *Clinical Science* **84**, 565–571.

Greenway, F.L. (1992) Clinical studies with phenylpropanolamine: a metaanalysis. *American Journal of Clinical Nutrition* **55**, 203S–205S.

Grivetti, L.E., Applegate, E.A., Clarkson, P.M., Grandjean, A.C., McDonald, R.B. & Tipton, C.M. (1996) From ancient Olympia to modern Atlanta: celebration of the Olympic Centennial. *Nutrition Today* **31**, 241–249.

Guy-Grand, B. (1992) Clinical studies with *d*-fenfluramine. *American Journal of Clinical Nutrition* **55**, 173S–176S.

Guy-Grand, B., Apfelbaum, M., Crepaldi, G., Gries, A., Lafebvre, P. & Turner, P. (1989) International trial of long-term dexfenfluramine in obesity. *Lancet* **ii**, 1142–1145.

Haldi, H. & Wynn, W. (1946) Action of drugs on efficiency of swimmers. *Research Quarterly* **17**, 96–101.

Hanna, J.M. (1970) The effects of coca chewing on exercise in the Quechua of Peru. *Human Biology* **42**, 1–11.

Hanna, J.M. (1971) Further studies on the effects of coca chewing on exercise. *Human Biology* **43**, 200–209.

Harris, R.C., Soderlund, K. & Hultman, E. (1992) Elevation of creatine in resting and exercised muscle of normal subjects by creatine supplementation. *Clinical Science* **83**, 367–374.

Haupt, H.A. (1989) Drugs in athletics. *Clinics in Sports Medicine* **8**, 561–582.

Haupt, H.A. & Rovere, G.D. (1984) Anabolic steroids: a review of the literature. *American Journal of Sports Medicine* **12**, 469–484.

Heinonen, O.J. (1996) Carnitine and physical exercise. *Sports Medicine* **22**, 109–132.

Horowitz, J.F., Mora-Rodriquez, R. & Coyle, E.F. (1995) The effect of pre-exercise medium-chain triglyceride ingestion on muscle glycogen utilization during high-intensity exercise. *Medicine and Science in Sports and Exercise* **27** (Suppl.), S203.

Horswill, C.A. (1994) Physiology and nutrition for wrestling. In D.R. Lamb, H.G. Knuttgen & R. Murray (eds) *Perspectives in Exercise Science and Sports Medicine, Vol. 7. Physiology and Nutrition for Competitive Sport*, pp. 131–180. Cooper Publishing Group, Carmel, Indiana.

Horton, T.J. & Geissler, C.A. (1991) Aspirin potentiates the effect of ephedrine on the thermogenic response to a meal in obese but not lean women. *International Journal of Obesity* **15**, 359–366.

Hough, D.O. (1990) Anabolic steroids and ergogenic aids. *American Family Physician* **41**, 1157–1164.

Hultman, E., Söderlund, K., Timmons, J.A., Cederblad, G. & Greenhaff, P.L. (1996) Muscle creatine loading in men. *Journal of Applied Physiology* **81**, 232–237.

Imhof, P.R., Blaatter., K., Fuccella, M. & Turri, M. (1969) Beta-blockade and emotional tachycardia; radiotelemetric investigations in ski jumpers. *Journal of Applied Physiology* **27**, 366–369.

James, I.M., Griffith, D.N.W., Pearson, R.M. & Newbury, P. (1977) Effect of oxyprenolol on stage-fright in musicians. *Lancet* **ii**, 952–954.

Jenkins, R.R. (1993) Exercise, oxidative stress, and

antioxidants: a review. *International Journal of Sports Nutrition* 3, 356–375.

Jeukendrup, A.E., Saris, W.H.M., Schrauwen, P., Brouns, F. & Wagenmarkers, A.J.M. (1995) Metabolic availability of medium-chain triglycerides coingested with carbohydrate during prolonged exercise. *Journal of Applied Physiology* 79, 756–762.

Johnson, R.C., Young, S.K., Cotter, R., Lin, L. & Rowe, W.B. (1990) Medium-chain-triglyceride lipid emulsion: metabolism and tissue distribution. *American Journal of Clinical Nutrition* 52, 502–508.

Kanter, M.M. & Williams, M.H. (1995) Antioxidants, carnitine, and choline as putative ergogenic aids. *International Journal of Sports Nutrition* 5, S120–S131.

Karlsson, J. (1997) *Antioxidants and Exercise.* Human Kinetics Publishers, Champaign, Illinois.

Karlsson, J., Diamant, B., Edlund, P.O., Lund, B., Folkers, K. & Theorell, H. (1992) Plasma ubiquinone, alpha-tocopherol and cholesterol in man. *International Journal for Vitamin and Nutrition Research* 62, 160–164.

Karlsson, J., Lin, L., Sylven, C. & Jansson, E. (1996) Muscle ubiquinone in healthy physically active males. *Molecular and Cellular Biochemistry* 156, 169–172.

Karpovich, P.V. (1959) Effect of amphetamine sulfate on athletic performance. *Journal of the American Medical Association* 170, 558–561.

Keith, R.E., O'Keeffe, K.A., Blessing, D.L. & Wilson, G.D. (1991) Alterations in dietary carbohydrate, protein, and fat intake and mood state in trained female cyclists. *Medicine and Science in Sports and Exercise* 23, 212–216.

Korkia, P. (1996) Use of anabolic steroids has been reported by 9% of men attending gymnasiums. *British Medical Journal* 313, 1009.

Kruse, P., Ladefoged, J., Nielsen, U., Paulev, P.-E. & Sørensen, J.P. (1986) β-Blockade used in precision sports: effect on pistol shooting performance. *Journal of Applied Physiology* 61, 417–420.

Laaksone, R., Fogelholm, M., Himberg, J.J., Laakso, J. & Salorinne, Y. (1995) Ubiquinone supplementation and exercise capacity in trained young and older men. *European Journal of Applied Physiology* 72, 95–100.

Lamb, D.R. (1984) Anabolic steroids in athletics: how well do they work and how dangerous are they? *American Journal of Sports Medicine* 12, 31–38.

Landsberg, L. & Young, J.B. (1993) Sympathoadrenal activity and obesity: physiological rationale for the use of adrenergic thermogenic drugs. *International Journal of Obesity* 17, S29–S34.

Laties, V.G. & Weiss, B. (1981) The amphetamine margin in sports. *Federation Proceedings* 40, 2689–2692.

Lehmann, M., Huonker, M., Dimeo, F. *et al.* (1995)

Serum amino acid concentrations in nine athletes before and after the 1993 Colmar Ultra Triathlon. *International Journal of Sports Medicine* 16, 155–159.

Lemmer, J.T., Fleck, S.J., Wallach, J.M. *et al.* (1995) The effects of albuterol on power output in non-asthmatic athletes. *International Journal of Sports Medicine* 16, 243–249.

Lemon, P.W.R. (1995) Do athletes need more protein and amino acids? *International Journal of Sports Nutrition* 5, S39–S61.

Lombard, K.A., Olson, A.L., Nelson, S.E. & Rebouche, C.J. (1989) Carnitine status of lactoovovegetarians and strict vegetarian adults and children. *American Journal of Clinical Nutrition* 50, 301–306.

Lombardo, J.A. (1986) Stimulants and athletic performance (Part 2): cocaine and nicotine. *Physician and Sportsmedicine* 14, 85–90.

Lombardo, J.A., Hickson, R.C. & Lamb, D.R. (1991) Anabolic/androgenic steroids and growth hormone. In D.R. Lamb & M.H. Williams (eds) *Perspectives in Exercise Science and Sports Medicine, Vol. 4. Ergogenics: Enhancement of Performance in Exercise and Sport,* pp. 249–284. Wm. C. Brown Publishers, Dubuque, Iowa.

Macintyre, J.G. (1987) Growth hormone and athletes. *Sports Medicine* 4, 129–142.

McKenzie, D.C., Rhodes, E.C., Stirling, D.R. *et al.* (1983) Salbutamol and treadmill performance in non-atopic athletes. *Medicine and Science in Sports and Exercise* 15, 520–522.

Malm, C., Svensson, M., Sjöberg, B., Ekblom, B. & Sjödin, B. (1996) Supplementation with ubiquinone-10 causes cellular damage during intense exercise. *Acta Physiologica Scandinavica* 157, 511–512.

Maltin, C.A., Delday, M.I., Watson, J.S. *et al.* (1993) Clenbuterol, a β-adrenoceptor agonist, increases relative muscle strength in orthopaedic patients. *Clinical Science* 84, 651–654.

Maresh, C.M., Gabaree, C.L., Hoffman, J.R. *et al.* (1994) Anaerobic power responses to amino acid nutritional supplementation. *International Journal of Sports Nutrition* 4, 366–377.

Martineau, L., Horan, M.A., Rothwell, N.J. & Little, R.A. (1992) Salbutamol, a β$_2$-adrenoceptor agonist, increases skeletal muscle strength in young men. *Clinical Science* 83, 615–621.

Massey, L.K. & Wise, K.J. (1992) Impact of gender and age on urinary water and mineral excretion responses to acute caffeine doses. *Nutrition Research* 12, 605–612.

Massicotte, D., Peronnet, F., Brisson, G.R. & Hillaire-Marcel, C. (1992) Oxidation of exogenous medium-chain free fatty acids during prolonged exercise: comparison with glucose. *Journal of Applied Physiology* 73, 1334–1339.

Maughan, R.J. (1995) Creatine supplementation and

exercise performance. *International Journal of Sports Nutrition* **5**, 94–101.

Meeusen, R. & De Meirleir, K. (1995) Exercise and brain neurotransmission. *Sports Medicine* **20**, 160–188.

Meeuwisse, W.H., McKenzie, D.C., Hopkins, S.R. & Road, J.D. (1992) The effect of salbuterol on performance in elite nonasthmatic athletes. *Medicine and Science in Sports and Exercise* **24**, 1161–1166.

Morton, A.R. & Fitch, K.D. (1992) Asthmatic drugs and competitive sport: an update. *Sports Medicine* **14**, 228–242.

Morton, A.R., Joyce, K., Papalia, S.M., Carroll, N.G. & Fitch, K.D. (1996) Is salmeterol ergogenic? *Clinics in Sports Medicine* **6**, 220–225.

Mujika, I., Chatard, J., Lacoste, L., Barale, F. & Geyssant, A. (1996) Creatine supplementation does not improve sprint performance in competitive swimmers. *Medicine and Science in Sports and Exercise* **28**, 1435–1441.

Munro, J.F., Scott, C. & Hodge, J. (1992) Appraisal of the clinical value of serotoninergic drugs. *American Journal of Clinical Nutrition* **55**, 189S–192S.

NCAA (1997) *NCAA Study of Substance Use and Abuse Habits of College Student Athletes*. National Collegiate Athletic Association.

Nicklas, B.J., Hackney, A.C. & Sharp, R.L. (1989) The menstrual cycle and exercise: performance, muscle glycogen, and substrate response. *International Journal of Sports Medicine* **10**, 264–269.

O'Connor, H.T., Richman, R.M., Steinbeck, K.S. & Caterson, I.D. (1995) Dexfenfluramine treatment of obesity: a double blind trial with post trial follow up. *International Journal of Obesity* **19**, 181–189.

Odland, L.M., MacDougall, J.D., Tarnopolsky, M.A., Elorriaga, A. & Borgmann, A. (1997) Effect of oral creatine supplementation on muscle [Pcr] and short-term maximum power output. *Medicine and Science in Sports and Exercise* **29**, 216–219.

Pasquali, R. & Casimirri, F. (1993) Clinical aspects of ephedrine in the treatment of obesity. *International Journal of Obesity* **17**, S65–S68.

Pasquali, R., Cesari, M.P., Melchionda, N., Stefani, C., Raitano, A. & Labo, G. (1987) Does ephedrine promote weight loss in low-energy-adapted obese women? *International Journal of Obesity* **11**, 163–168.

Pasquali, R., Casimirri, F., Melchionda, N. *et al.* (1992) Effects of chronic administration of ephedrine during very-low-calorie diets on energy expenditure, protein metabolism and hormone levels in obese subjects. *Clinical Science* **82**, 85–92.

Phillips, S.M., Atkinson, S.A., Tarnopolsky, M.A. & MacDougall, J.D. (1993) Gender differences in leucine kinetics and nitrogen balance in endurance athletes. *Journal of Applied Physiology* **75**, 2134–2141.

Porter, D.A., Costill, D.L., Zachwieja, J.J. *et al.* (1995) The effect of oral coenzyme Q_{10} on the exercise toler-

ance of middle-aged, untrained men. *International Journal of Sports Medicine* **16**, 421–427.

Redondo, D.R., Dowling, E.A., Graham, B.L., Almada, A.L. & Williams, M.H. (1996) The effect of oral creatine monohydrate supplementation on running velocity. *International Journal of Sports Nutrition* **6**, 213–221.

Rudman, D., Feller, A.G., Nagraj, H.S. *et al.* (1990) Effects of human growth hormone in men over 60 years old. *New England Journal of Medicine* **323**, 1–6.

Schwenk, T.L. (1997) Psychoactive drugs and athletic performance. *Physician and Sportsmedicine* **25**, 32–46.

Sherman, W.M. (1991) Carbohydrate feedings before and after exercise. In D.R. Lamb & M.H. Williams (eds) *Perspectives in Exercise Science and Sports Medicine, Vol. 4. Ergogenics: Enhancement of Performance in Exercise and Sport*, pp. 1–27. Wm C. Brown Publishers, Ann Arbor, Michigan.

Sherman, W.M. (1995) Metabolism of sugars and physical performance. *American Journal of Clinical Nutrition* **62** (Suppl.), 228S–241S.

Sherman, W.M. & Wimer, G.S. (1991) Insufficient dietary carbohydrate during training: does it impair athletic performance? *International Journal of Sports Nutrition* **1**, 28–44.

Sidney, K.H. & Lefcoe, N.M. (1978) Effects of tedral upon exercise performance: a double-blind cross-over study. In F. Landry & W.A.R. Organ (eds) *Sports Medicine*, pp. 297–299. Symposium Specialists, Miami.

Signorile, J.F., Kaplan, T.A., Applegate, B. & Perry, A.C. (1992) Effects of acute inhalation of the bronchodilator, albuterol, on power output. *Medicine and Science in Sports and Exercise* **24**, 638–642.

Signorile, J.F., Banovac, K., Gomez, M., Flipse, D., Caruso, J.F. & Lowensteyn, I. (1995) Increased muscle strength in paralyzed patients after spinal cord injury: effect of beta-2 adrenergic agonist. *Archives of Physical Medicine and Rehabilitation* **76**, 55–58.

Siitonen, L., Sonck, T. & Jänne, J. (1977) Effect of beta-blockade on performance: use of beta-blockade in bowling and in shooting competitions. *Journal of International Medical Research* **5**, 359–366.

Silverstone, T. & Goodall, E. (1992) Centrally acting anoretic drugs: a clinical perspective. *American Journal of Clinical Nutrition* **55**, 211S–214S.

Smith, G.M. & Beecher, H.K. (1959) Amphetamine sulfate and athletic performance. *Journal of the American Medical Association* **170**, 542–557.

Smith, G.M. & Beecher, H.K. (1960) Amphetamine, secobarbital, and athletic performance. *Journal of the American Medical Association* **172**, 1502–1514.

Snider, I.P., Bazzarre, T.L., Murdoch, S.D. & Goldfarb, A. (1992) Effects of coenzyme athletic performance system as an ergogenic aid on endurance performance to exhaustion. *International Journal of Sports Nutrition* **2**, 272–286.

Spann, C. & Winter, M.E. (1995) Effect of clenbuterol on athletic performance. *Annals of Pharmacotherapy* **29**, 75–77.

Spielvogel, H., Caceres, E., Koubi, H., Sempore, B., Sauvain, M. & Favier, R. (1996) Effects of coca chewing on metabolic and hormonal changes during graded incremental exercise to maximum. *Journal of Applied Physiology* **80**, 643–649.

Spriet, L.L. (1995) Caffeine and performance. *International Journal of Sports Nutrition* **5**, S84–S99.

Spriet, L.L. (1997) Ergogenic aids: recent advances and retreats. In D.R. Lamb & R. Murray (eds) *Perspectives in Exercise Science and Sports Medicine, Vol. 10. Recent Advances in the Science and Medicine of Sport*, pp. 185–234. Cooper Publishing Group, Carmel, Indiana.

Steen, S.N. (1991) Nutrition considerations for the low-body-weight athlete. In J.R. Berning & S.N. Steen (eds) *Sports Nutrition for the 90s: The Health Professional's Handbook*, pp. 153–174. Aspen Publishers Inc., Gaithersburg, Maryland.

Stinson, J.C., Murphy, C.M., Andrews, J.F. & Tomkin, G.H. (1992) An assessment of the thermogenic effects of fluoxetine in obese subjects. *International Journal of Obesity* **16**, 391–395.

Strauss, R.H. & Yesalis, C.E. (1991) Anabolic steroids in the athlete. *Annual Review of Medicine* **42**, 449–457.

Strauss, R.H., Liggett, M.T. & Lanese, R.R. (1985) Anabolic steroid use and perceived effects in ten weight-trained women athletes. *Journal of the American Medical Association* **253**, 2871–2873.

Swift, L.L., Hill, J.O., Peters, J.C. & Greene, H.L. (1990) Medium-chain fatty acids: evidence for incorporation into chylomicron triglycerides in humans. *American Journal of Clinical Nutrition* **52**, 834–836.

Taaffe, D.R., Pruitt, L., Reim, J. *et al.* (1994) Effect of recombinant human growth hormone on the muscle strength response to resistance exercise in elderly men. *Journal of Clinical Endocrinology and Metabolism* **79**, 1361–1366.

Tarnopolsky, J.T., MacDougall, J.D., Atkinson, S.A., Tarnopolsky, M.A. & Sutton, J.R. (1990) Gender differences in substrate for endurance exercise. *Journal of Applied Physiology* **68**, 302–308.

Tarnopolsky, M.A. (1994) Caffeine and endurance performance. *Sports Medicine* **18**, 109–125.

Tarnopolsky, M.A., Atkinson, S.A., Phillips, S.M. & MacDougall, J.D. (1995) Carbohydrate loading and metabolism during exercise in men and women. *Journal of Applied Physiology* **78**, 1360–1368.

Tennant, F.S. (1984) Dealing with cocaine use by athletes. *Sport Medicine Digest* **6**, 1–3.

Terney, R. & McLain, L.G. (1990) The use of anabolic steroids in high school students. *American Journal of Diseases of Children* **144**, 99–103.

Tesch, P.A. (1985) Exercise performance and β-blockade. *Sports Medicine* **2**, 389–412.

Thornton, G.R., Holck, H.G.O. & Smith, E.L. (1939) The effect of benzedrine and caffeine upon performance in certain psychomotor tasks. *Journal of Abnormal and Social Psychology* **34**, 96–113.

Tsintzas, K., Liu, R., Williams, C., Campbell, I. & Gaitanos, G. (1993) The effect of carbohydrate ingestion on performance during a 30-km race. *International Journal of Sports Nutrition* **3**, 127–139.

Van Hall, G., Raaymakers, J.S.H., Saris, W.H.M. & Wagenmakers, A.J.M. (1995) Ingestion of branched-chain amino acids and tryptophan during sustained exercise in man: failure to affect performance. *Journal of Physiology* **486**, 789–794.

Van Zyl, C.G., Lambert, E.V., Hawley, J.A., Noakes, T.D. & Dennis, S.C. (1996) Effects of medium-chain triglyceride ingestion on fuel metabolism and cycling performance. *Journal of Applied Physiology* **80**, 2217–2225.

Varnier, M., Sarto, P., Martines, D. *et al.* (1994) Effects of infusing BCAA during incremental exercise with reduced muscle glycogen content. *European Journal of Applied Physiology* **69**, 26–31.

Videman, T., Sonck, T. & Jänne, J. (1979) The effect of beta-blockade in ski-jumpers. *Medicine and Science in Sports and Exercise* **11**, 266–269.

Vukovich, M.D., Costill, D.L. & Fink, W.J. (1994) Carnitine supplementation: effect on muscle carnitine and glycogen content during exercise. *Medicine and Science in Sports and Exercise* **26**, 1122–1129.

Wagenmaker, A.J.M. (1991) L-Carnitine supplementation and performance in man. In F. Brouns (ed.) *Advances in Nutrition and Top Sport*. Medicine and Sport Science, Vol. 32, pp. 110–127. Karger, Basel.

Wagner, J.C. (1989) Abuse of drugs used to enhance athletic performance. *American Journal of Hospital Pharmacy* **46**, 2059–2067.

Wagner, J.C. (1991) Enhancement of athletic performance with drugs. *Sports Medicine* **12**, 250–265.

Walberg-Rankin, J. (1995) Dietary carbohydrate as an ergogenic aid for prolonged and brief competitions in sport. *International Journal of Sports Nutrition* **5**, S13–S28.

Welle, S., Thornton, C., Statt, M. & McHenry, B. (1996) Growth hormone increases muscle mass and strength but does not rejuvenate myofibrillar protein synthesis in healthy subjects over 60 years old. *Journal of Clinical Endocrinology and Metabolism* **81**, 3239–3243.

Williams, M.H. (1991) Alcohol, marijuana and beta blockers. In D.R. Lamb and M.H. Williams (eds) *Perspectives in Exercise Science and Sports Medicine, Vol. 4. Ergogenics: Enhancement of Performance in Exercise and Sport*, pp. 331–372. Brown and Benchmark, Carmel, Indiana.

Williams, M.H. & Thompson, J. (1973) Effect of variant dosages of amphetamine upon endurance. *Research Quarterly* **44**, 417–421.

Wilmore, J.H. (1988) Exercise testing, training, and beta-adrenergic blockade. *Physician and Sportsmedicine* **16**, 45–50.

Wirth, V.J. & Gieck, J. (1996) Growth hormone: myths and misconceptions. *Journal of Sport Rehabilitation* **5**, 244–250.

Wise, S.D. (1992) Clinical studies with fluoxetine in obesity. *American Journal of Clinical Nutrition* **55**, 181S–184S.

Wyndham, C.H., Rogers, G.G., Benade, A.J.S. & Strydom, N.B. (1971) Physiological effect of amphetamine during exercise. *South African Medical Journal* **45**, 247–252.

Yarasheski, K.E., Campbell, J.A., Smith, K., Rennie, M.J., Holloszy, J.O. & Bier, D.M. (1992) Effect of growth hormone and resistance exercise on muscle growth in young men. *American Journal of Physiology* **262**, E261–E267.

Yarasheski, K.E., Zachwieja, J.J., Angelopoulos, T.J. & Bier, D.M. (1993) Short-term growth hormone treatment does not increase muscle protein synthesis in experienced weight lifters. *Journal of Applied Physiology* **74**, 3073–3076.

Yarasheski, K.E., Zachwieja, J.J., Campbell, J.A. & Bier, D.M. (1995) Effect of growth hormone and resistance exercise on muscle growth and strength in older men. *American Journal of Physiology* **268**, E268–E276.

Chapter 23

Sexual Harassment and Abuse

CELIA BRACKENRIDGE

Introduction

Women athletes will only optimize their potential in sport if they are able to train and compete in conditions of complete safety. However, many females in sport endure less than safe conditions and, as a result, suffer pain, illness or injury. The major focus of this chapter is on the consequences for the female athlete when her personal safety is violated by others in the course of interpersonal relations in sport, through either harassment or abusive behaviour. Such potentially dangerous relationships include those between the athlete and her coach (usually male) or other authority figures (S. Kirby & L. Greaves, unpublished observation), as well as those between the athlete and her peers (Kane & Disch, 1993; Pike Masteralexis, 1995). The violation of personal safety within such relationships has serious outcomes for mental health. However, it is clear that a medical perspective alone cannot resolve the multifarious issues surrounding harassment and abuse of women in sport. A more complete understanding of the social and political context in which these actions occur is necessary.

This chapter sets out the current research knowledge about the incidence and prevalence of harassment and abuse of women in sport, the clinical therapy perspectives on the effects of such experiences, and known risk factors for the coach/athletic leader, athlete and sport context. A new model for risk analysis is proposed, drawing from existing clinical, therapeutic and social work approaches. Risk analysis and subsequent risk management is suggested as one practical method for securing better personal safety for the female athlete. However, the limitations of this approach are also acknowledged and a future research agenda is set out that might generate a better information base. This, in turn, should facilitate the development and implementation of more effective policy and practice in protecting the athlete from sexual harassment and abuse.

According to the National Society for the Prevention of Cruelty to Children in the UK, abuses takes four major forms: sexual, physical, emotional and neglect (Crouch, 1995). Clearly, combinations of these abuses frequently occur, for example where an athlete suffers emotional blackmail or physical damage as well as sexual exploitation. However, the focus of the rest of this chapter is on the psychological determinants and correlates of *sexual* harassment and abuse.

Sexual violations against the female athlete

Origins of research into sexual violations against women in sport

Whilst legal and constitutional changes towards sex equity in society at large had been secured by the women's movement in many western industrial nations during the 1970s (e.g. Title IX in the USA in 1972, the Sex Discrimination Act in the

UK in 1975 and the Charter of Rights and Freedoms, Constitution Act 1982 in Canada), it became apparent to those advocates of women's right within the world of sport that discriminatory behaviour was a persistent, deep-seated and resilient male habit that would take some time to change. Research mapping the extent of institutional discrimination preceded that on personal sexism and abuse (Acosta & Carpenter, 1985, 1990; White & Brackenridge, 1985) but provided an important platform of statistical evidence about vertical and horizontal sex segregation on which later interpersonal studies subsequently developed.

It is only since the late 1980s that research studies about interpersonal harassment and sexual abuse in sport have started to appear (Brackenridge, 1987, 1991, 1994, 1997a; Lackey, 1990; Lenskyj, 1992a; T. Crosset, unpublished observation). Specific knowledge about the extent and types of violations of personal and sexual safety in sport is comparatively sparse since systematic research into the issue began so late. However, literature from cognate fields such as women's studies, the sociology of violence, clinical therapy, and psychiatry were available and theories and models from these fields gave sports researchers a set of tools with which to begin investigating sexual harassment and abuse. The original stimulus for such work came not from medicine, even though clinical symptoms of harassment and abuse were evident amongst some female athletes, but as an extension of research into discriminatory practices and equal opportunities (Lenskyj, 1986; Theberge, 1987; Hall, 1988). It was but a short step from the study of sex discrimination to the study of sexual harassment (Table 23.1).

Table 23.1 The sexual violence continuum. (From Brackenridge, 1997b with permission)

Sex discrimination	Sexual harassment	Sexual abuse
Institutional	Personal	Personal
'The chilly climate'	*'Unwanted attention'*	*'Groomed or coerced'*
Vertical and horizontal job segregation	Written or verbal abuse or threats	Exchange of reward or privilege for sexual favours
Lack of harassment policy and/or officer or reporting channels	Sexually oriented comments	Rape
Lack of counselling or mentoring systems	Jokes, lewd comments or sexual innuendoes, taunts about body, dress, marital situation or sexuality	Anal or vaginal penetration by penis, fingers or objects
Differential pay or rewards or promotion prospects on the basis of sex	Ridiculing of performance	Forced sexual activity
Poorly/unsafely designed or lit venues	Sexual or homophobic graffiti	Sexual assault
Absence of security	Practical jokes based on sex	Physical/sexual violence
	Intimidating sexual remarks, propositions, invitations or familiarity	Groping
	Domination of meetings, play space or equipment	Indecent exposure
	Condescending or patronizing behaviour undermining self-respect or work performance	Incest
	Physical contact, fondling, pinching or kissing	
	Vandalism on the basis of sex	
	Offensive phone calls or photos	
	Bullying based on sex	

Definitions of sexual harassment and abuse

There is no universally accepted set of definitions of sexual harassment or sexual abuse. Even though these behaviours may be defined *objectively* it is important to recognize that they are experienced *subjectively*; thus the personal and psychological impact of the same behaviour may be vastly different depending on the individual female athlete's background and perceptions. However, if we accept a relativist position on sexual abuse (i.e. what constitutes abuse is in the eye/experience of the beholder) then we are also in danger of permitting exploitative behaviour to continue to undermine the sport experience for countless millions of women.

It is necessary therefore to agree on working definitions of abuse and harassment in order to facilitate a debate in sport about safe and unsafe interpersonal boundaries. In Table 23.1 sexual harassment and abuse are represented as the middle and extreme points along a continuum of sexual violence, and sets of behaviours are listed to exemplify each term. Whilst this conceptualization of behaviours separates each type, it is important to stress again that individual victims may experience them in an undifferentiated way; indeed, the nuances of definitional distinctions are completely irrelevant to the victim at the time of her experience. However, the model does offer us a means of approaching preventative work with authority figures in sport and may also facilitate variations in treatments and curative work.

There is an especially important distinction between sexual harassment, defined as unwanted behaviour or approaches on the basis of sex, and sexual abuse, defined as groomed or coerced collaboration in sexual acts. The grooming process, long recognized within clinical literature, is at the heart of the abusive relationship. The athlete gains trust in the coach or authority figure because he offers not only tangible extrinsic rewards for good performance (team selection, the chance to win competitions, representative honours and medals) but also because he nurtures and protects the athlete in a parent-like relationship, providing a mixture of discipline and affection upon which the athlete gradually becomes reliant. Grooming is a conscious process on the part of the abuser. The athlete, on the other hand, is an unwitting, sometimes nervously accepting, other times enthusiastically cooperating party to the gradual erosion of boundaries between her and the coach.

The power afforded the coach in his position of authority offers an effective camouflage for grooming and abuse. Incremental shifts in the **boundary between the coach and athlete** go **unnoticed, unrecognized or unreported by the** athlete until the point when she has become entirely trapped and is unable to resist his sexual advances. Disclosure is enormously difficult for the athlete, who risks uncertain support from her teammates and sport administrators and may even lose her athletic career by speaking out. Any rejection of grooming by an athlete or any challenge to the authority of the perpetrator carry the risk of sanctions such as withdrawal of privileges or his coaching expertise, even exclusion from the team or squad. Since the *raison d'être* of the talented young athlete is to succeed in her chosen sport, she feels virtually powerless to challenge the one individual who can help her achieve that success. For this reason, the athlete with potential talent is at higher risk of being targeted for sexual abuse than either the recreational athlete, who can leave the sport or club to find another, or the already successful athlete, who is no longer so dependent on her coach. For the athlete on the brink of top level success the stakes are highest of all and the pressures to collude with unsafe behaviours felt most keenly.

Recognizing the athlete at risk of sexual abuse

General statistics for non-sport settings indicate that around one in three or four girls experience sexual abuse, however defined, before reaching adulthood (Russell, 1984). Most of these cases occur within the familial setting, although extra-familial abuse comprises a small but significant proportion of the total recorded (LaFontaine,

1990). These figures suggest therefore that large numbers of girls and young women enter sports clubs and programmes already having experienced the stresses and trauma of sexual abuse in the family. These individuals are likely to be especially vulnerable to approaches by unscrupulous coaches. Research on small populations of female athlete survivors of abuse (Brackenridge, 1997a) indicates that a distant relationship with the parents, especially the father, may well be a risk factor for sexual abuse in sport. Whether having experienced sexual abuse in the home increases the susceptibility of the individual to abuse in sport is not known but it seems that this is highly likely.

Women athletes who present with signs of disordered eating (extreme weight loss, amenorrhoea, eroded tooth enamel, etc.) may also be showing the symptoms of sexual abuse. According to the literature on eating disorders, there is a proven link between anorexia and bulimia and sexual victimization (Johnson, 1994). One suggested explanation for this link is that the athlete is trying to desexualize her body in order to take back control over the sexual advances of her abuser. Certainly, the links between disordered eating and sexual abuse, within both sport and family settings, bear further examination. Other overt signs of sexual abuse and neglect include cuts or bruises to the body, vaginal soreness, unusual knowledge of or interest in sexual matters for a particular age, depression and social withdrawal, refusal to eat, or sudden changes in mood or routine behaviour.

Risk factors for sexual abuse in sport associated with the coach, the athlete and the sport have been extrapolated from both qualitative research (Brackenridge, 1997b) and quantitative research (S. Kirby & L. Greaves, unpublished observation) (Fig. 23.1 & Table 23.2). The risks of sexual exploitation in sport are particularly increased for young girls, for women and girls suffering physical disabilities or learning difficulties, and for those for whom communication or access to others is difficult.

Perpetrators of sexual abuse in sport appear to demonstrate at least two cycles of behaviour,

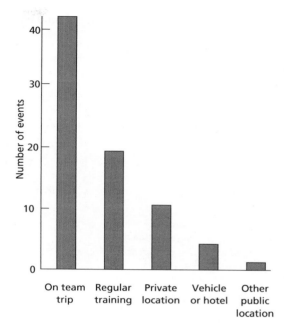

Fig. 23.1 Location of incidents of sexual abuse involving female athletes. $n = 146$. (Adapted from S. Kirby & L. Greaves, unpublished observations.)

one being the paedophile cycle (S.C. Wolf, cited in Fisher, 1994) and the other termed the 'predator' by Brackenridge (unpublished observation) (Fig. 23.2.). These two cycles bear theoretical resemblance to the child molester and rapist typologies developed in clinical psychology (see, for example, Knight & Prentky, 1990); however, the predator cycle has yet to be verified on data from a large sample.

Whilst it is tempting to focus analysis of risk entirely on perpetrator motivations and behaviours, this is also a dangerous strategy. Sexual abusers have proved notoriously difficult to classify and evidence from social work and therapy has repeatedly shown that they cross social and demographic categories (Russell, 1984; Waterhouse, 1993; Whetsell-Mitchell, 1995). No clear link with socioeconomic status, ethnicity or region has been proven, although it has been suggested that the silence veiling the incest taboo has been more effectively maintained by those from the wealthier classes

Table 23.2 Risk factors for sexual abuse in sport. (From Brackenridge, 1997b with permission)

Coach variables	Athlete variables	Sport variables
Sex (male)	Sex (female)	Amount of physical handling required for coaching
Age (older)	Age (younger)	Individual/team sport
Size/physique (larger/stronger)	Size/physique (smaller/weaker)	Location of training and competitions
Accredited qualifications (good)	Rank/status (potentially high)	Opportunity for trips away
Rank/reputation (high)	History of sexual abuse (unknown/none)	Dress requirements
Previous record of sexual harassment (unknown/ignored)	Level of awareness of sexual harassment (low)	Employment/recruitment controls and/or vetting (weak/none)
Trust of parents (strong)	Self-esteem (low)	**Regular evaluation, including athlete screening and cross-referencing to medical data**
Standing in the sport/ club/community (high)	Relationship with parents (weak)	Education and training on sexual harassment and abuse (none)
Chances to be alone with athletes in training, at competitions and away on trips (frequent)	Medical problems, especially disordered eating (medium/high)	Use of national and sport-specific codes of ethics or sport-specific codes of ethics and conduct (weak)
Commitment to sport/national coaches association codes of ethics and conduct (weak/none)	Devotion to coach (complete)	Existence of athlete and parent contracts (none)
Use of car to transport athletes (frequent)		Climate for debating sexual harassment (poor/nonexistent)

Comments in parentheses are based on trends from unstructured interviews with 12 survivors of sexual abuse in sport. Where there is no comment, further research is required.

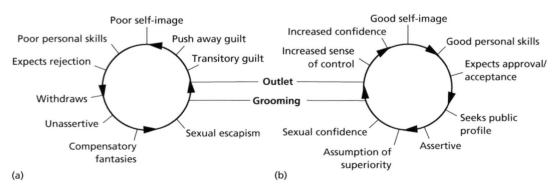

Fig. 23.2 Two cycles of sexual abuse in sport: (a) paedophile and (b) predator. (From C. Brackenridge, unpublished observations.)

(Doyle, 1994). A singular focus on perpetrators also distracts from other potentially useful areas of risk analysis and management, notably the athlete and the sport.

Not surprisingly, known athlete risk factors in sport match those recognized in other, non-sport settings. However, the added physical nature of sport, coupled with the requirements for extreme dedication and social, physical and emotional sacrifice at a relatively young age, all combine to increase risk. For the athlete who has low self-esteem or a weak relationship with her 'natural' parents, especially the father, there appear to be greater risks. Susceptibility to the close attention and interest of a parent substitute, the coach, can lead to close emotional attachment, infatuation and even love. Indeed, many survivors of sexual abuse in sport articulate mixed emotions about their abusers, perhaps even years or decades later, and blame themselves for falling prey to sexual exploitation.

The sport context represents another set of potential risks of sexual abuse for the female athlete (see Table 23.2). Organizations that have no formal policies or procedures for recruiting, checking, inducting or monitoring employees, whether paid or volunteer, are an especially easy target for the paedophile. This is particularly the case in the lower ranks of a sport or at the recreational level, where volunteer labour is often welcomed with little or no screening. Whether or not rules about requirements for dress or the amount of physical touching necessary for coaching influence the level of risk of sexual exploitation is unclear from research. However, sports in which it is possible for individuals to be isolated in or from the main training venue or taken on trips away from home clearly have a responsibility to implement rigorous safety procedures.

For the female athlete the consequences of experiencing sexual abuse are devastating and may be enduring. Many suffer psychological disorders for years afterwards and most have great difficulty summoning up the courage to report what has happened to them (Table 23.3).

Table 23.3 Feelings of abuse victims

Suspicious, unable to trust others
Afraid, unable to stand up for own opinion
Blames self for everything bad that happens
Feels guilty and ashamed even when there is no reason
Withdraws, does not want to spend time with others
Feels 'different' from others
Feels hurt by others a lot of the time
Lonely, bored and empty inside
Suicidal
Feels like a perfectionist, cannot tolerate mistakes
Constantly feels sorry for self
Feels angry all the time
Closes off feelings, unable to tolerate emotional pain
Not caring about appearance
Feels out of control of life
Depressed and sad
Afraid of change
Feels trapped, like nobody understands
Feels stupid, less capable than others
Ashamed of sexual feelings

Major research contributions

Researchers in several countries have taken different approaches to this topic and have built on different disciplinary foundations.

Celia Brackenridge (UK) has used pre-existing models from social work and sociology in the USA and the UK to help analyse female athletes' testimonies of abuse (Brackenridge, 1997b) and has suggested possible descriptions of offender profiles and risk factors for sexual harassment and abuse in sport (Brackenridge, 1997a). An extension of her risk factor model is currently being tested amongst a small group of sexually abused female athletes in The Netherlands in a study by Marian Cense commissioned by The Netherlands Olympic Committee. The Norwegian Confederation of Sport and the Norwegian Olympic Committee are also planning a study that will explore the incidence of sexual harassment and abuse among a sample of 600 élite sportswomen and seek to test a possible relationship between disordered eating and sexual abuse. Brackenridge has also developed workshop materials for groups of administrators, coaches and policy-makers that explore how to maintain safe boundaries between coaches and female athletes.

Todd Crosset and Lisa Pike Masteralexis (USA) have studied the legal status of women wishing to confront their abusers (Crosset *et al.*, 1995) and the extent of sexual violence to women amongst college athletes in campus populations (Pike Masteralexis, 1995). Crosset (unpublished observation) has also developed awareness-raising workshop materials for use with male coaches.

Sandra Kirby and Lorraine Greaves (Canada) are feminist researchers using quantitative and qualitative social research methods to build an analysis that defines harassment and abuse in sport as extensions of sexual violence towards women (S. Kirby, unpublished observation; S. Kirby & L. Greaves, unpublished observation). Sandra Kirby has also advised on the development of an information pack on sexual harassment for the Canadian Association for the Advancement of Women and Sport (1994), conducted a media analysis of coverage of cases of sexual abuse in sport, and begun to develop

policy approaches for the sports community based on the 'duty of care'.

Helen Lenskyj (Canada) is another feminist researcher whose research with and for women has also been drawn from a radical critique of violent gender relations (Lenskyj, 1992a); she has also helped to develop practical guidelines for the prevention of harassment of women in sport (Lenskyj, 1992b).

Don Sabo and Carole Oglesby (USA) have led a task force for the United States Women's Sports Foundation that has developed a set of training materials for administrators and sports organizations on abuse prevention and athletes' rights (Women's Sports Foundation, 1994). Don has also collaborated with Mike Messner on issues of masculinity, violence, sexuality and sport (Messner & Sabo, 1990).

Karin Volkwein (USA) has completed a large-scale survey of the incidence of sexual harassment and abuse amongst college athletes (K. Volkwein, unpublished observation).

Liv Kolnes (Norway) and Ilkay Yorganci (UK) are the first two researchers to complete doctoral theses on the topic of sexual harassment

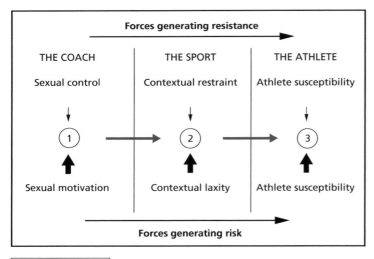

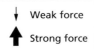

Weak force

Strong force

Fig. 23.3 Contingency model of risk of sexual abuse in sport. 1, sexual motivation of the coach/authority figure is stronger than his sexual self-control; 2, the sport's contextual restraints are weak or absent; 3, the athlete is susceptible to a sexual approach. (From C. Brackenridge, unpublished observations.)

and abuse in sport (Kolnes, 1992; Yorganci, 1994).

Recommendations for future research

The greatest impediment to future research into sexual abuse of athletes is access to the community of sport. Very few sport organizations are yet persuaded of the importance of the issue or of the need to gather more data. Even those working towards policies for improving athlete safety in this regard are reluctant to open themselves to the gaze of the researcher and to risk the possibility of uncovering 'bad news'. However, only with the systematic collection and analysis of large datasets, both quantitative and qualitative, and comparison with data outside the sport setting will the scale and dynamics of this issue become known. In the mean time, researchers continue to piece together data from purposive samples and from small surveys. The development of a contingency theory of sexual abuse in sport, which combines the perspectives of the athlete, the coach/abuser and the sport context, should enable sport organizations to assess risk in a given setting (Fig. 23.3). The most valuable research will identify the causes rather than just the symptoms of sexual abuse and therefore assist us in making sport a safer place for women.

Acknowledgements

Thanks are due to Dr Sandra Kirby, University of Winnipeg, and Lorraine Greaves, Centre for Research on Violence Against Women and Children, University of Western Ontario, for giving permission for their data to be quoted. Marian Cense of Transact, employed as a researcher by The Netherlands Olympic Committee to investigate sexual abuse in sport, has been especially supportive and is developing and extending the previous work on risk factors.

References

Acosta, R.V. & Carpenter, L.J. (1985) Women in sport. In D. Chu, J.O. Segrave & B.J. Becker (eds) *Sport and Higher Education*, pp. 313–325. Human Kinetics Publishers, Champaign, Illinois.

Acosta, R.V. & Carpenter, L.J. (1990) *Women in Intercollegiate Sport: A Longitudinal Study 1977–1990*. Brooklyn College, Brooklyn.

Brackenridge, C.H. (1987) Ethical problems in women's sport. *Coaching Focus* 6, 5–7.

Brackenridge, C.H. (1991) Cross-gender coaching relationships: myth, drama or crisis? *Coaching Focus* 16, 12–14.

Brackenridge, C.H. (1994) Fair play or fair game: child sexual abuse in sport organisations. *International Review for the Sociology of Sport* 29, 287–299.

Brackenridge, C.H. (1997a) 'He owned me basically . . .' Women's experiences of sexual abuse in sport. *International Review for the Sociology of Sport* 32, 115–130.

Brackenridge, C.H. (1997b) Researching sexual abuse in sport. In G. Clarke & B. Humberstone (eds) *Researching Women in Sport*, pp. 126–141. Macmillan, London.

Canadian Association for the Advancement of Women and Sport (1994) *What Sport Organisations Need to Know about Sexual Harassment*. Canadian Association for the Advancement of Women and Sport, Ottawa.

Crosset, T., Benedict, J. & McDonald, M. (1995) Male student-athletes reported for sexual assault: a survey of campus police departments and judicial affairs offices. *Journal of Sport and Social Issues* May, 126–140.

Crouch, M. (1995) *Protecting Children: A Guide for Sportspeople*. National Society for the Prevention of Cruelty to Children/National Coaching Foundation, Leeds.

Doyle, C. (1994) *Child Sexual Abuse: A Guide for Health Professionals*. Chapman & Hall, London.

Fisher, D. (1994) Adult sex offenders: Who are they? Why and how do they do it? In T. Morrison, M. Erooga & R.C. Beckett (eds) *Sexual Offending Against Children: Assessment and Treatment of Male Abusers*, p. 19. Sage, London.

Hall, M.A. (1988) The discourse of gender and sport: from femininity to feminism. *Sociology of Sport Journal* 5, 330–340.

Johnson, M. (1994) Disordered eating. In R. Agostini (ed.) *Medical and Orthopaedic Issues of Active and Athletic Women*, pp. 143–151. Mosby, St Louis.

Kane, M.J. & Disch, L.J. (1993) Sexual violence and the reproduction of male power in the locker room: 'The Lisa Olsen incident'. *Sociology of Sport Journal* 10, 331–352.

Kolnes, L. (1992) Coaches, athletes and gender relations: questions of power control and self-identity. Paper presented to the Pre-Olympic Scientific Congress on Sport and Quality of Life, Malaga, Spain, July 1992.

Knight, R.A. & Prentky, R.A. (1990) Classifying sexual offenders: the development and corroboration of taxonomic models. In W.L. Marshall, D.R. Laws & H.E. Barbaree (eds) *Handbook of Sexual Assault: Issues, Theories and Treatment of the Offender*, pp. 23–49. Plenum Press, New York.

Lackey, D. (1990) Sexual harassment in sports. *Physical Educator* **47**, 22–26.

LaFontaine, J. (1990) *Child Sexual Abuse*. Polity, London.

Lenskyj, H. (1986) *Out of Bounds: Women, Sport and Sexuality*. Women's Press, Toronto.

Lenskyj, H. (1992a) Unsafe at home base: women's experiences of sexual harassment in university sport and physical education. *Women in Sport and Physical Activity Journal* **1**, 19–34.

Lenskyj, H. (1992b) Sexual harassment: female athletes' experiences and coaches' responsibilities. *Sport Science Periodical on Research and Technology in Sport* 12, 6, Special Topics B-1.

Messner, M. & Sabo, D. (eds) (1990) *Sport, Men and the Gender Order*. Human Kinetics Publishers, Champaign, Illinois.

Pike Masteralexis, L. (1995) Sexual harassment and athletics: legal and policy implications for athletic departments. *Journal of Sport and Social Issues* May, 141–156.

Russell, D.E.H. (1984) *Sexual Exploitation: Rape, Child Sexual Abuse and Workplace Harassment*. Sage, London.

Theberge, N. (1987) Sport and women's empowerment. *Women's Studies International Forum* **10**, 387–393.

Waterhouse, L. (1993) *Child Abuse and Child Abusers: Protection and Prevention*. Jessica Kingsley, London.

Whetsell-Mitchell, J. (1995) *Rape of the Innocent: Understanding and Preventing Child Sexual Assault*. Taylor & Francis, London.

White, A.C. & Brackenridge, C.H. (1985) Who rules sport? Gender divisions in the power structure of British sporting organisations from 1960. *International Review for the Sociology of Sport* **20/21**, 95–107.

Women's Sports Foundation (1994) *Prevention of Sexual Harassment in Athletic Settings: An Educational Resource Kit for Athletic Administrators*. Women's Sports Foundation, New York.

Yorganci, I. (1994) *Gender, sport and sexual harassment*. PhD Thesis, University of Brighton.

PART 6

THE FEMALE ATHLETE TRIAD

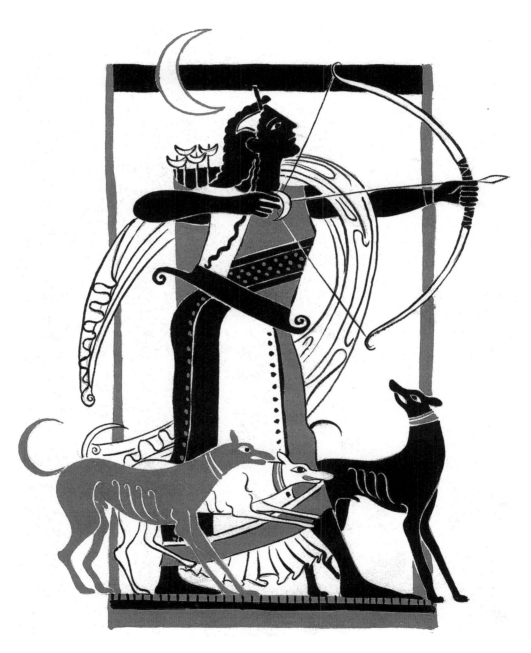

Chapter 24

Body Composition

WENDY M. KOHRT

Introduction

In a global context, body composition undoubtedly has a strong bearing on the performance of many physical activities. Aesthetics aside, the performance of skills that are the essence of such activities as gymnastics, figure skating and ballet dancing requires considerable muscle mass and strength. A high lean to fat mass ratio is obviously desirable for athletes who participate in these activities, as well as in others that involve lifting, or moving the body mass. It is not surprising, therefore, that reducing fat mass to improve performance can often lead to success in such sports. However, weight loss does not necessarily result in improved sports performance and may, in fact, lead to worsened performance and/or adverse health outcomes. The latter concern has emerged in recent years as the number of girls and women taking part in competitive sports has grown and as health professionals have become increasingly aware of the pernicious nature of the female athlete triad.

The term 'triad' refers to the clustering of disordered eating, amenorrhoea and premature osteoporosis that tends to occur in female athletes participating in sports where successful performance is dependent on, physiologically and/or aesthetically, a low body fat content (Yeager et al., 1993). Each of these disorders is discussed in greater detail in subsequent chapters. However, a separate discussion of body composition is warranted, as the desire to attain the ideal body composition for optimal athletic performance is probably the principal driving force behind the development of the female athlete triad. Several issues regarding the role of body composition in the female athlete triad are addressed.

Body composition and sports performance

Cross-sectional comparisons of non-athletes and athletes of different calibres

Comparisons of physiological profiles of élite and non-élite athletes often reveal characteristics that are related to superior performance. Table 24.1 summarizes results from some of the studies that have measured body composition of élite sportswomen. In many cases, comparison groups of competitive or recreational athletes or non-athletic controls were included. This is important not only for comparing groups within a study but also for making relative comparisons across studies, since different methods of assessing body composition may not yield equivalent results. Across sports, it is obvious that body composition is an important determinant of successful sports performance. Relative body fat levels tend to be lower among athletes participating in individual rather than team sports, and lowest in sports that require moving or lifting the body mass (e.g. running, jumping, gymnastics, etc.). Within a sport, élite sportswomen tend to have lower relative body fat levels than non-

353

Table 24.1 Examples of body composition of young female athletes

Reference (method of determination of body composition)	Activity	Level	No. of athletes	Height (cm)	Weight (kg)	Fat (%)	Fat-free mass (kg)
Fleck (1983)	Swimming	Élite	41		62.0	19.5	49.9
(hydrodensitometry)	Handball	Élite	17		68.8	19.0	55.7
	Rowing	Élite	19		67.4	18.4	55.0
	Speed skating	Élite	20		56.3	17.8	46.3
	Volleyball	Élite	36		69.4	15.8	58.4
	Running	Élite	28		50.5	13.8	43.5
	Sprinting	Élite	21		56.7	13.7	48.9
	Jumping	Élite	22		60.3	13.2	52.3
Graves et al. (1987)	Running	Élite	15	161	47.2	14.3	40.4
(hydrodensitometry)		Competitive	12	162	49.4	16.8	41.1
Alway et al. (1990)	Weight-	Élite	5	167	62.2	18.0	51.0
(total body volume)	lifting	Recreational	8	167	58.8	21.6	46.1
Schulz et al. (1992) (hydrodensitometry)	Running	Élite	9	163	52.4	12.0	46.1
Slemenda &	Figure	Élite	22	158	50.3	18.7	40.9
Johnston (1993) (dual-energy X-ray absorptiometry)	skating	Control	22	160	53.1	24.3	40.2
Koutedakis et al. (1994) (total body potassium)	Rowing	Élite	6		58.4	11.5	51.7
Creagh & Reilly	Orienteering	Élite	12	168	56.3	20.4	44.8
(1995) (skinfold		Competitive	11	170	57.7	21.8	45.1
thickness)		Control	20	167	63.4	26.6	46.5
Evans et al. (1995) (hydrodensitometry)	Running	Competitive	10	165	53.1	15.0	45.1
Fehling et al. (1995)	Volleyball	Collegiate	8	182	76.3	24.2	57.8
(hydrodensitometry)	Swimming	Collegiate	7	171	65.6	23.9	49.9
	Gymnastics	Collegiate	13	161	55.6	19.0	45.0
	Control	Collegiate	17	163	58.6	27.5	42.1
Hetland et al. (1995)	Running	Élite	28		57.2	13.3	49.6
(dual-energy X-ray		Competitive	89		62.1	20.8	49.2
absorptiometry)		Recreational	88		62.2	24.1	47.2
Nichols et al. (1995)	Basketball	Collegiate	14	172	66.4	29.0	47.1
(dual-energy X-ray	Volleyball	Collegiate	13	176	69.5	27.1	50.7
absorptiometry)	Gymnastics	Collegiate	13	160	53.9	22.6	41.7
	Tennis	Collegiate	6	166	59.8	30.2	41.7
	Control	Collegiate	12	165	60.6	30.6	42.1
Pacy et al. (1995) (hydrodensitometry)	Rowing	Élite	15	178	72.6	20.7	57.6

élite competitors, and athletes tend to have less fat than non-athletes regardless of the activity (Graves et al., 1987; Alway et al., 1990; Slemenda & Johnston, 1993; Creagh & Reilly, 1995; Fehling et al., 1995; Hetland et al., 1995; Nichols et al., 1995). Although these cross-sectional comparisons provide useful descriptions of élite sportswomen, they do not provide information regarding the extent to which changes in body composition affect performance level.

Effects of weight loss on performance

The observation of lower body fat levels in élite compared with non-élite athletes within a sport raises the question of the extent to which body composition can be manipulated to enhance performance. Could competitive runners who have a body fat content of 17–21% of body weight (Graves *et al.*, 1987; Hetland *et al.*, 1995) become élite runners if they reduced their fat content to the level characteristic of élite runners, i.e. 12–14% (Fleck, 1983; Graves *et al.*, 1987; Schulz *et al.*, 1992; Hetland *et al.*, 1995)? This is a difficult question to answer and one that does not have a definitive answer. There is a considerable body of literature on the effects of rapid weight loss (i.e. to make a weight requirement for competition) on measures of physiological function in male wrestlers (Fogelholm, 1994; American College of Sports Medicine, 1996). In general, rapid weight loss does not appear to have beneficial effects and may in fact have adverse effects on muscle strength, anaerobic power and endurance capacity.

There is a paucity of data on the effects of gradual weight loss on physiological function and performance in athletes who are already relatively lean, particularly women (Fogelholm, 1994). From the few controlled studies that have been conducted, it appears that the protective effect of exercise on the maintenance of lean body mass that occurs during diet-induced weight loss in overweight people (Ballor & Poehlman, 1994) does not occur in athletes who are relatively lean. In male and female athletes who lost weight at rates of 0.3–0.8 kg·week^{-1} over 7–16 weeks, 26–58% of the reduction was lean tissue (Widerman & Hagan, 1982; Horswill *et al.*, 1990; Inger & Sundgot-Borgen, 1991; Manore *et al.*, 1993; Koutedakis *et al.*, 1994). Whether the reduction in lean mass counteracts any potential benefits of reduced fat mass on performance is equivocal. In élite female skiers, Inger and Sundgot-Borger (1991) found that the training-induced increase in maximal aerobic power ($\dot{V}_{O_{2max}}$) that occurred in weight-stable athletes did not occur in athletes who reduced their body weight by 9% over 9 weeks; 26% of the weight loss was lean mass. Koutedakis *et al.* (1994) studied a group of élite oarswomen who underwent two different periods of weight reduction while continuing their usual exercise training. They reduced their body weight by 3.8 kg (6.0%) over 2 months and by 4.7 kg (7.4%) over 4 months; in both cases, approximately 50% of the reduction was lean mass. The 2-month weight-reduction period was associated with significant decreases in knee flexion peak torque and ventilatory threshold during a maximal rowing ergometer test, and non-significant decreases in $\dot{V}_{O_{2max}}$, knee extension peak torque and power output during an anaerobic power test. Conversely, in response to the 4-month weight-reduction period, there were significant increases in $\dot{V}_{O_{2max}}$, ventilatory threshold, knee flexion peak torque and peak power during the anaerobic power test. The investigators speculated that the longer weight-reduction period allowed more time for the biochemical and biomechanical adaptations to weight loss to occur, leading to improvements in measures of performance. What the investigators did not address, however, was the possibility that the 2-month weight-reduction period could have led to the same improvements in performance as the 4-month weight-reduction period if the athletes had been assessed after 4 months of training, i.e. 2 months after the weight-reduction period.

In such sports as running and gymnastics, athletes are often strongly encouraged by coaches and/or parents to attain very low body fat levels. The justification for this practice most likely stems from the theoretical benefit of a low body fat content on performance, coupled with the observation that élite performers tend to be very lean. From a scientific perspective, however, there is little or no evidence that weight reduction will enhance performance in already lean athletes. In fact, weight reduction in relatively lean athletes can result in a significant loss of lean mass and have an adverse effect on performance.

Body composition and health

It would be unethical to consider the effects of weight loss on the performance of competitive sportswomen without also considering the potential concomitant effects on health. It is common knowledge that being overweight increases the risk for many diseases, including coronary artery disease, diabetes mellitus and hypertension, and that weight loss is generally associated with improved health. However, being markedly underweight can also be unhealthy, and weight loss in an already lean individual may result in adverse health outcomes. Because a comprehensive overview of the effects on health of being underweight are beyond the scope of this chapter, discussion focuses on those aspects of health that are relevant to the female athlete triad.

Body composition and amenorrhoea

TOTAL BODY ADIPOSITY

An important question with regard to body composition and the female athlete triad is whether reducing fat mass below a certain level leads to amenorrhoea. It was once proposed that maintenance of normal menstrual function required a body fat content of at least 22% of body weight (Frisch & McArthur, 1974). This notion has been effectively dispelled, as many eumenorrhoeic athletes have been shown to have body fat levels less than 22% of body weight (Fisher et al., 1986; Kaiserauer et al., 1989; Crist & Hill, 1990; Snead et al., 1992; Wilmore et al., 1992; Myburgh et al., 1993; Rutherford, 1993). Moreover, no clear association between either relative or absolute body fat content and menstrual function of athletes has emerged (Table 24.2). Thus, there does not appear to be a critical level of adiposity, either absolute mass or relative fraction of body weight, below which menstrual irregularities occur. However, this does not rule out the possibility that amenorrhoea occurs as a result of changes in body composition. It is possible that there is a critical level of adiposity necessary for

normal menstrual function but that it varies widely among individuals. Careful monitoring of changes in body composition and changes in menstrual function in individual athletes is necessary to determine whether such thresholds exist.

REGIONAL ADIPOSITY

It has been suggested that critical levels of regional, rather than total, adiposity may be necessary for normal menstrual function (Brownell et al., 1987). The notion that regional differences in fat deposition can influence metabolism is indeed plausible. There is overwhelming evidence that accumulation of fat in the intra-abdominal region is more closely associated with the development of coronary artery disease, adult-onset diabetes mellitus and hypertension than is total degree of adiposity (Björntorp, 1992). Brownell et al. (1987) speculate that amenorrhoea may be triggered by depletion below a certain threshold of fat in the femoral region because of the importance of that site in providing energy for lactation and pregnancy.

Unfortunately, few studies have assessed regional fat distribution in athletes who differ in menstrual function. One comparison of amenorrhoeic and eumenorrhoeic runners found no significant differences in abdominal or leg fat content (i.e. percentage of total regional mass) measured by dual-energy X-ray absorptiometry (DXA) (Hetland et al., 1995). In another study, magnetic resonance imaging (MRI) was used to assess the total and regional fat content of 20 rowers, 12 of whom were anovulatory, and four amenorrhoeic runners (Frisch et al., 1993). There were no significant differences between eumenorrhoeic athletes and those with menstrual dysfunction in any of the fat regions that were assessed. Thus, there appears to be no evidence that regional adiposity plays a role in the development of amenorrhoea. However, these negative findings should be interpreted cautiously because of the small number of subjects that were assessed (Frisch et al., 1993) and the inability of DXA (Hetland et al., 1995) to distinguish between

Table 24.2 Body composition and/or lumbar spine bone mineral density of eumenorrhoeic and amenorrhoeic or oligomenorrhoeic athletes

Reference (method of determination of body composition)	Subjects	Status	No. of athletes	Weight (kg)	Fat (%)	Fat mass (kg)	Fat-free mass (kg)	Bone mineral density (g·cm^{-2})
Snead et al. (1992)	Runners	E	24	58.7	21.4	12.8	46.0	1.15
(hydrodensitometry)		A	11	59.6	19.8	12.1	47.5	1.02
Wilmore et al. (1992)	Runners	E	5	52.0	10.3	5.4	46.6	1.17
(hydrodensitometry)		A	8	51.4	10.8	5.6	45.8	1.16
Myburgh et al. (1993)	Athletes	E	9	53.2	20.3	10.8	42.4	1.05
(dual-energy X-ray absorptiometry)		A	12	52.9	16.7	8.8	44.1	0.93
Rutherford (1993)	Runners	E	16	60.1	14.7	8.8	51.3	1.18
(dual-energy X-ray absorptiometry)	and triathletes	A	15	55.3	10.9	6.0	49.3	1.07
Micklesfield et al.	Runners	E	15	58.3	28.5	16.6	41.7	1.09
(1995) (skinfold thickness)		O/A	10	57.2	29.0	16.6	40.6	0.95
Fisher et al. (1986)	Runners	E	24	56.3	21.3	12.0	44.3	
(hydrodensitometry)		A	11	58.0	22.1	12.8	45.2	
Kaiserauer et al. (1989)	Runners	E	9	54.2	10.7	5.8	48.4	
(hydrodensitometry)		A	8	49.3	11.8	5.8	43.5	
Crist & Hill (1990)	Runners	E	5	54.7	10.2	5.6	49.1	
(hydrodensitometry)		A	6	55.2	17.4	9.6	45.6	
Hetland et al. (1995)	Runners	E	93	61.6	22.2	13.7	47.9	
(dual-energy X-ray absorptiometry)		A	13	59.7	18.9	11.3	48.4	
Rencken et al. (1996)	Athletes	E	20	56.1				1.07
(dual-energy X-ray absorptiometry)		A	29	55.3				0.95
Robinson et al. (1995)	Runners	E	14					0.89
(dual-energy X-ray		O/A	6					0.86
absorptiometry)	Gymnasts	E	11					1.12
		O/A	10					1.05

A, amenorrhoeic; E, eumenorrhoeic; O/A, oligomenorrhoeic/amenorrhoeic.

subcutaneous fat and fat stores in intra-abdominal or intramuscular regions. The question of whether the relative depletion of specific fat depots triggers amenorrhoea should continue to be explored.

Body composition and osteoporosis

Low body weight is a risk factor for osteoporosis, while being overweight provides a degree of protection against osteoporosis (Lindsay, 1996). Total body weight, lean body mass and body fat content have been shown to be related to bone mineral density. Theoretically, each may have an independent effect on skeletal integrity. For most people, the majority of the loading forces acting on the skeleton on a day-to-day basis are introduced through ground reaction forces. Body weight is an important determinant of the magnitude of these forces, and peak loading forces are thought to play an important role in the bone modelling/remodelling process (Lanyon, 1992). Lean body mass, as a surrogate measure of muscle mass, may reflect the structural and functional link between muscle strength and bone strength. Men and women with a large muscle mass generally also have a large bone mass (Heinrich *et al.*, 1990; Karlsson *et al.*, 1993), and muscle strength has been shown to be a determinant of bone mineral density in the skeletal regions on which the muscles act (Bevier *et al.*, 1989; Pocock *et al.*, 1989). Finally, because androgens can be converted to oestrogen in adipose tissue, this source of oestrogen may provide protection against bone mineral loss when ovarian oestrogen production diminishes (Perel & Killinger, 1979).

The **relative influence** of fat and lean mass on **bone mineral density was evaluated** in 246 healthy women, aged 20–40 years, who were grouped into nine cells by tertiles of fat mass (low, <10.7 kg; high, >21.1 kg) and tertiles of lean mass (low, <42.5 kg; high, >47.4 kg) (Sowers *et al.*, 1992). Having a high lean body mass was associated with high bone mineral density at the femoral neck and trochanter sites, regardless of the body fat content. The bone mineral densities at these sites were similar in women in the high lean/low fat and high lean/high fat categories, despite a large difference in the average body weights of the two groups (67 and 91 kg respectively). Women in the low lean/low fat category (average body weight 49 kg) had the lowest bone mineral density values, 15–20% lower than those of women in the high lean/high fat group. Aloia *et al.* (1995a) also found that lean mass was a stronger determinant of bone mass than was fat mass among 164 women aged 24–79 years.

It would seem therefore that the relatively high lean body mass levels of athletes (see Tables 24.1 & 24.2) are protective against osteoporosis even when body fat levels are low. Given that lumbar spine bone mineral density is often lower in amenorrhoeic compared with eumenorrhoeic athletes matched for body composition (see Table 24.2), it is likely that hormonal status, rather than body composition, plays a primary role in the premature osteoporosis characteristic of the female athlete triad. However, the low lean body mass of athletes who maintain a very low body weight may contribute to their risk for osteoporosis.

Assessment of body composition

Methodological considerations

All the issues discussed thus far regarding the effects of body composition on performance and health of young female athletes must be interpreted cautiously as there is no guarantee, even in the most carefully conducted studies, that measures of body composition are accurate. All methods for assessing body composition of humans are indirect and are therefore reliant on certain assumptions. Error within a method occurs when the underlying assumptions are violated, and it is usually possible to make only theoretical estimates of the degree of error that may occur.

For example, the principal assumption of the reference method for assessing body composition, hydrostatic weighing (Fig. 24.1), is that the density of the fat-free mass is constant. This implies that the constituents of fat-free mass (i.e. water, protein and minerals) are present in the same proportion in all individuals. With respect to the female athlete triad, a specific reduction in only the bone mineral fraction of fat-free mass in amenorrhoeic athletes would theoretically result in a systematic overestimation of body fat content by hydrodensitometry. Based on hypothetical calculations, a 15% reduction in osseous mineral mass in an athlete with a body fat content of 12.0% of body weight, independent of any other changes in body composition, would result in the body fat level being erroneously estimated as 14.3% rather than 12.1%. Thus, if amenorrhoea causes a disproportionate loss of bone mineral, it is possible that all comparisons of densitometrically determined body composition of eumenorrhoeic and amenorrhoeic athletes are inherently flawed. Alternatively, it is possible that reductions in bone mineral in response to oestrogen deficiency do not occur independently but rather that proportional reductions occur in other constituents of fat-free mass (Aloia *et al.*, 1991, 1995b; Poehlman *et al.*, 1995), resulting in little or no error in estimating body composition from body density.

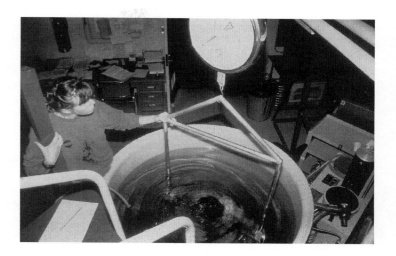

Fig. 24.1 Hydrostatic weighing: the gold standard for estimation of body fat.

Another concern regarding the assessment of body composition is that different methods can yield highly variable results. In nine élite female distance runners (Schulz *et al.*, 1992), body fat content assessed by hydrodensitometry, total body water and bioelectrical impedance averaged $12 \pm 3\%$, $11 \pm 4\%$ and $17 \pm 3\%$ of body weight, respectively. Pacy *et al.* (1995) evaluated body composition of 15 élite heavyweight oarswomen by hydrodensitometry, total body potassium counting, two commercially available bioelectrical impedance analysers, two equations to predict body fat content from skinfold thicknesses and three equations to predict fatness from body mass index (BMI, i.e. weight in kilograms divided by height in metres). The average body fat levels as a percentage of body weight ranged from 15.7% (total body potassium) to 28.5% (BMI); the average using hydrodensitometry was 20.7%. Although using BMI to estimate fatness was the simplest of the methods, requiring measurements only of weight and height, the three BMI equations yielded the highest estimates (26.8–28.5% of body weight). There was considerable variability even for a given method. For example, the two bioelectrical impedance analysers measured body fat as 16.7% and 20.9% of body weight. For individual athletes, the differences between the highest and lowest estimates of fatness ranged from 11.3% to 24.0% of body weight. Even when the estimates from BMI were disregarded, the differences between the highest and lowest values ranged from 4.0% to 20.7% of body weight. Importantly, it cannot be determined which of the methods, if any, yielded an accurate estimate of body composition.

Is there a valid method of assessing body composition in humans? Computed tomography (CT) provides objective measures of adipose-tissue and lean-tissue areas in cross-sectional images of body regions. Serial CT images of the entire body should therefore yield accurate measures of adipose-tissue and lean-tissue volumes. However, CT is not a feasible method for total body assessments because it involves exposure to ionizing radiation. Even if technological advances should make it possible to reduce the radiation exposure to acceptable levels, the conversion of adipose-tissue and lean-tissue areas to fat and fat-free masses would require certain assumptions that could introduce error. Although Frisch *et al.* (1993) have suggested that valid measures of fat and lean masses can be obtained by MRI, a soft-tissue imaging procedure that does not involve radiation exposure, this is not the case. MRI is subject to the same errors as CT that result when fat and fat-free masses are estimated from adipose-tissue and lean-tissue areas. Furthermore, unlike CT, the MRI signal intensity for adipose tissue is not homogeneous within a cross-section or between serial cross-sectional images. The quantification of adipose-tissue and lean-tissue areas therefore requires subjective input from the person analysing the image, which is an obvious source of variability.

Another procedure that has received considerable attention as a possible reference method for the assessment of body composition is DXA (Roubenoff et al., 1993; Kohrt, 1995). DXA provides a precise measure of bone mineral content and can further distinguish non-bone tissue into fat and lean components. Although some investigators have already endorsed DXA as a valid means of assessing body composition (Formica et al., 1993), this is premature for two reasons. First, it is inappropriate to speak in general terms of the validity of DXA per se, as there is incongruity among the different manufacturers of DXA instruments with regard to methods of calibration, data acquisition and data analysis. The issue of the validity of body composition assessment by DXA must therefore be specific to the manufacturer of the instrument, the instrument model, the mode of operation and the version of the software analysis program.

The second reason it is premature to endorse DXA as a valid method of assessing body composition is that there is convincing evidence that it is not accurate in some circumstances. Because the X-ray attenuation properties of lard are such that it appears to be 98% fat by DXA analysis, this material can be used to manipulate fat mass experimentally and determine whether DXA accurately assesses such manipulations. Snead et al. (1993) assessed body composition with a Hologic QDR-1000/W instrument and version 5.5 of the enhanced whole body software when packets of lard were positioned over central regions of the body or over the thighs. Compared to the control condition, DXA accurately assessed the composition of the added mass as 96% fat when it was positioned over the thighs. However, when it was positioned over the abdomen and chest, the additional mass was estimated to be only 55% fat. Similar results were obtained by Milliken et al. (1996) using a Lunar DPX-L instrument and software version 1.3y. It is likely that the source of the error lies in the method of data analysis rather than acquisition. In fact, an updated version of the Hologic enhanced whole body software program (version 5.64) now appears to assess exogenous fat accurately when it is positioned over central or peripheral regions of the body (Kohrt, 1998).

As with other methods of assessing body composition, DXA is dependent on some assumptions that will always make it vulnerable to a certain degree of error. However, if that degree of error can be quantified and is found to be within acceptable limits, there would be advantages to using DXA to assess body composition in sportswomen susceptible to the female athlete triad of disorders. The most obvious advantage, which is important because of the risk for premature osteoporosis, is that changes in total bone mineral content and density can be monitored simultaneously with changes in fat and fat-free mass. Another advantage is that relatively large fluctuations in hydration status, which are not uncommon in athletes who train vigorously or restrict their energy intake, have a negligible effect on the assessment of fat mass by DXA (Horber et al., 1992; Formica et al., 1993; Going et al., 1993; Kohrt, 1995).

Assessment of body composition to establish weight goals

Given the methodological problems associated with the assessment of body composition, the judiciousness of using such information to establish body weight goals for the purpose of optimizing sports performance is highly questionable. It is not difficult to imagine how an overestimation of fatness could lead coaches, parents and/or athletes to set unrealistic goals for weight loss and initiate behavioural changes that could have adverse effects on physical and/or psychological health. The suggestion to establish an acceptable range of values, rather than a specific degree of fatness, for athletes in a particular sport is certainly a more conservative approach (Brownell *et al.*, 1987). However, given that some of the common methods of assessing body composition yield estimates of fatness that vary within an individual by 20% of body weight or more (Pacy *et al.*, 1995), the range of values would have to be generous indeed to encompass this degree of methodological variability.

Because body composition is an important determinant of performance in many sports, the assessment of body composition for the purpose of determining ideal weight is a practice that will undoubtedly continue whether or not there are established guidelines. It is important therefore that acceptable ranges of body fat levels, based on sound scientific principles, be established within given sports and that the ranges be specific to the method of assessment of body composition. Furthermore, there should be an ongoing effort to evaluate the appropriateness of such guidelines, with the principal focus being the overall health of the athlete. At a minimum, it is recommended that records of body weight, menstrual function and training level be maintained to assist individual athletes in finding the ideal body weight for health and performance. Raising the level of consciousness of athletes and their coaches, parents and physicians with regard to the disorders that comprise the female athlete triad, and the role that striving to achieve a low body weight may play in its development, is certainly paramount to the prevention and treatment of the disorders.

Recommendations for future research

For such sports as wrestling, where athletes often repeatedly strive to achieve a certain weight limit for competition, there has been considerable research on the effects of weight loss on physiological measures of performance and health (American College of Sports Medicine, 1996). However, since weight loss for such sports is typically accomplished rapidly and is transient, it is unlikely that findings are applicable to athletes such as gymnasts or distance runners, who strive to maintain a low body weight for a prolonged period of time. To learn more about the potential effects of weight loss on the health and performance of athletes and to better understand the role that body composition plays in the development of the female athlete triad, the following are some of the issues that must continue to be explored.

• Does weight loss in already lean athletes result in a disproportionate loss of lean mass? Is the loss of lean mass affected by the method of achieving weight loss (e.g. fast vs. slow, increased energy expenditure vs. reduced energy intake)?

• In relatively lean athletes, what is the effect of weight loss on physiological measures of performance? Does the method of achieving weight loss affect the changes in performance?

• Within individual athletes, is there a critical body fat level necessary for maintaining normal menstrual function?

• In eumenorrhoeic and amenorrhoeic athletes matched for body composition and performance level, are there differences in the regional accumulation of fat?

• Is there a negative effect of weight loss, independent of menstrual dysfunction, on bone mineral density in athletes? Is a reduction in non-bone lean mass accompanied by a proportional reduction in bone mass?

References

Aloia, J.F., McGowan, D.M., Vaswani, A.N., Ross, P. & Cohn, S.H. (1991) Relationship of menopause to skeletal and muscle mass. *American Journal of Clinical Nutrition* **53**, 1378–1383.

Aloia, J.F., Vaswani, A., Ma, R. & Flaster, E. (1995a) To what extent is bone mass determined by fat-free or fat mass? *American Journal of Clinical Nutrition* **61**, 1110–1114.

Aloia, J.F., Vaswani, A., Russo, L., Sheehan, M. & Flaster, E. (1995b) The influence of menopause and hormonal replacement therapy on body cell mass and body fat mass. *American Journal of Obstetrics and Gynecology* **172**, 896–900.

Alway, S.E., Stray-Gundersen, J., Grumbt, W.H. & Gonyea, W.J. (1990) Muscle cross-sectional area and torque in resistance trained subjects. *European Journal of Applied Physiology* **60**, 86–90.

American College of Sports Medicine (1996) Position

stand: weight loss in wrestlers. *Medicine and Science in Sports and Exercise* **28**, ix–xii.

Ballor, D.L. & Poehlman, E.T. (1994) Exercise-training enhances fat-free mass preservation during diet-induced weight loss: a meta-analytical finding. *International Journal of Obesity and Related Metabolic Disorders* **18**, 35–40.

Bevier, W.C., Wiswell, R.A., Pyka, G., Kozak, K.C., Newhall, K.M. & Marcus, R. (1989) Relationship of body composition, muscle strength, and aerobic capacity to bone mineral density in older men and women. *Journal of Bone and Mineral Research* **4**, 421–432.

Björntorp, P. (1992) Abdominal fat distribution and disease: an overview of epidemiologic data. *Annals of Medicine* **24**, 15–18.

Brownell, K.D., Nelson Steen, S. & Wilmore, J.H. (1987) Weight regulation practices in athletes: analysis of metabolic and health effects. *Medicine and Science in Sports and Exercise* **19**, 546–556.

Creagh, U. & Reilly, T. (1995) A multivariate analysis of kinanthropometric profiles of elite female orienteers. *Journal of Sports Medicine and Physical Fitness* **35**, 59–66.

Crist, D.M. & Hill, J.M. (1990) Diet and insulinlike growth factor I in relation to body composition in women with exercise-induced hypothalamic amenorrhea. *Journal of the American College of Nutrition* **9**, 200–204.

Evans, S.L., Davy, K.P., Stevenson, E.T. & Seals, D.R. (1995) Physiological determinants of 10-km performance in highly trained female runners of different ages. *Journal of Applied Physiology* **78**, 1931–1941.

Fehling, P.C., Alekel, L., Clasey, J., Rector, A. & Stillman, R.J. (1995) A comparison of bone mineral densities among female athletes in impact loading and active loading sports. *Bone* **17**, 205–210.

Fisher, E.C., Nelson, M.E., Frontera, W.R., Turksoy, R.N. & Evans, W.J. (1986) Bone mineral content and levels of gonadotropins and estrogens in amenorrheic running women. *Journal of Clinical Endocrinology and Metabolism* **62**, 1232–1236.

Fleck, S.J. (1983) Body composition of elite American athletes. *American Journal of Sports Medicine* **11**, 398–403.

Fogelholm, M. (1994) Effects of bodyweight reduction on sports performance. *Sports Medicine* **18**, 249–267.

Formica, C., Atkinson, M.G., Nyulasi, I., McKay, J., Heale, W. & Seeman, E. (1993) Body composition following hemodialysis: studies using dual-energy X-ray absorptiometry and bioelectrical impedance analysis. *Osteoporosis International* **3**, 192–197.

Frisch, R.E. & McArthur, J.W. (1974) Menstrual cycles: fatness as a determinant for minimum weight or height necessary for their maintenance or onset. *Science* **185**, 949–951.

Frisch, R.E., Snow, R.C., Johnson, L.A., Gerard, B., Barbieri, R. & Rosen, B. (1993) Magnetic resonance imaging of overall and regional body fat, estrogen metabolism, and ovulation of athletes compared to controls. *Journal of Clinical Endocrinology and Metabolism* **77**, 471–477.

Going, S.B., Massett, M.P., Hall, M.C. et al. (1993) Detection of small changes in body composition by dual-energy X-ray absorptiometry. *American Journal of Clinical Nutrition* **57**, 845–850.

Graves, J.E., Pollock, M.L. & Sparling, P.B. (1987) Body composition of elite female distance runners. *International Journal of Sports Medicine* **8**, 96–102.

Heinrich, C.H., Going, S.B., Pamenter, R.W., Perry, C.D., Boyden, T.W. & Lohman, T.G. (1990) Bone mineral content of cyclically menstruating female resistance and endurance trained athletes. *Medicine and Science in Sports and Exercise* **22**, 558–563.

Hetland, M.L., Haarbo, J. & Christiansen, C. (1995) Body composition and serum lipids in female runners: influence of exercise level and menstrual bleeding pattern. *European Journal of Clinical Investigation* **25**, 553–558.

Horber, F.F., Thomi, F., Casez, J.P., Fonteille, J. & Jaeger, P. (1992) Impact of hydration status on body composition as measured by dual energy X-ray absorptiometry in normal volunteers and patients on haemodialysis. *British Journal of Radiology* **65**, 895–900.

Horswill, C.A., Park, S.H. & Roemmich, J.N. (1990) Changes in the protein nutritional status of adolescent wrestlers. *Medicine and Science in Sports and Exercise* **22**, 599–604.

Inger, F. & Sundgot-Borgen, J. (1991) Influence of body weight regulation on maximal oxygen uptake in female elite athletes. *Scandinavian Journal of Medicine and Science in Sports* **1**, 141–146.

Kaiserauer, S., Snyder, A.C., Sleeper, M. & Zierath, J. (1989) Nutritional, physiological, and menstrual status of distance runners. *Medicine and Science in Sports and Exercise* **21**, 120–125.

Karlsson, M.K., Johnell, O. & Obrant, K.J. (1993) Bone mineral density in weight lifters. *Calcified Tissue International* **52**, 212–215.

Kohrt, W.M. (1995) Body composition by DXA: tried and true? *Medicine and Science in Sports and Exercise* **27**, 1349–1353.

Kohrt, W.M. (1998) Preliminary evidence that DEXA provides an accurate assessment of body composition. *Journal of Applied Physiology* **84**, 372–377.

Koutedakis, Y., Pacy, P.J., Quevedo, R.M. et al. (1994) The effects of two different periods of weight-reduction on selected performance parameters in elite lightweight oarswomen. *International Journal of Sports Medicine* **15**, 472–477.

Lanyon, L.E. (1992) The success and failure of the adaptive response to functional load-bearing in averting bone fracture. *Bone* **13**, S17–S21.

Lindsay, R. (1996) Prevention of osteoporosis. In M.J. Favus (ed.) *Primer on the Metabolic Bone Diseases and Disorders of Mineral Metabolism*, 3rd edn, pp. 256–261. Lippincott–Raven Publishers, Philadelphia.

Manore, M.M., Thompson, J. & Russo, M. (1993) Diet and exercise strategies of a world-class bodybuilder. *International Journal of Sports Nutrition* **3**, 76–86.

Micklesfield, L.K., Lambert, E.V., Fataar, A.B., Noakes, T.D. & Myburgh, K.H. (1995) Bone mineral density in mature, premenopausal ultramarathon runners. *Medicine and Science in Sports and Exercise* **27**, 688–696.

Milliken, L.A., Going, S.B. & Lohman, T.G. (1996) Effects of variations in regional composition on soft tissue measurements by dual-energy X-ray absorptiometry. *International Journal of Obesity and Related Metabolic Disorders* **20**, 677–682.

Myburgh, K.H., Bachrach, L.K., Lewis, B., Kent, K. & Marcus, R. (1993) Low bone mineral density at axial and appendicular sites in amenorrheic athletes. *Medicine and Science in Sports and Exercise* **25**, 1197–1202.

Nichols, D.L., Sanborn, C.F., Bonnick, S.L., Gench, B. & DiMarco, N. (1995) Relationship of regional body composition to bone mineral density in college females. *Medicine and Science in Sports and Exercise* **27**, 178–182.

Pacy, P.J., Quevedo, M., Gibson, N.R., Cox, M., Koutedakis, Y. & Millward, J. (1995) Body composition measurement in elite heavyweight oarswomen: a comparison of five methods. *Journal of Sports Medicine and Physical Fitness* **35**, 67–74.

Perel, E. & Killinger, D.W. (1979) The interconversion and aromatization of androgens by human adipose tissue. *Journal of Steroid Biochemistry* **10**, 623–627.

Pocock, N., Eisman, J., Gwinn, T. *et al.* (1989) Muscle strength, physical fitness, and weight but not age predict femoral neck bone mass. *Journal of Bone and Mineral Research* **4**, 441–448.

Poehlman, E.T., Toth, M.J. & Gardner, A.W. (1995) Changes in energy balance and body composition at menopause: a controlled longitudinal study. *Annals of Internal Medicine* **123**, 673–675.

Rencken, M.L., Chesnut, C.H. III. & Drinkwater, B.L. (1996) Bone density at multiple skeletal sites in amenorrheic athletes. *Journal of the American Medical Association* **276**, 238–240.

Robinson, T.L., Snow-Harter, C., Taaffe, D.R., Gillis, D., Shaw, J. & Marcus, R. (1995) Gymnasts exhibit higher bone mass than runners despite similar prevalence of amenorrhea and oligomenorrhea. *Journal of Bone and Mineral Research* **10**, 26–35.

Roubenoff, R., Kehayias, J.J., Dawson-Hughes, B. & Heymsfield, S.B. (1993) Use of dual-energy X-ray absorptiometry in body composition studies: not yet a 'gold standard'. *American Journal of Clinical Nutrition* **58**, 589–591.

Rutherford, O.M. (1993) Spine and total body bone mineral density in amenorrheic endurance athletes. *Journal of Applied Physiology* **74**, 2904–2908.

Schulz, L.O., Alger, S., Harper, I., Wilmore, J.H. & Ravussin, E. (1992) Energy expenditure of elite female runners measured by respiratory chamber and doubly labeled water. *Journal of Applied Physiology* **72**, 23–28.

Slemenda, C.W. & Johnston, C.C. (1993) High intensity activities in young women: site specific bone mass effects among female figure skaters. *Bone and Mineral* **20**, 125–132.

Snead, D.B., Weltman, A., Weltman, J.Y. *et al.* (1992) Reproductive hormones and bone mineral density in women runners. *Journal of Applied Physiology* **72**, 2149–2156.

Snead, D.B., Birge, S.J. & Kohrt, W.M. (1993) Age-related differences in body composition by hydrodensitometry and dual-energy X-ray absorptiometry. *Journal of Applied Physiology* **74**, 770–775.

Sowers, M.F., Kshirsagar, A., Crutchfield, M.M. & Updike, S. (1992) Joint influence of fat and lean body composition compartments on femoral bone mineral density in premenopausal women. *American Journal of Epidemiology* **136**, 257–265.

Widerman, P.M. & Hagan, R.D. (1982) Body weight loss in a wrestler preparing for competition: a case report. *Medicine and Science in Sports and Exercise* **14**, 413–418.

Wilmore, J.H., Wambsgans, K.C., Brenner, M. *et al.* (1992) Is there energy conservation in amenorrheic compared with eumenorrheic distance runners? *Journal of Applied Physiology* **72**, 15–22.

Yeager, K.K., Agostini, R., Nattiv, A. & Drinkwater, B. (1993) The female athlete triad: disordered eating, amenorrhea, osteoporosis. *Medicine and Science in Sports and Exercise* **25**, 775–777.

Chapter 25

Eating Disorders

JORUNN SUNDGOT-BORGEN

Introduction

Disordered eating comprises a wide spectrum of harmful and often ineffective eating behaviours used in attempts to lose weight. These behaviours range from mild caloric restriction to the clinical disorders of anorexia nervosa and bulimia nervosa. Symptoms of both disordered eating and eating disorders are more prevalent among female athletes than non-athletes. Specific risk factors for the development of eating disorders occur in some sport settings. For example, athletes competing in sports where leanness or a specific weight are considered important for performance are at increased risk of developing eating disorders.

Psychological, biological and social factors interrelate to produce the clinical picture of eating disorders. The diagnosis of an eating disorder in female athletes can easily be missed unless coaches, trainers and team physicians are aware of the problem and alert to the symptoms. For a number of reasons, there is a strong pattern of denial and a standardized scale or a diagnostic interview specific for female athletes must be used to identify those at risk. If left untreated, eating disorders can have long-lasting physiological and psychological effects and may even be fatal. This chapter reviews the definitions, diagnostic criteria, prevalence and risk factors for the development of eating disorders in sport. The identification and treatment of eating-disordered athletes and the need for future research are also discussed.

Definitions and diagnostic criteria

According to the third edition of the *Diagnostic and Statistical Manual of Mental Disorders* (American Psychiatric Association, 1987), eating disorders are characterized by gross disturbances in eating behaviour. However, athletes constitute a unique population and special diagnostic considerations should be taken into account when working with this group (Szmuckler *et al.*, 1985; Sundgot-Borgen, 1993; Thompson & Trattner-Sherman, 1993). An attempt has been made to describe athletes who show significant symptoms of eating disorders but who do not meet all the criteria for anorexia nervosa or bulimia nervosa. The term *anorexia athletica* has been suggested for athletes who have a subclinical eating disorder (Sundgot-Borgen, 1994). As many cases of anorexia nervosa and bulimia nervosa may begin as subclinical variants of these disorders, early identification and treatment may prevent development of the full disorder (Bassoe, 1990). Finally, subclinical cases are more prevalent among athletes than those meeting the formal diagnostic criteria for anorexia nervosa and bulimia nervosa (Grange *et al.*, 1994).

Diagnosis

Tables 25.1 and 25.2 summarize the diagnostic criteria for anorexia nervosa and bulimia nervosa specified in the fourth edition of the *Diagnostic and Statistical Manual of Mental Disorders* (American Psychiatric Association, 1994). These new cri-

Table 25.1 Diagnostic criteria for anorexia nervosa. (Reprinted with permission from the *Diagnostic and Statistical Manual of Mental Disorders*, 4th edn. © 1994 American Psychiatric Association)

A Refusal to maintain body weight at or above a minimally normal weight for age and height (e.g. weight loss leading to maintenance of body weight less than 85% of that expected; or failure to make expected weight gain during period of growth, leading to body weight less than 85% of that expected)

B Intense fear of gaining weight or becoming fat, even though underweight

C Disturbance in the way in which one's body weight or shape is experienced, undue influence of body weight or shape on self-evaluation, or denial of the seriousness of the current low body weight

D In postmenarcheal females, amenorrhoea, i.e. the absence of at least three consecutive menstrual cycles (a woman is considered to have amenorrhoea if her periods occur only following hormone, e.g. oestrogen, administration)

Specify type
Restricting type: during the episode of anorexia nervosa, the person has not regularly engaged in binge-eating or purging behaviour (i.e. self-induced vomiting or the misuse of laxatives, diuretics or enemas)
Binge-eating/purging type: during the current episode of anorexia nervosa, the person has regularly engaged in binge-eating or purging behaviour (i.e. self-induced vomiting or the misuse of laxatives, diuretics or enemas)

Table 25.2 Diagnostic criteria for bulimia nervosa. (Reprinted with permission from the *Diagnostic and Statistical Manual of Mental Disorders*, 4th edn. © 1994 American Psychiatric Association)

A Recurrent episodes of binge-eating. An episode of binge-eating is characterized by both of the following: (i) eating, in a discrete period of time (e.g. within any 2-hour period), an amount of food that is definitely larger than most people would eat during a similar period of time in similar circumstances; and (ii) a sense of lack of control over eating during the episode (e.g. a feeling that one cannot stop eating or control what or how much one is eating)

B Recurrent inappropriate compensatory behaviour in order to prevent weight gain, such as self-induced vomiting, misuse of laxatives, diuretics or other medications, fasting or excessive exercise

C The binge-eating and inappropriate compensatory behaviours both occur, on average, at least twice a week for 3 months

D Self-evaluation is unduly influenced by body shape and weight

E The disturbance does not occur exclusively during episodes of anorexia nervosa

Specify type
Purging type: the person regularly engages in self-induced vomiting or the misuse of laxatives, diuretics or enemas
Non-purging type: the person uses other inappropriate compensatory behaviours, such as fasting or excessive exercise, but does not regularly engage in self-induced vomiting or the misuse of laxatives, diuretics or enemas

teria formalize overlapping conventions for subtyping anorexia nervosa into restricting and binge-eating/purging types based on the presence or absence of binge-eating and/or purging (i.e. self-induced vomiting or the misuse of laxatives or diuretics). Most athletes, depending on the sport they represent, move between these two subtypes of eating disorders. However, it is the author's experience that chronicity leads to an accumulation of eating-disordered athletes in the binge-eating/purging subgroup. The category 'eating disorder not otherwise specified' is for disorders of eating that do not meet the criteria for any specific eating disorder. This category

acknowledges the existence and importance of a variety of eating disturbances.

The term 'anorexia athletica' was first introduced by Pugliese *et al.* (1983). The main feature of anorexia athletica is an intense fear of gaining weight or becoming fat even though an individual is already lean (at least 5% less than expected normal weight for age and height for the general female population). Weight loss is accomplished by a reduction in energy intake, often combined with extensive or compulsive exercise. Restrictive eaters have an energy intake below that required to maintain the energy requirements of the high training volume (Sundgot-

Table 25.3 Diagnostic criteria for anorexia athletica. (From Sundgot-Borgen, 1994 with permission)

Weight loss > 5% of expected body weight	+
Delayed puberty (no menstrual bleeding at age 16, i.e. primary amenorrhoea)	(+)
Menstrual dysfunction (primary amenorrhoea, secondary amenorrhoea and oligomenorrhoea)	(+)
Gastrointestinal complaints	(+)
Absence of medical illness or affective disorder explaining the weight reduction	+
Distorted body image	(+)
Excessive fear of becoming obese	+
Restriction of food [< 5040 kJ (1200 kcal) daily]	+
Use of purging methods (self-induced vomiting, laxatives and diuretics	(+)
Binge-eating	(+)
Compulsive exercise	(+)

+, Absolute criteria; (+), relative criteria.

Borgen, 1993). In addition to normal training to enhance performance in sport, athletes with anorexia athletica exercise excessively or compulsively in order to purge their bodies of the effect of eating. These athletes frequently report binge-eating and the use of vomiting, laxatives or diuretics. The binge-eating is usually planned and included in a strict training and study schedule. The criteria for anorexia athletica listed in Table 25.3 include a modification of the original criteria introduced by Pugliese *et al.* (1983).

Prevalence of eating disorders in athletes

Data on the prevalence of eating disorders in athletic populations are limited and equivocal. Most studies have looked at the symptoms of eating disorders, such as preoccupation with food and weight, disturbed body image or the use of pathogenic methods for weight control. Estimates of the prevalence of the symptoms of eating disorders and true eating disorders among female athletes range from < 1% to as high as 75% (Gadpalle

Table 25.4 Athletes competing in five endurance events who met the eating disorder criteria

	No. of athletes	Percentage with eating disorders (CI)
Cross-country skiing	22	33.3 (31.4–34.5)
Middle- and long-distance running	15	27.2 (26.1–28.1)
Cycling	10	20.0 (17.5–22.5)
Swimming	20	15.0 (14.2–15.7)
Orienteering	13	0
Average	80	20.0 (19.9–20.1)

CI, confidence interval.

et al., 1987; Warren *et al.*, 1990; Sundgot-Borgen, 1994).

Methodological weaknesses, such as small sample size, failure to define the competitive level and type of sport(s) and the method of data collection, characterize most of the studies that have attempted to investigate the prevalence of eating disorders (Sundgot-Borgen, 1994). In addition, eating disorders are known to be secretive activities and many athletes do not admit they have a problem. Only one study has used a clinical evaluation and applied the criteria specified in the *Diagnostic and Statistical Manual of Mental Disorders* (1987) to both athletes and controls (Sundgot-Borgen, 1994). The prevalence of anorexia nervosa (1.3%) appeared to be within the same range as that reported in non-athletes (Andersen, 1990), whereas bulimia nervosa (8.2%) and subclinical eating disorders (8%) appeared to be more prevalent among athletes than non-athletes (Sundgot-Borgen, 1994). Furthermore, the prevalence of eating disorders was significantly higher among athletes competing in aesthetic and weight-dependent sports compared with athletes competing in sports where leanness is considered less important (Fig. 25.1). Further analysis revealed a significant difference in the prevalence of eating disorders between the sports included in the endurance group (Table 25.4 & Fig. 25.2).

The frequency of eating disorder problems

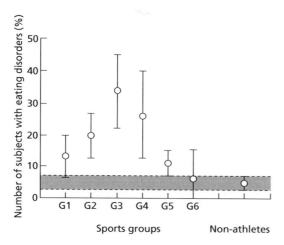

Fig. 25.1 Prevalence of eating disorders in female élite athletes representing technical sports (G1; $n=98$), endurance sports (G2; $n=119$), aesthetic sports (G3; $n=64$), weight-dependent sports (G4; $n=41$), ball games (G5; $n=183$), power sports (G6; $n=17$) and non-athletes ($n=522$). The data are shown as mean and 95% confidence intervals. The shaded area is the 95% CI for the control group of non-athletes. (From Sundgot-Bergen, 1993 with permission.)

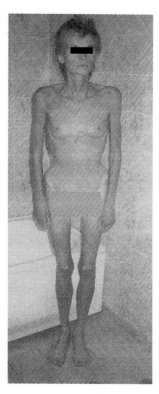

Fig. 25.2 This endurance athlete reduced her weight by a few kilograms and felt that she had enhanced her performance level. Those few kilograms were the beginning of years of anorexia nervosa.

when determined by questionnaire is much higher than the frequency reported when athletes have been evaluated clinically (Rosen & Hough, 1988; Rucinski, 1989). Despite the methodological weaknesses, existing studies are consistent in showing that symptoms of eating disorders and pathogenic methods of weight control are more prevalent in female athletes compared with non-athletes and more prevalent in sports in which leanness or a specific weight are considered important compared with sports where these factors are considered less important (Rosen et al., 1986; Dummer et al., 1987; Sundgot-Borgen & Corbin, 1987; Hamilton et al., 1988; Rosen & Hough, 1988; Wilmore, 1991; Sundgot-Borgen, 1993; O'Connor et al., 1995).

Self-report vs. clinical interview

In questionnaires, élite athletes have been found to under-report the use of purging methods (e.g. laxatives, diuretics and vomiting) and the pres-

ence of an eating disorder and over-report the use of binge-eating (Sundgot-Borgen & Larsen, 1993). In spite of the high sensitivity observed in the subtests of the Eating Disorder Inventory as a predictor of eating disorders (Sundgot-Borgen, 1994), it is the author's opinion that determining whether an athlete actually suffers from any of the eating disorders described above requires an interview with a clinician in order to assess the athlete's physical and emotional condition and whether this interferes with everyday functioning.

Effect of skill level

It is assumed that some risk factors (e.g. intense pressure to be lean, increased training volume and perfectionism) are more pronounced in élite athletes. However, Hamilton *et al.* (1988) found that in the USA less-skilled dancers reported significantly more eating problems than more skilful dancers. On the other hand, Garner *et al.* (1987) found that dancers at the highest performance level had a higher prevalence of eating disorders than dancers at a lower level. Thus, firm conclusions about the prevalence at different skill levels cannot be drawn without longitudinal studies with careful classification and description of the calibre of the athletes investigated.

Risk factors for the development of eating disorders

Psychological, biological and social factors are implicated in the development of eating disorders (Katz, 1985; Garfinkel *et al.*, 1987). It has been claimed that female athletes appear to be more vulnerable to eating disorders than the general female population because of additional stresses associated with the athletic environment (Wilmore, 1991). Other factors specific to sport may also play a role, as listed below.

• It has been suggested that sport attracts individuals who are anorectic, at least in attitude if not in behaviour or weight, before they start participating in sport (Sacks, 1990; Thompson & Trattner-Sherman, 1993).

• A biobehavioural model of activity-based anorexia nervosa has been proposed in a series of studies (Epling *et al.*, 1983; Epling & Pierce, 1988). Indeed, there are some studies indicating that an increased training load may induce caloric deprivation in endurance athletes, which in turn may elicit biological and social reinforcements leading to the development of eating disorders (Sundgot-Borgen, 1994). Longitudinal studies in athletes representing different sports with close monitoring of a number of sport-specific factors, such as volume, type and intensity of training, are needed before the the role played by different sports in the development of eating disorders can be determined.

• Starting sport-specific training at a prepubertal age may prevent athletes from choosing the sport most suitable for their adult body type. Athletes with eating disorders have been shown to start sport-specific training at an earlier age than athletes who do not meet the criteria for eating disorders (Sundgot-Borgen, 1994).

• In addition to the pressure to reduce weight, athletes are often pressed for time: they have to lose weight rapidly to make or stay on the team. As a result they often experience frequent periods of restrictive dieting or weight cycling (Sundgot-Borgen, 1994). Such periods have been suggested as important risk or trigger factors for the development of eating disorders in athletes (Brownell *et al.*, 1987; Sundgot-Borgen, 1994) (Fig. 25.3).

• The characteristics of a sport (e.g. emphasis on

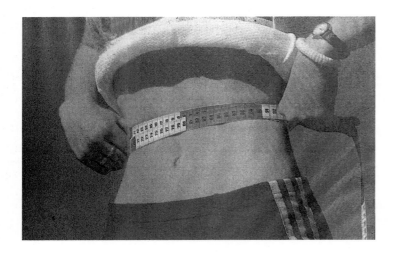

Fig. 25.3 Periods of restrictive dieting and weight cycling are risk factors for the development of eating disorders.

leanness or individual competition) may interact with the personality traits of the athlete to initiate and perpetuate an eating disorder (Wilson & Eldredge, 1992).

Athletes have reported that they developed eating disorders as a result of an injury or illness that left them temporarily unable to continue their normal level of exercise (Katz, 1985; Sundgot-Borgen, 1994). An injury can curtail the athlete's exercise and training habits. As a result of weight gain due to less energy expenditure, the athlete may develop an irrational fear of weight gain and begin to diet as a means of compensating (Thompson & Trattner-Sherman, 1993). Thus, the loss of a coach or unexpected illness or injury can be regarded as traumatic events similar to those described as trigger mechanisms for eating disorders in non-athletes (Bassoe, 1990).

Pressure to reduce weight has been the general explanation for the increased prevalence of eating-related problems among athletes. It is not necessarily dieting *per se* but the situation in which the athlete is told to lose weight, the words used and whether the athlete receives guidance or not is important. The different reasons for the development of eating disorders reported by high-level athletes are presented in Table 25.5. Most researchers agree that coaches do not cause eating disorders in athletes, although the problem may be triggered or exacerbated in

Table 25.5 The different reasons for the development of eating disorders reported by eating-disordered athletes. (From Sundgot-Borgen, 1994 with permission)

Prolonged periods of dieting	37%
New coach	30%
Injury/illness	23%
Casual comments	19%
Leaving home/failure at school/work	10%
Problem in relationship	10%
Family problems	7%
Illness/injury to family members	7%
Death of significant others	4%
Sexual abuse (by coach)	4%

Multiple answers were allowed; 15% did not give any specific reason.

vulnerable individuals through inappropriate coaching (Wilmore, 1991). In most cases the role of coaches in the development of eating disorders in athletes should be seen as part of a complex interplay of factors.

Medical issues

Eating disorders can result in serious medical problems and can even be fatal. It is the author's experience that signs and symptoms of eating disorders in competitive athletes are often ignored or trivialized. Whereas most complications of anorexia nervosa occur as a direct or indirect result of starvation, the complications of bulimia nervosa occur as a result of binge-eating and purging (Thompson & Trattner-Sherman, 1993). Johnson and Connor (1987), Hsu (1990) and Mitchell (1990) all provide information on the medical problems encountered in eating-disordered patients.

Studies have reported mortality rates of <1% to as high as 18% in patients with anorexia nervosa in the general population (Thompson & Trattner-Sherman, 1993). Death is usually attributable to fluid and electrolyte abnormalities or suicide (Brownell & Rodin, 1992). Mortality in bulimia nervosa is less well studied but deaths do occur, usually secondary to the complications of the bingeing–purging cycle or suicide. Mortality rates of eating disorders among athletes are not known. However, a number of deaths of top-level athletes, representing gymnastics, running, cross-country, alpine skiing and cycling, have been reported in the media. Of those diagnosed in the Norwegian study (Sundgot-Borgen, 1994), five (5.4%) reported that they had tried to commit suicide.

For years, athletes have used and abused drugs in order to control weight (Thompson & Trattner-Sherman, 1993). Some athletes use dieting, bingeing, vomiting, sweating and fluid restriction for weight control. It is clear that many of these behaviours represent health hazards for the athlete. Laxatives, diet pills and diuretics are probably the type of drugs most commonly abused by athletes, while eating-disordered dancers also report the use of marijuana, cocaine, tranquillizers and amphetamines (Holderness *et al.*, 1994). Of the Norwegian élite athletes suffering from eating disorders, 8% reported use of diuretics (Sundgot-Borgen, 1994). It should be noted that diet pills often contain drugs in the stimulant class and that both these and diuretics are banned by the International Olympic Committee.

Long-term health effects

The long-term effects of body weight cycling and eating disorders in athletes are not clear. Biological maturation and growth have been investigated in girl gymnasts before and during puberty; these studies provide sufficient data to conclude that young female gymnasts are smaller and mature later than females competing in sports that do not require extreme leanness, e.g. swimming (Mansfield & Emans, 1993; Theintz *et al.*, 1993). However, it is difficult to separate the effects of physical strain, energy restriction and genetic predisposition on delayed puberty. Athletes with frequent or long periods of amenorrhoea fail to achieve normal peak bone mass and may be at risk for premature osteoporosis (see Chapter 27). More longitudinal data on rapid and gradual body weight reduction and cycling in relation to health and performance parameters in different groups of athletes are clearly needed.

Identifying athletes with eating disorders

Most individuals with anorexia athletica do not realize that they have a problem and therefore do not seek treatment on their own. Only if these athletes see that their performance level is impaired might they consider seeking help. The physical and psychological characteristics listed in Tables 25.6 and 25.7 may indicate the presence of anorexia nervosa or anorexia athletica.

Most athletes suffering from bulimia nervosa are at, or near, normal weight. Bulimic athletes usually try to hide their disorder until they feel that they are out of control or when they realize that the disorder is affecting sport performance

Table 25.6 Physical symptoms of athletes with anorexia nervosa or anorexia athletica. (Modified from Thompson & Trattner-Sherman, 1993)

Significant weight loss beyond that necessary for adequate sport performance
Amenorrhoea or menstrual dysfunction
Dehydration
Fatigue beyond that normally expected in training or competition
Gastrointestinal problems (i.e. constipation, diarrhoea, bloating, postprandial distress)
Hyperactivity
Hypothermia
Bradycardia
Lanugo
Muscle weakness
Overuse injuries
Reduced bone mineral density
Stress fractures

Table 25.7 Psychological and behavioural characteristics of athletes with anorexia nervosa and anorexia athletica. (From Thompson & Trattner-Sherman, 1993; Sundgot-Borgen, 1994 with permission)

Anxiety, both related and unrelated to sport performance
Avoidance of eating and eating situations
Claims of 'feeling fat' despite being thin
Resistance to weight gain or maintenance recommended by sport support staff
Unusual weighing behaviour (i.e. excessive weighing, refusal to weigh, negative reaction to being weighed)
Compulsiveness and rigidity, especially regarding eating and exercise
Excessive or obligatory exercise beyond that required for a particular sport
Exercising while injured despite prohibitions by medical and training staff
Restlessness: relaxing is difficult or impossible
Social withdrawal from team-mates and sport support staff, as well as from people outside sports
Depression
Insomnia

negatively. Therefore, the team staff must be able to recognize the physical symptoms and psychological characteristics listed in Tables 25.8 and 25.9. It should be noted that the presence of some

Table 25.8 Physical symptoms of athletes with bulimia nervosa. (From Thompson & Trattner-Sherman, 1993 with permission)

Callus or abrasion on back of hand from inducing vomiting
Dehydration, especially in the absence of training or competition
Dental and gum problems
Oedema, complaints of bloating, or both
Electrolyte abnormalities
Frequent and often extreme weight fluctuations (i.e. mood worsens as weight goes up)
Gastrointestinal problems
Low weight despite eating large volumes
Menstrual irregularity
Muscle cramps, weakness, or both
Swollen parotid glands

Table 25.9 Psychological and behavioural characteristics of athletes with bulimia nervosa. (From Thompson & Trattner Sherman, 1993 with permission)

Binge-eating
Agitation when bingeing is interrupted
Depression
Dieting that is unnecessary for appearance, health or sport performance
Evidence of vomiting unrelated to illness
Excessive exercise beyond that required for the athlete's sport
Excessive use of the rest room
Going to the rest room or 'disappearing' after eating
Self-critical, especially concerning body, weight and sport performance
Secretive eating
Substance abuse: legal, illegal, prescribed or over-the-counter drugs, medications or other substances
Use of laxatives, diuretics (or both) that is unsanctioned by medical or training staff

of the characteristics listed in Tables 25.6–25.9 do not necessarily indicate the presence of the disorder. However, the likelihood of the disorder being present increases as the number of characteristics increases (Thompson & Trattner-Sherman, 1993). The laboratory investigations recommended for all eating-disordered patients, those indicated for particular patients and those of academic interest with expected findings are discussed by Beumont *et al.* (1993).

Effect of eating disorders on sports performance

The nature and the magnitude of the effect of eating disorders on sports performance are influenced by the severity and chronicity of the eating disorder and the physical and psychological demands of the sport.

Aerobic endurance

Loss of endurance due to dehydration impairs exercise performance (Fogelholm, 1994). Reduced plasma volume, impaired thermoregulation and nutrient exchange, decreased glycogen availability and decreased buffer capacity in the blood are plausible explanations for reduced performance in aerobic, anaerobic and muscle

endurance work, especially after rapid weight reduction (Fogelholm, 1994). Absolute maximal oxygen uptake (litres per minute) may be unchanged or decreased after rapid body weight loss, although maximal oxygen uptake expressed in relation to body weight may increase after gradual body weight reduction (Ingjer & Sundgot-Borgen, 1991; Fogelholm, 1994).

Anaerobic performance, muscle strength and coordination

Anaerobic performance and muscle strength are typically decreased after rapid weight reduction with or without 1–3 hours of rehydration. When tested after 5–24 hours of rehydration, performance is maintained at euhydrated levels (Klinzing & Karpowicz, 1986; Fogelholm *et al.*, 1993). Loss of coordination due to dehydration is also reported to impair exercise performance (Fogelholm, 1994).

Psychological effects

Studies on the psychological effect of dieting and weight cycling are lacking in female athletes; however, it is reported that many young wrestlers experience mood alterations (increased fatigue, anger or anxiety) when attempting to lose body weight rapidly (Brownell *et al.*, 1987).

Treatment of eating disorders

Few authors have discussed the specific issue of the treatment of eating disorders in athletes. Therefore, the comments here rely primarily on the experiences described by Thompson and Trattner-Sherman (1993) and Clark (1993), and the author's own experiences in treating élite athletes suffering from eating disorders.

• Admitting to an eating disorder is more threatening for the athlete with bulimia nervosa or bulimic symptoms than for those suffering from anorexia nervosa or anorexia athletica.

• Eating-disordered athletes seem more likely to accept the idea of a consultation than the prospect of prolonged treatment. Persuading the athlete to accept a referral for evaluation is sometimes a significant accomplishment in itself; persuading her to participate in formal treatment may be another challenge entirely.

• The formal treatment of athletes with eating disorders should be undertaken only by qualified healthcare professionals. Ideally, these individuals should also be familiar with, and have an appreciation for, the sport environment (Clark, 1993; Thompson & Trattner-Sherman, 1993).

• The success of the treatment plan must be based on establishing a trusting relationship between the athlete and the care providers. This includes respecting the athlete's desire to be lean for athletic performance and expressing a willingness to work together to help the eating-disordered athlete be lean and healthy.

• The treatment team needs to listen to the athlete's fears and irrational thoughts about food and weight and then present a rational approach for achieving self-management of a healthy diet, weight and training programme (Clark, 1993).

The athlete's family may be involved in the process of persuading the athlete to begin treatment. One factor affecting this involvement is the athlete's age: the younger the athlete, the more the family's involvement is recommended. For the athlete who agrees to participate, treatment can involve a variety of types and modes and may vary with regard to goals, duration and intensity.

Training and competition

Once an athlete has begun treatment, an important question is whether she should be allowed to continue to train and compete while recovering from the disorder. Generally, it is not recommended that athletes compete during treatment. However, in some cases it may be permissible for the athlete to continue competing before successfully completing treatment. However, several important issues must be considered, the most important of which include diagnosis, the severity of the disorder, the type of sport and competitive level. In addition, allowing an athlete to compete while affected by an eating disorder may give her the message that sport performance is more important than her health.

For an anorectic athlete the medical risks of competition are considerable; this is usually also true for athletes suffering from bulimia nervosa. In certain circumstances it may be acceptable for some athletes with milder symptoms, such as anorexia athletica or eating disorder not otherwise specified, to compete before they have completed treatment. The athlete who is being considered for competition while in treatment must undergo extensive medical and psychological evaluations. These must indicate that the athlete is not at risk medically and that competition will not increase her risk either medically or psychologically (Thompson & Trattner-Sherman, 1993).

If the athlete is allowed to continue competing and training, Thompson and Trattner-Sherman (1993) believe minimal criteria must be set.

• The athlete must agree to comply with all treatment strategies as best she can.

• She must genuinely want to compete.

• She must be closely monitored on an ongoing basis by the medical and psychological healthcare professionals handling her treatment and by the sport-related personnel who are working with her in her sport.

• The treatment must always take precedence over the sport.

• If any question arises at any time regarding whether the athlete is meeting, or is able to meet, the preceding criteria, competition is not to be considered a viable option while the athlete is in treatment.

Some athletes should be allowed to compete while in aftercare, if not medically or psychologically contraindicated. However, it is extremely important to examine whether the athlete really wants to go back to competitive sport. If so and if she is in good health, she should be allowed to return as soon as she feels ready after finishing treatment (Thompson & Trattner-Sherman, 1993).

Limited training while in treatment

If the above-mentioned criteria for returning to competition cannot be met, or if competition rather than physical exertion is a problem, some athletes may still be allowed to engage in limited training. The same criteria that are used to assess the safety of competition apply here as well (i.e. diagnosis, severity of problem, type of sport, competitive level and health maintenance) (Thompson & Trattner-Sherman, 1993). Some athletes in treatment will be encouraged by the opportunity to continue training; thus if the athlete is recovering from her disorder and if she is determined to continue competing in her sport after treatment, allowing her to continue with her sport can increase her motivation and enhance the effect of treatment. It is the author's experience that a total suspension is not a good solution. Therefore, if no medical complications are present, she should be allowed to train but at a lower volume and at a decreased intensity.

Inpatient vs. outpatient

Treatment for an eating disorder can involve either inpatient or outpatient treatment, or both. Generally, most individuals with anorexia nervosa require at least some inpatient treatment, although the healthcare provider may try outpatient treatment if the individual's weight is stable and not extremely low and if she is not purging (Hsu, 1990). Conversely, most athletes with anorexia athletica or bulimia nervosa can and should be treated on an outpatient basis.

Types of treatment

Whether the athlete is in inpatient or outpatient treatment, she is likely to be involved in several modes of treatment. Typically these include individual, group and family therapy. Nutritional counselling and pharmacotherapy may also be included as adjuncts to the treatment regimen. The different types of treatment strategies have been described in detail by Thompson and Trattner-Sherman (1993).

Treatment goals and expectations

The primary focus of treatment is normalizing weight, eating behaviour and exercise behaviour, modifying unhealthy thought processes that maintain the disorder and dealing with the emotional issues in the individual's life. Athletes have the same general concerns as non-athletes about gaining weight, but they also have concerns from a sporting point of view. What they think is an ideal competitive weight, one that they believe helps them to be successful in their sport, may be significantly lower than their treatment goal weight. As a result, athletes may have concerns about their ability to perform in their sport following treatment. It is the author's experience that most athletes are willing to allow a coach or other support staff only minimal contact with the therapist, while some athletes want the coach involved and view this as evidence of caring and concern on the part of the coach.

Health maintenance standards

If the athlete is permitted to train or compete during treatment, 'bottom-line' standards regarding health maintenance must be imposed to protect the athlete. The treatment staff determine these and individually tailor them according to the athlete's particular condition. These standards may vary between individual athletes or by sport. At a minimum, athletes should maintain a weight of no less than 90% of 'ideal' weight, not sport related but health related. The athlete should eat at least three balanced meals a day, consisting of enough calories to sustain the pre-established weight standard the dietitian has proposed. Athletes who have been amenorrhoeic for 6 months or more should undergo a gynaecological examination in order to consider hormone replacement therapy. In addition, bone mineral density should be assessed and results should be within the normal range.

Prevention of eating disorders in athletes

Since the exact causes of eating disorders are unknown, it is difficult to draw up preventive strategies. Coaches should realize that they can greatly influence their athletes. Coaches or others involved with young athletes should not comment on an individual's body size or demand weight loss in young and still growing athletes. Without nutritional guidance, dieting may result in unhealthy eating behaviour or eating disorders in highly motivated and uninformed athletes (Eisenman et al., 1990). Early intervention is also important, since eating disorders are more difficult to treat the longer they progress. However, most important of all is the prevention of circumstances or factors that could lead to an eating disorder. Therefore, professionals working with athletes should be informed about the possible risk factors for the development, early signs and symptoms of eating disorders, the medical, psychological and social consequences of these disorders, how to approach the problem if it occurs, and what treatment options are available.

Weight loss recommendations

A change in body composition and weight loss can be achieved safely if the goal weight is realis-

tic and based on body composition rather than weight-for-height standards.

• The weight loss programme should start well before the season begins.

• Athletes must consume regular meals with sufficient calories and nutrients to avoid menstrual irregularities, loss of bone mass, loss of muscle tissue and the experience of compromised performance.

• The healthcare personnel should set realistic goals that address methods of dieting, rate of weight change and a reasonable target range of weight and body fat.

• Change in body composition should be monitored on a regular basis to detect any continued or unwarranted losses or fluctuations in weight.

• Measurements of body composition should be made in private in order to reduce the stress, anxiety and embarrassment of public assessment.

• A registered dietitian who knows the demands of the specific sport should be involved in the planning of individual nutritionally adequate diets. Throughout this process, the role of overall good nutrition practices in optimizing performance should be emphasized.

• If the athlete exhibits symptoms of an eating disorder, the athlete should be counselled about the possible problem.

• Coaches should not try to diagnose or treat eating disorders but should be specific about their suspicions and talk with the athlete about the fears or anxieties she may be having about food and performance. They should encourage medical evaluation and support the athlete.

• The coach should assist and support the athlete during treatment.

Conclusion and recommendations for future research

• The prevalence of eating disorders is higher among female athletes than non-athletes, but the relationship to performance or training level is unknown. Additionally, athletes competing in sports where leanness or a specific weight are considered important are more prone to eating disorders than athletes competing in sports where these factors are considered less important.

• It is not known whether eating disorders are more common among élite athletes than among less-successful athletes. Therefore, it is necessary to examine anorexia nervosa, bulimia nervosa and subclinical eating disorders, and the range of behaviours and attitudes associated with eating disturbances, in athletes representing different sports and competitive levels in order to learn how these clinical and subclinical disorders are related.

• Clinical interview seems to be superior to self-report for determining the prevalence of eating disorders. However, because of methodological weaknesses in the existing studies (e.g. deficient description of the populations investigated and procedures of data collection) the best instrument or interview method is not known. Therefore, there is a need to validate self-report and interview methods with athletes and identify the conditions under which self-reporting of eating disturbances is most likely to be accurate.

• Interesting suggestions have been made about possible sport-specific risk factors for the development of eating disorders in athletes, but large-scale longitudinal studies are needed in order to learn more about risk factors and the aetiology of eating disorders in athletes at different competitive levels and within different sports.

• The formal treatment of athletes with eating disorders should be undertaken only by qualified healthcare professionals. Ideally, these individuals should also be familiar with, and have an appreciation for, the sport environment.

• More knowledge is needed about the short-term and long-term effects of weight cycling and eating disorders on the health and performance of athletes.

References

American Psychiatric Association (1987) *Diagnostic and Statistical Manual of Mental Disorders*, 3rd edn, pp. 65–69. APA, Washington, DC.

American Psychiatric Association (1994) *Diagnostic and Statistical Manual of Mental Disorders*, 4th edn, pp. 1–2. APA, Washington, DC.

Andersen, A.E. (1990) Diagnosis and treatment of males with eating disorders. In A.E. Andersen (ed.) *Males With Eating Disorders*, pp. 133–162. Brunner/Mazel, New York.

Bassoe, H.H. (1990) Anorexia/bulimia nervosa: the development of anorexia nervosa and of mental symptoms. Treatment and the outcome of the disease. *Acta Psychiatrica Scandinavica* **82**, 7–13.

Beumont, P.J., Russell, J.D. & Touyz, S.W. (1993) Treatment of anorexia nervosa. *Lancet* **341**, 1635–1640.

Brownell, K.D. & Rodin, J. (1992) Prevalence of eating disorders in athletes. In K.D. Brownell, J. Rodin & J.H. Wilmore (eds) *Eating, Body Weight and Performance in Athletes*, pp. 128–143. Lea and Febiger, Philadelphia.

Brownell, K.D., Steen, S.N. & Wilmore, J.H. (1987) Weight regulation practices in athletes: analysis of metabolic and health effects. *Medicine and Science in Sports and Exercise* **19**, 546–560.

Clark, N. (1993) How to help the athlete with bulimia: practical tips and case study. *International Journal of Sports Nutrition* **3**, 450–460.

Dummer, G.M., Rosen, L.W. & Heusner, W.W. (1987) Pathogenic weight-control behaviors of young competitive swimmers. *Physician and Sportsmedicine* **5**, 75–86.

Eisenman, P.A., Johnson, S.C. & Benson, J.E. (1990) *Coaches Guide to Nutrition and Weight Control*, 2nd edn. Leisure Press, Champaign, Illinois.

Epling, W.F. & Pierce, W.D. (1988) Activity based anorexia nervosa. *International Journal of Eating Disorders* **7**, 475–485.

Epling, W.F., Pierce, W.D. & Stefan, L. (1983) A theory of activity based anorexia. *International Journal of Eating Disorders* **3**, 27–46.

Fogelholm, M. (1994) Effects of bodyweight reduction on sports performance. *Sports Medicine* **4**, 249–267.

Fogelholm, G.M., Koskinen, R. & Laakso, J. (1993) Gradual and rapid weight loss: effects on nutrition and performance in male athletes. *Medicine and Science in Sports and Exercise* **25**, 371–377.

Gadpalle, W.J., Sandborn, C.F. & Wagner, W.W. (1987) Athletic amenorrhea, major affective disorders and eating disorders. *American Journal of Psychiatry* **144**, 9399–9443.

Garfinkel, P.E., Garner, D.M. & Goldbloom, D.S. (1987) Eating disorders: implications for the 1990's. *Canadian Journal of Psychiatry* **32**, 624–631.

Garner, M.D., Garfinkel, P.E., Rockert, W. & Olmsted, M.P. (1987) A prospective study of eating disturbances in the ballet. *Psychotherapy and Psychosomatics* **48**, 170–175.

Grange, D.L., Tibbs, J. & Noakes, T. (1994) Implications of a diagnosis of anorexia nervosa in a ballet school. *International Journal of Eating Disorders* **4**, 369–376.

Hamilton, L.H., Brocks-Gunn, J., Warren, M.P. & Hamilton, W.G. (1988) The role of selectivity in the pathogenesis of eating problems in ballet dancers. *Medicine and Science in Sports and Exercise* **20**, 560–565.

Holderness, C.C., Brooks-Gunn, J. & Warren, M.P. (1994) Eating disorders and substance use: a dancing vs. nondancing population. *Medicine and Science in Sports and Exercise* **26**, 297–302.

Hsu, L.K.G. (1990) *Eating Disorders*. Guilford Press. New York.

Ingjer, F. & Sundgot-Borgen, J. (1991) Influence of body weight reduction on maximal oxygen uptake in female elite athletes. *Scandinavian Journal of Medicine and Science in Sports* **1**, 141–146.

Johnson, C. & Connor, S.M. (1987) *The Etiology and Treatment of Bulimia Nervosa*. New York Basic Books, New York.

Katz, J.L. (1985) Some reflections on the nature of the eating disorders. *International Journal of Eating Disorders* **4**, 617–626.

Klinzing, J.E. & Karpowicz, W. (1986) The effect of rapid weight loss and rehydration on a wrestling performance test. *Journal of Sports Medicine and Physical Fitness* **26**, 149–156.

Mansfield, M.J. & Emans, S.J. (1993) Growth in female gymnasts: should training decrease during puberty? *Pediatrics* **122**, 237–240.

Mitchell, J.E. (1990) *Bulimia Nervosa*. University of Minnesota Press, Minneapolis.

O'Connor, P.J., Lewis, R.D. & Kirchner, E.M. (1995) Eating disorder symptoms in female college gymnasts. *Medicine and Science in Sports and Exercise* **27**(4), 550–555.

Pugliese, M.T., Lifshitz, F., Grad, G., Fort, P. & Marks-Katz, M. (1983) Fear of obesity. A cause of short stature and delayed puberty. *New England Journal of Medicine* **309**, 513–518.

Rosen, L.W. & Hough, D.O. (1988) Pathogenic weight-control behaviors of female college gymnasts. *Physician and Sportsmedicine* **16**(9), 141–144.

Rosen, L.W., McKeag, D.B. & Hough, D.O. (1986) Pathogenic weight-control behaviors in female athletes. *Physician and Sportsmedicine* **14**, 79–86.

Rucinski, A. (1989) Relationship of body image and dietary intake of competitive ice skaters. *Journal of the American Dietetic Association* **89**, 98–100.

Sacks, M.H. (1990) Psychiatry and sports. *Annals of Sports Medicine* **5**, 47–52.

Sundgot-Borgen, J. (1993) Prevalence of eating disorders in female elite athletes. *International Journal of Sports Nutrition* **3**, 29–40.

Sundgot-Borgen, J. (1994) Risk and trigger factors for the development of eating disorders in female elite athletes. *Medicine and Science in Sports and Exercise* **26**(4), 414–419.

Sundgot-Borgen, J. & Corbin, C.B. (1987) Eating disorders among female athletes. *Physician and Sportsmedicine* **2**(15), 89–95.

Sundgot-Borgen, J. & Larsen, S. (1993) Nutrient intake and eating behavior of female elite athletes suffering from anorexia nervosa, anorexia athletica and bulimia nervosa. *International Journal of Sports Nutrition* **3**, 431–442.

Szmuckler, G.I., Eisler, I., Gillies, C. & Hayward, M.E. (1985) The implications of anorexia nervosa in a ballet school. *Journal of Psychiatric Research* **19**, 177–181.

Theintz, M.J., Howald, H. & Weiss, U. (1993) Evidence of a reduction of growth potential in adolescent female gymnasts. *Journal of Pediatrics* **122**, 306–313.

Thompson, R.A. & Trattner-Sherman, R. (1993) *Helping Athletes with Eating Disorders*. Human Kinetics Publishers, Champaign, Illinois.

Warren, B.J., Stanton, A.L. & Blessing, D.L. (1990) Disordered eating patterns in competitive female athletes. *International Journal of Eating Disorders* **5**, 565–569.

Wilmore, J.H. (1991) Eating and weight disorders in female athletes. *International Journal of Sports Nutrition* **1**, 104–117.

Wilson, T. & Eldredge, K.L. (1992) Pathology and development of eating disorders: implications for athletes. In K.D. Brownell, J. Rodin & J.H. Wilmore (eds) *Eating, Body Weight and Performance in Athletes: Disorders of Modern Society*, pp. 115–127. Lea & Febiger, Philadelphia.

Chapter 26

Amenorrhoea

LORNA A. MARSHALL

Introduction

Of the three disorders in the female athlete triad, amenorrhoea, or the absence of menstrual bleeding, was the first to be recognized. Several reports in the 1970s suggested an association between exercise and delayed puberty or secondary amenorrhoea (Feicht *et al.*, 1978; Malina *et al.*, 1978). By the 1980s, the association of exercise with amenorrhoea was well recognized, especially in ballet dancers (Frisch *et al.*, 1980; Warren *et al.*, 1986) and long-distance runners. Shangold and Levine (1982) showed an increased incidence of oligomenorrhoea and amenorrhoea with the onset of marathon training, suggesting a causal relationship between exercise and amenorrhoea.

Initially, many individuals viewed menstrual dysfunction as a benign consequence of strenuous exercise. Gradually, the association of amenorrhoea with osteoporosis and disordered eating was recognized, and the concept of the female athlete triad was formulated (Yeager *et al.*, 1993). Amenorrhoea continues to be the problem that first brings a female athlete to medical attention. Its presence should prompt the physician or trainer to search for underlying disordered eating and consider the possibility of osteoporosis.

Amenorrhoea is a relatively common disorder, with an estimated prevalence of 2–5% in the general female population and as high as 8.5% in an unselected adolescent population (Johnson & Whitaker, 1992). The prevalence of amenorrhoea in female athletes has been difficult to determine, with estimates based on descriptive cross-sectional studies. In addition, the definition of amenorrhoea has varied between investigations. Glass *et al.* (1987) showed that 19% of women in Olympic marathon trials were amenorrhoeic. In various studies 3.4–66% of certain groups of the athletic population have been estimated to be amenorrhoeic (Feicht *et al.*, 1978; Frisch *et al.*, 1981; Warren, 1992).

Physiology of the menstrual cycle

A basic understanding of the physiology of the normal menstrual cycle will help the clinician evaluate the athlete with amenorrhoea or other menstrual cycle abnormalities. In the absence of pregnancy and lactation, a menstrual period should occur every 21–35 days from menarche to menopause. To achieve this, the hypothalamus, pituitary gland and ovaries must function in a coordinated manner to allow the normal production of female reproductive hormones. In addition, a uterus and vagina must be present to allow the endometrial growth and vaginal bleeding that occurs in the course of a menstrual cycle.

Hypothalamic production of gonadotrophin-releasing hormone

Gonadotrophin-releasing hormone (GnRH) must be produced by the hypothalamus in sufficient quantity and must be secreted in a regular pulsatile pattern. GnRH is released into the portal vessels, through which it travels down the pituitary stalk to affect the cells in the pituitary gland that produce luteinizing hormone (LH) and follicle-stimulating hormone (FSH). Amenorrhoea results when the GnRH pulses that reach the pituitary gland decrease below a critical frequency or concentration, or are disordered (Liu, 1990). There are many neurohormones, including endorphins and catecholamines, that modulate GnRH production (Plosker et al., 1990). Physical and emotional stresses are believed to result in 'hypothalamic amenorrhoea' by affecting such neurohormones. In addition, the GnRH-producing cells in the hypothalamus can be damaged or congenitally deficient, or the pituitary stalk can be traumatized, resulting in amenorrhoea.

Pituitary production of LH and FSH

The cells in the pituitary gland that produce LH and FSH must be intact and functional. LH and FSH are necessary to initiate the maturation of the egg, stimulate ovulation and support the corpus luteum after ovulation. Large pituitary tumours or ischaemia may compromise or destroy these cells. Prolactin is also secreted by the pituitary gland; when prolactin levels are high from any cause, LH and FSH secretion falls and amenorrhoea may follow.

Ovarian production of oestrogen and progesterone

The ovaries must produce oestrogen and progesterone in a sequential manner. This depends on the presence of oocytes (eggs), their maturation and the appropriate development of a corpus luteum after ovulation. Oestrogen stimulates the endometrium to develop, and the withdrawal of both oestrogen and progesterone results in menstrual shedding. 'Ovarian failure' or 'menopause' means that there are few or no functional oocytes remaining, and despite normal pituitary and hypothalamic function the ovary cannot produce significant oestrogen or progesterone. When oestrogen is present but not progesterone (as in chronic anovulation or polycystic ovarian syndrome), the endometrium develops but will usually bleed erratically and infrequently.

Genital outflow tract

A uterus, a normal endometrial lining and a tract connecting the uterine cavity with the external genitalia must be present for menstrual bleeding to be observed. A normal uterus with an obstructed outflow tract may result in the uterus, vagina and peritoneal cavity distended with menstrual blood, and amenorrhoea will be reported.

Overview of menstrual dysfunction

Amenorrhoea

Amenorrhoea usually refers to the absence of menstrual bleeding for 6 months or for a length of time equal to the sum of three previous menstrual cycles. Women who have not had any menstrual bleeding by 16 years of age, or by 14 years of age in the absence of sexual development, are also considered to be amenorrhoeic. Definitions of amenorrhoea vary greatly from study to study and should be noted when comparing findings in athletes with amenorrhoea. To standardize future reports, the International Olympic Committee has defined amenorrhoea as one period or less in a year.

Primary amenorrhoea refers to women who have never had menstrual bleeding; secondary amenorrhoea refers to those who have had at least one episode of menstrual bleeding before amenorrhoea. Many reproductive disorders can result in either primary or secondary amenorrhoea, so their evaluation is almost identical.

Delayed menarche

Delayed menarche refers to the onset of menses after the age of 16. For practical purposes this is a retrospective diagnosis used, for example, to profile the athlete with secondary amenorrhoea.

The young female athlete who presents with primary amenorrhoea may eventually be diagnosed with delayed menarche, but should be evaluated and treated like any other woman with primary amenorrhoea.

Oligomenorrhoea

There is a spectrum of menstrual dysfunction that seems to occur with greater frequency in the female athlete, including oligomenorrhoea and luteal phase defect as well as amenorrhoea (Shangold *et al.*, 1990). Oligomenorrhoea refers to menstrual cycles longer than 35 days and is usually, but not always, associated with anovulation. Oligomenorrhoea can be associated with normal or high levels of oestrogen but no progesterone. Alternatively, both oestrogen and progesterone levels may be low.

Luteal phase defect

The luteal phase is the period from ovulation to the first day of the next menses, usually about 12–14 days. A luteal phase defect or inadequate luteal phase is defined as a lag of more than 2 days in histological development of the endometrium. It is difficult to diagnose since menstrual periods may occur regularly. The diagnosis requires two abnormal endometrial biopsies for its strict definition (Speroff *et al.*, 1994). A luteal phase of less than 10 days is usually associated with an inadequate luteal phase. It is very difficult to identify women with luteal phase defects when large numbers of women are being studied. The prevalence of luteal phase defects in the general female population or in athletes is unknown. Shangold *et al.* (1979) have shown that runners with regular menstrual cycles have decreased peak progesterone levels during training periods compared with control periods. Salivary progesterone levels have also been used to suggest a luteal phase defect in runners (Ellison & Lager, 1986). However, a single progesterone measurement in the luteal phase is an inaccurate method for determining the presence or absence of a luteal phase defect. Multiple measurements of progesterone in one menstrual cycle, with determination of the area under the curve or measurement of progesterone in a pooled sample, are much more accurate determinants of a luteal phase defect.

Causes of amenorrhoea and other menstrual dysfunctions

When an athlete presents with amenorrhoea, the clinician should not assume that the causative factor is exercise; 'exercise-associated' or 'athletic' amenorrhoea is a diagnosis of exclusion. All other causes of amenorrhoea should be considered and an appropriate evaluation initiated.

Pregnancy

Pregnancy is the most common cause of amenorrhoea and *must* be considered first in all women. It should even be considered in sexually active women recovering from long-standing amenorrhoea; the first ovulation can occur before the first menses. It can sometimes be devastating for the athlete to delay the diagnosis of pregnancy.

Hypothalamic dysfunction

Except for pregnancy, hypothalamic dysfunction is the most common cause of secondary amenorrhoea. Hypothalamic amenorrhoea is also associated with primary amenorrhoea or delayed menarche (Liu, 1990). Exercise-associated amenorrhoea is generally considered to be a subset of hypothalamic amenorrhoea. In hypothalamic amenorrhoea, pulsatile GnRH is deficient, absent or inappropriately secreted by the hypothalamus. Psychological/physical stress may affect the neurohormones that modulate GnRH and is most commonly implicated as a cause of hypothalamic amenorrhoea. Rarely, congenital abnormalities or destructive processes such as trauma or a tumour, may affect GnRH secretion.

Several subtypes of hypothalamic amenorrhoea have been characterized. Isolated gonadotrophin deficiency refers to a developmental defect in the GnRH-producing centres and often in the hypothalamic olfactory centres as well. Acute weight loss has been associated with amenorrhoea. Frisch and McArthur (1974) proposed that a critical percentage of body fat is necessary for the initiation and maintenance of reproductive function, although others (Bronson & Manning, 1991) have argued strongly against this theory. Anorexia nervosa is invariably associated with amenorrhoea, presumably from the profound weight loss. Marked weight fluctuations and binge–purge behaviour, especially in adolescents, have been associated with a higher incidence of amenorrhoea (Johnson & Whitaker, 1992). Stressful life events, such as divorce or the death of a family member, have been associated with a variable period of 'psychogenic amenorrhoea'. An individual's perception of such events, her coping skills and perhaps the resiliency of her individual reproductive system may determine whether or not menstrual dysfunction will occur. Exercise-associated amenorrhoea is generally discussed separately from psychogenic or weight-loss amenorrhoea.

The onset of hypothalamic amenorrhoea may be abrupt or gradual. If gradual, a luteal phase defect and then oligomenorrhoea may precede amenorrhoea. Often, the recovery from amenorrhoea is much more prolonged than its onset: it may be months or years after the causative stress is relieved before normal menses resume. However, some athletes have reported resumption of menses within 1 or 2 months of an injury or period of reduced activity (Warren, 1980).

Women with hypothalamic amenorrhoea may have symptoms of vaginal atrophy but do not usually have vasomotor symptoms. They have normal prolactin levels, normal or low LH and FSH levels, low oestrogen levels and no withdrawal bleeding after a progestin challenge. Peripheral blood GnRH determinations do not reflect hypothalamic secretion and serve no clinical purpose. A pituitary tumour should be considered and excluded to confirm the diagnosis of hypothalamic amenorrhoea. Although the athlete who presents with amenorrhoea will most likely have exercise-associated amenorrhoea, other diagnoses must first be considered. Abnormalities of menstrual function can result from dysfunction at all levels of the reproductive system.

Pituitary causes of amenorrhoea

The most common pituitary abnormality that can result in amenorrhoea is a prolactin-secreting adenoma. Galactorrhoea occurs in only one-third of women who present with these tumours, so its absence does not exclude the diagnosis. However, a normal prolactin level does exclude the diagnosis. The measurement of serum prolactin levels should be part of every evaluation for amenorrhoea.

Ovarian causes of amenorrhoea

Ovarian failure can occur at any time during the reproductive years, or even before the first menstrual period is expected. The average age of ovarian failure, or menopause, is 51, although it is normal for a woman to undergo menopause any time after the age of 40. Most women whose ovaries fail after normal menses have been established experience vasomotor symptoms or hot flashes. A high FSH ($>40\,IU\cdot l^{-1}$) is diagnostic. Women aged less than 40 with amenorrhoea and elevated FSH levels should be referred to a gynaecologist or reproductive endocrinologist for further evaluation. Oestrogen replacement therapy or oral contraceptive pills are recommended for treating vasomotor symptoms and preventing osteoporosis.

Polycystic ovarian disease refers to women who have chronic anovulation associated with excessive androgen secretion. Most of these women present with irregular or infrequent menses since menarche, and menstruate after the administration of progestins. Occasionally, androgen levels are high enough to result in endometrial atrophy and failure to bleed after a progestin challenge. Similarly, athletes who self-administer androgenic hormones may become oligomenorrhoeic or amenorrhoeic.

Outflow tract abnormalities

Abnormalities of the reproductive tract may occasionally result in amenorrhoea. Congenital discontinuities of the reproductive tract should be considered when an athlete presents with primary amenorrhoea and normal sexual development.

Pathophysiology of exercise-associated amenorrhoea

Exercise is generally considered to be one cause of hypothalamic amenorrhoea. Whether exercise-associated amenorrhoea is a disorder separate from weight-loss or psychogenic amenorrhoea is controversial (Schwartz et al., 1981). In fact, the recognition of the female athlete triad has revived this controversy. The strong association of eating disorders with amenorrhoea in the athlete suggests that weight loss or marked fluctuations in weight may explain many cases of amenorrhoea, and exercise per se may not be a significant causative factor.

Numerous studies on exercise-associated amenorrhoea provide a profile of the athlete at highest risk and afford clues to the pathophysiology. The athlete may present with primary or secondary amenorrhoea. Competitive long-distance runners, gymnasts and professional ballet dancers seem to be at highest risk (Feicht et al., 1978; Frisch et al., 1980; Glass et al., 1987). Cyclists, rowers and swimmers also seem to be at risk. Walberg and Johnston (1991) found that 30% of recreational weight-lifters and 86% of competitive body-builders were amenorrhoeic or oligomenorrhoeic. Other groups of athletes may also be at risk for menstrual dysfunction but have not been subjected to systematic study.

The athlete with exercise-associated amenorrhoea often has an inadequate nutritional status. Compared with athletes with normal menses, she is likely to weigh less and to have lost more weight after the onset of vigorous physical activity (Schwartz et al., 1981). Most studies have shown that amenorrhoeic athletes have a lower percentage body fat (Schwartz et al., 1981; Glass

et al., 1987), although some studies have demonstrated that amenorrhoeic athletes have the same percentage body fat as athletes with normal cycles (Sanborn et al., 1987). If her weight has been stable, total calorie intake may be less than that of eumenorrhoeic athletes and inadequate to meet energy demands (Frisch & McArthur, 1974; Marcus et al., 1985); however, Baer and Taper (1992) could not find any differences in energy intake between amenorrhoeic and eumenorrhoeic runners. Frequently, the percentage of protein in her diet is low. Vegetarian athletes have a higher incidence of amenorrhoea (Slavin et al., 1984).

True eating disorders are common with deliberate attempts to decrease weight (see Chapter 25). Eating disorders are especially common in adolescents (Johnson & Whitaker, 1992) and highly competitive athletes (Weight & Noakes, 1987). Major affective disorders are occasionally associated with eating disorders in athletes (Gadpaille et al., 1987).

In some studies athletes with secondary amenorrhoea have a higher incidence of delayed menarche or other menstrual abnormalities prior to vigorous training (Shangold & Levine, 1982). In other studies the age of menarche was the same in eumenorrhoeic runners as in those with secondary amenorrhoea (Glass et al., 1987). In addition, athletes who began training before menarche have been reported to have a higher incidence of amenorrhoea than those who began training after menarche.

Exercise intensity is high in amenorrhoeic athletes and is more likely to have been increased rapidly (Bullen et al., 1985). Feicht et al. (1978) found a direct correlation between training mileage in runners and the prevalence of amenorrhoea. In addition, these athletes tend to associate training with a higher level of stress compared with eumenorrhoeic athletes (Schwartz et al., 1981). The return of menses during intervals of rest even without weight gain or increase in body fat has been reported, suggesting that low body fat or weight is probably not the single cause of amenorrhoea (Warren, 1980).

Assuming that exercise-associated amenorrhoea is a distinct entity, its pathophysiology is probably complex. Most likely the aetiology is heterogeneous, with weight loss, lowered body fat, emotional stress and physical stress all contributing differently in individual athletes. Not all thin, competitive runners become amenorrhoeic, suggesting that there are individual variations in the resiliency of the reproductive system. Some researchers have even postulated that those thin women who may be genetically at risk for delayed maturation or secondary amenorrhoea may be attracted to sports such as running or gymnastics. Most theories agree that exercise somehow results in hypothalamic dysfunction. By some mechanism, hypothalamic secretion of GnRH is diminished, resulting in decreased pulsatile LH and FSH (Cumming *et al.*, 1985; Veldhuis *et al.*, 1985; Loucks *et al.*, 1989). Egg development and ovulation are not appropriately stimulated and the ovaries secrete inadequate oestrogen and progesterone. Reproductive potential is therefore suspended, perhaps to prevent an individual with inadequate energy stores from undergoing the additional stress of pregnancy.

A currently popular theory is that the athletes most likely to become amenorrhoeic consume inadequate calories for their apparent levels of energy use (Nelson, 1990). The high incidence of eating disorders in exercise-associated amenorrhoea supports this theory as a major mechanism. Multiple studies have shown daily caloric intakes of 5250–9030 kJ (1250–2150 kcal) in amenorrhoeic athletes with expected daily caloric expenditures of 9660–12 600 kJ (2300–3000 kcal) (Wilmore *et al.*, 1992). In some way the hypothalamus senses the energy drain, output of GnRH is reduced and amenorrhoea results. The mechanism by which this occurs is unclear, but interest has centred on insulin as a mediator of fuel availability. One recently proposed metabolic signal is insulin-like growth factor-binding protein 1, which was reported to be higher in those Olympic athletes and professional ballet dancers who were amenorrhoeic (Crist & Hill, 1990; Jenkins *et al.*, 1993).

It has been proposed that the stress associated with 'overreached' athletes is responsible for exercise-associated amenorrhoea. Athletes who are amenorrhoeic are more likely to take part in performance sports and associate training with a high level of stress. Many studies have shown that exercise induces the release of cortisol; however, Loucks and Horvath (1984) found that acute exercise in amenorrhoeic runners released less stress hormones such as cortisol compared with eumenorrhoeic runners. Other mediators of this stress response have been proposed, including corticotrophin-releasing hormone and catecholoestrogens. In the latter theory, catecholamines released by the adrenal glands in response to the stress of exercise are converted to catecholoestrogens, which are thought to be inhibitors of GnRH secretion (Russell *et al.*, 1984).

Another hypothesis states that increased endogenous opioids directly suppress the frequency and amplitude of GnRH pulses, resulting in exercise-associated amenorrhoea (Carr *et al.*, 1981). Exercise appears to stimulate endogenous opioid secretion more than any single stimulus. However, endogenous opioids apparently suppress GnRH secretion most effectively in an environment of high oestrogen and/or progesterone (Plosker *et al.*, 1990). This does not support a prominent role of opioids in the hypooestrogenic amenorrhoeic athlete. Furthermore, opioid blockade with naloxone does not increase GnRH release in amenorrhoeic athletes (Samuels *et al.*, 1991). Other changes in neurohormones have been noted in various studies (Botticelli *et al.*, 1992).

Evaluation of the amenorrhoeic athlete

All women need a complete evaluation to determine the cause of amenorrhoea, no matter how clearly the history seems to indicate exercise as the causative factor.

Medical interview

A review of pubertal milestones is essential when evaluating the athlete with primary amenorrhoea. Normal breast and pubic hair development for age not followed by menarche suggests a structural abnormality of the reproductive organs. Lack of any pubertal development may occur with hypothalamic dysfunction, pituitary abnormalities or primary ovarian failure.

A thorough history of previous menstrual patterns should be elicited from any athlete who presents with secondary amenorrhoea. It is particularly useful to elicit a detailed history of the athlete's menses in the year prior to the onset of amenorrhoea. If the onset was abrupt, the relationship between stresses such as weight loss and amenorrhoea may be drawn more readily.

A history of sexual activity, contraception and previous pregnancies should be taken. Women on birth control pills may stop having monthly withdrawal bleeding and do not need to be evaluated for amenorrhoea if pregnancy is excluded. If menses do not resume within 6 months of stopping oral contraceptives, an evaluation should be initiated. 'Postpill amenorrhoea' is no longer felt to be a valid diagnosis.

An attempt should be made to quantify physical activity. The type, frequency and intensity of exercise needs to be documented, with particular attention paid to changes in activity that may have occurred near the onset of amenorrhoea. It is important to note the duration of training, since athletes who have trained hard for many years have been reported to be at greater risk of amenorrhoea (Frisch *et al.*, 1981).

A careful nutritional history is very important in evaluating the amenorrhoeic athlete. Weight gain or loss in the year prior to amenorrhoea should be recorded. Determination of fluctuations in weight over shorter intervals of time is also important. Recording the athlete's nutritional intake over the past 2–3 days helps the clinician quantify the caloric intake. The percentage of protein, fat and carbohydrate should also be estimated. It is especially important to elicit any history suggestive of an eating disorder, such as self-induced vomiting, use of laxatives or diet pills, or periods of fasting. If an eating disorder is suspected from the initial history, it is useful to arrange a consultation with a nutritionist and psychologist or psychiatrist.

An attempt should be made to assess the athlete's association of training and competition with stress. In addition, inquiries into stresses at home, work, school and in social situations should be made. Her support systems and methods of coping with stress should be noted.

A history of athletic injuries should be taken. The degree of trauma that resulted in a fractured bone should be elicited. A general review of systems should be completed with particular attention paid to symptoms that might suggest a cause for amenorrhoea. Vaginal dryness and dyspareunia suggest oestrogen deficiency. Vasomotor symptoms or hot flushes are specific for ovarian failure. Symptoms of androgen excess include a history of coarse facial, chest or abdominal hair, or acne. Virilization, including temporal balding or deepening of the voice, may occur with exposure to very high levels of androgens. A history of galactorrhoea (spontaneous secretion of milk) should be elicited.

The athlete should be questioned carefully about the use of medications and other drugs. The administration of anabolic steroids may result in amenorrhoea and signs of androgen excess.

Physical examination

The physical examination of the amenorrhoeic athlete should include blood pressure, pulse, height and weight. Skeletal proportions should be determined in women with primary amenorrhoea; arm span is greater than height in eunuchoid individuals.

Determination of hair distribution is an important part of the examination. For the young woman with primary amenorrhoea, pubic hair should be staged according to Marshall and Tanner (1969). The absence of axillary and pubic hair in the presence of breast development suggests complete androgen sensitivity, a cause of primary amenorrhoea. Androgen excess or administration is suggested by coarse facial or chest hair or hair along the linea alba or above the inverse triangle. Acne may also suggest androgen excess.

The clinician should search for signs of disordered eating. Signs of bulimia include parotid swelling ('chipmunk cheeks'), erosion of tooth enamel and Russell's sign (finger and nail changes on the first and second digits of the dominant hand). Some athletes with anorexia have yellowing of the skin secondary to hypercarotaemia.

The thyroid should be palpated and the breast examined for Tanner staging and galactorrhoea. Galactorrhoea should be excluded by gently compressing the nipples during breast examination. White secretions appear as fat globules microscopically. Pigmented abdominal striae in nulliparous women suggest Cushing's syndrome.

A careful pelvic examination should be done. A normal clitoris should measure less than 1 cm. The vagina should be moist and greyish pink, with a rugose surface. In women with atrophic vaginitis, the vagina is dry and thin with decreased or flattened rugae. Abundant cervical mucus is associated with oestrogen production. Abnormalities of the cervix and vagina, such as a vaginal septum, may suggest a structural cause for primary amenorrhoea. The uterus and ovaries should be palpated using a bimanual technique. An apparently normal uterus does not exclude an early pregnancy. Rarely, ovarian tumours are associated with amenorrhoea.

Laboratory evaluation and other testing

Pregnancy testing should be ordered liberally in the amenorrhoeic athlete. Studies on the impact of high-intensity training on thyroid hormone secretion have yielded conflicting results. Loucks *et al.* (1992) have shown normal thyroid-stimulating hormone (TSH) measurements but a slight reduction in all circulating thyroid hormones in female athletes with amenorrhoea compared with those having normal menses. However, other studies have shown no significant thyroid hormone changes, and it is unlikely that measurement of thyroid hormones helps make the diagnosis of exercise-associated amenorrhoea. A TSH measurement is recommended for identifying the occasional athlete with overt hypothy-

roidism as a cause of amenorrhoea. A prolactin level should be determined in order to exclude a prolactin-secreting pituitary adenoma. Measurement of FSH is recommended in all women with amenorrhoea in order to exclude ovarian failure.

Other laboratory tests may be used selectively in evaluating the amenorrhoeic athlete. A karyotype should be performed on all women under 30 with an elevated FSH and on all women with an absent uterus. Measurement of serum oestradiol is rarely helpful in managing the amenorrhoeic athlete. The androgenic hormones testosterone and dehydroepiandrosterone should be measured in women with signs of androgen excess.

Hormonal challenges are sometimes useful for indirectly assessing the adequacy of oestrogen production or the normalcy of the genital outflow tract. However, many clinicians feel that the need for these tests is limited when a thorough history and physical examination have been performed along with a selective hormonal evaluation. In a progestin challenge, medroxyprogesterone acetate 10 mg is administered orally for 5 days; alternatively, another oral progestin or a single intramuscular injection of progesterone-in-oil 100–200 mg may be given. A pregnancy test must be confirmed as negative prior to progestin administration. Any vaginal bleeding within 10 days of the injection or the last pill is considered a positive response to a progestin challenge and suggests that the uterine lining is sufficiently prepared by endogenous oestrogens (equivalent to 40–50 pg·ml^{-1}). A negative response is usually consistent with an abnormal or obstructed outflow tract, severe hypo-oestrogenaemia from any cause, pregnancy or, occasionally, an excessive androgen effect on the endometrium.

If the FSH level is low and no withdrawal bleeding occurs after a progestin challenge test, pituitary imaging should be carefully considered. It may not always be necessary when the relationship between onset of amenorrhoea and a marked increase in exercise intensity or weight loss is obvious. When the prolactin level is elevated, the pituitary is best evaluated with magnetic resonance imaging (MRI). Pituitary tumours that cause amenorrhoea but do not secrete prolactin are often large and can usually be excluded using imaging tests that are less expensive than MRI, such as computed tomography.

Bone mineral density determinations are sometimes helpful in the management of the amenorrhoeic athlete. Dual-energy X-ray absorptiometry (DXA) can accurately measure bone mineral density at several sites in a very short period of time. It can be used to determine how much bone has been lost when hypo-oestrogenic amenorrhoea has been prolonged. The success of therapy can be determined with serial measurements. When an amenorrhoeic woman is resisting oestrogen therapy, an abnormal bone mineral density may help convince her of the need for therapy. However, there are many limitations of the clinical use of bone density determinations. Oestrogen therapy is intended to prevent not treat osteoporosis. A normal bone density may give false reassurance that therapy is not needed. This test has limited use in the adolescent age group, where normal values are not well established.

Body fat measurements may be helpful in assessing nutritional status. Body fat can be determined with one of the many simple methods, such as calipers or underwater weighing. However, body fat determinations in the amenorrhoeic patient may be overestimated with underwater weighing if she is osteopenic. DXA can accurately measure body fat and lean body mass, as well as bone density, but its clinical utility is limited by its higher cost. MRI can measure overall and regional body fat directly, although its use is still considered investigational (Frisch et al., 1993).

Other imaging tests are occasionally useful. Sonography is a good screening test to confirm the presence or absence of a uterus and ovaries. MRI can often clearly identify a reproductive tract abnormality. Bone age determinations should be made when pubertal development as well as menarche are delayed.

Treatment of the amenorrhoeic athlete

The treatment guidelines for diagnoses other than athletic amenorrhoea are beyond the scope of this chapter. If appropriate, referral to a gynaecologist or reproductive endocrinologist should be initiated.

General principles of treatment

Management decisions should depend on the currently recognized short-term and long-term consequences of the disorder. The athlete may find the absence of menstrual bleeding desirable in the short term and may resist any recommendations for treatment that will result in the return of menstrual bleeding. In one study, exercise performance, as measured by oxygen uptake, minute ventilation, heart rate, respiratory exchange ratio, rating of perceived exertion and time to fatigue, was identical for amenorrhoeic and eumenorrhoeic runners (DeSouza et al., 1990). Kanaley et al. (1992) showed that energy substrate utilization is the same in amenorrhoeic and eumenorrhoeic athletes. According to these results, amenorrhoeic athletes do not experience any disadvantages or advantages in performance because of their menstrual function. However, musculoskeletal injuries have been shown to be increased in athletes with menstrual irregularities (Lloyd et al., 1986), in part because of osteopenia. As detailed in Chapter 27, bone mineral content is decreased (Drinkwater et al., 1984) and the incidence of stress fractures increased in amenorrhoeic athletes as a consequence of long-term oestrogen deprivation.

The long-term consequences of untreated exercise-associated amenorrhoea are less clear. When there is no other underlying menstrual dysfunction, exercise-associated amenorrhoea seems to be reversible. Reproductive function is usually re-established with the onset of normal menses. An individual's peak bone mass is nearly attained as early as mid-adolescence and is fully attained by the end of an individual's third decade. It is unknown whether maximal bone mass can be achieved after this time period or whether women who are amenorrhoeic in mid-adolescence can later 'make up' for bone not gained during those years. Drinkwater *et al.* (1986) showed that, in spite of lifestyle changes that restored normal menses, previously amenorrhoeic athletes could not regain bone density to the level seen in control eumenorrhoeic athletes. Exercise-associated amenorrhoea may diminish peak bone mass, possibly increasing the risk of osteoporosis in the postmenopausal years. Rencken *et al.* (1996) have shown that multiple sites of bone loss occur in amenorrhoeic athletes, including sites with maximum weight-bearing. There is no evidence that these athletes with a history of amenorrhoea have an increased risk of heart disease, despite data showing that the associated oestrogen deficiency has an adverse effect on the lipid profile (Lamon-Fava *et al.*, 1989).

Several other considerations are important when treating the athlete with exercise-associated amenorrhoea. Usually, the recreational athlete will consider a reduction in exercise intensity if appropriate, but the élite competitive athlete often will not. The anticipated time span of intense exercise may influence the clinician's recommendations concerning hormone replacement therapy. An athlete planning to retire from competitive sports within a few months may be treated less aggressively than one who expects many more years of intensive conditioning. An athlete's sexual activity and current desire for pregnancy clearly influence the treatment plan. Most clinicians manage the adolescent athlete differently from the adult, especially if adult height has not yet been attained.

All amenorrhoeic athletes need additional calcium intake and supplementation to reach a target of 1500 mg daily is recommended. Vitamin D intake should be approximately 400–600 IU daily.

Recommendations for the adult with exercise-associated amenorrhoea

For the woman who does not desire conception, nutrition, weight and exercise intensity should be optimized and hormone replacement recommended. A dietitian may be useful in evaluating and counselling about dietary intake. Caloric intake should approximately equal expenditure. If the woman is sexually active, she should be counselled about contraceptive options. The first ovulation after amenorrhoea often occurs prior to the first episode of menstrual bleeding. A decrease in exercise intensity or a 2–3% increase in weight should be encouraged. Weight as well as menstrual history is important in determining bone mineral density.

The clinician should recommend that oestrogen replacement therapy be initiated soon after the diagnosis of amenorrhoea is made. Whether or not the athlete is sexually active, oral contraceptive pills are probably the best source of oestrogen. Hormone replacement therapy, using a combination of 625 μg conjugated oestrogens or its equivalent and a progestin, has been shown to prevent bone loss and reduce fractures in postmenopausal women. The same regimens have been shown not to preserve or improve bone density in premenopausal women with hypo-oestrogenic amenorrhoea. In one randomized trial, this dose of oestrogen plus 10 mg medroxyprogesterone acetate administered for 10 days every month was equivalent to 1200 mg calcium in its ability to preserve bone density for 2 years (Emans *et al.*, 1990). Such regimens should be used only when women have significant side-effects or contraindications to oral contraceptive pills.

Oral contraceptives are usually better accepted than postmenopausal hormone replacement. However, amenorrhoeic women who have been accustomed to the hypo-oestrogenic state often have marked symptoms, such as breast tenderness and bloating, as they readjust to a normal oestrogenic state. The clinician should reassure the athlete that these symptoms are expected and transitory. The athlete should be advised that oral contraceptives do not correct the underlying problem even though they may result in cyclic bleeding. Amenorrhoea usually resumes after the drugs are discontinued. For athletes who find it desirable to avoid menses, monophasic oral contraceptives can sometimes be given without the usual placebo week.

Reassessment of the athlete every 3–6 months is recommended in order to follow dietary intake, weight and body fat, exercise intensity and menstrual pattern. If the amenorrhoeic athlete has refused hormone replacement therapy, is taking less than an optimal dose of oestrogen or if abnormal bone density has been documented, follow-up bone density examinations are recommended at intervals of 1–2 years.

Recommendations for the adolescent with exercise-associated amenorrhoea

The appropriate management of exercise-associated amenorrhoea in the adolescent female is more controversial. Delayed menarche or amenorrhoea after one or more menstrual periods may occur in the adolescent athlete. The long-term consequences of untreated amenorrhoea are very poorly understood in this group. Eating disorders are particularly prevalent in the adolescent athlete with amenorrhoea, and dietary patterns need to be carefully followed. Nutritional intake, including calcium supplementation, should be optimized. A decrease in exercise intensity or modification of the exercise programme should be strongly encouraged, especially for the adolescent athlete anticipating many years of vigorous athletic participation.

The American Academy of Pediatrics (1989) has recommended that amenorrhoeic athletes within 3 years of menarche should be counselled to decrease the intensity of exercise and improve nutritional intake. The Academy has not recommended hormonal therapy for younger girls. However, oestrogen supplementation is suggested, possibly in the form of oral contraception, for the amenorrhoeic athlete more than 3 years past menarche or over the age of 16. In addition, this treatment is recommended for the younger athlete with a history of stress fractures. Dietary supplements should be given to ensure a calcium intake of at least 1200–1500 mg daily.

The appropriate time to initiate oestrogen replacement remains controversial, with many clinicians recommending a more aggressive approach than the American Academy of Pediatrics. In order to prevent premature closure of the epiphyses, linear growth should be completed before initiation of therapy. Hormone replacement should be prescribed in the form of oral contraceptives because of their greater protection against bone loss, even when contraception is not necessary. No studies have shown that hormone replacement therapy is effective in the standard postmenopausal protocols as protection against osteoporosis. Careful follow-up is very important in this age group, with visits at least every 3–6 months to ensure that training and dietary modifications are being followed.

Recommendations for the athlete desiring conception

When a female athlete wishes to conceive, the clinician's approach is very different. The athlete should be strongly advised to decrease her exercise intensity in an attempt to allow spontaneous restoration of ovulation and menses. Nutritional intake, including calcium, should be optimized. Women attempting pregnancy should take a standard prenatal vitamin with folic acid.

A variety of medications are available for the induction of ovulation in this group of women. However, when an underlying eating disorder is not treated or a compulsive exercise programme is not modified, these women have been shown to have a higher risk of delivering low-birth-weight babies (Abraham et al., 1990). The clinician must be very certain that nutritional intake is optimized and any disordered eating is addressed prior to prescribing medications to induce ovulation.

When a decrease in exercise intensity does not result in restoration of normal menses, and the clinician is satisfied that nutrition has been optimized, induction of ovulation is offered. First, other causes of infertility should be excluded. A semen analysis should be performed on the sexual partner, and evaluation of tubal function with a hysterosalpingogram should be considered. If any bleeding occurs after a progestin challenge, clomiphene citrate may be successful; 25–50 mg clomiphene citrate should be given for 5 days to initiate oocyte development. If clomiphene citrate is unsuccessful, pulsatile GnRH administered via an infusion pump results in ovulation in more than 90% of women with hypothalamic amenorrhoea (Leyendecker *et al.*, 1980). Alternatively, gonadotrophin preparations with both LH and FSH are also very successful in achieving ovulation but are associated with a higher chance of multiple pregnancies than the GnRH pump.

Recommendations for the athlete with oligomenorrhoea or luteal phase defect

It remains speculative whether athletes with other degrees of menstrual dysfunction need to be treated. The female athlete with infrequent menses may be hypo-oestrogenic and at risk for bone loss. Certainly, a careful medical interview should be taken. Early modifications of diet or training programme may reverse these changes or prevent progression to amenorrhoea. Birth control pills should be recommended liberally for contraception, dysmenorrhoea and other gynaecological disorders since they may also provide some protection against bone loss. It is impractical to screen athletes for a luteal phase defect in any clinical practice. Recommendations for any treatment of this group of patients must await further studies in which the diagnosis is made rigorously and long-term follow-up is available.

Prevention is the best approach to any disorder. Prepartication evaluation for female competitive athletes should include an assessment of menstrual pattern and diet. Athletes, coaches, athletic trainers and parents should be counselled about the possible consequences of overtraining and poor nutritional habits. They should be educated to recognize and discourage binge–purge behaviour and other disordered eating. Athletes should learn to develop healthy attitudes towards nutrition and weight while realizing their athletic potential.

Recommendations for future research

There is an immediate need for more research concerning exercise-associated amenorrhoea in order to make appropriate treatment recommendations.
• The short-term, mid-term and long-term effects of athletic amenorrhoea in adolescence clearly need further research. The possibility that peak bone density is nearly attained in mid-adolescence suggests that more aggressive treatment of young women with athletic amenorrhoea may be indicated. Current studies are small and cross-sectional. Larger, longitudinal studies are clearly needed.
• The role of nutritional intervention and behavioural modification in reversing amenorrhoea needs to be evaluated. Whether or not these interventions can act quickly enough to restore reproductive function before irreversible bone loss occurs needs to be established.
• The long-term consequences of other types of menstrual dysfunction, such as oligomenorrhoea and luteal phase defect, need to be studied further in order to allow appropriate recommendations to be given to these athletes.
• The mechanism by which the hypothalamus is signalled to decrease GnRH secretion needs to be established.

References

Abraham, S., Mira, M. & Llewellyn-Jones, D. (1990) Should ovulation be induced in women recovering from an eating disorder or who are compulsive exercisers? *Fertility and Sterility* **53**, 566–568.

American Academy of Pediatrics (1989) Amenorrhea in adolescent athletes. *Pediatrics* **84**, 394–395.

Baer, J. & Taper, L. (1992) Amenorrheic and eumenorrheic adolescent runners: dietary intake and exercise training status. *Journal of the American Dietetic Association* **92**, 89–91.

Botticelli, G., Bacchi Modena, A., Bresciani, D. *et al.* (1992) Effect of naltrexone treatment on the treadmill exercise-induced hormone release in amenorrheic women. *Journal of Endocrinological Investigation* **15**, 839–847.

Bronson, F. & Manning, J. (1991) The energetic regulation of ovulation: a realistic role for body fat. *Biology of Reproduction* **44**, 945–950.

Bullen, B., Skrinar, G., Beitins, I., Von Mering, G., Turnbull, B. & McArthur, J. (1985) Induction of menstrual disorders by strenuous exercise in untrained women. *New England Journal of Medicine* **312**, 1349–1353.

Carr, D., Bullen, B., Skrinar, G. *et al.* (1981) Physical conditioning facilitates the exercise-induced secretion of beta-endorphin and beta-lipotropin in women. *New England Journal of Medicine* **305**, 560–563.

Crist, D. & Hill, J. (1990) Diet and insulinlike growth factor I in relation to body composition in women with exercise-induced hypothalamic amenorrhea. *Journal of the American College of Nutrition* **9**, 200–204.

Cumming, D., Vickovic, M., Wall, S. & Fluker, M. (1985) Defects in pulsatile LH release in normally menstruating runners. *Journal of Clinical Endocrinology and Metabolism* **60**, 810–812.

DeSouza, M., Maguire, M., Rubin, K. & Maresh, C. (1990) Effects of menstrual phase and amenorrhea on exercise performance in runners. *Medicine and Science in Sports and Exercise* **22**, 575–580.

Drinkwater, B., Nilson, K., Chesnut, C., Bremner, W., Shainholtz, S. & Southworth, M. (1984) Bone mineral content of amenorrheic and eumenorrheic athletes. *New England Journal of Medicine* **311**, 277–281.

Drinkwater, B., Nilson, K., Ott, S. & Chesnut, C. (1986) Bone mineral density after resumption of menses in amenorrheic women. *Journal of the American Medical Association* **256**, 380–382.

Ellison, P. & Lager, C. (1986) Moderate recreational running is associated with lowered salivary progesterone profiles in women. *American Journal of Obstetrics and Gynecology* **154**, 1000–1003.

Emans, S., Grace, E., Hoffer, F., Gundberg, C., Ravnikar, V. & Woods, E. (1990) Estrogen deficiency in adolescent young adults: impact on bone mineral content and effects of estrogen replacement therapy. *Obstetrics and Gynecology* **76**, 585–592.

Feicht, C., Johnson, T., Martin, B., Sparkes, K. & Wagner, W. (1978) Secondary amenorrhoea in athletes. *Lancet* **ii**, 1145–1146.

Frisch, R. & McArthur, J. (1974) Menstrual cycles: fatness as a determinant of minimum weight for height necessary for their maintenance or onset. *Science* **185**, 949–951.

Frisch, R., Wyshak, G. & Vincent, L. (1980) Delayed menarche and amenorrhea in ballet dancers. *New England Journal of Medicine* **303**, 17–19.

Frisch, R., Gotz-Welbergen, A. & McArthur, J. (1981) Delayed menarche and amenorrhea of college athletes in relation to age of onset of training. *Journal of the American Medical Association* **246**, 1559–1563.

Frisch, R., Snow, R., Johnson, L., Gerard, B., Barbieri, R. & Rosen, B. (1993) Magnetic resonance imaging of overall and regional body fat, estrogen metabolism, and ovulation of athletes compared to controls.

Journal of Clinical Endocrinology and Metabolism **77**, 471–477.

Gadpaille, W., Sanborn, C. & Wagner, W. (1987) Athletic amenorrhea, major affective disorders, and eating disorders. *American Journal of Psychiatry* **144**, 939–942.

Glass, A., Deuster, P., Kyle, S., Yahiro, J., Vigersky, R. & Schoomaker, E. (1987) Amenorrhea in Olympic marathon runners. *Fertility and Sterility* **48**, 740–745.

Jenkins, P., Ibanez-Santos, X., Holly, J. *et al.* (1993) IGFBP-1: a metabolic signal associated with exercise-induced amenorrhoea. *Neuroendocrinology* **57**, 600–604.

Johnson, J. & Whitaker, A. (1992) Adolescent smoking, weight changes, binge–purge behavior: associations with secondary amenorrhea. *American Journal of Public Health* **82**, 47–54.

Kanaley, J., Boileau, A., Bahr, A., Misner, J. & Nelson, R. (1992) Substrate oxidation and GH responses to exercise are independent of menstrual phase and status. *Medicine and Science in Sports and Exercise* **24**, 873–880.

Lamon-Fava, S., Fisher, E. & Nelson, M. (1989) Effect of exercise and menstrual cycle status on plasma lipids, low density lipoprotein particle size, and apolipoproteins. *Journal of Clinical Endocrinology and Metabolism* **68**, 17–21.

Leyendecker, G., Wildt, L. & Hansmann, M. (1980) Pregnancies following chronic intermittent (pulsatile) administration of GnRH by means of a portable pump (Zyklomat): a new approach in the treatment of infertility in hypothalamic amenorrhea. *Journal of Clinical Endocrinology and Metabolism* **51**, 1214–1216.

Liu, J. (1990) Hypothalamic amenorrhea: clinical perspectives, pathophysiology, and management. *American Journal of Obstetrics and Gynecology* **163**, 1732–1736.

Lloyd, T., Triantafyllou, S., Baker, E. *et al.* (1986) Women athletes with menstrual irregularity have increased musculoskeletal injuries. *Medicine and Science in Sports and Exercise* **18**, 374–379.

Loucks, A. & Horvath, S. (1984) Exercise-induced stress responses of amenorrheic and eumenorrheic runners. *Journal of Clinical Endocrinology and Metabolism* **59**, 1109–1120.

Loucks, A., Mortola, J., Girton, L. & Yen, S. (1989) Alterations in the hypothalamic–pituitary–ovarian and hypothalamic–pituitary–adrenal axes in athletic women. *Journal of Clinical Endocrinology and Metabolism* **68**, 402–411.

Loucks, A., Laughlin, G., Mortola, J., Girton, L., Nelson, J. & Yen, S. (1992) Hypothalamic–pituitary–thyroidal function in eumenorrheic and amenorrheic athletes. *Journal of Clinical Endocrinology and Metabolism* **75**, 514–518.

Malina, R., Spirduso, W., Tate, C. & Baylor, A. (1978) Age at menarche and selected menstrual characteristics in athletes at different competitive levels and in different sports. *Medicine and Science in Sports and Exercise* **10**, 218–222.

Marcus, R., Cann, C., Madvig, P. *et al.* (1985) Menstrual function and bone mass in elite women distance runners. *Annals of Internal Medicine* **102**, 158–163.

Marshall, W.A. & Tanner, J.M. (1969) Variations in pattern of pubertal changes in girls. *Archives of Disease in Childhood* **44**, 291–296.

Nelson, M., Fisher, E., Catsos, P. *et al.* (1990) Diet and bone status in amenorrheic runners. *American Journal of Clinical Nutrition* **43**, 910–916.

Plosker, S., Marshall, L., Martin, M. & Jaffe, R. (1990) Opioid, catecholamine, and steroid interactions in prolactin and gonadotropin regulation. *Obstetrical and Gynecological Survey* **45**, 441–453.

Rencken, M., Chesnut, C. & Drinkwater, B. (1996) Bone density at multiple skeletal sites in amenorrheic athletes. *Journal of the American Medical Association* **276**, 238–240.

Russell, J., Mitchell, D. & Musey, P. (1984) The role of β-endorphins and catechol estrogens on the hypothalamic–pituitary axis in female athletes. *Fertility and Sterility* **42**, 690–695.

Samuels, M., Sanborn, C., Hofeldt, F. & Robbins, R. (1991) The role of endogenous opiates in athletic amenorrhea. *Fertility and Sterility* **55**, 507–512.

Sanborn, C., Albrecht, B. & Wagner, W. (1987) Athletic amenorrhea: lack of association with body fat. *Medicine and Science in Sports and Exercise* **19**, 207–211.

Schwartz, B., Cumming, D., Riordan, E., Selye, M., Yen, S. & Rebar, R. (1981) Exercise-associated amenorrhea: a distinct entity? *American Journal of Obstetrics and Gynecology* **141**, 662–670.

Shangold, M. & Levine, H. (1982) The effect of marathon training upon menstrual function. *American Journal of Obstetrics and Gynecology* **143**, 862–869.

Shangold, M., Freeman, R., Thysen, B. & Gatz, M. (1979) The relationship between long-distance running, plasma progesterone, and luteal phase length. *Fertility and Sterility* **31**, 130–133.

Shangold, M., Rebar, R., Wentz, A. & Schiff, I. (1990) Evaluation and management of menstrual dysfunction in athletes. *Journal of the American Medical Association* **263**, 1665–1669.

Slavin, J., Lutter, J. & Cushman, S. (1984) Amenorrhoea in vegetarian athletes (letter). *Lancet* **i**, 474.

Speroff, L., Glass, R. & Kase, N. (1994) *Clinical Gynecologic Endocrinology and Infertility*, 5th edn. Williams & Wilkins, Baltimore.

Veldhuis, J., Evans, W., Demers, L., Thorner, M., Wakat, D. & Rogol, A. (1985) Altered neuroendocrine regulation of gonadotropin secretion in women distance runners. *Journal of Clinical Endocrinology and Metabolism* **61**, 557–563.

Walberg, J. & Johnston, C. (1991) Menstrual function and eating behavior in female recreational weightlifters and competitive body builders. *Medicine and Science in Sports and Exercise* **23**, 30–36.

Warren, M. (1980) The effect of exercise on pubertal progression and reproductive function in girls. *Journal of Clinical Endocrinology and Metabolism* **51**, 1150–1156.

Warren, M. (1992) Amenorrhea in endurance runners. *Journal of Clinical Endocrinology and Metabolism* **75**, 1393–1397.

Warren, M., Brooks-Gunn, J., Hamilton, L., Warren, L. & Hamilton, W. (1986) Scoliosis and fractures in young ballet dancers: relation to delayed menarche and secondary amenorrhea. *New England Journal of Medicine* **314**, 1348–1353.

Weight, L. & Noakes, T. (1987) Is running an analog of anorexia? A survey of the incidence of eating disorders in female distance runners. *Medicine and Science in Sports and Exercise* **18**, 213–217.

Wilmore, J., Wambsgans, K., Brenner, C., Paijmans, I., Volpe, J. & Wilmore, K. (1992) Is there energy conservation in amenorrheic compared with eumenorrheic distance runners? *Journal of Applied Physiology* **72**, 15–22.

Yeager, K., Agostini, R., Nattiv, A. & Drinkwater, B. (1993) The female athlete triad: disordered eating, amenorrhea, osteoporosis. *Medicine and Science in Sports and Exercise* **25**, 775–777.

Chapter 27

Osteoporosis

JANE GIBSON

Introduction

The relationship between exercise and bone mineral density (BMD) is marked in athletes (Heinrich *et al.*, 1990; Risser *et al.*, 1990; Wolman *et al.*, 1991; Slemenda & Johnston, 1993) and at one time it was assumed that the more intense the exercise, the greater the skeletal response. However, during the last 10 years it has become clear that in some young women intensive athleticism is associated with amenorrhoea (see Chapter 26) and low BMD. In some regions of the skeleton, for instance the vertebral bodies, BMD may be as much as 25% lower in amenorrhoeic women compared with their eumenorrhoeic peers. In the short term, musculoskeletal injuries are more common and concern has arisen that in the long term there may be a risk of clinical osteoporosis and fracture.

Effects of menstrual irregularity on bone metabolism

In the normal hormonal milieu, bone resorption and formation are 'coupled' so that appropriate remodelling can occur as required. In the presence of low levels of oestrogen and progesterone bone resorption increases and, since bone formation is insufficiently augmented to compensate, there is a net loss of bone mineral. Not only is the rate of resorption altered when oestrogen levels are low, but the ratio of live to dead cells may be reduced and this may influence the integrity of bone in other ways. For instance,

a reduction in viable osteocytes to the levels seen in elderly women has been noted in the hypo-oestrogenic state associated with gonadotrophin-releasing hormone (GnRH) agonist treatment for endometriosis in young women (Tomkinson *et al.*, 1997). These non-viable osteocytes appear to have undergone apoptosis, although whether this is a direct or indirect effect of oestrogen suppression is not clear. The reduction in the number of live osteocytes may increase bone fragility or impair the ability of bone to adapt to mechanical loading. In paediatric calvarial bone, there appears to be preferential bone remodelling in areas high in apoptotic osteocytes, possibly due to the release of local signals during apoptosis (Noble *et al.*, 1997), and this is a putative mechanism by which bone fragility is increased in the hypo-oestrogenic state.

There is less direct evidence that low progesterone levels can lead to bone loss, although it is known that progesterone can directly stimulate osteoblast proliferation *in vitro* (Tremollieres *et al.*, 1992). It has been suggested that even asymptomatic disturbances of ovulation such as anovulation or short luteal phase, which are associated with low progesterone levels, can lead to bone mineral losses of up to 4% per year (Prior *et al.*, 1990), although this finding has not been confirmed by De Souza *et al.* (1997). In this recent study, menstrual function was assessed by daily measurement of urinary sex steroid hormones and their metabolites over three consecutive menstrual cycles. Urinary markers of bone turnover such as collagen cross-links and osteocalcin were measured weekly; bone density of total body, lumbar spine and proximal femur was assessed using dual-energy X-ray absorptiometry (DXA). Comparison was made between ovulatory sedentary women, ovulatory exercising women and exercising women with luteal phase defects. There were no statistical differences between the groups at any site. Additionally, there were no differences in levels of urinary markers reflecting bone turnover. As De Souza *et al.* (1997) suggest, the conflict in findings may be due to flaws in the determination of the ovulatory state made in the study by Prior *et al.* (1990).

Many female athletes have more severe disruption of their menstrual cycle, sometimes resulting in complete amenorrhoea, and this has now been recognized to have profound effects on bone mineral content. Trabecular bone has a higher rate of turnover than cortical bone and losses in bone mineral are first observed in skeletal areas with a high percentage of trabecular bone, such as the vertebral bodies, distal radius, neck of femur and neck of humerus.

Few athletes are willing to undergo bone biopsy and so the changes in bone occurring at the microscopic level in amenorrhoeic athletes are little studied. However, Warren *et al.* (1990) performed a bone biopsy on a 20-year-old dancer with longstanding anorexia and primary amenorrhoea who suffered collapse of a femoral head. She was known to have lumbar BMD that was more than two standard deviations below the normal mean for her age. On microscopy, femoral cortical bone was markedly reduced in thickness and increased in porosity. At the trabecular level, the resorption surfaces were greatly increased, although the formation surface was normal. It is unknown whether such changes occur in all amenorrhoeic athletes, at what rate they might occur, or whether they are reversible with resumption of menses or treatment with appropriate hormones.

Menstrual irregularity and bone density in athletes

Bone density of non-weight-bearing bones

During the last decade several studies have examined the effect of menstrual irregularity on BMD in athletes. Studies on amenorrhoeic runners compared with either eumenorrhoeic runners or sedentary controls have been consistent in showing lumbar BMD to be 10–20% lower in those with amenorrhoea (Cann *et al.*, 1984; Drinkwater *et al.*, 1984; Lindberg *et al.*, 1984; Marcus *et al.*, 1985; Nelson *et al.*, 1986; Wolman *et al.*, 1990). In the largest study of its kind, Drinkwater *et al.* (1990) demonstrated a linear relationship between vertebral BMD and lifetime menstrual history in 97 active women. Those who had a long history of amenorrhoea/oligomenorrhoea had a mean BMD 17% lower than those who had always had regular periods (Fig. 27.1). The linear relationship between degree of menstrual dysfunction and vertebral bone density has also been shown in British

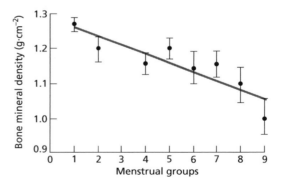

Fig. 27.1 Regression of vertebral (L1–L4) bone density on menstrual history for 97 active women. The mean ± SE is shown for each of the following groups: 1, R (*n* = 21); 2, R/O (*n* = 7); 3, O/R (*n* = 2); 4, O/O (*n* = 5); 5, R/A (*n* = 22); 6, A/R (*n* = 9); 7, O/A (*n* = 10); 8, A/O (*n* = 10); 9, A/A (*n* = 11). A, amenorrhoeic; O, oligomenorrhoeic; R, regular menstruation; the terminology (e.g. A/A) describes current status/history. (From Drinkwater *et al.*, 1990 with permission.)

national and international standard endurance runners. Wilson *et al.* (1994a) analysed the BMD of 50 runners, of whom 24 were amenorrhoeic (zero to three cycles per year), 9 oligomenorrhoeic (four to nine menses per year) and 17 eumenorrhoeic. Bone density of the lumbar spine was 15.6% lower in amenorrhoeic and 10.1% lower in oligomenorrhoeic runners compared with eumenorrhoeic peers.

In most studies no relationship has been found between levels of oestradiol and lumbar BMD, although Nelson *et al.* (1986) did demonstrate a positive correlation between these two measurements in small groups of amenorrhoeic and eumenorrhoeic runners. They measured oestradiol levels in eumenorrhoeic runners between days 5 and 7 of the menstrual cycle (the early follicular phase), whereas other workers have not specified menstrual phase. This difference in protocol may explain the contrast in findings.

Much of the work on BMD in athletes has concentrated on distance runners. This group of athletes have a fairly defined type of training that is usually at least 90% running, an activity which places little direct muscular stress on the vertebral bodies. The stimulus for bone remodelling and subsequent increases in bone density in the spine is probably less than in other sports and it is therefore unsurprising that BMD is low at this site in amenorrhoeic runners. Additionally, the vertebral bodies have a high percentage of trabecular bone and might be expected to show changes in bone mineral early in low-oestrogen states. The effect of hypo-oestrogenism may not be as marked in other athletes as in runners. Young *et al.* (1994) found a small but significant reduction of only 3.5% in the lumbar spine of ballet dancers, with slightly greater reductions of 5–6% in ribs, arms and skull compared with non-dancers with regular menstrual cycles. Robinson *et al.* (1995) showed that runners had lumbar BMD values 12% lower than controls, whereas values in gymnasts were 5.5% higher than controls despite a similar prevalence of oligomenorrhoea in the two athletic groups. The gymnasts were much stronger generally than the runners

or controls and it is possible that the greater muscular stresses applied to the spine in gymnasts and dancers help to offset any reduction in bone mineral due to menstrual dysfunction. Certainly in rowers this seems to be the case. Wolman *et al.* (1990) found that, in a group of élite athletes, rowers with prolonged amenorrhoea had higher lumbar bone density than non-rowers, and rowers with or without menstrual dysfunction had significantly greater back strength than amenorrhoeic runners.

Bone density of weight-bearing bones

It has been proposed that muscular stresses and ground reaction forces in the weight-bearing bones may offset any effect of hypo-oestrogenaemia and indeed it has been shown that amenorrhoeic athletes have higher BMD than sedentary amenorrhoeic anorexic women (Young *et al.*, 1994). Until recently there have been conflicting reports on the effect of amenorrhoea on weight-bearing bones in athletes compared with eumenorrhoeic athletes and sedentary controls. Reduction in femoral shaft BMD in amenorrhoeic active women has been noted by one study (Drinkwater *et al.*, 1990), although Wolman *et al.* (1991) found no difference in femoral shaft BMD between amenorrhoeic and eumenorrhoeic runners, rowers and dancers. Femoral neck, calcaneal and total leg BMD have also been shown to be well maintained despite amenorrhoea (Drinkwater *et al.*, 1990; Harber *et al.*, 1991; Myerson *et al.*, 1992; Snead *et al.*, 1992; Young *et al.*, 1994).

One of the problems encountered in many studies is the scarcity of athletes who are truly amenorrhoeic, defined by most authors as fewer than three menstrual cycles in 12 months or no menstrual cycles in the last 6 months. Therefore some authors have combined athletes with oligomenorrhoea and amenorrhoea in order to achieve reasonable numbers. If trabecular bone in the femur is affected by hypo-oestrogenaemia in a similar manner to the spine, then combining different menstrual groups will obscure any linear relationship between degree of menstrual irregularity and BMD. For instance, Robinson *et al.* (1995) found lower femoral neck BMD in a group of 20 runners, of whom 30% were oligomenorrhoeic, compared with eumenorrhoeic sedentary controls. When analysed according to more detailed menstrual history, there was a 17% difference between those runners who had always had regular menstrual cycles and those who had had prolonged amenorrhoea, a percentage difference very similar to that found in the spine by other studies; unfortunately, numbers in each group were too small for more elaborate analysis.

However, there is further support for low BMD in the femur of amenorrhoeic athletes. Despite small numbers, Myburgh *et al.* (1993) found significantly lower bone density in all areas of the proximal femur as well as the femoral mid-shaft in 12 amenorrhoeic athletes compared with nine eumenorrhoeic peers. A study with relatively large numbers of amenorrhoeic athletes (29

runners with no more than two menstrual cycles in the previous 12 months) was performed by Rencken *et al.* (1996). Bone density of lumbar spine, proximal femur (neck, trochanteric regions and Ward's triangle), femoral shaft, tibia and fibula was measured by DXA, with significantly lower BMD noted in amenorrhoeic athletes compared with eumenorrhoeic peers at all sites except the fibula (Fig. 27.2), refuting findings from their earlier study (Drinkwater *et al.*, 1990) when BMD was assessed by the less precise dual photon absorptiometry (DPA).

In the study of runners by Wilson *et al.* (1994b), BMD was 16.5% and 19.5% lower in the femoral neck and trochanteric regions, respectively, in the amenorrhoeic group compared with the eumenorrhoeic group. Results also suggested a linear relationship between menstrual group and bone density, similar to that seen in the spine, with BMD in the oligomenorrhoeic athletes lying midway between that of the amenorrhoeic and eumenorrhoeic groups (Fig. 27.3).

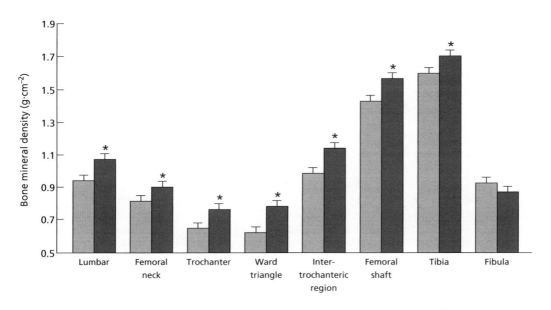

Fig. 27.2 Bone mineral density of the lumbar spine and lower limb in amenorrhoeic athletes (▨; $n = 29$) and eumenorrhoeic athletes (■; $n = 20$). Athletes were required to exercise for 45 min four times per week for enrolment in the study. The majority were runners and average age was 26.3 years. *, $P < 0.01$; error bars indicate SE. (From Rencken *et al.*, 1996 with permission.)

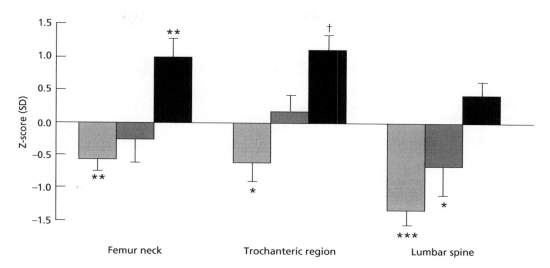

Fig. 27.3 Bone mineral density (BMD) of the proximal femur in national and international standard middle- and long-distance runners, with an average age of 26.5 years. The average training distance per week was 78 km. BMD was compared with the age-matched European reference range (expressed as the Z-score, i.e. number of standard deviations above or below the age-matched mean). In all regions measured, the BMD was lower in the groups with menstrual irregularity: amenorrhoeic vs. eumenorrhoeic, $P<0.001$; oligomenorrhoeic vs. eumenorrhoeic, $P<0.01$. ▨, amenorrhoeic ($n=24$); ▨, oligomenorrhoeic ($n=9$); ■, eumenorrhoeic ($n=17$). Asterisks show comparison of mean Z-score with the European reference range: *, $P<0.05$; **, $P<0.005$; †, $P<0.001$. (Based on data from Wilson et al., 1994a.)

Effect of body weight on bone density in amenorrhoeic athletes

Controversy has arisen about whether bone density should be expressed according to body weight. Most population studies have shown that body mass is a significant independent predictor of bone density: those who are lightest have the lowest bone density. This is of particular relevance in athletes, who in general are lighter than their sedentary peers. Amenorrhoeic athletes tend to be even lighter. Some authors have therefore analysed their data after adjustment for body mass. Myerson et al. (1992), Young et al. (1994) and Robinson et al. (1995) all found that previously noted differences between amenorrhoeic and eumenorrhoeic athletes were eliminated when this method was used. Only Drinkwater et al. (1990) found a continuing trend towards reduced lumbar spine BMD even when adjusted for weight. Whether this is relevant to

future risks of osteoporosis is unknown, although it seems unlikely given that BMD *per se* is the best predictor of future fracture.

Consequences of low bone density in athletes

A number of studies have examined the consequences of low bone density in athletes (Table 27.1).

Stress fractures

Lloyd et al. (1986) reviewed the medical records of 207 collegiate athletes and found fractures confirmed by X-ray (type of fracture not defined) in 9% of regularly menstruating women and 24% of women with irregular or absent menses. In dancers, two studies reported a relationship between bone injuries or stress fractures and amenorrhoea (Warren et al., 1986; Benson et al.,

Table 27.1 Musculoskeletal consequences of athletic amenorrhoea

Increased frequency and duration of musculoskeletal injury
Increased risk of stress fractures
Low bone mineral density
Increased risk of fractures, particularly osteoporotic fractures
Risk of early osteoporosis after the menopause

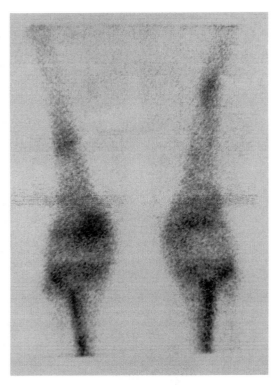

Fig. 27.4 ⁹⁹ᵐTc-methylene diphosphonate bone scan of the femurs in a female 10 000 m runner. This athlete had been amenorrhoeic for more than 10 years and had a bone mineral density of the hip and spine more than two standard deviations below that expected for her age. She complained of 'pulled hamstrings' unresponsive to physiotherapy. The bone scan reveals bilateral areas of increased uptake reflecting stress fractures.

1990) and a survey of 240 female athletes showed a higher incidence of stress fractures in those with fewer than five menses per year (49%) compared with those having 10 or more menses per year (29%) (Barrow & Saha, 1988). Lindberg *et al.* (1984) found that 49% of the amenorrhoeic runners in their study had experienced stress fractures in the previous year, whereas none of the eumenorrhoeic runners had suffered such injuries. However, two reports found no significant relationship between menstrual history and stress fractures, although both contained small numbers of subjects and so lacked statistical power (Frusztajer *et al.*, 1990; Grimston *et al.*, 1990).

Stress fractures of the femur seem to be particularly common in amenorrhoeic runners and are sometimes bilateral (Fig. 27.4). They present as a muscular type of pain that is poorly localized and, because of the inaccessibility of the femur to direct palpation, the diagnosis can be missed. These fractures may be treated for many weeks as a soft tissue injury before being referred for further investigation. A high index of suspicion of stress fractures in amenorrhoeic women is important because delay in diagnosis can result in full-thickness fracture (Leinberry *et al.*, 1992).

It remains unclear whether the increased rate of stress fractures in amenorrhoeic athletes is related to low BMD. Myburgh *et al.* (1990) found that in athletes with similar training habits those with stress fractures were more likely to have lower femoral neck and spinal bone density, lower dietary calcium intake, current menstrual irregularity and lower oral contraceptive use. However, Carbon *et al.* (1990) assessed élite female runners with and without stress fractures and found no difference in the femoral BMD between the two groups. Others have also described a lack of association between tibial BMD and stress fractures in military recruits (Milgrom *et al.*, 1989). It is likely that the association between amenorrhoea and stress fractures is due to impaired microfracture healing in the absence of adequate levels of oestrogen rather than decreased mechanical integrity. In hypooestrogenic states, such as after the menopause or during amenorrhoea, the increase in programmed cell death (apoptosis) of osteocytes (Tomkinson *et al.*, 1997) may affect the ability of bone to transduce mechanical forces and to initiate the repair of microscopic cracks, which occur even under normal circumstances in spinal trabeculae and the femoral head and neck from at least middle age onwards. If oestrogen suppression during athletic amenorrhoea leads to osteocyte apoptosis, there may be a consequent disruption of the signalling pathways responsible for microfracture repair, leading to crack enlargement and the development of a clinical stress fracture.

Musculoskeletal injuries

Stress fractures may not be the only injury more prevalent in amenorrhoeic athletes. Participants in a 10-km race who responded to a questionnaire were more likely to have taken time off training due to any form of musculoskeletal injury if they had irregular menses (Lloyd *et al.*, 1986). Benson *et al.* (1990) studied 49 female dancers and found that those with abnormal menses had more 'bone injuries' (mean 15.0) than normally menstruating dancers (mean 5.0) ($P < 0.05$). Additionally, dancers with a low body mass index ($< 19.0\,kg\cdot m^{-2}$) had a greater duration of low-grade musculoskeletal injury (mean 24.1 days) than those with a higher body mass index (mean 11.6 days) ($P < 0.05$).

More severe bone injuries also occur in amenorrhoeic athletes. In dancers, scoliosis was found to be more common in those with delayed menarche and in whom anorectic behaviour was more prevalent (Warren *et al.*, 1986). Warren *et al.* (1990) later described a 20-year-old ballet dancer with longstanding anorexia nervosa, primary amenorrhoea and low BMD who suffered femoral head collapse. In 1994, Wilson and Wolman reported an osteoporotic fracture in the neck of the humerus of a 30-year-old marathon runner with a history of anorexia and low bone density (see Case history below). Stress fractures and osteoporotic fractures are reported in other young women with long-term amenorrhoea, most notably in anorexia nervosa (Rigotti *et al.*, 1991; Laban *et al.*, 1995; Maugars *et al.*, 1996), and it is likely that the incidence of fracture in athletes is much higher than appears from the published literature.

CASE HISTORY

A 30-year-old marathon runner (with a personal best time of 2 hours 53 min) had been training seriously for 8 years (up to $96\,km\cdot week^{-1}$) and developed amenorrhoea within 6 months of starting this schedule. Prior to this time she had been eumenorrhoeic since her menarche at age 13. After 6 years of amenorrhoea, she was 164 cm tall, weighed 47 kg and had a body mass index of $17.47\,kg\cdot m^{-2}$ (expected for age, $22.9\,kg\cdot m^{-2}$). Percentage body fat was 15.2%. Eating habits were assessed by questionnaires, which revealed subclinical anorexia nervosa and the presence of mildly disordered compulsive eating, binge-eating and a preoccupation with being thinner. Calcium intake, derived from a dietary calcium questionnaire, was 587 mg daily.

She developed a stress fracture of the left pubic ramus and was unable to train for 8 months. During this time there was a significant weight gain of 11 kg, an increase in body fat (15.9% to 23%) and menstruation returned. She then restarted training at a lower level ($40\,km\cdot week^{-1}$) but within 2 months developed right thigh pain that isotope bone scanning confirmed to be a stress fracture of the shaft of the right femur. A month later she slipped at the side of a swimming pool, fell on to her left side and sustained a fracture of the neck of the left humerus. Bone densities at this time (measured by DXA) of lumbar spine and femoral neck were 2.0 and 1.8 standard deviations below the age-matched mean respectively.

She was treated with rest in a sling and made an uncomplicated recovery. Since then she has returned to marathon training, is running up to $80\,km\cdot week^{-1}$ and has once more ceased to menstruate. Her bone mineral density has continued to decline by 1% to 7% per year since menstruation stopped again.

Long-term consequences

Amenorrhoeic athletes may be at risk of premature osteoporosis and fractures but as yet there are few long-term data on these women. As bone mass peaks at 20–30 years of age, athletes should have attained their peak BMD during their most athletic years. Eumenorrhoeic athletes have higher peak BMD than the mean for the population. However, if amenorrhoeic athletes fail to attain their maximum potential peak BMD at this age, it is unknown whether they are able to 'catch up' later in life. If the lifetime risk of hip fracture is related to peak bone mass, eumenorrhoeic athletes are likely to be at reduced risk of osteoporotic fracture whereas amenorrhoeic athletes may always be at a relative disadvantage.

Whether BMD recovers when menstruation returns in these athletes remains unclear. Drinkwater et al. (1986) followed nine amenorrhoeic athletes over a 15.5-month period; seven of the women had regained menses and two had remained amenorrhoeic. Lumbar BMD increased by 6.3% in the previously amenorrhoeic women whilst decreasing a further 0.3% in those who had remained amenorrhoeic. Small increases in BMD were also seen in the radius. These results are very similar to those of Lindberg et al. (1987) who retested seven amenorrhoeic runners at 15 months. Four had recovered menses and showed an improvement of 6.5% in lumbar BMD, while the other three remained amenorrhoeic and showed no improvement in BMD. J.H. Wilson et al. (unpublished observations) followed 13 amenorrhoeic runners (mean age 26 years) receiving no treatment. Over the first year of follow-up, five became eumenorrhoeic and BMD increased by 2.4% in the neck of femur and 1.7% in the lumbar spine. The remaining eight athletes had no menstrual cycles at all during the first year and BMD fell by 5.1% and 3.7%, respectively, in neck of femur and lumbar spine.

More recently, Keen and Drinkwater (1997) returned to 29 of their original cohort of female athletes after an interval of 8.1 years and compared bone densities in three subgroups according to their menstrual status at the first study:

those who had always been regular menstruators (R/R), those who had regular cycles interspersed with oligomenorrhoea (R/O/A) and those who were oligomenorrhoeic and who had never had regular cycles (O/A). Of the 11 women in the O/A group, eight regained regular menstruation within 1 year of the previous study, one regained menstruation a year later and one took the oral contraceptive pill after a further 7 years of amenorrhoea. Despite the return of menstruation, bone density of the lumbar spine remained at 84.4% of the R/R value compared with 84.8% at the time of the first study. Those with intermittent oligomenorrhoea remained at an intermediate position of 94.7% of the R/R mean. These results strongly suggest that early intervention is necessary to prevent irreversible bone loss at this age, although more studies with greater numbers of subjects are needed to confirm these findings.

Some data are also available from women with anorexia and amenorrhoea. Rigotti et al. (1991) followed cortical bone density of the radius in non-athletic patients with anorexia nervosa over a median of 25 months. Of the 27 women only six regained menses, although most gained some weight, took calcium supplements and exercised regularly. There were no significant changes in BMD in women who regained menses, received oestrogen therapy or who gained weight to more than 80% of their ideal weight. In addition there was a high incidence of vertebral compression fractures and non-spinal fractures. However, Bachrach et al. (1991) have shown that weight gain and either oestrogen therapy or return of menses are associated with improvements in spinal BMD in women with anorexia. Studies on women recovered from anorexia also suggest that total body BMD may return towards normal for the age (Treasure et al., 1987; Bachrach et al., 1991).

Thus, although all the short-term studies suggest that small improvements in BMD may occur in some regions of the skeleton, particularly those high in trabecular bone such as the spine, when menstruation returns these gains may be short-lived. If sufficient trabeculae are lost, it may be impossible fully to recalcify these areas of bone.

The studies discussed above have of course focused on young premenopausal athletic women. However, cross-sectional studies of populations of older premenopausal and post-menopausal women have also highlighted the importance of gynaecological and obstetric parameters in the determination of bone density. A greater number of pregnancies, early menarche and greater number of days bleeding have all been correlated with higher radial BMD (Fox *et al.*, 1993). In this study, for each decade of menstruation, radial BMD was 2% higher but there was no association with length of the menstrual cycle or previous history of irregularity. This contrasts with findings by Georgiou *et al.* (1989) who found that bone mineral content of the forearm in postmenopausal women had a better linear correlation with the total number of menstrual cycles than with age or years since the menopause.

In a study of mature premenopausal athletes aged 29–39 years of age, Micklesfield *et al.* (1995) found that bone density of lumbar spine but not proximal femur was correlated with menstrual history index. Low BMD was noted in those athletes with a history of oligomenorrhoea despite

return of menstruation. In a study of slightly older premenopausal veteran runners (aged 40 years and over), BMD of lumbar spine and proximal femur were measured in a group of 13 runners with a history of menstrual dysfunction and compared with peers who had always had regular menstruation (Wilson *et al.*, 1994b). Bone density was similar in all femoral regions measured but was lower in the lumbar spine in those with previous menstrual irregularity (Fig. 27.5). These results suggest that for the femur, if menstruation returns, continued weight-bearing exercise may be sufficient to offset any bone mineral loss incurred at a younger age through amenorrhoea but that there may be long-lasting effects on other parts of the skeleton. These findings are consistent with the long-term prospective study by Keen and Drinkwater (1997).

Treatment of reduced bone density in athletes

The studies and observations described above suggest that bone density at a variety of sites may increase in the short term provided menstruation returns, although it appears to be unlikely that there is a total return to expected values. Prevention of substantial loss of bone mineral is there-

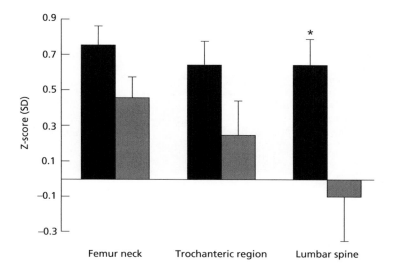

Fig. 27.5 Bone mineral density (BMD) of premenopausal veteran athletes aged 40 years and over. ■, always eumenorrhoeic ($n=37$); ▨, at least 2 years of prior oligomenorrhoea although currently eumenorrhoeic ($n=13$). BMD is expressed as the Z-score (number of standard deviations above or below the age-matched European reference range). The BMD is lower in all areas but only reaches significance in the lumbar spine (*, $P<0.05$). (Based on data from Wilson *et al.*, 1994b.)

fore of paramount importance and the most natural way of acheiving this goal is the resumption of normal menstruation. However, in the studies by Drinkwater *et al.* (1986) and Lindberg *et al.* (1987) return of menses required a reduction in training volume or intensity and a concomitant increase in weight. Not all athletes are willing to alter training habits in order to resume menstruation. For many, menstruation would be a nuisance and for some it might interfere with performance. In such athletes treatment to **prevent further bone mineral** loss or to **improve low bone density despite amenorrhoea would be** of interest. It is thought that demineralization of the skeleton occurs early in amenorrhoea, as it does after the menopause, and intervention is advised if menstrual disturbance lasts longer than 6 months.

Treatment regimens used in women with secondary amenorrhoea have included calcium supplementation, various forms of hormone treatment and intranasal calcitonin (Table 27.2). In a survey of physician members of the American Society for Sports Medicine, 92% of respondents supported the use of sex steroid supplementation, 87% would prescribe additional oral calcium, 64% advised increased caloric intake, 57% would reduce exercise intensity, 43% would aim for weight gain and 26% advised vitamin supplementation (Haberland *et al.*, 1995). Thus despite very little in the way of

Table 27.2 Treatment options for athletic amenorrhoea

Oral contraceptive pill
Hormone replacement therapy (combined oestrogen and progestogen)
Calcium supplementation
? Cyclic medroxyprogesterone
? Intranasal calcitonin

The most appropriate management strategy is to encourage resumption of the normal menstrual cycle by reduction of precipitating risk factors. Should normal menstruation not resume with adoption of this strategy, treatment should commence within 6 months of onset of amenorrhoea to avoid rapid loss of bone mineral

published evidence for the efficacy of such treatments, many physicians faced with an amenorrhoeic athlete would elect for some form of oestrogen/progestin replacement.

Combined oral contraceptive pill

Cross-sectional population studies have suggested that the oral contraceptive pill (OCP) may protect against low bone density. In a population-based study of young women Lindsay *et al.* (1986) determined that vertebral bone density was increased by approximately 1% per year of exposure to the OCP. Further studies have confirmed the dose-related protective effect of oestrogens on bone density and suggest that the optimal dosage appears to be 25–35 µg of ethinyloestradiol. Formulations such as the 'mini-pill', which contain lower doses of oestradiol, may therefore not be as effective.

In a 2-year non-randomized study of 85 premenopausal women with amenorrhoea due to a variety of causes, BMD of the lumbar spine was seen to increase in all patients treated with either synthetic or natural oestrogens in various forms. After an interval of 19.6 months of treatment, BMD increased from 0.85 to 0.89 g·cm^{-2}, equivalent to a gain of 2.1% per year (Gulekli *et al.*, 1994). The impact of this study is reduced by its non-randomization and the diversity of diagnoses treated, but does suggest that the OCP or standard-formulation hormone replacement therapy would be suitable treatments for athletes.

It would be expected that OCP use would be protective against bone mineral loss in athletes by maintaining oestrogen levels even in those who, without treatment, would have become amenorrhoeic. Lindholm *et al.* (1995) compared 19 former élite gymnasts with 21 women of comparable age who had not trained vigorously. Of the gymnasts 14 had been or were currently using the OCP; the remainder were currently eumenorrhoeic. Despite a mean delay in menarche of 2.7 years, the former gymnasts had similar total body and spinal bone density compared with the controls. The authors suggest that this shows either 'catch-up' on return of menstruation or a protective effect of the OCP.

De Cree *et al.* (1988) used 2 mg cyproterone acetate and 50 µg ethinyloestradiol as a combined OCP in seven amenorrhoeic athletes. During 8 months of treatment, BMD in the lumbar spine increased by 9.5% compared with a control group of four athletes in whom BMD increased by only 1.6%. Very little change occurred in the radius in either group. It is difficult to assess the effect of cyproterone acetate on bone density; indeed the increase may have been solely due to the relatively high dose of oestrogen used. In a study of 15 non-athletic women with primary and secondary amenorrhoea, Haenggi *et al.* (1994) showed increases of 2.5% and 2.9% per year in lumbar spine and Ward's triangle, respectively, when treated with an OCP containing 30 µg ethinyloestradiol and 150 µg desogestrel. Non-significant increases in BMD were observed in the femoral neck and tibia, suggesting that the greatest effects occur at sites high in trabecular bone.

However, treatment with oestrogen and progestins in patients with anorexia nervosa with proven low spinal trabecular BMD has given conflicting results. Only those with body weight less than 70% of ideal appeared to derive benefit from treatment, in that further bone loss was prevented compared with controls. The greatest changes were seen in those controls who regained menses, in whom there was a 19.4% increase in BMD (Klibanski *et al.*, 1995).

Progesterone-only treatment

Studies on non-athletic premenopausal and postmenopausal women suggest that treatment with medroxyprogesterone only, either as a depot oral contraceptive or to protect against bone loss in the postmenopausal period, is associated with lower than expected bone mineral in premenopausal users (Cundy *et al.*, 1991) and fails to protect against bone mineral loss in postmenopausal users (Gallagher *et al.*, 1991). However, Prior *et al.* (1994) report that cyclic rather than continuous treatment with medroxy-progesterone in physically active women with menstrual cycle disturbance results in significant improvements in spinal BMD. They used cyclic medroxyprogesterone 10 mg daily for 10 days each cycle, either with or without calcium carbonate 1000 mg daily, in a 1-year, randomized, double-blind, placebo-controlled trial in 61 active women aged 21–45 years. In those receiving the active progestin, bone density of the lumbar spine increased by 1.7% (SE=±0.5%, P= 0.004) during the year, did not change significantly in those receiving calcium and declined in those receiving both placebos (–2.0±0.6%, P= 0.005). Oestrogen levels increased in all groups and were not related to changes in BMD. This study, although not replicated, suggests that cyclic treatment with medroxyprogesterone may protect the amenorrhoeic athlete against bone mineral loss.

Calcium

Bone mass is higher in children and adolescents with a high calcium intake (Chan, 1991; Sentipal *et al.*, 1991) and this may result in an increased bone mass in later life (Matkovic *et al.*, 1979). Work on healthy premenopausal women supports a role for dietary calcium in the development of bone, particularly when associated with exercise (Kanders *et al.*, 1988; Halioua & Anderson, 1989). The synergistic effect of calcium and exercise on bone has also been demonstrated in animal models (Lanyon, 1986).

A positive linear relationship between trabecular BMD in the lumbar spine and calcium intake in athletes has been demonstrated by Wolman *et al.* (1992), a finding that was independent of menstrual status and which has not been shown in other studies (Nelson *et al.*, 1986; Grimston *et al.*, 1990; Heinrich *et al.*, 1990). These differences may be due to methodology, particularly in assessment of calcium intake, or statistical confounding by another risk factor. Alternatively, the relationship between calcium intake and bone mineral content may not be linear. Kanders *et al.* (1988) showed a positive relationship between calcium intake and vertebral BMD in normal healthy eumenorrhoeic women but not above a daily intake of 800–1000 mg. Additionally, the ability of an individual to adapt to a low calcium intake may be genetically determined (Krall *et al.*, 1993; Ferrari *et al.*, 1995).

Low calcium intakes have been reported in many athletes (Rucinski, 1989; Benson *et al.*, 1990; Pate *et al.*, 1990; Bergen-Cico & Short, 1992; Delistraty *et al.*, 1992; Frederick & Hawkins, 1992; Stensland & Sobal, 1992), particularly in amenorrhoeic women. Low oestrogen levels are associated with decreased intestinal absorption of calcium and increased urinary loss (Nordin & Heaney, 1990) so dietary calcium requirements may be even higher in amenorrhoeic athletes. On theoretical grounds, therefore, calcium supplementation would be reasonable in such athletes.

Treatment with calcium has been suggested to be weakly effective by Prior *et al.* (1994) in their study of 61 active women, although no effect has been shown by others. Baer *et al.* (1992) treated seven adolescent amenorrhoeic runners with 1200 mg calcium carbonate and 400 IU vitamin D daily. During a 12-month period the subjects consumed an average of 2400 mg calcium daily but BMD of the lumbar spine did not increase and in two subjects it declined further. In larger population-based studies, calcium supplementation does appear to have a small but significant effect on BMD, particularly before or at the menopause and even in those with established osteoporosis (Elders *et al.*, 1994). Supplementation with calcium and vitamin D_3 can also reduce fracture rates in high-risk elderly women (Chapuy *et al.*, 1992). Larger studies on amenorrhoeic athletes may show more evidence of benefit than has been demonstrated hitherto, although it is unlikely that the effect will be as great as can be gained with oestrogen supplementation.

Intranasal calcitonin

In non-athletes with menstrual abnormalities, intranasal calcitonin has been used. In seven women with primary amenorrhoea who completed 6 months of treatment with either intranasal calcitonin or combined oestrogen/ progesterone therapy, BMD of the lumbar spine increased by 4.1% in the former group and by 9.2% in the latter group (Biberoglu *et al.*, 1990). Unlike oestrogen replacement or bisphosphonate therapy, there is much less population-based data on the use of intranasal calcitonin in low oestrogen states. A recent consensus statement from Canada on the use of calcitonin in osteoporosis advised that current evidence for the long-term use of calcitonin in the prevention of osteoporosis is limited and that it should not be used as a first-line treatment (Siminoski & Josse, 1996).

Bisphosphonates

As yet there are no studies on the effect of bisphosphonates on low bone density in amenorrhoeic athletes. Animal studies suggest that bisphosphonates may adversely affect the outcome of pregnancy and therefore are not recommended for women of child-bearing age.

Effect on performance

Although these studies mentioned the incidence of side-effects with treatment, no reference was made to effects of treatment on sports performance. The side-effects associated with hormone therapy, such as breast tenderness, weight gain and emotional lability, are unlikely to be tolerated by runners and are particularly common in women who have not been exposed to oestrogen for a long time. Commencing treatment at half doses and building up slowly may reduce the incidence of these side-effects. Calcium in high doses may also cause troublesome gastrointestinal upsets in a minority of women.

Conclusion

Menstrual irregularity in athletes is common and often overlooked. Its profound effects on skeletal integrity are no longer in doubt and great efforts must be made to ensure that all those who care for young athletes are aware of the problem and familiar with its management. Athletes too must be educated so that they no longer see loss of menstruation as a bonus but appreciate its implications and know where to seek help. If the causes and consequences of menstrual irregularity are managed sympathetically with a multidisciplinary approach, treatment need not interfere with athletic performance.

However, there is still much that is unknown about this disorder. In particular, the long-term effects of prolonged amenorrhoea on bone mineralization must be delineated and this requires careful follow-up over decades, an aim that may not be achievable. Also, therapeutic strategies must be investigated in prospective randomized trials, a project likely to require multicentre collaboration in order to achieve a substantial cohort.

References

Bachrach, L.K., Katzman, D.K., Litt, I.F., Guido, D. & Marcus, R. (1991) Recovery from osteopenia in adolescent girls with anorexia nervosa. *Journal of Clinical Endocrinology and Metabolism* **72**, 602–606.

Baer, J.T., Taper, L.J., Gwazdauskas, F.G. *et al.* (1992) Diet, hormonal and metabolic factors affecting bone mineral density in adolescent amenorrheic and eumenorrheic female runners. *Journal of Sports Medicine and Physical Fitness* **32**, 51–58.

Barrow, G.W. & Saha, S. (1988) Menstrual irregularity and stress fractures in collegiate female distance runners. *American Journal of Sports Medicine* **16**, 209–214.

Benson, J.E., Allemann, Y., Theintz, G.E. & Howald, H. (1990) Eating problems and calorie intake levels in Swiss adolescent athletes. *International Journal of Sports Medicine* **11**, 249–252.

Bergen-Cico, D.K. & Short, S.H. (1992) Dietary intakes, energy expenditures, and anthropometric characteristics of adolescent female cross-country runners. *Journal of the American Dietetic Association* **92**, 611–612.

Biberoglu, K., Yildiz, A., Gursoy, R., Kandemir, O. & Bayhan, H. (1990) Bone mineral content in young women with primary amenorrhoea. In C. Christiansen & K. Overgaard (eds) *Osteoporosis 1990*, pp. 712–714. Osteopress, Copenhagen, Denmark.

Cann, C.E., Martin, M.C., Genant, H.K. & Jaffe, R.B. (1984) Decreased spinal mineral content in amenorrheic women. *Journal of the American Medical Association* **251**, 626–629.

Carbon, R., Sambrook, P.N., Deakin, V. *et al.* (1990) Bone density of elite female athletes with stress fractures *Medical Journal of Australia* **153**, 373–376.

Chan, G.M. (1991) Dietary calcium and bone mineral status of children and adolescents. *American Journal of Diseases of Children* **145**, 631–634.

Chapuy, M.C., Arlot, M.E., Duboeuf, F. *et al.* (1992) Vitamin D3 and calcium to prevent hip fractures in elderly women. *New England Journal of Medicine* **327**, 1637–1642.

Cundy, T., Evans, M., Roberts, H., Wattie, D., Ames, R. & Reid, I. (1991) Bone density in women receiving depot medroxyprogesterone acetate for contraception. *British Medical Journal* **303**, 13–16.

De Cree, C., Lewin, R. & Ostyn, M. (1988) Suitability of cyproterone acetate in the treatment of osteoporosis associated with athletic amenorrhoea. *International Journal of Sports Medicine* **9**, 187–192.

Delistraty, D.A., Reisman, E.J. & Snipes, M. (1992) A physiological and nutritional profile of young female figure skaters. *Journal of Sports Medicine and Physical Fitness* **32**, 149–155.

De Souza, M.J., Miller, B.E., Sequenzia, L.C. *et al.* (1997) Bone health is not affected by luteal phase abnormalities and decreased ovarian progesterone production in female runners. *Journal of Clinical Endocrinology and Metabolism* **82**, 2867–2876.

Drinkwater, B.L., Nilson, K., Chesnut, C.H., Bremner, W.J., Shainholtz, S. & Southworth, M.B. (1984) Bone mineral content of amenorrheic and eumenorrheic athletes. *New England Journal of Medicine* **311**, 277–281.

Drinkwater, B.L., Nilson, K., Ott, S. & Chesnut, C.H. (1986) Bone mineral density after resumption of menses in amenorrheic athletes. *Journal of the American Medical Association* **256**, 380–382.

Drinkwater, B.L., Bruemner, B. & Chesnut, C.H. (1990) Menstrual history as a determinant of current bone density in young athletes. *Journal of the American Medical Association* **263**, 545–548.

Elders, P.J., Lips, P., Netelenbos, J.C. *et al.* (1994) Long-term effect of calcium supplementation on bone loss in perimenopausal women. *Journal of Bone and Mineral Research* **9**, 963–970.

Ferrari, S., Rizzoli, R., Chevalley, T., Slosman, D., Eisman, J.A. & Bonjour, J.-P. (1995) Vitamin D receptor gene polymorphisms and change in lumbar spine bone mineral density. *Lancet* **345**, 423–424.

Fox, K.M., Magaziner, J., Sherwin, R. *et al.* (1993) Reproductive correlates of bone mass in elderly women. *Journal of Bone and Mineral Research* **8**, 901–908.

Frederick, L. & Hawkins, S.T. (1992) A comparison of nutrition knowledge and attitudes, dietary practices, and bone densities of postmenopausal women, female college athletes, and non-athletic women. *Journal of the American Dietetic Association* **92**, 299–305.

Frusztajer, N.T., Dhuper, S., Warren, M.P., Brooks-Gunn, J. & Fox, R.P. (1990) Nutrition and the incidence of stress fractures in ballet dancers. *American Journal of Clinical Nutrition* **51**, 779–883.

Gallagher, J.C., Kable, W.T. & Goldgar, D. (1991) Effect of progestin therapy on cortical and trabecular bone: comparison with oestrogen. *American Journal of Medicine* **90**, 171–178.

Georgiou, E., Ntalles, K., Papageorgiou, A., Korkotsidis, A. & Proukakis, C. (1989) Bone mineral loss related to menstrual history. *Acta Orthopaedica Scandinavica* **60**, 192–194.

Grimston, S.K., Engsberg, J.R., Kloiber, R.M. & Hanley, D.A. (1990) **Menstrual, calcium, and training history: relationship to bone health in female runners.** *Clinics in Sports Medicine* **2**, 119–128.

Gulekli, B., Davies, M.C. & Jacobs, H.S. (1994) Effect of treatment on established osteoporosis in young women with amenorrhoea. *Clinical Endocrinology* **41**, 275–281.

Haberland, C.A., Seddick, D., Marcus, R. & Bachrach, L.K. (1995) A physician survey for exercise-associated amenorrhoea: a brief report. *Clinical Journal of Sports Medicine* **5**, 246–250.

Haenggi, W., Casez, J.-P., Birkhaeuser, M.H., Lippuner, K. & Jaeger, P. (1994) Bone mineral density in young women with long-standing amenorrhoea: limited effect of hormone replacement therapy with ethinyl-oestradiol and desorgestrel. *Osteoporosis International* **4**, 99–103.

Halioua, L. & Anderson, J.J.B. (1989) Lifetime calcium intake and physical activity habits: independent and combined effects on the radial bone of healthy premenopausal Caucasian women. *American Journal of Clinical Nutrition* **49**, 534–541.

Harber, V.J., Webber, C.E., Sutton, J.R. & MacDougall, J.D. (1991) The effect of amenorrhoea on calcaneal bone density and total bone turnover in runners. *International Journal of Sports Medicine* **12**, 505–508.

Heinrich, C.H., Going, S.B., Pamenter, R.W., Perry, C.D., Boyden, T.W. & Lohman, T.G. (1990) Bone mineral content of cyclically menstruating female resistance and endurance-trained athletes. *Medicine and Science in Sports and Exercise* **22**, 558–563.

Kanders, B., Dempster, D.W. & Lindsay, R. (1988) Interaction of calcium, nutrition and physical activity on bone mass in young women. *Journal of Bone and Mineral Research* **3**, 145–149.

Keen, A.D. & Drinkwater, B.L. (1997) Irreversible bone loss in amenorrheic athletes. *Osteoporosis International* **7**, 311–315.

Klibanski, A., Biller, B.M.K., Schoenfield, D.A., Herzog, D.B. & Saxe, V.C. (1995) The effects of estrogen administration on trabecular bone loss in young women with anorexia nervosa. *Journal of Clinical Endocrinology and Metabolism* **80**, 898–904.

Krall, E.A. & Dawson-Hughes, B. (1993) Heritable and lifestyle determinants of bone mineral density. *Journal of Bone and Mineral Research* **8**, 1–9.

Laban, M.M., Wilkinns, J.C., Sackeyfio, A.H. & Taylor, R.S. (1995) Osteoporotic stress fractures in anorexia nervosa: etiology, diagnosis and review of four cases. *Archives of Physical Medicine and Rehabilitation* **76**, 884–887.

Lanyon, L.E. (1986) Modulation of bone loss during calcium insufficiency by controlled dynamic loading. *Calcified Tissue International* **38**, 209–216.

Leinberry, C.F., McShane, R.B., Stewart, W.G. & Hume, E.L. (1992) A displaced subtrochanteric stress fracture in a young amenorrheic athlete. *American Journal of Sports Medicine* **20**, 485–487.

Lindberg, J.S., Fears, W.B., Hunt, M., Powell, M.R., Boll, D. & Wade, C.E. (1984) Exercise-induced amenorrhea and bone density. *Annals of Internal Medicine* **101**, 647–648.

Lindberg, J.S., Powell, M.R., Hunt, M.M., Ducey, D.E. & Wade, C.E. (1987) Increased vertebral bone mineral in response to reduced exercise in amenorrheic runners. *Western Journal of Medicine* **146**, 39–42.

Lindholm, C., Hagenfeldt, K. & Ringertz, H. (1995) Bone mineral content of young former gymnasts. *Acta Paediatrica Scandinavica* **84**, 1109–1112.

Lindsay, R., Tohme, J. & Kanders, B. (1986) The effect of oral contraceptive use on vertebral bone mass in pre- and post-menopausal women. *Contraception* **34**, 333–340.

Lloyd, T., Triantafyllou, S.J., Baker, E.R. *et al.* (1986) Women athletes with menstrual irregularity have increased musculoskeletal injuries. *Medicine and Science in Sports and Exercise* **18**, 374–379.

Marcus, R., Cann, C., Madvig, P. *et al.* (1985) Menstrual function and bone mass in elite women distance runners. *Annals of Internal Medicine* **102**, 158–163.

Matkovic, V., Kostial, K., Simonovic, I., Buzina, R., Brodarec, A. & Nordin, B.E.C. (1979) Bone status and fracture rates in two regions of Yugoslavia. *American Journal of Clinical Nutrition* **32**, 540–549.

Maugars, Y., Bertholet, J.M., Lalande, S., Charlier, C. & Prost, A. (1996) Osteoporotic fractures revealing anorexia nervosa in five females. *Revue du Rhumatisme* (English edn) **63**, 201–206.

Micklesfield, L.K., Lambert, E.V., Fataar, A.B., Noakes, T.D. & Myburgh, K.H. (1995) Bone mineral density in mature premenopausal ultramarathon runners. *Medicine and Science in Sports and Exercise* **27**, 688–696.

Milgrom, C., Giladi, M., Simkin, A. *et al.* (1989) The area moment inertia of the tibia: a risk factor for stress fractures. *Journal of Biomechanics* **22**, 1243–1248.

Myburgh, K.H., Hutchins, J., Fataar, A.B., Hough, S.F. & Noakes, T.D. (1990) Low bone density is an etiological factor for stress fractures in athletes. *Annals of Internal Medicine* **113**, 754–759.

Myburgh, K.H., Bachrach, L.K., Lewis, B., Kent, K. & Marcus, R. (1993) Low bone density at axial and appendicular sites in amenorrheic athletes. *Medicine and Science in Sports and Exercise* **25**, 1197–1202.

Myerson, M., Gutin, B., Warren, M.P., Wang, J., Lichtman, S. & Pierson, R.N. (1992) Total body bone density in amenorrheic runners. *Obstetrics and Gynecology* **79**, 973–978.

Nelson, M.E., Fisher, E.C., Catsos, P.D., Meredith, C.N., Turksoy, R.N. & Evans, J.E. (1986) Diet and bone status in amenorrheic runners. *American Journal of Clinical Nutrition* **43**, 910–916.

Noble, B.S., Stevens, H., Loveridge, N. & Reeve, J. (1997) Identification of apoptotic changes in normal and pathological human bone. *Bone* **20**, 273–282.

Nordin, B.E.C. & Heaney, R.P. (1990) Calcium supplementation of the diet: justified by present evidence. *British Medical Journal* **300**, 1056–1060.

Pate, R.R., Sargent, R.G., Baldwin, C. & Burgess, M.L. (1990) Dietary intake of women runners. *International Journal of Sports Medicine* **11**, 461–466.

Prior, J.C., Vigna, Y.M., Schechter, M.T. & Burgess, A.E. (1990) Spinal bone loss and ovulatory disturbance. *New England Journal of Medicine* **323**, 1221–1227.

Prior, J.C., Vigna, Y.M., Barr, S.I., Rexworthy, C. & Lentle, B.C. (1994) Cyclic medroxyprogesterone treatment increases bone density: a controlled trial in active women with menstrual cycle disturbances. *American Journal of Medicine* **96**, 521–530.

Rencken, M.L., Chesnut, C.H. & Drinkwater, B.L. (1996) Bone density at multiple skeletal sites in amenorrheic athletes. *Journal of the American Medical Association* **276**, 238–240.

Rigotti, N.A., Neer, R.M., Skates, S.J., Herzog, D.B. & Nussbaum, S.R. (1991) The clinical course of osteoporosis in anorexia nervosa. *Journal of the American Medical Association* **265**, 1133–1138.

Risser, W.L., Lee, E.J., Leblanc, A., Poindexter, J.M.H. & Schneider, V. (1990) Bone density in eumenorrhoeic female college athletes. *Medicine and Science in Sports and Exercise* **22**, 570–574.

Robinson, T.L., Snow-Harter, C., Taaffe, D.R., Gillis, D., Shaw, J. & Marcus, R. (1995) Gymnasts exhibit higher bone mass than runners despite similar prevalence of amenorrhoea and oligomenorrhoea. *Journal of Bone and Mineral Research* **10**, 26–34.

Rucinski, A. (1989) Relationship of body image and dietary intake of competitive ice-skaters. *Journal of the American Dietetic Association* **89**, 98–100.

Sentipal, J.M., Wardlaw, M., Mahan, J. & Matkovic, V. (1991) Influence of calcium intake and growth indexes on vertebral bone mineral density in young females. *American Journal of Clinical Nutrition* **54**, 425–428.

Siminoski, K. & Josse, R.G. (1996) Prevention and management of osteoporosis: consensus statements from the Scientific Advisory Board of the Osteoporosis Society of Canada. 9. Calcitonin in the treament of osteoporosis. *Canadian Medical Association Journal* **155**, 962–965.

Slemenda, C.W. & Johnston, C.C. (1993) High intensity activities in young women: site specific bone mass effects among female figure skaters. *Bone and Mineral* **20**, 125–132.

Snead, D.B., Weltman, A., Weltman, J.Y. et al. (1992) Reproductive hormones and bone mineral density in women runners. *Journal of Applied Physiology* **72**, 2149–2156.

Stensland, S.H. & Sobal, J. (1992) Dietary practices of ballet, jazz, and modern dancers. *Journal of the American Dietetic Association* **92**, 319–324.

Tomkinson, A., Reeve, J., Shaw, R. & Noble, B. (1997) The death of osteocytes via apoptosis accompanies oestrogen withdrawal in human bone. *Journal of Clinical Endocrinology and Metabolism* **82**, 3128–3135.

Treasure, J.L., Russell, J.F.M., Fogelman, I. & Murby, B. (1987) Reversible bone loss in anorexia nervosa. *British Medical Journal* **295**, 474–475.

Tremollieres, F.A., Strong, D.D., Baylink, D.T. & Mohan, S. (1992) Progesterone and promegestone stimulate human bone cell proliferation and insulin-like human growth factor 2 production. *Acta Endocrinologica* **126**, 329–337.

Warren, M.P., Brooks-Gunn, J., Hamilton, L.H., Warren, L.F. & Hamilton, W.G. (1986) Scoliosis and fractures in young ballet dancers. *New England Journal of Medicine* **314**, 1348–1353.

Warren, M.P., Shane, E., Lee, M.J. et al. (1990) Femoral head collapse associated with anorexia nervosa in a 20-year-old ballet dancer. *Clinical Orthopaedics and Related Research* **251**, 171–176.

Wilson, J.H. & Wolman, R.L. (1994) Osteoporosis and fracture complications in an amenorrheic athlete. *British Journal of Rheumatology* **33**, 480–481.

Wilson, J.H., Reeve, J. & Harries, M.G. (1994a) Determinants of bone mineral density in female athletes. *Bone* **15**, 450.

Wilson, J.H., Harries, M.G. & Reeve, J. (1994b) Bone mineral density in premenopausal veteran female athletes and the influence of menstrual irregularity. *Clinical Science* **86**, 2p.

Wolman, R.L., Clark, P., McNally, E., Harries, M. & Reeve, J. (1990) Menstrual state and exercise as determinants of spinal trabecular bone density in female athletes. *British Medical Journal* **301**, 516–518.

Wolman, R.L., Faulmann, L., Clark, P., Hesp, R. & Harries, M.G. (1991) Different training patterns and bone mineral density of the femoral shaft in elite, female athletes. *Annals of the Rheumatic Diseases* **50**, 487–489.

Wolman, R.L., Clark, P., McNally, E., Harries, M. & Reeve, J. (1992) Dietary calcium as a statistical determinant of spinal trabecular bone density in amenorrheic and oestrogen-replete athletes. *Bone and Mineral* **17**, 415–423.

Young, N., Formica, C., Szmukler, G. & Seeman, E. (1994) Bone density at weight-bearing and non-weight-bearing sites in ballet dancers: the effects of exercise, hypogonadism, and body weight. *Journal of Clinical Endocrinology and Metabolism* **78**, 449–454.

PART 7

PSYCHOSOCIAL ISSUES

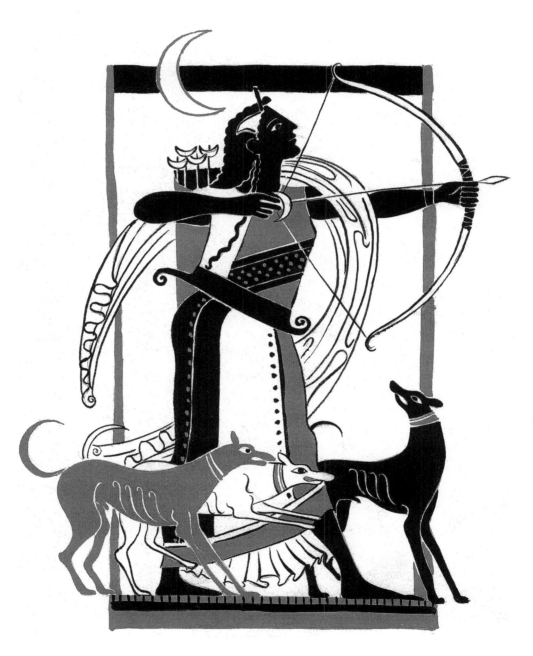

Chapter 28

The Young Élite Athlete: the Good, the Bad and the Ugly

MAUREEN R. WEISS, ANTHONY J. AMOROSE AND
JUSTINE B. ALLEN

Introduction

I am not suggesting that gymnastics and figure skating in and of themselves are destructive . . . both sports are potentially wonderful and enriching . . . the average child can develop a sense of mastery, self-esteem, and healthy athleticism . . . it's about the elite child athlete and the American obsession with winning that has produced a training environment wherein results are bought at any cost, no matter how devastating. It's about how our cultural fixation on beauty and weight and youth has shaped both sports and driven the athletes into a sphere beyond the quest for physical performance (Ryan, 1995, p. 5).

Ever since the 1930s, when public elementary schools relinquished their hold over children's competitive sport in the USA (Wiggins, 1996), independent sports organizations such as national youth agencies (e.g. YMCA), national youth sport organizations (e.g. Little League baseball) and national governing bodies (e.g. USA Gymnastics, USA Swimming) have contributed to the dramatic onslaught of millions of children and teenagers involved in competitive, and often very intense, participation. The numbers of children and teenagers involved in competitive sport today are staggering: an estimated 20–35 million in non-school agency-sponsored sports and another 10 million in high-school sports (Ewing & Seefeldt, 1996; Weiss & Hayashi, 1996).

Along with this astronomical increase in the numbers of young people participating in competitive sport is the equity afforded young girls and women. Since the passage of Title IX of the Educational Equity Act in 1972, the latent benefits of this legal action are only now being realized in the opportunities available for participation; the quality of training, equipment and coaching; and the potential for college scholarships and sport-related careers. For example, half of non-school sport participants are female and in 1995 2.1 of the 5.6 million interscholastic athletes were female. By the end of 1997 there were two women's professional basketball leagues and a women's professional softball league, women's ice hockey was made a new Olympic event for the 1998 Winter Games in Nagano and, inevitably, there was enhanced attention in the media; just some of the many 'firsts' formerly reserved for male athletes. With these changes for female youth emerged both advocates and critics.

On the positive side, advocates argue that girls and young women now have the same opportunities to develop lifelong skills and attributes as their brothers have always had. These include the development of a variety of motor and physical skills, leadership and follower qualities, physical fitness and social relationships with adults and peers, the benefits alluded to in the first part of Joan Ryan's quote at the beginning of this chapter. In contrast, critics question the costs of the sudden and steep incline in competitive and material opportunities, disadvantages implied by the second half of Joan Ryan's quote. Poor self-esteem and high levels of competitive anxiety and stress may result from the increased pressure to win. In turn, these changes in attitudes may manifest themselves in such behaviours as injuries, burnout, eating disorders and substance abuse.

Whether the advocates or critics are right is a moot point. Children's competitive sport, and at highly intense levels, is here to stay, as are the increased opportunities and rewards available for female athletes. These are good things. However, the world of sport does not occur in isolation but within a social context, one governed and controlled by significant adults such as parents, coaches and administrators, as well as by the participants themselves. Together they determine the attitudes and behaviours condoned by the subculture of that specific sport (Iversen, 1990; Coakley, 1992; Brustad & Ritter-Taylor, 1996). Thus 'good', 'bad' and 'ugly' are all possible outcomes of sport involvement. Bonnie Blair is a prime example of the good. Starting in competitive speed skating at an early age, Blair's perspective on sport participation and winning was shaped by a strong social support network, including her parents, siblings, friends and coach. Mary Pierce, professional tennis player, might be an example of the bad. Although a highly successful player on the tour, her father has been banned from tournaments for his verbally abusive behaviour. Finally, an easy example of the ugly is Tonya Harding's role in the physical assault on Nancy Kerrigan, who stood in her way of making the Olympic figure-skating team.

As we ponder the role of high-level competitive sport in the development of young females, there are no black and white answers to many questions. At what age should girls start specializing? Should certain sports (e.g. gymnastics, boxing) be discouraged for girls? How much is too much—number of sports, time commitment, financial investment? These are difficult to answer at a superficial level. However, research and experiential evidence can help us make informed decisions about how to structure com-

petitive sport, evaluate and recommend the best coaching styles, and encourage parenting roles and responsibilities so that young female athletes can maximize the good, minimize the bad and sidestep the ugly.

The purpose of this chapter is to address several issues concerning the social and psychological ramifications of the participation of young females in high-level competitive sport. First, we highlight the key psychosocial outcomes of competitive youth sport, including the good, bad and ugly. Next, we synthesize what the scientific research says about psychosocial issues across a number of specific sports. Third, we present what the anecdotal literature says, sampling the perspectives of journalists who have been granted greater access to child sport stars. Fourth, we summarize common themes from the scientific and anecdotal literatures. Finally, we offer recommendations to national governing bodies, coaches and parents for maximizing the good, minimizing the bad and avoiding the ugly in competitive sport for girls and young women.

Psychosocial outcomes of competitive youth sport

Positive and negative outcomes of sporting competition are equally possible (Table 28.1). Educators and researchers often refer to this as the 'double-edged sword' of sport participation (Martens, 1978). On the one hand, competitive participation affords opportunities for developing positive self-perceptions (e.g. self-esteem, self-confidence), emotions/affect (e.g. pride, enjoyment, excitement) and motivation (i.e. the intrinsic desire to continue participating). Positive outcomes can also include achievement behaviours (e.g. effort and persistence in the face of challenges, attaining personal performance goals), moral and social development (e.g. sportspersonship, interpersonal skills with adults and peers), a positive attitude towards the value of physical activity for health-related behaviours and the ability to cope with competitive stress (Weiss & Glenn, 1992; Weiss, 1993).

Table 28.1 Positive and negative psychosocial outcomes of high-level sport. (Data from Gould, 1993; Weiss, 1993)

Positive	Negative	Ugly
Self-perceptions	Self-perceptions	Injuries
Self-esteem	Self-esteem	Burnout
Self-confidence	Self-confidence	Eating disorders
Affect	Affect	Substance abuse
Enjoyment	Anxiety	Parental control
Motivation	Motivation	Coach abuse
Intrinsic	Extrinsic	Unidimensional
High achievement	Low achievement	self-identity
Character	'Characters'	Loss of enjoyment
Interpersonal skills	Maladaptive social	Poor self-image
Positive attitude	skills	Lost childhood
Cope with stress	Negative attitude	Politics of the sport
	Experience stress	

However, when the sword is wielded recklessly, competitive participation can contribute to: low self-esteem and low levels of self-confidence; negative emotions, such as anxiety, disappointment and shame; and a dependence on extrinsic forms of motivation, such as feeling that participation is compulsory rather than voluntary, which may eventually lead to burnout (Gould, 1993). This undesirable type of motivation may be driven by coercion from parents or coaches, by internal guilt about the money invested by parents or by an emphasis on winning fame, status and fortune through élite-level participation. This 'win at all costs' mentality unfortunately takes its toll in a most unbecoming way on a young athlete's psychological core, her self-esteem. Other negative outcomes that mirror the positive ones are achievement behaviour (e.g. low performance accomplishment), low levels of moral development (e.g. cheating to gain an advantage), poor interpersonal skills (e.g. poor anger management skills, disrespect for coaches and team-mates), a negative attitude towards sport and physical activity, and high levels of competitive stress that, if not corralled early, may escalate to overtraining, staleness or psychological burnout.

When an overemphasis on winning gets out of hand, high-level competitors start to exhibit some rather ugly consequences. Because élite-level sport emphasizes performance enhancement rather than the overall social and psychological development of the young athlete, it may be easy for these undesirable behaviours to emerge: injuries which, if ignored, may result in disabilities (e.g. bone loss, arthritis) that carry lifelong health implications; burnout, which is most often defined as the physical, psychological and emotional withdrawal of a once enjoyable activity due to excessive stress; and eating disorders (bulimia and anorexia), which young females adopt in order to conform to the aesthetic image expected, albeit unrealistically, of athletes in their sport or as a means of controlling something in their life because adults control everything else about their competitive sport world (Nash, 1987).

There are other potentially ugly consequences for females participating at élite levels of competitive sport. Substance abuse may be adopted as a means of coping with the undue levels of stress and anxiety of competition, to gain a competitive edge over similarly talented opponents or to dull the feelings of low self-image or helplessness prevalent during training regimens designed to pursue high status and financial pay-offs. Another hazard of high-level competition is the abusive coach or parent, who may see the potential for fame, glory and monetary gain as vicarious reward for their prodigy/daughter's performances. This abuse is most commonly psychological abuse, such as name-calling, withdrawal of love and affection, and intangible pressure placed on the young athlete as a result of the expectations placed on their performance (Donnelly, 1993; Ryan, 1995).

In addition to these ugly consequences, Coakley (1992) warns that young athletes may be prone to a unidimensional self-identity. This self-identity is one in which the young athlete's view of herself is totally as an athlete (e.g. gymnast or tennis player or swimmer) and not as a normal multidimensional being who holds academic, social and artistic goals as well as athletic dreams. This proneness towards a unidimensional athletic identity, Coakley laments, may leave young female athletes with nothing to fall back on when their sport is no longer there, for example when they decide to retire or if they are forced out. This may lead to a 'crash and burn' period that may prove devastating to normal growth and development as a child and teenager if not handled immediately and professionally.

This overview of the good, the bad and the ugly is meant to communicate the potential for the sword to swing in either positive or negative directions. The traditional role of sport has been believed to lie in the development of virtues such as honesty and fair play, as well as being an arena in which to learn life skills such as coping with stress and developing self-confidence. In order for these virtues and skills to outplay their negative alter ego (i.e. unethical behaviour, low self-esteem, excessive stress), it is crucial to understand how the positives and negatives may be nurtured in the same environment and what we can do to ensure that the benefits outweigh the costs of participation. Thus, we start with an in-depth look at the scientific literature in order to determine the effects of frequency and intensity of sport participation on these psychosocial outcomes.

Scientific research

Given the potential for intense competitive sport to produce positive or negative outcomes, a number of studies have been conducted over the last 20 years to understand more fully the conditions under which this can occur. Many studies have examined children's participation from a psychosocial perspective, the large majority of which have been on children and teenagers in organized agency-sponsored competitive sport, such as 'select' soccer, age-group swimming, club gymnastics and Little League baseball. Although these levels are not considered élite *per se*, they can be quite competitive in their own right. Only a handful of studies have been conducted on élite, high-level young athletes. A good reason for this is access; researchers are often unable to gain permission from parents and coaches to survey or interview young athletes about their experiences. If scientific research on élite young athletes is to advance, it is necessary for national governing bodies to be willing to look inwards at their own sport and grant access to researchers. After all, both researchers and practitioners are involved in this field for the same reason: the positive development of the young female through sport participation and competition.

We focus our discussion on those studies that have investigated élite young female athletes, although we also include results from studies of highly competitive but not élite athletes where appropriate. They can provide a window through which to understand the potential of sport to contribute positively or negatively to youth psychosocial development. There are a number of characteristics about the literature that should be kept in mind. First, most of the studies have been conducted on both female and male athletes. In the mixed samples, in many cases, the differential responses of females and males have not been teased out. Thus it is possible that the combined results may be skewed in a more positive or negative direction than if separate analyses had been conducted. Second, most of these studies have investigated children in high-level individual sports, such as gymnastics, skating, swimming, wrestling and running. Although generalization to team sports is inappropriate, individual sports are more likely to place athletes in the limelight who are most susceptible to negative stressors. Finally, several studies have used retrospective, rather than prospective, research designs. This means that adults who were once élite youth competitors were asked to reflect upon their childhood experiences. Although some believe that this approach contains problems, such as memory inaccuracy, we believe that there are strong and compelling reasons why this type of design offers unique opportunities for understanding youth sport experiences. Among these reasons are language articulation skills (children do not usually have the vocabulary to express experiences as vividly as adults), motivation (adults enjoy being asked about their experiences and see the value of giving back to their sport) and emotional maturity, which is essential given the sensitive topics that are likely to be discussed (e.g. disordered eating, coach and parent styles, playing with pain).

Gymnastics

There is no doubt that Olga Korbut in 1972 and Nadia Comaneci in 1976 changed the face of women's gymnastics forever. Following their dramatic Olympic performances, droves of young girls in the USA were enrolled in gymnastics by their parents, many of whom were eager to shape or drive their daughters to become champions. Ryan (1995) reports that the 1976 US Olympic gymnasts were, on average, 17.5 years old, 161.3 cm tall and weighed 48 kg; in 1992, these averages were 16 years old, 144.8 cm and 37.6 kg—a year and a half younger, 16.5 cm shorter and 10.4 kg lighter. A subculture was born, one in which long hours of training, lithe bodies fortified by shallow calories and competing in pain are accepted as 'normal' practices in this sport (Ryan, 1995; Brustad & Ritter-Taylor, 1996; Krane et al., 1997). It is no surprise, then, that interest in the perceptions of these young athletes was sought by educators and researchers.

When one of the authors (M.R.W.) was at the University of Oregon, a series of studies was con-

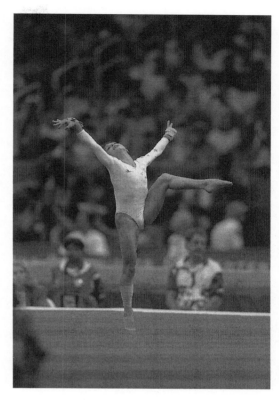

Fig. 28.1 Young gymnast performing a floor routine at the 1996 Olympics. (© Allsport / Doug Pensinger.)

ducted on young élite gymnasts who occupied two Olympic-development academies (Klint, 1985; Klint & Weiss, 1986, 1987; Weiss et al., 1989; Weiss & Hayashi, 1995). These investigators questioned young athletes about their reasons for participating in, and discontinuing, gymnastics, the sources of stress in competitive gymnastics and the perceptions of athletes and parents of the parent–child relationship through gymnastics.

This series of studies uncovered several positive as well as negative issues. Klint and Weiss (1986) sought to understand the reasons for continued participation as well as reasons for attrition in current (n=21 females, 22 males) and former (n=27 females, 10 males) highly competitive gymnasts. Current gymnasts ranged in age from 7 to 18 (mean 12.4) years and practised for an average of 23.9 (SD 8.9) h·week^{-1}. Former gymnasts ranged in age from 10 to 25 (mean 16.7) years and reported an average of 31.4 (SD 11.9) h·week^{-1} of practice/competition when they were still involved. Reasons for participation were quite similar for both groups of competitors: action (e.g. excitement), team atmosphere (e.g. being on the team), social recognition (e.g. popular with others), challenge (e.g. learning new skills) and friends (e.g. being with or meeting new friends). When queried about why they had left gymnastics after investing an average of 4 (SD 1.8) years of competition, former participants cited being injured as the most important (18.9%), followed by not having enough fun (13.5%), not liking the pressure (10.8%) and taking up too much time (10.8%).

At first glance, 'being injured' may appear to be a neutral reason for discontinuing involvement. However, subsequent interviews with these former competitors indicated that they recognized when they were no longer happy with their involvement but found making the decision to leave very difficult, often taking 2 months and sometimes a year before finally departing. Many reported that they were afraid to leave because of the stigma of being labelled a 'quitter', not knowing what to do with their extra time or losing contact with their friends in gymnastics. All the interviewees indicated that they were waiting for a 'good enough' reason to leave; two confided that they 'caused' the injury, allowing them a socially acceptable reason to leave the sport gracefully. The notion that being injured is perceived as a legitimate reason for leaving or as a viable alternative to high-pressure competition has been echoed by Nash (1987), who goes on to say that young gymnasts often linger over their injuries well beyond normal healing time as a way of avoiding competitive pressure.

In contrast to some of these negatives, the study also showed that 35 of the 37 former élite gymnasts had continued their athletic involvement in other organized sports or gymnastics at a lower level of intensity (i.e. high-school team). Thus, although they have dropped out of élite-level gymnastics and could be potentially viewed as quitters, they have not given up sport participation completely. Rather a dropout is most likely to be a 'sport transfer', who shifts to other activities that demand less time commitment, more opportunities for playing time and more exposure to social relationships in different contexts. Thus, once a young athlete leaves a particular sport it appears likely that she will seek out another sport that aligns with her interests and motives rather than dropping out of sports completely (Weiss & Petlichkoff, 1989).

The interviews also helped glean information about different categories of athletes leaving gymnastics. Three categories of leaver were identified in this study: reluctant, voluntary and resistant. Reluctant leavers were characterized by gymnasts who had incurred bona fide injuries that prevented them from continuing, by those for whom the cost of gymnastic continuation was prohibitive for their parents or by those who had moved away from the area and thus no longer had the opportunity to practise at the gymnastic club. Voluntary leavers were those who insisted that they wanted to try other things, including sports, academic clubs or other activities such as music or theatre; these youngsters felt that the time and energy commitment required of them in gymnastics forced them to miss other types of social opportunities.

In contrast to these neutral or acceptable reasons for gymnastics attrition, which suggest a continued valuing of their gymnastic experience, the third classification of leaver was not as positive. Resistant leavers were individuals who were unhappy with their gymnastics experience but felt that personal unhappiness was not a good enough reason to leave. They had the most difficulty making the decision to leave the sport because of outside pressures from parents and coaches to stay and because of the fear of losing gym friendships. Unfortunately, gymnastics had ceased to be a fun endeavour or one in which they felt they were developing or demonstrating their skills. Some of these gymnasts disclosed that they caused their own injury as a legitimate means of escaping their dilemma.

As part of the interview, the gymnastic leavers

Table 28.2 Athlete-recommended changes to Olympic-development gymnastic programmes. (Data from Klint & Weiss, 1986)

Decrease the number of practice hours/make practice more efficient
Have more organized social time together
Less segregation according to ability
Less pressure from the coaches
More shared decision-making between athlete and coach
More understanding and empathy from coaches
More encouragement from coaches
Less emphasis on weight control

---

were also asked what they felt they had gained from gymnastics, as well as what advice they would give to gymnastics organizers for making positive changes to the programme (Table 28.2). The former gymnasts felt that their training gave them confidence, discipline and independence, taught them how to set realistic challenging goals and helped them achieve in their other sport activities. Thus, their participation in gymnastics was not necessarily viewed as a negative phenomenon. Rather the stigma attached to leaving by coaches was internalized by the athletes themselves and most likely led to the difficult process of deciding to leave and the associated behaviours (i.e. causing an injury). In summary, this study allowed researchers access to a group of high-level young gymnasts, and their responses offered a rich and insightful look at both the positives and negatives of the sport.

In a thoughtful reflection of her own experience as an élite gymnast, Iversen (1990) offers a compelling look at the psychosocial correlates of delayed puberty in young élite female gymnasts. Because the female adolescent athlete faces two completely different social contexts, that of her school environment and the one in the gym, different sets of rules or norms dictate what attitudes and behaviours are acceptable and condoned by significant adults (parents, coaches) and peers in each environment. The competitive gymnast's body is in synchrony with her cohorts in the gym but out of step with her peers of the same age at school. Menarche, a normal developmental marker for girls, is looked upon as an abnormal or deviant occurrence in the social context of gymnastics. This normal maturation can lead to potentially traumatic consequences and experiences for the young gymnast, who may now be cast as an outsider from a once stable social support network (parents, coaches, team-mates). Iversen emphasizes the crucial role of the gymnast's support network in promoting healthy physical and psychological development during the critical period of puberty.

Figure skating

Dubbed the 'ice princesses of the winter games' (Ryan, 1995), the awe of skaters in the USA that started with such stars as Peggy Fleming and Dorothy Hamill continues to grow. However, recent attention has turned from the glory and glamour to the politics and pressure of the sport. This may be attributable in part to events such as the insurmountable pressure placed on Debi Thomas in the 1988 Calgary Olympics as the first African-American skater in line to win a gold medal and of course the outrageous tactics of Tonya Harding in her pursuit of an Olympic berth. Studies of young élite figure skaters have used a retrospective approach, in which current athletes and coaches reflected upon their sources of enjoyment and positive experiences in skating (Scanlan et al., 1989a,b; Gould et al., 1993a), negative experiences and sources of stress (Scanlan et al., 1991; Gould et al., 1993b) and coping strategies they used to deal with the excessive demands of the sport (Gould et al., 1993c). These studies have shed insight on what skaters find enjoyable about their sport and why they endure the pressure in pursuit of winning performances.

Scanlan et al. (1989a,b, 1991) interviewed 26 former élite figure skaters who had competed at national championships and who at the time were coaching the sport in southern California. This sample had averaged four visits to nationals. In addition eight went on to compete at the world championships and five of these eight were former Olympians. At the time of the interview, skaters ranged in age from 22 to 49 (mean 35.1) years and included 15 male and 11 female participants. The female skaters began skating on average at 6.1 years of age compared with 10.6 years for the male skaters. Former skaters were interviewed concerning the most competitive phase of their skating career (about ages 13–19 for the females), one in which they devoted their greatest commitment to the sport, skating 5.5 hours a day, 6 days a week and 50 weeks a year.

Table 28.3 reveals the sources of enjoyment of these skaters during the most competitive, and thus potentially most stressful, time of their career. The most frequently cited source of enjoyment was social and life opportunities, defined as forming meaningful relationships with significant adults and peers (e.g. friendship opportunities), as well as having broader experiences outside the boundaries of sport (e.g. opportuni-

ties afforded by touring). Perceived competence was another source of enjoyment and was defined as personal perceptions of competence derived from one's autonomous and/or social achievement in sport (e.g. mastery, competitive achievement). A third contributor to skaters' enjoyment was social recognition of competence, defined as receiving recognition for having skating ability through acknowledgement of one's performances and achievement by others. The act of skating itself provided such qualities as the movement sensations of skating and self-expression/creativity. Two final sources of enjoyment included a sense of specialness due to personal perceptions of being highly talented, and coping through skating such as using skating to escape from non-skating-related problems or to gain a sense of personal competence or control. These results illuminate the multifaceted

Table 28.3 Sources of enjoyment and stress in élite figure skaters. (Data from Scanlan, 1989b, 1991)

Sources of enjoyment	Sources of stress
Social and life opportunities (92%)	Negative aspects of competition (81%)
Friendship opportunities	Worries about competition
Going to competitions and touring	Competitive failure
Family/coach relationships	Preparation for competition
Perceived competence (88%)	Competitive hurdles
Mastery	Negative significant-other relationships (77%)
Competitive achievement	Interpersonal conflict
Performance achievement	Performance expectations
Demonstration of athletic ability	Skating politics
Social recognition of competence (81%)	Psychological warfare
Achievement recognition	Demands or costs of skating (69%)
Performance recognition	Financial demands or costs
Act of skating (65%)	Time demands or costs
Movement and sensations	Personal costs
Self-expression/creativity	Personal struggles (65%)
Athleticism of skating	Physical or mental difficulties
Flow/peak experiences	Self-doubts about talent
Special cases (50%)	Perfectionism
Sense of specialness	Dealing with homosexuality
Coping through skating	Traumatic experiences (19%)
	Family disturbances

Numbers in parentheses denote percentage of sample that cited this source of enjoyment or stress.

nature of sources of enjoyment in élite skating and illustrate the potential benefits of competition at this level.

These same former élite skaters were also interviewed about the sources of stress experienced during their most intense period of commitment to the sport (Scanlan et al., 1991). Five major sources of stress were cited (see Table 28.3): (i) negative aspects of competition (e.g. worries about failure); (ii) negative relationships with significant others (e.g. performance expectations of others); (iii) demands or costs of skating (e.g. financial and time demands); (iv) personal struggles (e.g. weight problems, perfectionism); and (v) traumatic experiences such as death of a loved one or family problems. Some of these sources of stress, most notably negative aspects of competition, personal struggles and negative interactions with significant others, had been seen previously from a different perspective as positive sources of participation (i.e. as sources of enjoyment in the form of social opportunities, social recognition of competence and perceived competence). Thus, the notion that competitive sport can be a double-edged sword emerges once again: some of the same sources that were implicated as *enjoyable* also emerged as *stressors* when observed from a different perspective. The problem is how to maximize the positive or enjoyable aspects of skating and minimize the negative or stressful aspects.

Gould et al. (1993b) extended Scanlan et al.'s research on sources of stress for figure skaters in several ways. First, all 17 (10 female, 7 male) of their participants were former national champions. In addition, the sample included three world champions and seven medallists at world championships or Olympics. The interviewees were about 25 years of age (range 18–33 years) with 13 years of skating experience at the time of interview. They were asked to reflect upon two phases of their skating career: phase 1 covered the time from when they first began skating at a senior level until they won a national championship; and phase 2 covered the time between winning a national championship and the present interview or at the time of their retire-

ment. Thus a comparison of sources of stress at two different points in their skating career could be made.

Several common sources of stress occurred at phase 1 and 2 according to the skaters. These included the physical demands of skating (e.g. maintaining weight, injury), environmental demands (e.g. media exposure, skating politics) and psychological demands (e.g. competitive anxiety, self-doubts). High performance expectations were also common, although in phase 1 this had more to do with expected potential while in phase 2 concerns revolved around living up to previous performance standards. Concerns about relationships or stressors related to significant other were common to both phases, including conflicts with coach and skating partner and stress on the family. Concern about life direction was a stressor in phase 2 but not phase 1; this involved thinking about the end of their careers (i.e. 'What next?'). Finally, the majority of athletes (71%) indicated that they felt more stress after, rather than before, winning their national title. The increased stress resulted from increased media attention, more criticism, pressure to please judges, increased expectations and being in the 'big time.' In summary, physical, psychological and relationship sources of stress dominated the life of the élite young skater.

Tennis

Andrea Jaeger, Tracy Austin, Mary Pierce, Jennifer Capriati: the one thing these women have in common is that they entered professional tennis at the ripe old age of 14 or 15 years; and shortly after attaining success and even high status at one or more of the grand slam events of their era, these 'women' disappeared from the sport. Whether these disappearances were attributable to injury, burnout or social distractions, the rather consistent entry of young female players into the professional tennis world at the age of 14 has raised some eyebrows and calls for documented data to substantiate recommendations for change.

To assess the extent to which burnout is a

problem in junior elite tennis, Gould *et al.* (1996a,b, 1997) investigated factors related to burnout in élite young players (mean 16.4 years, SD 2.4). The study participants were ranked in the top five in their state, the top six in their region and the top 55 in the nation for their age group. In this study, burnout was defined as the psychological, emotional and physical withdrawal from a formerly pursued and enjoyable activity because of chronic stress. In a quantitative assessment of burnout vs. control subjects (24 females, 36 males), a number of demographic, **personality, psychological** and coping variables differentiated the two groups. The strongest differences between the two groups, as assessed by size of effect, were that players with burnout reported less input into their training and tournament schedules, a greater number of years 'playing up' in age category, more parental criticism, more concern over mistakes and less constructive coping skills.

In a qualitative follow-up assessment of 10 players (6 females, 4 males) who scored highest on the burnout and perfectionism scales, several interesting findings were uncovered. Factors leading to burnout included physical concerns (e.g. injured, overtraining, poor play), logistical concerns (e.g. time demands, travel, adjusting to school), social interpersonal concerns (e.g. dissatisfaction with social life, negative parent or coach interactions) and psychological concerns (e.g. unfulfilled expectations, lack of enjoyment, pressure from self, coach and parents). This type of in-depth reporting made it possible to 'walk a mile in the heads' (Scanlan *et al.*, 1989a) of these young athletes in order to understand why they left the sport they once loved. One of the more encouraging findings from Gould *et al.*'s assessments (1996a,b, 1997) was that of the 30 burned-out athletes who participated in the study, 17 (55%) later returned to tennis, usually at a lower intensity of competition (e.g. high-school team). **Finally, a section of the interview allowed the** athlete to offer advice to other players, parents and coaches in dealing with the stresses of competitive tennis. These recommendations are summarized in Table 28.4.

To acknowledge the unique attributes of each individual's experiences, Gould *et al.* (1997) presented case studies of three burned-out young athletes (a 13-year-old female who burned out at 12, an 18-year-old male who burned out at 17 and a 21-year-old female who burned out at 17). Although each identified a number of physical, logistical, social interpersonal and psychological concerns reflective of the earlier content analysis, each case was unique in the most salient motives that impelled their withdrawal from the sport of tennis. The younger female cited pressure from her mother, who continually compared her with

Table 28.4 Advice by junior élite tennis players to other players, parents and coaches. (Data from Gould *et al.*, 1996b)

Other players	Parents	Coaches
Play for your own reasons	Recognize optimal amount of	Cultivate personal involvement
Balance tennis with other things	'pushing' needed	with player
No fun—do not play	Lessen involvement	Have two-way communication
Try to make it fun	Reduce importance of	Use player input
Relax	outcome	Understand player feelings
Take time off	Show support/empathy	Other
Other	Parent–coach role separation	Coach at your right level
Have goal structure	Solicit player input	Foster right atmosphere
Leave things on court	Other	Talk to pressuring parents
Let people know how you feel	Do non-tennis activities	
Make lots of friends	with children	
	Allow children to be children	

her older sister and with other better players, as well as her desire to be more social and spend time with her friends, none of whom were tennis players. The older female, in contrast, indicated that the most important factor for her was placing too much pressure on herself to attain high but unrealistic expectations, which in turn led her to overtrain (average 5 hours daily for 7 days a week), resulting in a back injury that made it harder to play and thus less fun.

In summary, while Gould and colleagues noted a number of individual factors related to burnout (physical, logistical concerns), this phenomenon occurred within a social context in which the structure of tennis, with its emphasis on performance outcome, combined with parental expectations and demands, the need for and importance of having friends to maintain motivation, and coaching communication styles and behaviours played a big role in these athletes' perceptions of their tennis experiences. The results of this series of studies substantiated the age eligibility rule for women's tennis (see Chapter 37).

Swimming

Like gymnastics, figure skating and tennis, highly competitive swimmers start their sport at an early age and thus overtraining, staleness or burnout is imminent if not carefully monitored. In addition the intense pressure to win is heightened by the fact that thousandths of seconds can separate winners from losers, thus leading in recent years to substance abuse in young élite swimmers. However, until recently very little information has been gleaned from young competitive swimmers to understand what factors contribute to their enjoyment, as well as the perceived pressures, of the sport.

Two studies of age-group swimmers have been reported that focus upon a number of salient factors present in swimming (Black & Weiss, 1992; Raedeke, 1997). The study by Black and Weiss (1992) was inspired by Black's own climb through the age-group system to qualify for the fateful Olympics of 1980. Her memories were that she succeeded despite the insensitive coaching she received as a youngster, a style that drove all her friends from the sport. The study investigated 312 swimmers (168 females, 144 males) who ranged in age from 10 to 18 years and represented 11 USA Swimming registered teams. The sample represented levels from novice to junior national status. Swimmers rated their coaches with regard to frequency of giving praise, encouragement, instruction and criticism, and these ratings were correlated with the swimmers' perceptions of competence, enjoyment and motivation for trying challenging skills.

The results were analysed separately by gender. Coaches who were perceived as giving more frequent praise combined with instruction following good performances and encouragement plus instruction following unsuccessful performances were associated with young female swimmers who rated themselves higher in swim success, swim ability, enjoyment of their swimming experience, perceived effort and challenge motivation. In contrast, those swimmers who reported that their coaches engaged less frequently in these behaviours reported lower perception of ability, enjoyment and motivation. Interestingly for males, results were quite similar in perceived coaching behaviours and psychosocial outcomes. These results suggest that a positive coaching style predominated by praise, instruction and encouragement is related to positive self-perceptions and motivation among highly competitive young female swimmers.

Raedeke (1997) conducted a rather extensive examination of the determinants of burnout levels in senior swimmers, the highest level for age-group swimmers, who participated on club teams under the auspices of USA Swimming. The sample consisted of 145 female and 84 male swimmers who ranged in age from 13 to 18 years (mean 15.5, SD 1.5). These swimmers reported working out 10.6 months a year, 14 hours a week, 7.2 sessions a week and 36 500 m per week; indeed a high level of investment in their sport. Raedeke adopted a commitment perspective in order to understand the phenomenon of burnout; this perspective contends that individuals may be committed to continuing an activity either because they 'want to' stay involved (i.e. attraction to the sport) or because they feel they 'have to' stay involved (i.e. feel entrapped or obligated to stay based on pressure by others). Raedeke hypothesized that swimmers who are committed because of attraction to swimming should show low levels of burnout, while swimmers who feel entrapped in swimming should show high levels of burnout.

To test his predictions, Raedeke assessed the swimmers on a number of psychological constructs that help determine commitment types: perceptions of enjoyment, benefits and costs of swimming, attractiveness of alternative activities, personal investments (i.e. time, energy), social constraints (i.e. pressure from parents, team-mates, coaches), swim identity, and control or choice over swim-related activities. A cluster analysis identified four distinct profiles of swimmers who varied in their pattern of scores on measured constructs (Table 28.5). 'Malcontent' swimmers ($n=26$) perceived their swim involvement comparatively negatively in relation to other profiles. They were characterized by low enjoyment, low benefits and high costs, low investments in swimming and felt that other activities were more attractive than swimming. In addition, they felt pressured by, or obligated

to, others to remain involved in swimming and perceived little choice about their participation in swimming or about decisions regarding their swim workouts.

In contrast to the malcontents, 'enthusiastic' swimmers ($n=104$) reported favourable impressions of their swim involvement. This was indicated by their comparatively high scores on enjoyment and benefits; low costs, low social constraints and attractive alternatives; and high investments, perceived choice and swim identity. The third profile, dubbed the 'obligated' swimmers ($n=40$), were distinguished by their high social constraints, low perceived choice and high investments. Moreover, they reported moderately low enjoyment and benefits and moderately high costs and attractive alternatives. Finally, the 'indifferent' swimmers ($n=66$) scored comparatively low on swim investments and swim identity. Moreover, scores for enjoyment, benefits and social constraints were moderately low.

In summary, enthusiastic swimmers characterized the 'want to' or attraction-based commitment profile, while malcontent and obligated swimmers were notable for a more 'have to' or entrapment form of commitment to swimming. Finally indifferent swimmers appeared to be neither attracted nor entrapped by their swim

Table 28.5 Commitment profiles of swimmers and scores on burnout dimensions. (Data from Raedeke, 1997)

Variable	Malcontent	Enthusiastic	Obligated	Indifferent
Enjoyment	Lower	Higher	Average	Average
Benefits	Lower	Higher	Average	Moderately lower
Costs	Higher	Lower	Moderately higher	Average
Attractive alternatives	Higher	Lower	Average	Average
Investments	Lower	Higher	Moderately higher	Lower
Social constraints	Higher	Moderately lower	Higher	Moderately lower
Swim identity	Lower	Higher	Moderately higher	Lower
Perceived control	Lower	Higher	Lower	Average
Emotional/physical exhaustion	Higher	Lower	Higher	Average
Reduced swim accomplishment	Higher	Lower	Moderately higher	Average
Swim devaluation	Higher	Lower	Moderately higher	Average

involvement; these swimmers may be candidates for giving up the sport because of their unremarkable scores on any of the positive (e.g. enjoyment) or negative (e.g. social constraints) variables.

These four rather distinct swimmer profiles were then compared on levels of burnout. In this study burnout was defined as a psychological syndrome of physical and emotional exhaustion, devaluation of swimming and perceptions of reduced swim accomplishments. As Raedeke predicted, enthusiastic swimmers, who displayed attraction-based commitment, recorded the lowest scores on all three burnout dimensions (see Table 28.5). In contrast, malcontent swimmers, who characterized entrapment-based commitment, scored highest on all burnout dimensions. Obligated swimmers, who also resembled entrapment-based commitment, scored high on exhaustion and moderately high on swim devaluation and reduced swim accomplishment dimensions. The indifferent swimmers registered average scores on all three burnout dimensions.

Based on the results of this study, the swimmer profiles were distinguished from one another by a set of consistent variables, including enjoyment, benefits and costs, social constraints and perceived choice. Although Raedeke adopted a different framework to examine burnout to that used by Gould *et al.* (1996a,b, 1997), in both sets of studies there are common findings regarding élite young tennis players and swimmers: (i) social psychological factors, in the form of perceived support or pressure from significant adults and peers; and (ii) psychological characteristics, such as enjoyment or lack of enjoyment, input or lack of input into training schedules, and high or low motivation.

Across-sport findings

Peter Donnelly (1993) conducted in-depth interviews with 45 retired Canadian élite athletes who were asked to reflect upon their childhood high-level sport participation (i.e. national team, nationally ranked). Athletes included 29 females and 16 males who ranged in age from 19 to 35 years of age at the time of interview and who represented a variety of sports: artistic and rhythmic gymnastics, figure skating, swimming (including synchronized), skiing, ice hockey, tennis, track and field, football, martial arts, rowing and wrestling. Female athletes were represented in all but skiing, field events, football, martial arts and wrestling. The purpose of the study was to determine if common problems were associated across a variety of sports and for both female and male athletes.

Athletes were asked to recall the positive and negative aspects of their childhood athletic careers. A number of positive experiences were noted, such as opportunities to travel, gain prestige, make lifelong friendships and the sheer enjoyment of the sport. However, respondents spent much more time expounding their negative experiences. Among the problems reported were troubled family relationships (e.g. parental pressure, missing a part of family life, sibling jealousy), problems in social relationships (e.g. no time for friends, missing out on activities like 'hanging out', peer pressure), athlete–coach relationships (e.g. physical and mental abuse, dependence, domination), educational problems (e.g. balancing school and sport), and physical and psychological problems (e.g. overtraining, illness, lack of sleep, burnout).

Female athletes predominated in problems regarding the athlete–coach relationship. The majority of female athletes had male coaches and several incidents of sexual encounters and abuse were cited. Problems regarding the relationship with coaches were rarely raised by the male athletes. Sexual abuse and sexual harassment of young female athletes have been much publicized recently with a shocking article about Rick Butler, a USA volleyball coach of a top-level youth team, who has been indicted for sexual misconduct with several of his former players when they were under the age of 18 years (Howard & Munson, 1997). The greater frequency of abusive coach–athlete relationships has resulted in a call for national governing bodies to develop, endorse and implement a code of conduct for coaches that would spell out the rights of athletes and the responsibilities of coaches, and the consequences for coaches who violate the code (Donnelly, 1993).

Several other negative experiences were noted by these athletes. Excessive behaviours (e.g. binge-eating and drinking, vandalism), use of performance-enhancing drugs, dietary problems (e.g. eating disorders), politics of the sport (e.g. team selection, judging, poorly trained coaches) and retirement from competition (e.g. adjustment difficulties) were other issues the athletes cited as difficult to cope with during childhood. Of these problems, the majority of females cited problems with diet and body image that led in many cases to excessive dieting or eating disorders. These problems were not reported by the male athletes.

Donnelly implicated three major factors that contributed to the negative experiences reported by these athletes: the organizational structure of the sport; large time commitments at such an early age; and gender. Donnelly's analysis of the data suggests that the negative experiences were far more serious and far-reaching for the female compared with the male athletes. In citing specific examples, he indicated that dietary problems seem to be brought on by the pursuit of beauty, image and delayed puberty, which were perceived as requirements for success in certain sports like gymnastics and figure skating. Moreover, the girls' struggle to fight off natural growth contrasted starkly with the boys' embrace of natural growth that allows them to become bigger and stronger and to extend their careers as professional athletes.

Other sports

Studies of psychosocial factors related to élite or highly competitive young athletes in sports other than gymnastics, figure skating, tennis and swimming have also been conducted. These include studies of young distance runners (Rowland & Walsh, 1985; Feltz & Albrecht, 1986; Seefeldt & Steig, 1986; Vogel, 1986; Feltz et al., 1992), wrestlers (Gould et al., 1983a,b, 1991), ice

hockey players (Ewing et al., 1988) and speed skaters (Gutmann et al., 1984, 1986). These studies are not reviewed here because they primarily described personality characteristics or included only young male athletes. However, it is clear that considerably more research is needed on young, élite female athletes across a number of diverse sports so that we can better understand, explain and predict behaviours that occur within the sport context or because of their sport experiences.

Anecdotal literature

Over the last 15 years a number of books have been written by journalists and athletes about the child susperstar athlete (Greenspan, 1983; Stabiner, 1986; Joravsky, 1995; Louganis, 1995; Ryan, 1995). These works are notable because they include exclusive interviews with, and observations of, élite young athletes, their parents and coaches in sports such as gymnastics, tennis, figure skating, swimming, diving, basketball and distance running. The ability to get 'up close and personal' with the major 'players' of the élite child's world provides a unique perspective on her perceptions, social environment and the pressures and demands of the sport.

Each of these books adopts a slightly different slant on the topic. For example, *Little Winners* (Greenspan, 1983) includes many different types of individual sports and examines well-known as well as little-known names (i.e. those who did not 'cut it') in sports. *Courting Fame* (Stabiner, 1986) looks exclusively at the world of the women's professional tennis tour and the challenges and barriers involved in attempting to rise up the ranks. *Hoop Dreams* (Joravsky, 1995), made into an award-winning documentary, magnifies the lives of two young superstar boy basketball players in the city of Chicago and the widely different roads they travelled based on their growth and development patterns and their coach's expectations. In *Breaking the Surface* (Louganis, 1995), eight-time gold medal winner in Olympic diving Greg Louganis provides a birds-eye view of his formative years, focusing on several of the barriers to success in his early and later life such as a learning disability, conflicts with his father, ethnic discrimination and attitudes toward his homosexuality. Finally, *Little Girls in Pretty Boxes* (Ryan, 1995), perhaps the book to make the biggest impact on public opinion, challenges the subculture in élite women's gymnastics and figure skating by calling it 'celebrated child abuse'. Through numerous interviews with former and current athletes, coaches, parents and team-mates, Ryan documents mostly the horrors of what the élite-level young athlete faces day in and day out in a social context that condones working out in pain, unhealthy weight-management techniques and coaches who simulate dictators in their control over their athletes' lives.

Despite the unique contribution each book makes to our understanding of élite young athletes, these books also communicate strikingly similar messages. One consistent theme is the adoption and internalization of behaviours that are accepted in the subculture of many individual sports, such as disordered eating, substance abuse (e.g. laxatives) and competing with serious injuries. Another theme is the controlling and often abusive behaviours adopted by coaches and parents in their vicarious pursuit of fame and glory, pressuring young athletes to attempt developmentally difficult skills and to train for an exorbitant number of hours. Some of the chapter titles of Ryan's (1995) book encompass these issues: 'Whatever it takes: coaches' and 'We all became junkies: parents'. Joan Ryan recounts the comments of Elaine Zayak, national figure-skating champion at age 15, when she decided she wanted to quit the sport. Her parents told her that she had no say in the decision and that they had scrimped to pay the prohibitive skating fees each year; finally, they exerted their control by taking away her new car, which her father drove himself.

A third theme that emerged was the politics inherent in the sport, especially in gymnastics and figure skating, where the difference in order of placing and thus amount of prize money

usually depends on 'image' (i.e. femininity), costume (i.e. 'attractive' or gaudy), weight ('be thin and win'), development ('boobs and hips'), ability to charm the judges or simply predetermined expectations of performance. Two other themes run through all these journalists' accounts: the development of one-dimensional athletic identities and the notion of lost childhoods. Time and again the athletes interviewed identified themselves exclusively as 'gymnasts', 'tennis players' or 'figure skaters' without other avenues of achievement to balance their days, weeks and years consumed with training and competing in their sport. When their careers ended, often prematurely from developing bodies betraying them, these young, talented athletes often had a difficult time adjusting or adapting to the 'normal' life of a child or teenager. In a similar vein, young athletes lamented 'lost childhoods' because of the demanding schedules and pressures of their sport. They expressed a longing for hanging out with friends, participating in normal school activities and living the unhurried, relatively hassle-free life of a child or teenager.

Counteracting these negative experiences are the almost unanimous comments by athletes of the positive learning experiences and psychological attributes they gained from élite sport participation and the special status they held among sporting and non-sporting peers. The majority of athletes in Donnelly's (1993) study indicated that they would repeat their careers and would involve their children in the sport if they could. These affirmative responses were dependent, at least in part, upon resolution of some of the current problems in the sport. However, these responses and those of athletes in other studies (Klint & Weiss, 1986; Scanlan *et al.*, 1989a,b, 1991; Coakley, 1992) highlight that the time, energy and financial costs of competing at the élite level also come with unique benefits or opportunities that may be difficult to attain in other domains. Thus, with some convergence between scientific and journalistic research we now turn to the question of what these findings mean and what national governing bodies, coaches and parents can do to maximize positive experiences in high-level competitive young female athletes.

What do these findings mean?

One theme that has emerged consistently from the research-based and anecdotal findings is the importance of sport as a source of enjoyment for high-level athletes. Recall that the results of Scanlan *et al.* (1989b) showed that social and life opportunities, perceived competence, social recognition and the act of skating were most frequently cited as sources of enjoyment in figure skating. Similarly, it was shown that a lack of enjoyment may lead to withdrawal or burnout. Many of the gymnastic leavers in the study by Klint and Weiss (1986) indicated 'not having enough fun' as a major reason, and their advice to organizers included providing opportunities for more organized social time. In the studies by Gould *et al.* (1996a,b) lack of enjoyment was cited as a psychological concern leading to burnout, and in the study by Raedeke (1997) malcontent swimmers scored low in enjoyment and high in burnout. Clearly, the enjoyment, pleasure and fun experienced by élite young athletes are crucial factors for their involvement in the sport. However, it should be emphasized that 'enjoyment' does not mean frivolous play and lack of focus. Rather, as indicated by Klint and Weiss (1986), Scanlan *et al.* (1989) and Raedeke (1997), mastering difficult skills and strategies, working hard to attain realistic but challenging goals, feeling a sense of competence and accomplishment, and expressing oneself and being creative through the movements of the sport all constitute sources of enjoyment for young, top-level athletes.

A second common theme that emerges from the data is the young athlete's need and desire for control and autonomy over her involvement in sport. This view is bolstered by the research data: in the investigation by Klint and Weiss (1986), gymnasts advised organizers to urge athletes to become involved in decision-making; in Raedeke's (1997) report, the perceptions of swimmers that they had little choice or control

was related to higher levels of burnout; and in the research by Gould *et al.* (1996a), the tennis players advised other athletes to play for their own reasons and urged parents and coaches to solicit player input. The anecdotal literature is replete with examples of controlling or coercive behaviours on the part of coaches and parents to exhort young athletes to higher levels of performance. It is clear that high-level competitive young athletes want control over their actions and choice in their training schedules and routines. It would appear, then, that a balance in coaching and parenting styles that allows young athletes to have an input in decision-making and choice of activities would be of paramount importance for positive consequences.

A third implication of the findings is the importance of emphasizing social *support* over social *constraints*. Social support refers to the encouragement, personal concern for the athlete as a human being, empathy and unconditional affection that coaches and parents can provide for élite young females who are faced with tough demands and expectations. A young athlete's sense of worth or value as a person should not be contingent on good performances or winning medals. Social constraints, in contrast, refer to the emphasis on pressure, guilt trips, unrealistically high expectations and the sense of obligation that coaches and parents place on young athletes to force them to stick to their training. Although this latter set of methods certainly succeeds in most cases, the child and teenager comes to resent these tactics and strives to detach herself at the first possible opportunity. This not only makes common sense but is also sound from a developmental perspective, as early adolescence marks a period where youngsters are motivated to establish a sense of independence from adults.

The data support the necessity of maximizing social support and minimizing social constraints: the gymnasts in the study by Klint and Weiss (1986), who suggested less pressure, more sympathy and more understanding from coaches; the tennis players in the studies by Gould *et al.* (1996a,b, 1997), who requested that parents and coaches engage in an optimal amount of 'pushing', 'mellowing out', more support and empathy and 'being there' in tennis and outside the sport; the swimmers in the study by Raedeke (1997), who reported that high social constraints were a risk for higher levels of burnout; and the skaters in the study by Scanlan *et al.* (1991), who reported negative relationships with significant others as a major source of stress.

Finally, a multidimensional self-identity is a characteristic that is essential for a balanced lifestyle inside and outside of one's sporting existence. This topic raises the issue of how young or at what age youngsters should specialize in their sport and the risks of doing so. On the one hand, focused training from a young age is likely to give a young female the competitive edge over others who started later. On the other hand, the potential for injury, staleness and lack of a normal childhood may contribute to 'burn out' the light in a young athlete's passion for the sport. The tennis players in the studies by Gould *et al.* (1996a,b, 1997) were most likely referring to this attribute when they acknowledged social interpersonal concerns (e.g. dissatisfaction with social life) and logistical concerns (e.g. 'gave up all my time for tennis', 'tennis overwhelmed life', 'sole tennis focus', 'conflicting interests'). Also, Donnelly's (1993) élite sample commented on problems in social relationships (e.g. no time for friends, missing out on activities) and on balancing school and sport.

Coakley (1992) cautions that the structure of sport for high-level adolescent athletes demands a sole or unidimensional focus on athletic achievements. Also, this structure exerts a great deal of control over the athlete's life in and out of sport. These structural qualities of élite sport, Coakley contends, contribute strongly to an athlete's stress reactions, maladaptive behaviours and burnout. Thus in light of the scientific data and the anecdotal findings, and the convergence of these sources, it is clear that structural changes to the sport (e.g. code of conduct for coaches) as well as individual interventions (e.g. support systems for athletes) are necessary to avoid the negative outcomes that can emerge (Coakley, 1992; Donnelly, 1993; Nielsen, 1994).

What can national governing bodies, coaches and parents do?

The behaviours and norms adopted within élite child sports can be easily subjected to a number of psychologically based remedies, such as stress management skills for athletes, educating coaches on child development, and shared goal-setting sessions for coach and athlete. However, the structure or organization of sport is a larger entity that condones the types of activities that may lead to heightened stress, overtraining, burnout and excessive behaviours. Therefore, it is important to consider both sociologically or structure-based and psychologically or individual-based strategies for change (Coakley, 1992; Donnelly, 1993; Gould, 1993; Gould *et al.*, 1996a).

Structural changes

Coakley (1992) suggests that changes to the structure and organization of sport programmes can 'empower' young athletes so that they have control over their lives inside and outside of sport. This, he believes, offers the child athlete the best chance of healthy social and psychological development. One way in which the structure of sport can be changed is through laws governing adult control of young athletes. Coakley (cited in Nielsen, 1994) and Donnelly (1993) contend that child labour laws and laws regulating children in entertainment emerged to protect children from the control of employers, agents and parents. They raise the analogy: Should there be child athlete labour laws? In today's world of child athletic superstars, some families depend upon their child's earnings from endorsements and winnings to sustain their family income and a comfortable lifestyle. Thus the potential for control and conflict may occur because parents, coaches and agents stand to gain from the talents of young athletes.

Coakley (1992) and Donnelly (1993) argue that it is time to establish laws for élite child athletes. These would include the maximum number of hours of training per day, number of days per week children can practise and compete, amount of time elapsed between performances, amount of time devoted to compulsory education, protection of income in trust funds, and health and safety regulations guaranteed in the gym (pool, field). To date, only the trust fund for young athletes is in effect. Because of the increased business and corporate nature of amateur and professional sports, Coakley's and Donnelly's advice is not as sensational as one might at first think. Perhaps a code of conduct for coaches in specific sports is an idea that would be more immediately embraced. Coakley (cited in Nielsen, 1994) outlines the crucial qualities that should characterize such codes, which should include a number of goals and guidelines (Table 28.6). In addition, athletes in Donnelly's (1993) study echoed many of the same goals when asked to make recommendations for improving their sport. Foremost among these goals is prioritizing what children and adolescents want from their coaches, including the following (Nielsen, 1994).

• Competence: to know the sport and be able to communicate this knowledge to children.
• Approachability: to be open to what young athletes have to say and be willing to take criticism and admit to errors.
• Fairness and consistency: to recognize and treat young athletes according to their unique needs.

Table 28.6 Goals and guidelines for a coach's code of conduct. (Data from Coakley cited in Nielsen, 1994)

Prioritize what athletes want from their coaches
Identify realistic developmental goals
Create support systems for athletes
Provide a sound education for young athletes
Code should be part of coaching qualifications
Reorganize and regulate high-level sport to promote overall athlete development
Facilitate athlete informed choices about participation
Ensure that children do not lose their childhood in high-level sport
Prevent sexual abuse and sexual harassment
Outline models of constructive coach–athlete relationships

• Confidence: to use a clear set of principles to guide themselves and their athletes.
• Motivation: to be excited about their sport, their athletes and their team.
• Personal concern: to be concerned about them as children first and as athletes second.
• Support: to recognize and praise their good performances and constructively instruct them on skill errors.

In addition to providing caring and competent coaches, other crucial qualities of a code of conduct entail several issues previously discussed in this chapter. Most notable are the issues related to healthy and constructive coach–athlete relationships and the importance of developmental goals for young athletes, including physical (skill development, injury free), social (friendships, moral development) and psychological (self-confidence, coping with stress) goals. Recently the International Olympic Committee and the US Olympic Committee have developed codes of conduct for coaches. Now the challenge is to launch the codes of conduct into action and hold governing bodies, administrators and coaches accountable for adhering to the code.

Individual change strategies

Both ego-involved (i.e. social comparison, winning) and task-involved (i.e. learning, improving, fun) goals coexist in the highly competitive world of youth sport. The key is how to keep a perspective on winning so that it does not dominate all other goals. Therefore, a number of individual-centred or psychological-change strategies can be offered based on the literature reviewed in this chapter.

A consistent finding is that the potential for undue levels of stress exists in the competitive context. Thus, young athletes should be educated about what causes stress and how they can cope with it in practice and competition. Both Orlick and McCaffrey (1991) and Weiss (1991) suggest a number of self-regulated learning strategies, such as relaxation, imagery, self-talk and goal-setting, that young athletes can learn and improve with practice. These skills can also be transferred to other social situations, such as academic tests, public speaking and music or dance performance.

Other individual-orientated strategies derive from advice by élite young athletes (Klint & Weiss, 1986; Gould *et al.*, 1996a) or from factors that they believed contribute to continued motivation in their sport (Raedeke, 1997). The advice and reasons for motivation revolve around the consistent themes outlined in this chapter: the need for a multidimensional identity (i.e. balancing sport with other activities), having choice and control over sport involvement (e.g. input on decision-making), experiencing fun and enjoyment (e.g. achievement-related and non-achievement-related areas) and the need for social support not social constraints (e.g. seeking and requesting positive coach–athlete and parent–athlete relationships).

Conclusion

It is clear that considerably more research is needed on the élite young female athlete from a psychosocial perspective in order to make informed conclusions about sport participation and recommendations for change. For researchers, this means being granted more opportunities for access to young athletes so that they can be interviewed about their experiences in a setting that is non-threatening and protected from negative adult consequences (i.e. anonymous, group data reported). To empower athletes it is important to give them a voice so that they can provide input about what they want from their experiences, their coaches and the governing body that oversees their particular sport.

It is important to note that both positive and negative aspects were recognized and acknowledged by the élite young athletes in the studies reviewed. Athletes understand and appreciate the unique benefits of being a talented young performer and realize that their experiences travelling, competing, being recognized by audiences and occupying centre stage are events

reserved for first-rate skilled individuals. On the other hand, they also recognize that they missed out on many normal activities that colour most children's lives: hanging out with friends, eating and sleeping at normal hours, joining school clubs and achieving in other domains, and just being a kid. The cost–benefit trade-off is one that still needs to be examined and resolved if young, highly competitive, female athletes are to mature physically, psychologically and socially.

References

Black, S.J. & Weiss, M.R. (1992) The relationship among perceived coaching behaviors, perceptions of ability, and motivation in competitive age-group swimmers. *Journal of Sport and Exercise Psychology* **14**, 309–325.

Brustad, R.J. & Ritter-Taylor, M. (1996) Applying social psychological perspectives to the sport psychology consulting process. *Sport Psychologist* **11**, 107–119.

Coakley, J. (1992) Burnout among adolescent athletes: a personal failure or social problem? *Sociology of Sport Journal* **9**, 271–285.

Donnelly, P. (1993) Problems associated with youth involvement in high-performance sport. In B.R. Cahill & A.J. Pearl (eds) *Intensive Participation in Children's Sports*, pp. 95–126. Human Kinetics Publishers, Champaign, Illinois.

Ewing, M.E. & Seefeldt, V. (1996) Patterns of participation and attrition in American agency-sponsored youth sports. In F.L. Smoll & R.E. Smith (eds) *Children in Sport: A Biopsychosocial Perspective*, pp. 31–45. Brown & Benchmark, Indianapolis.

Ewing, M.E., Feltz, D.L., Schultz, T.D. & Albrecht, R.R. (1988) Psychological characteristics of competitive young hockey players. In E.W. Brown & C.F. Branta (eds) *Competitive Sports for Children and Youths*, pp. 49–61. Human Kinetics Publishers, Champaign, Illinois.

Feltz, D.L. & Albrecht, R.R. (1986) Psychological implications of competitive running. In M.R. Weiss & D. Gould (eds) *Competitive Sport for Children and Youths*, pp. 225–230. Human Kinetics Publishers, Champaign, Illinois.

Feltz, D.L., Lirgg, C.D. & Albrecht, R.R. (1992) Psychological implications of competitive running in elite young distance runners: a longitudinal analysis. *Sport Psychologist* **6**, 128–138.

Gould, D. (1993) Intensive sport participation and the prepubescent athlete: competitive stress and burnout. In B.R. Cahill & A.J. Pearl (eds) *Intensive Participation in Children's Sport*, pp. 19–38. Human Kinetics Publishers, Champaign, Illinois.

Gould, D., Horn, T. & Spreeman, J. (1983a) Competitive anxiety in junior elite wrestlers. *Journal of Sport Psychology* **5**, 58–71.

Gould, D., Horn, T. & Spreeman, J. (1983b) Sources of stress in junior elite wrestlers. *Journal of Sport Psychology* **5**, 159–171.

Gould, D., Eklund, R., Petlichkoff, L., Peterson, K. & Bump, L. (1991) Psychological predictors of state anxiety and performance in age-group wrestlers. *Pediatric Exercise Science* **3**, 198–208.

Gould, D., Jackson, S.A. & Finch, L.M. (1993a) Life at the top: the experience of U.S. national champion figure skaters. *Sport Psychologist* **7**, 354–374.

Gould, D., Jackson, S.A. & Finch, L.M. (1993b) Sources of stress in national champion figure skaters. *Journal of Sport and Exercise Psychology* **15**, 134–159.

Gould, D., Finch, L.M. & Jackson, S.A. (1993c) Coping strategies used by national champion figure skaters. *Research Quarterly for Exercise and Sport* **64**, 453–468.

Gould, D., Tuffey, S., Udry, E. & Loehr, J. (1996a) Burnout in competitive junior tennis players: II. A qualitative analysis. *Sport Psychologist* **10**, 341–366.

Gould, D., Udry, E., Tuffey, S. & Loehr, J. (1996b) Burnout in competitive junior tennis players: I. A quantitative analysis. *Sport Psychologist* **10**, 322–340.

Gould, D., Tuffey, S., Udry, E. & Loehr, J. (1997) Burnout in competitive junior tennis players: III. Individual differences in the burnout experience. *Sport Psychologist* **11**, 257–276.

Greenspan, E. (1983) *Little Winners: Inside the World of the Child Sports Star*. Little, Brown and Company, Boston.

Gutmann, M.C., Pollock, M.L., Foster, C. & Schmidt, D. (1984) Training stress in Olympic speed skaters: a psychological perspective. *Physician and Sportsmedicine* **12**, 45–57.

Gutmann, M.C., Knapp, D.N., Foster, C., Pollock, M.L. & Rogowski, B.L. (1986) Age, experience, and gender as predictors of psychological response to training in Olympic speedskaters. In D.M. Landers (ed.) *Sport and Elite Performers*, pp. 97–102. Human Kinetics Publishers, Champaign, Illinois.

Howard, J. & Munson, L. (1997) Betrayal of trust: the case against a top volleyball coach focuses attention on the sexual abuse of young athletes. *Women/Sport* **1**, 66–77.

Iversen, G. (1990) Behind schedule: psychosocial aspects of delayed puberty in the competitive female gymnast. *Sport Psychologist* **4**, 155–167.

Joravsky, B. (1995) *Hoop Dreams*. Turner Publishing, Atlanta.

Klint, K.A. (1985) *Participation motives and self-perceptions of current and former athletes in youth gymnastics*. Master's thesis, University of Oregon, Eugene.

Klint, K.A. & Weiss, M.R. (1986) Dropping in and dropping out: participation motives of current and former youth gymnasts. *Canadian Journal of Applied Sport Sciences* **11**, 106–114.

Klint, K.A. & Weiss, M.R. (1987) Perceived competence and motives for participating in youth sports: a test of Harter's competence motivation theory. *Journal of Sport Psychology* **9**, 55–65.

Krane, V., Greenleaf, C.A. & Snow, J. (1997) Reaching for gold and the price of glory: a motivational case study of an elite gymnast. *Sport Psychologist* **11**, 53–71.

Louganis, G. (1995) *Breaking the Surface*. Random House, New York.

Martens, R. (1978) *Joy and Sadness in Children's Sports*. Human Kinetics Publishers, Champaign, Illinois.

Nash, H.L. (1987) Elite child-athletes: how much does victory cost? *Physician and Sportsmedicine* **15**, 129–133.

Nielsen, W.V. (1994) Ethics in coaching: it's time to do the right thing. *Olympic Coach* **4**, 2–5.

Orlick, T. & McCaffrey, N. (1991) Mental training with children for sport and life. *Sport Psychologist* **5**, 322–334.

Raedeke, T.D. (1997) Is athlete burnout more than just stress? A sport commitment perspective. *Journal of Sport and Exercise Psychology* **19**, 396–417.

Rowland, T.W. & Walsh, C.A. (1985) Characteristics of child distance runners. *Physician and Sportsmedicine* **13**, 45–53.

Ryan, J. (1995) *Little Girls in Pretty Boxes: The Making and Breaking of Elite Gymnasts and Figure Skaters*. Doubleday, New York.

Scanlan, T.K., Ravizza, K. & Stein, G.L. (1989a) An in-depth study of former figure skaters: I. Introduction to the project. *Journal of Sport and Exercise Psychology* **11**, 54–64.

Scanlan, T.K., Stein, G.L. & Ravizza, K. (1989b) An in-depth study of former elite figure skaters: II. Sources of enjoyment. *Journal of Sport and Exercise Psychology* **11**, 65–83.

Scanlan, T.K., Stein, G.L. & Ravizza, K. (1991) An in-depth study of former elite figure skaters: III. Sources of stress. *Journal of Sport and Exercise Psychology* **13**, 103–120.

Seefeldt, V. & Steig, P. (1986) Introduction to an interdisciplinary assessment of competition on elite young distance runners. In M.R. Weiss & D. Gould (eds) *Competitive Sport for Children and Youths*, pp. 213–218. Human Kinetics Publishers, Champaign, Illinois.

Stabiner, K. (1986) *Courting Fame: The Perilous Road to Women's Tennis Stardom*. Harper & Row, San Francisco.

Vogel, P. (1986) Training and racing involvement of elite young runners. In M.R. Weiss & D. Gould (eds)

Competitive Sport for Children and Youths, pp. 219–224. Human Kinetics Publishers, Champaign, Illinois.

Weiss, M.R. (1991) Psychological skill development in children and adolescents. *Sport Psychologist* **5**, 335–354.

Weiss, M.R. (1993) Psychological effects of intensive sport participation on children and youth: self-esteem and motivation. In B.R. Cahill & A.J. Pearl (eds) *Intensive Participation in Children's Sports*, pp. 39–69. Human Kinetics Publishers, Champaign, Illinois.

Weiss, M.R. & Glenn, S.D. (1992) Psychological development and females' sport participation: an interactional perspective. *Quest* **44**, 138–157.

Weiss, M.R. & Hayashi, C.T. (1995) All in the family: parent–child socialization influences in competitive youth gymnastics. *Pediatric Exercise Science* **7**, 36–48.

Weiss, M.R. & Hayashi, C.T. (1996) The United States. In P. De Knop, L.M. Engstrom, B. Skirstad & M.R. Weiss (eds) *Worldwide Trends in Child and Youth Sport*, pp. 43–57. Human Kinetics Publishers, Champaign, Illinois.

Weiss, M.R. & Petlichkoff, L.M. (1989) Children's motivation for participation in and withdrawal from sport: identifying the missing links. *Pediatric Exercise Science* **1**, 195–211.

Weiss, M.R., Wiese, D.M. & Klint, K.A. (1989) Head over heels with success: the relationship between self-efficacy and performance in youth gymnastics. *Journal of Sport and Exercise Psychology* **11**, 444–451.

Wiggins, D.K. (1996) A history of highly competitive sport for American children. In F.L. Smoll & R.E. Smith (eds) *Children in Sport: A Biopsychosocial Perspective*, pp. 15–30. Brown & Benchmark, Indianapolis.

Chapter 29

Ethical Issues

ANGELA SCHNEIDER

Introduction

The ethical story of women's participation in sport in general, and Olympic sport in particular, is the story of two ideals in apparent conflict. From inception, the ideal of the Olympic Games and the ideal Olympic athlete applied specifically and exclusively to men. In de Coubertin's ideal the goals to be achieved by the athletes through participation in the Olympic Games were not appropriate for women (de Coubertin, 1986). It is this basic idea, that sport (or sometimes even physical activity) and particularly high-level competitive sport is somehow incompatible with what women are or what they should be, that dominates any discussion of ethical issues for women in sport. The notions of ideal Olympic sport and ideal women lie behind many of the discussions in modern sport: whether to permit women to compete, the types of sport in which women can compete, the development of judging standards for adjudicated as opposed to refereed sports (contrast gymnastics and basketball), attitudes to aggression and competition, and indeed the very existence of women's sport as a separate entity at all.

Before examining some of these issues in detail, it is worth making a distinction at the outset. Many of the moral issues that arise in sport arise equally for men and women. At the personal level, the decision whether or not to cheat, what attitude you will take to your opponents or the unearned win are moral problems any athlete must face. At the institutional level,

decisions about rules prohibiting drug use or equipment limitations designed to improve participant safety should apply equally to women and men. Thus, those moral problems common to the realm of sport, important as they are, are more appropriately discussed elsewhere (Schneider, 1992, 1993; Butcher & Schneider, 1993; Schneider & Butcher, 1993, 1994, 1998). However, this chapter is devoted to the moral issues that arise because it is women who are the athletes. Thus the discussion that follows focuses on gender, ethics and sport, and the interrelationships amongst them.

How to approach ethical issues for women in sport and sport medicine

There are three standard elements of a methodology that attempts to deal with ethics and women in sport and sport medicine (this methodology was first identified by Tong (1995) in the field of bioethics). The first involves asking what was originally referred to as 'the woman question' and is now called by some researchers 'the gender biased question' (Tuttle, 1986). This question challenges the supposed objectivity of scientific research findings regarding the nature of woman and the objectivity of the profession of medicine based on that research (Dreifus, 1977; Corea, 1985; Schiebinger, 1989, 1993; Okruhlik, 1995). Underpinning this question is the claim that many of the 'facts' about female 'nature' actually result from values founded on biased social constructions (Ehrenreich & English, 1979;

Fausto-Sterling, 1992). The precepts and practices of medicine can be and are misshaped by gender bias (Sherwin, 1992; Tong, 1995). This gender bias works almost unconsciously and occurs when decision-makers in sport and physicians in sport medicine treat all athletes, all human bodies, as if they were all male athletes and male bodies. They then view athletes or their bodies as dysfunctional if they fail to function like male bodies or express little or no curiosity or interest in the problems unique to women. There are issues in sport medicine that are, for the most part, unique to women, e.g. the female athlete triad (eating disorders, amenorrhoea and osteoporosis), gender verification, reproductive control and pregnancy, sexual harassment, etc. There are issues unique to men. There are issues unique to certain sports. There are common issues for participants across regions, sports and particular quadrennial cycles. Sport medicine, as a profession, and sport organizers need to be aware of sex/gender similarities and differences in order to deal adequately with ethical issues.

The second part of this methodology is that of consciousness-raising. This requires that women be invited to contribute their personal experiences to sport and sport medicine so that it has wider meaning for all women. To a certain extent this kind of invitation was issued by the International Olympic Committee when it held the First World Conference on Women and Sport in October 1996. For example, women who share experiences of sexual stereotyping or sexual harassment in sport often come to realize that their feeling of having been treated as a girl rather than as a woman is not unique to them but common to most women. Such women, if given the opportunity, routinely gain the courage and confidence to challenge those who presume to know what is best for them as they become increasingly convinced that it is not they but the sport 'system' that is crazy. The purpose of this consciousness-raising is to achieve fundamental changes by connecting the personal experiences of women to developments in sport and sport medicine. Consciousness-raising suggests that women, sharing among themselves, will become

empowered and able to take on some of the responsibility for changing the sport world.

The last part of this methodology is based on three philosophical moral theorists: Aristotle, Rawls and Mill. It is an attempt to gain a Rawlsian reflective equilibrium between principles, rules, ideals, values and virtues on the one hand, and actual cases in which moral decisions must be made on the other. Aristotelian practical reasoning assumes that moral choices are made, for the most part, between several moral agents rather than isolated within one individual. Mill's views on the importance of listening, as well as speaking, in the course of a moral dialogue is stressed. Since the practice of ethics requires communication, corroboration and collaboration, we are not alone when we grapple with applying ethics to sport and sport medicine. Accepting our limited ability to explain and justify our decisions and actions to each other, while simultaneously insisting that we try harder to find the appropriate words, is a necessary part of this practical reasoning.

Using this three-part methodology we can discover mutually agreeable ways to weaken patterns of human domination and subordination in the realm of sport and sport medicine and, in particular, patterns of male domination and female subordination. This type of discussion requires the adoption of a particular stance and the development of a particular set of questions. The answers to these questions must be dealt with and understood within the context of women's experiences in sport. If we truly seek understanding of these issues, we must understand the perspective and thus the social, psychological and political predispositions that we ourselves bring to the discussion. For example, I am a white, female, well-educated, socially/politically advantaged, Canadian, agnostic, heterosexual, mother, former Olympic silver medallist, etc., and I am going to bring a different perspective and context to the questions of gender, ethics and sport than someone who has a different race, gender, education, social/political position, nationality, religion, sexuality, etc. This does not mean that we cannot reach some agreement on important issues, but it does mean that we must be willing to listen and give due respect to differing perspectives in our search for justice. This search for justice also requires an understanding of where the power to make changes lies and the willingness of those who hold it to share that power.

The Olympic ideal and women athletes

Although there are competing interpretations of de Coubertin's conception of Olympism (Lowe, 1977; Rioux, 1986; Segrave, 1988; Loland, 1994), there is general agreement on some of the dominant themes. The values that seem to have the greatest support are those deemed to have defined Olympism for most of this century: (i) education; (ii) international understanding (peace); (iii) equal opportunity; (iv) fair and equal competition; (v) cultural expression; (vi) independence of sport; (vii) excellence; and (viii) amateurism until fairly recently. On the face of it, there seems to be no reason whatsoever that any of these values be exclusive to male athletes or males in general. However, it is equally clear that women athletes have not been given the same opportunities as male athletes, from the ancient Greek Olympics through the 19th century until current times. It would now seem rather obvious that the value of equal opportunity would logically entail women athletes.

Equal opportunity

Baron de Coubertin intended his vision of sport to be universal and available to all classes (Segrave & Chu, 1988; Loland, 1994) but there are interesting gaps in the scope of his late-19th century vision in that he does not include just over half the population—women. However, de Coubertin's views on women in sport were not atypical for the late 19th century: 'Throughout his writings, he expressed his views against women in sport. He did not think well of women perspiring in public, assuming positions he deemed ungainly, and appearing in public riding

horses, skiing or playing soccer' (Spears, 1988). Several discussions of de Coubertin's position on women and sport include the following quotation from the *Olympic Review* of 1912 as evidence of his gender-biased view of the Olympic Games: '[as] the solemn and periodic exaltation of male athleticism, with internationalism as a base, loyalty as a means, art for its setting, and female applause as reward' (Leigh, 1974; Spears, 1988; De Frantz, 1993). De Coubertin, and many others in the Olympic Movement, believed that sport was the proper preserve of men. Women were somehow unsuited to sport and should, for their own good, be excluded (Veblen, 1953). This is one area where the attitudes and values of Olympism have shown steady (albeit slow) development.

Ideal woman

It should be clear that the battles which represent the ethical issues for women in Olympic sport will be fought over conceptions of women: their bodies and their minds. The traditional ideals of woman upheld during the ancient Olympic Games and during the revival of the modern Olympic Games (up to and including some current ideals) are intimately tied to a particular view of woman's body. Some of these characteristics are soft, graceful, weak and beautiful. The desirable qualities for a woman in the time of the ancient Olympics can generally be summarized as beauty, chastity, modesty, obedience, inconspicuous behaviour, a good wife and a good mother (Lefkowitz & Fant, 1982) (Fig. 29.1). Of course, these characteristics are tied to the roles of wife, mother and daughter. These characteristics are not similar to those of the traditional ideal of man as hard, powerful, strong and rational, which are tied to the roles of leader, warrior and father. More importantly, if we examine the underlying characteristics of the traditional ideal athlete, in particular the Olympian hero, we can plainly see that the ideal man and the ideal Olympian are very similar, particularly in the role of warrior (for a current personal account of the relationship between masculinity and sport in North America see Messner & Sabo, 1994).

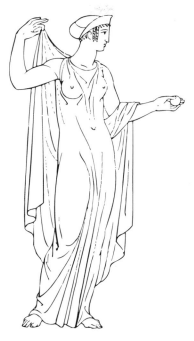

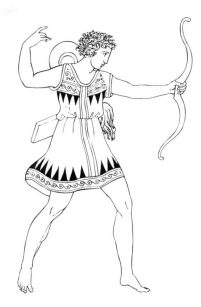

Fig. 29.2 Amazon. (Adapted from Mercatante, 1988.)

Fig. 29.1 Venus (Aphrodite). (Adapted from Mercatante, 1988.)

Conversely, we can plainly see that during the times of the ancient Olympic Games and during the rebirth of the modern Olympic Games the ideal woman and the traditional ideal Olympian athlete are almost opposites, so much so that women were hardly ever mentioned in conjunction with sport.

'In contrast to these infrequent and casual references to women's sport, accounts of men's sport and athletics abound in ancient Greek literature. Homer vividly describes events from chariot racing to boxing. Pausanias furnishes a detailed account of the Olympic Games, and Herodotus, Thucydides, and other Greek authors refer to the Olympic Games and athletic festivals such as the Pythian, Isthmian, and Nemean Games' (Spears, 1988).

One might argue that since the ancient athletic festivals did not embrace women, why should de Coubertin, in his attempt to successfully revive them, do so? One response is that de Coubertin had an ideal in mind and he selected what he wanted from the ancient games and rejected aspects that did not fit his ideal (Spears, 1988). He also had some exceptional counter-examples from ancient Greece in the writings of Plato, even though it is unlikely that de Coubertin knew that girls did compete in athletic festivals in ancient Greece. Plato argued that women should be accorded the right to attain the highest rank he could conceive of in human excellence—the philosopher ruler—and to be equally educated in the gymnasium by exercising naked with the men (Bluestone, 1987). Other exceptional counter-examples from ancient Greece that stress physicality and a warrior nature for woman are the archetypes of Artemis, Atalanta and the Amazons, who all rejected the traditional role for women (Creedon, 1994) (Fig. 29.2). However, de Coubertin apparently never saw women as having central roles in Olympism; he preferred them as spectators and medal bearers for the presentation to the victors.

The fundamental ethical issue in this entire discussion is who decides which images of woman are permitted, desired or pursued in

Olympic sport. The primary ethical question for women in sport is inextricably linked to the question of power and autonomy. At the institutional level, if men decide what sports women are permitted to attempt, the standards of physical perfection that are to be met in adjudicated sports or the levels of funding accorded women's as opposed to men's sport, then women have a legitimate grievance of not being treated with due respect. Just as it is the responsibility of each male to decide for himself the type of body and the type of life he wishes to pursue, moral or otherwise, it is the responsibility and right of each woman to deal with the challenges with which the female athlete must contend.

Paternalism and autonomy

The *Oxford Dictionary of Philosophy* defines 'paternalism' as 'government as by a benign parent'. Paternalism is not necessarily sexist, although it often has been in sport and sport medicine, and is often well-meaning. It occurs when one person makes a decision on behalf of, or speaks for, another that he or she takes to be in the latter person's best interest. In the case of children, this is a necessary part of the parenting process until the child becomes an adult. Paternalism is also morally acceptable in cases where the person concerned is unable, for good reason, to speak or make decisions for himself or herself. It is morally troubling when it occurs on behalf of competent adults.

The concept of autonomy in ethical decision-making is very important. In the *Oxford Dictionary of Philiosophy* autonomy is defined as the 'capacity for self-government'; furthermore, 'agents are autonomous if their actions are truly their own'. The crucial point here is that an essential part of being human is having the right and the capacity to make the choices and decisions that most affect oneself. Each competent human adult has the right to choose to pursue the projects and endeavours that he or she most cares about. That right is naturally limited by the rights of others to pursue their own desires and interests, but what the concept of autonomy

takes for granted is that no one is entitled to speak on another's behalf without that person's permission.

Sport paternalism and women's participation

Is there any reason why women should not participate in sports that men have traditionally played? It is instructive to look at what could possibly count as a morally acceptable answer. If there was a sport practised by men that was physiologically impossible for women, this would count as a reason for the non-participation of women. However, there is no such sport. To qualify, the sport would probably have to primarily involve male genitalia and there is no institutionally sanctioned sport of this type. A second possibility would be if there was a sport played by men that no women in the world actually wanted to play. It is possible that a sport might be invented that not one woman would want to play, but then the reason the women would not be playing would be that *they* had chosen not to play, not that someone else had decided that they should not. Morally unacceptable answers for prohibiting women from playing sport include 'it would be bad for women to participate' or 'there is not enough money to allow women to participate'. Let us look at each of these answers in turn.

'It would be bad for women to participate' is the standard line that has been used throughout the history of sport. The exact nature of the harm that would befall women changes: it could be that participation 'defeminizes', which might mean that it would make some women less attractive in the eyes of some men, either physically or mentally, or that it would be harmful for women such that they or their yet unborn children would suffer some physiological damage (for a good discussion of these points see Schneider, 1993; Cahn, 1994). There are two points to be made here. The first is practical: the assertions that women are harmed and men are not harmed by strenuous physical exertion are simply not true. However, it is the second point that is more important: women have the right, just as men do, to decide what risks of harm they will run. Subject to the normal limitations on every person's freedom, it is immorally paternalistic to decide on behalf of another competent adult what personal risks he or she can choose to accept.

The argument that 'there is not enough money' can be a more difficult case to answer. It cannot be morally required to do the impossible. However, 'there is not enough money' often masks an inequitable distribution of the resources that are available. If there is money available for anyone to participate in sport, then that money must be available on an equitable basis for both women and men. Men's sport is not intrinsically more important or more worthwhile than women's sport and therefore has no automatic right to majority funding.

Challenges to women athletes

In this section, some of the challenges that women athletes face are examined from a moral point of view. Some of these challenges are a result of the institutional climate for women in sport (e.g. biased, resistant and 'chilly'), which will require policy and practice changes. Other challenges, physical, mental and indeed spiritual, occur at a personal level. From a physical perspective these challenges may include, but are not limited to, body composition and development issues related to the health and well-being of the athlete. Some of these problems are a direct result of the demands of participation in sport. For example, many élite-level sports have a high risk of injuries and, generally speaking, élite-level training produces fit but not necessarily healthy athletes. The results of those pressures can be, and in many cases are, different for men and women but the choice of whether or not to train and compete is the same. However, in those sports where performance is judged (e.g. gymnastics, diving, ice skating), the physical requirements and resulting risks are directly caused by decisions about what counts as an excellent performance (Suits, 1988). The judging criteria for these sports should be tailored so as to minimize the health risks they impose on the athlete.

Amenorrhoea and pregnancy are unique to women athletes and raise issues concerned with: (i) the implications all women face when reproductive aspects of their lives are designated as illness; and (ii) the tension between the two conflicting traditional ideals of woman and athlete. An essential part of the traditional ideal woman is fertility because it is necessary for child-bearing. Fertility and child-bearing are not only superfluous for the ideal athlete, they are antithetical to the role of athlete as warrior (e.g. Amazons). In many ways the Amazons were viewed as monstrosities because they rejected the primary biological role of woman.

Historically, some medical authorities have created a series of double binds (i.e. situations in which options for an oppressed group are reduced to a very few and all of them expose the group to penalty, censure or deprivation; Frye, 1983; Sherwin, 1992) for women because of the decision to view menstruation, pregnancy, menopause, body size and some feminine behaviours as diseases (Broverman et al., 1981; Martin, 1987; Lander, 1988). For the female athlete the situation is more complicated because she can be classified as even more abnormal when reproductive changes are evaluated in the context of the traditional male sports arena. For example, if the normal healthy woman is considered an unhealthy adult from a medical perspective, because the ideal healthy adult is based on being male (Broverman et al., 1981), the female athlete starts out as an unhealthy adult because she is a woman. Further, if the female athlete shows signs of masculinization, this is thought of as a further abnormality because it is not normal for a woman to have masculine characteristics. Following this kind of medical classification, when a woman bleeds she is ill ('Woman . . . is generally ailing at least one week out of four . . . woman is not only an invalid, but a wounded one'; Lander, 1988) and if she does not bleed (e.g. amenorrhoea, menopause and pregnancy) she is ill, because it is not normal for her to be unable to conceive and thus make successful use of her reproductive organs (Martin, 1987; Lander, 1988; Zita, 1988; Sherwin, 1992). Pregnancy constitutes a state of health for the traditional ideal woman and should not be treated as a disease requiring a significant amount of specialized treatment. However, throughout pregnancy women, and women athletes in particular, are not encouraged to think of themselves or their lifestyles as healthy. Serious charges of irresponsibility can be levelled when the relationship between a woman athlete and her fetus is characterized as adversarial. Most pregnant women athletes, who are falsely charged with harming their fetuses, face at least moral pressure based on the view that being pregnant and participating in sport is a socially unacceptable behaviour. However, genuine harm to the fetus may occur with participation in some sports, such as scuba diving. Rather than sanctioning interference with a female athlete's reproductive freedom that denies her interest in the health of her fetus and her role as an active independent moral agent, the focus should be on education.

The classification of these reproductive aspects as illnesses has led to wide-scale paternalistic medical management of women under the façade of beneficence (Sherwin, 1992). In sport, these so-called illnesses have been part of the basis for excluding women. This does not mean that serious complications requiring medical interventions cannot occur during a female athlete's reproductive life or life-cycle changes and ageing. There will be particular cases where the label of illness or disease is appropriate, provided that it does not lead to discrimination against women athletes from a sport policy perspective (e.g. banning them from participation rather than educating them about coping with their illness and participating in sport).

The female athlete must also face challenges regarding the mental requirements of sporting competition, i.e. aggression and violence. Male athletes also face these challenges, but it is considered 'normal' for men and 'abnormal' for women to engage in violence. Traditionally it has also been predominantly men who have committed sexual abuse against women and minors in sport. Some researchers suggest that this predominance may be linked to the socially and legally acceptable extreme levels of violence in some sports (S. Kirby & C. Brackenridge, unpublished observations). The control over, and moral responsibility for, violence, abuse, harassment and discrimination in and surrounding sport lies mainly in the hands of those in the sport community and is a concern for both men and women. Some women, weary of being ignored on these issues and for a host of other reasons, advocate completely separate sport for women as opposed to any integration at all.

One argument against integration is that women have to accept the current selection of sports that were primarily designed for and practised by men, with an established culture that rewards and recognizes values that most women do not hold (e.g. viewing sport as a battleground on which one conquers one's foes). Separation might allow women the freedom to create sport based on the values they choose (Lenskyj, 1984). In this argument, capacities viewed as unique to women are stressed: sharing, giving, nurturing, sympathizing, empathizing and, above all, connecting as opposed to dividing. Nevertheless, some would urge women to pay the high price of integration so that they can have the same opportunities, occupations, rights and privileges that men have. This drive for the uniformity of women with men has sometimes denied women's unique qualities and that these qualities might contribute very positively to sport and the study of sport medicine. The argument is that if women emphasize their differences from men, viewing these as biologically produced and/or culturally shaped, they will trap themselves in ghettos while men will continue as they have been.

If we think that women athletes must either act as men if they accept the male ideal or be separate and generate their own ideal, then the sport experience is highly gender specific. However, the two views of sport, i.e. sport as competition ('agonistic') or sport as connected co-questers searching and striving for excellence, may be logically independent of the gender of the athlete. The greatest tension arises for women if we have an agonistic view of sport and women are found to be inherently or 'essentially' caring and connected to others (Gilligan, 1982; Noddings, 1984). In such a model of sport, women may be required to disconnect from their embodied experience. This could be the basis for some form of alienation. It is probably the case that most athletes (male and female) find themselves torn between conflicting views of sport because pushing oneself to one's limits challenges even the strongest sense of self; because in their moments of agony and joy they tend to experience themselves as both radically alone, since no one else can really understand what they feel, and fundamentally united to their team-mates, their competitors and with all of humanity, particularly when this experience happens during competition in the Olympic Games.

The logic of gender verification

Entirely separate sport, even just separate women's events, inevitably leads to the question of the logic of gender verification. If there are to be separate sports or sporting events for women only, it must be possible to exclude any men that may wish, for whatever reason, to compete. This means that there must be a rule of eligibility that excludes men. Conversely, if we have such a rule for excluding men, should we, for consistency, have such a rule excluding women from men's events even if the women believed they would inevitably lose but wanted to take part anyway? This in turn requires that we have a test of gender and/or sex that can be applied fairly to any potential participant. There are at least three methods of applying such a test: (i) test all contestants; (ii) test random contestants; and (iii) test targeted individuals.

Before examining testing further, we must first deal with the response that we do not need to test because a man would never wish to compete in a women's event. 'Never' is a very strong word. It is not beyond the realm of imagination that a money-hungry promoter might decide that it was a great publicity stunt to enter a man in a

women's event. A male may even, with good intentions, choose to enter a women's event such as synchronized swimming as a form of protest against gender discrimination. Without a test to decide who is eligible, we could be forced to accept participants in women's events who were quite obviously and unashamedly male but who merely professed to be female.

One case which illustrates the conceptual and moral issues that litter the issue of gender verification is that of Renée Richards. In 1976 a new player, Renée Clarke, appeared on the US women's tennis circuit and 'soundly thrashed' the defending champion in the women's division. She was subsequently shown to be Renée Richards, who had recently undergone a sexchange operation and was previously an élite-level male tennis player (Birrell & Cole, 1994). The US Women's Tennis Federation wanted to exclude the player, who was genetically male but reconstructed physiologically and presumably psychologically as a female, as unfair competition. The United States Tennis Association, the Women's Tennis Association and the United States Open Committee therefore introduced the requirement that players take the Barr test (Birrell & Cole, 1994), a chromosomal test. Richards refused and went to court to demand the right to participate in women's events. In court she was deemed to be female on the basis of the medical evidence produced by the surgeons and medical professionals who had overseen her transformation from male to female. In the media this story played as an example of a courageous individual fighting for personal rights against an intransigent and uncaring 'system' (Birrell & Cole, 1994). There are other ways of viewing the story.

What makes a woman a woman? Is it chromosomes, genitalia, a way of life or set of roles, or a medical record? It is not clear why medical evidence of surgery and psychology should outweigh chromosomal evidence; in fact it is not clear why any one answer should be taken as categorically overriding any other. However, if the methodology outlined in the second section of this chapter is used, the process of arriving at a conclusion becomes clearer: (i) asking 'the woman or gender biased question'; (ii) raising consciousness by connecting the personal experiences of women to developments in gender verification in sport and sport medicine; and (iii) using practical reasoning that attempts to gain a reflective equilibrium and accepts our limited ability to explain and justify our decisions, while simultaneously insisting that we try harder to find the appropriate ways. Thus women themselves can, and need to, be the guardians and decision-makers concerning women's sport.

Some women argue that any gender or sex test is demeaning (especially visual confirmation of the 'correct' genitalia) and discriminates against women athletes if it is not also applied to men. Clearly the use of any test, given the complexity of human sex and gender, may lead to anomalies and surprises. Yet many women wish to have sporting competition that excludes men. The best result we can achieve will be one that arises through discussion, debate and consensus and thus will be the fairest we can arrive at.

Recommendations for future research

Dealing with instances of gender oppression or neglect in sport and sport medicine requires multiple combinations of social, biological, political, ontological and epistemological methods. This complex approach enables the development of an ethical framework that can provide the means for discerning and solving the problems regarding women and sport and requires the acknowledgement that there is no clear line between ethics and social/political concerns. Some of the most important moral questions to be asked in cases of gender oppression and neglect in sport and sport medicine are specifically about male domination and female subordination. A coherent understanding of the causes of women's subordination to men in sport, coupled with a refined programme of action designed to eliminate the systems and attitudes that oppress or cause neglect of women in sport, must guide this complex approach. A detailed analysis of the dis-

tribution of power in each case can identify a particular factor as the primary cause of women's subordinate status in sport, which for the most part has traditionally been based on biology. However, to adequately deal with these problems, researchers must also look at economics, law, education, national boundaries, language and so on, because all of these factors have contributed, more or less strongly, to the current status of women's sport and sport medicine pertaining to women athletes. Researchers can, and should, attempt to ascertain the actual status of both sexes in sport and the actual health of both sexes in sport medicine and determine how far that condition deviates from what justice prescribes.

The current conditions in sport and sport medicine may be made more objective by providing more facts, as opposed to myths or stereotypes, about women athletes, thus alleviating or even eliminating the past and ongoing injustices. The knowledge required to create good, just and rational sport practice and sport medicine practice can be acquired. It is a matter of discovering and acknowledging all the true facts. Unfortunately for women athletes, it may still be some time before all rational agents see the same thing when the facts stare them in the face. Women are now beginning to be credited with being able to recognize the realities of sport that men do not typically see (Messner & Sabo, 1990). The 'master's position' in any set of dominating social relations—the general position of men *vis-à-vis* women in sport—tends to produce distorted visions of the real regularities and underlying causal tendencies in social relations. Men experience their power over women as normal, even beneficial, but this is not women's experience. Women see systems of male domination and female subordination in sport and sport medicine as abnormal and harmful ways for men and women to relate to one another. Rather than being irrelevant, political and social position determines the way in which we see the facts, including fundamental facts, about the human body and mind. It is possible to find truth and justice for women in sport, but presently they are partial, provisional and changing in nature (as Tong (1995) has concluded in the area of bioethics). Everyone's knowledge about sport, sport science and the health and well-being of all athletes, including women athletes, is limited. If we wish to understand a broader experience than just the dominant one, we must talk to and take seriously as many athletes as possible. Truth and justice will emerge through these shared conversations.

Acknowledgements

I would like to thank Drs S. Kirby, K. Okruhlik, and S. Brennan for their informative input to this chapter. I would especially like to thank my partner Dr R.B. Butcher for the critical analysis and insights he contributed throughout this chapter and his patience, support and encouragement.

References

Aristotle (1941) Ethica Nicomachea (Nicomachean ethics). In R. McKeon (ed.) *The Basic Works of Aristotle*, pp. 935–1127. Random House, New York.

Birrell, S. & Cole, C.L. (1994) *Women, Sport, and Culture*. Human Kinetics Publishers, Champaign, Illinois.

Bluestone, N. (1987) *Women and the Ideal Society: Plato's Republic and Modern Myths of Gender*. University of Massachusetts Press, Amherst.

Broverman, I., Broverman, D., Clarkson, F., Rosenkrantz, P. & Vogel, S. (1981) Sex role stereotypes and clinical judgments of mental health. In E. Howell & M. Bayes (eds) *Women and Mental Health*, pp. 112–121. Basic Books, New York.

Butcher, R.B. & Schneider, A.J. (1993) *The Ethical Rationale for Drug-Free Sport*. Canadian Centre for Drug-free Sport, Ottawa, Ontario.

Cahn, S. (1994) *Coming on Strong: Gender and Sexuality in Twentieth-Century Women's Sport*. The Free Press, New York.

Corea, G. (1985) *The Hidden Malpractice: How American Medicine Mistreats Women*, revised edn. Harper Colophon Books, New York.

Creedon, P. (ed.) (1994) *Women, Media and Sport*. Sage Publications, California.

De Coubertin, P. (1986) Revue Olympique. In N. Muller (ed.) *Textes Choisis, Vol. II, Olympisme*, pp. 707–708. Weidmann, Zurich.

De Frantz, A. (1993) The Olympic Games: our birthright to sports. In G. Cohen (ed.) *Women in Sport:*

Issues and Controversies, pp. 185–193. Sage Publications, California.

Dreifus, C. (ed.) (1977) *Seizing Our Bodies: The Politics of Women's Health*. Vintage Books, Random House, New York.

Ehrenreich, B. & English, D. (1979) *For Her Own Good: 150 years of the Experts' Advice to Women*. Anchor Books, Garden City, New York.

Fausto-Sterling, A. (1992) *Myths of Gender: Biological Theories About Women and Men*, 2nd edn. Basic Books, New York.

Frye, M. (1983) *The Politics of Reality: Essays in Feminist Theory*. Crossing Press, Freedom, California.

Gilligan, C. (1982) *In a Different Voice: Psychological Theory and Women's Moral Development*. Harvard University Press, Cambridge, Massachusetts.

Lander, L. (1988) *Images of Bleeding: Menstruation as Ideology*. Orlando Press, New York.

Lefkowitz, M. & Fant, M. (1982) *Women's Life in Greece and Rome: A Source Book in Translation*. Johns Hopkins University Press, Baltimore.

Leigh, M. (1974) *The evolution of women's participation in the Summer Olympic Games, 1900–1948*. Doctoral dissertation, Ohio State University, Columbus.

Lenskyj, H. (1984) *Sport Integration or Separation*. Fitness and Amateur Sport, Ottawa.

Loland, S. (1994) Pierre de Coubertin's ideology of Olympism from the perspective of the history of ideas. In R.K. Barney & K.V. Meier (eds) *Critical Reflections on Olympic Ideology: Second International Symposium for Olympic Research*, pp. 26–45. Centre for Olympic Studies, University of Western Ontario, London, Ontario.

Lowe, B. (1977) *The Beauty of Sport: A Cross-disciplinary Inquiry*. Prentice-Hall, Englewood Cliffs, New Jersey.

Martin, E. (1987) *The Woman in the Body: A Cultural Analysis of Reproduction*. Beacon Press, Boston.

Mercatante, A.S. (1988) *The Facts on File: Encyclopedia of World Mythology and Legend*. Oxford University Press, New York.

Messner, M. & Sabo, D. (eds) (1990) *Sport, Men and the Gender Order: Critical Feminist Perspectives*. Human Kinetics Publishers, Champaign, Illinois.

Messner, M. & Sabo, D. (1994) *Sex, Violence and Power in Sports: Rethinking Masculinity*. Crossing Press, Freedom, California.

Mill, J. (1972) *Utilitarianism, On Liberty, and Considerations on Representative Government*. H. Acton (ed.). E.P. Dutton & Co., New York.

Noddings, N. (1984) *Caring: A Feminine Approach to Ethics and Moral Education*. University of California Press, Berkeley.

Okruhlik, K. (1995) Gender and the biological sciences. *Canadian Journal of Philosophy* **20**, 21–42.

Plato (1961) Republic. In E. Hamilton & H. Cairns (eds) *Plato: The Collected Dialogues*, pp. 575–844. Princeton University Press, Princeton.

Rawls, J. (1971) *A Theory of Justice*. Harvard University Press, Cambridge, Massachusetts.

Rioux, G. (1986) Propos liminaires: Pierre de Coubertin educateur (1863–1937). In G. Rioux (ed.) *Pierre de Coubertin, Textes Choisis, Tome I, Revelations*, pp. 19–21. Weidmann, Zurich.

Schiebinger, L. (1989) *The Mind Has No Sex? Women in the Origins of Modern Science*. Harvard University Press, Cambridge, Massachusetts.

Schiebinger, L. (1993) *Nature's Body: Gender in the Making of Modern Science*. Beacon Press, Boston.

Schneider, A.J. (1992) Harm, athletes' rights and doping control. In R.K. Barney & K.V. Meier (eds) *First International Symposium for Olympic Research*, pp. 164–172. Centre for Olympic Studies, University of Western Ontario, London, Ontario.

Schneider, A.J. (1993) Doping in sport and the perversion argument. In G. Gaebauer (ed.) *The Relevance of the Philosophy of Sport*, pp. 117–128. Academia Verlag, Berlin.

Schneider, A.J. (1995) Gender, sexuality and sport in America. *Journal of the Philosophy of Sport* **22**, 136–143.

Schneider, A.J. & Butcher, R.B. (1993) For the love of the game: a philosophical defense of amateurism. *Quest* **45**, 460–469.

Schneider, A.J. & Butcher, R.B. (1994) Why Olympic athletes should avoid the use and seek the elimination of performance-enhancing substances and practices in the Olympic Games. *Journal of the Philosophy of Sport* **20/21**, 64–81.

Schneider, A.J. & Butcher, R.B. Fair play as respect for the game. *Journal of the Philosophy of Sport* **25**, 1–22.

Segrave, J. (1988) Toward a definition of Olympism. In J. Segrave & D. Chu (eds) *The Olympic Games in Transition*, pp. 149–162. Human Kinetics Publishers, Champaign, Illinois.

Segrave, J. & Chu, D. (eds) (1988) *The Olympic Games in Transition*. Human Kinetics Publishers, Champaign, Illinois.

Sherwin, S. (1992) *No Longer Patient: Feminist Ethics and Health Care*. Temple University Press, Philadelphia.

Spears, B. (1988) Tryphosa, Melpomene, Nadia, and Joan: the IOC and women's sport. In J. Segrave & D. Chu (eds) *The Olympic Games in Transition*, pp. 365–374. Human Kinetics Publishers, Champaign, Illinois.

Suits, B. (1988) Tricky triad: games, play and sport. *Journal of the Philosophy of Sport* **13**, 1–9.

Tong, R. (1995) What's distinctive about feminist bioethics? In F. Baylis, J. Downie, B. Freedman, B. Hoffmaster & S. Sherwin (eds) *Health Care Ethics in Canada*, pp. 22–30. Harcourt Brace Canada, Toronto.

Tuttle, L. (1986) *Encyclopaedia of Feminism*. Longman, Harlow, Essex.

Veblen, T. (1953) *Theory of Leisure Class: An Economic Study of Institutions*. New American Library, New York.

Zita, J. (1988) The premenstrual syndrome: dis-easing the female cycle. *Hypatia* **3**, 77–99.

Chapter 30

Women's Role in National and International Sports Governing Bodies

KARI FASTING

Introduction

National and international sports governing bodies have one common characteristic: they are chaired primarily by men. This lack of women in the decision-making bodies of sport applies even to sports where the members are predominantly women. Whereas formerly there were separate sports organizations for women and men and women had a leadership role, today these organizations have merged. According to Dyer (1982), when sex-separated organizations have merged, men have taken over the leadership positions. The situation in the USA illustrates this point very clearly. As an effect of Title IX (a law requiring equal rights in school and college sport), many women's and men's athletic departments were merged. At about the same time the National Collegiate Athletic Association (NCAA) opened up for women; in practice the Association for Intercollegiate Athletics for Women (AIAW) was absorbed by the NCAA. Title IX produced an enormous increase in the number of female athletes in the USA, although there seems also to have been an 'unexpected' effect. American professor Joan H. Hult (1989) expressed it this way:

> The success of Title IX has led to male governance power in all amateur sports from high school competition through college, nonschool agencies, and the Olympic movement. Title IX has left untouched pervasive fundamental inequities in leadership, decision-making

authority, coaching systems and role models for girls in all athletic situations.

One other characteristic of sports governing bodies is that fewer women are found in the higher echelons of a hierarchical sports organization. Based on Canadian studies, Beamish (1985) writes that 'as sports executives become more encompassing and have more powerful mandates, women tend to be excluded'. On the positive side, however, during the last few years more and more national and international sports governing bodies have discussed the lack of women in decision-making positions and have decided on different approaches to increase the number of female sports leaders. In some countries, for example Sweden and Canada, this work has continued for about 20 years. Experience from these countries indicates that it is very difficult to reach a democratic representation based on the percentage of the female membership. Some of the reasons for this are outlined later in this chapter.

Research in the area of women in sports governing bodies is scarce. A search on the SPORT Discs SIRC database, combining women and sport with sports governing bodies, produced 98 references. Much of what has been written presents distributive statistics and/or the popular media presentation of women in sports organizations, with little empirical data or theoretical foundation. Other research presents the life stories of famous women, such as the female members of the Olympic Movement. The research and literature drawn on in this chapter are mostly from Europe or North America, which means that one must be very careful about generalizing to other parts of the world, such as Asia or Africa. It is relevant to mention here that Canada seems to be the country with the most research in this area, such as the work of Theberge (1984), Beamish (1985), Hall *et al.* (1989) and Whitson and MacIntosh (1989). An important source of information has also been a state of the art report on women in leadership positions published by the Swedish Sports Federation (Cederberg & Olofsson, 1996).

In the first part of this chapter some statistics on women in sports governing bodies are presented. Since the International Olympic Committee (IOC) is the most powerful sports organization in the world, special attention is focused on its engagement in this area. Based on an overview of the most important studies, the main part of the chapter attempts to answer the question: Why are there so few women in sports governing bodies? The answers to this question should also provide the direction for the most effective strategies needed to correct the current imbalance and also to determine what kind of future research needs to be done in this area.

Number of women in sports governing bodies

Until recently the Olympic Movement has been heavily dominated by men. However, the IOC is different from other sports organizations and therefore is not comparable with other sports governing bodies. This is due primarily to the fact that the IOC is a self-perpetuating body whose new members are elected by the existing members. According to Davenport (1988), IOC members do not represent their countries, they represent the IOC and are ambassadors of Olympism to their countries. The former Director of the IOC, Mme Berlioux, wrote in 1981 that:

National Olympic committees, national or international federations, regional organizations, organizing committees are all, in prac-

tice, run as 'all-male' clubs, in which women are tolerated only in small doses as guests.

For 87 years the IOC had only male members. In 1981 the first 'guests' were permitted, when Flor Isara Fonesca from Venezuela and Pirjo Häggman from Finland became the first female members. Since then nine more women have been appointed and one has retired. Today the number of women on the IOC is 10, which accounts for about 10% of the membership.

The IOC supports 22 commissions of which only one is chaired by a woman. Many commissions have no female members. One example is the Sport for All Commission which has no female members, in spite of the fact that large numbers of females around the world participate in recreational sports. Of the 34 international federations represented in the Olympic programme, only two are headed by a woman and two have female secretary generals (L. Darlison, unpublished observations). Of the 200 national Olympic committees, three have a female president and nine have female secretary generals (Women and Sport Bulletin, 1999).

Based on the different initiatives that the IOC has recently enacted it is hoped that this low female representation will change. At their Centennial Congress in Paris in 1994 the following recommendations (International Olympic Committee, 1994) were among those agreed.

• Increase the numbers of IOC members who are women, doubling the number by the year 2000.

• Increase the number of women who serve on IOC commissions, recommending the appointment of women when they are not nominated by international federations or national Olympic committees.

• Create incentives for each international federation, national federation and national Olympic committee to develop women as coaches and administrators.

Two years later the IOC appointed a working group on women and sport. At its initial meeting in March 1996 the following decisions were among those agreed.

• Increase the numbers of IOC members who

are women, doubling the number by the year 2000.

• More women must be appointed to commissions and working groups as well as to the international federations and national Olympic committees, recommending the appointment of women when they are not nominated by international federations or national Olympic committees.

• Seminars for women in administration and leadership, coaching and sports journalism should be organized every year.

• The Olympic Study Centre is encouraged to make studies on the role of women and sport.

These recommendations were followed up at the IOC's session in Atlanta 1996, where it was decided to establish the goal of ensuring that by the year 2000 at least 10% of all offices in the IOC's decision-making structures should be held by women; by 2005 it should be 20%. It was further decided that all the sports organizations belonging to the Olympic Movement should establish the goal of ensuring that similar developments take place (L. Darlison, unpublished observations).

The IOC also held its first conference on women and sport in October 1996. At the end of the three days of discussion the participants adopted a list of recommendations, of which the following concern women's role in sports governing bodies.

• Recognition that the Olympic ideal cannot be fully realized without, and until there is, equality for women within the Olympic Movement.

• The IOC, international federations and national Olympic committees should take into consideration the issue of gender equality in all their policies, programmes and procedures, and recognize the special needs of women so that they may play a full and active part in sport.

• All women involved in sport should be provided with equal opportunities for professional and personal advancement, whether as athletes, coaches or administrators, and that the international federations and national Olympic committees create special committees or working groups composed of at least 10% women to design and implement a plan of action with a view to promoting women in sport.

• Commissions dealing specifically with the issue of women in sport should be set up at national and international levels.

• Within Olympic solidarity a special fund should be earmarked for the promotion of women's sport at all levels, as well as for the training of women administrators, technical officials and coaches, particularly in developing countries.

• The IOC should organize each year, and on the five continents, a training course for women in one of the following areas: coaching, technical activity, administration or media/journalism.

During the 102 years that the IOC has existed, the last two years may be looked upon as a new era for the role of women in sport. The crucial point is whether, and in what way, these actions and recommendations will be put into practice. As discussed later, it may be difficult to gain equity for women in sports governing bodies without changing some fundamental structures of the sports organizations themselves, their values and the way they operate. The IOC has the power to do this, but the question is whether they want to.

The low number of women in decision-making positions in sports governing bodies has also been discussed in Europe. According to Delforge (1989), the point has been raised on various occasions by the Council of Europe, which has arranged two conferences on this theme, one in Dublin, Ireland in 1980 and one in Bisham Abbey, UK in 1989. One finding of the seminar in Dublin was that due to the low number of female sports leaders, 'decisions concerning women are taken by men without any real knowledge of women's true needs'. The Dublin seminar also decided upon several recommendations, such as 'that governments should encourage sports federations to consider new measures that would ensure, in line with their own regulations, the recruitment of women in leadership positions at local, national, and international levels'. European surveys were carried out in 1980 and 1989, the last one aimed at assessing the impact of the

Dublin recommendations. In the report where the results of this study were presented, Delforge (1989) stated that:

> most countries have a legal framework that provides for equal opportunities for men and women. Despite the legal framework, however, discrimination still exists at all levels and in particular in matters of sport (discriminating regulations applied by sports bodies, especially in certain disciplines; access to sports facilities, awkward opening and closing times, quality of the equipment; influence of certain cultural values, etc.).

Another conclusion was that the proportion of women in leadership positions seemed to be increasing in most countries, although fair representation was still a long way off. However, the proportion of women in leadership positions tended to increase as the focus shifted from the national to the regional and local levels, although the highest positions were generally occupied by men whatever the level (Delforge, 1989).

Some months after the meeting in the UK, another European sports body, the European Sports Conference, held its ninth conference in Bulgaria. Here a working group on the role of women in sport was set up. The overall aim proposed by the working group 2 years later was 'to increase the involvement of women in sport at all levels and in all functions and roles'. To fulfil this aim, three goals were suggested. One of them concerns the theme of this chapter: 'To increase the number of women coaches and women in advisory, decision making and administrative bodies at all levels' (Fasting, 1993). Twenty European countries participated in a monitoring study in 1993 and the gender representation on the executive boards was surveyed. The results demonstrated great variations inside Europe. Three countries did not have any female members in their highest decision-making organization; in others, the female representation was about 45%. However, the overall picture was that women seemed to be proportionally underrepresented on the executive boards (Fasting, 1993). Two years later a similar question was posed in another European survey. Countries were asked about the number of female board members in five significant sports federations (European handball, swimming, soccer, gymnastics and tennis). The proportion of countries that had female board members was 28% for gymnastics, 12% for swimming, 9% for European handball, 8% for tennis and only 3% for soccer. Three countries, Norway, Romania and Sweden, had female members on all the executive boards of these five sports federations (Fasting, 1995). These results confirm that even sports like gymnastics, which is strongly dominated by female members, are led or ruled by men.

Statistics available from different countries indicate large variations in the number of women in sports governing bodies at both regional and national levels. In addition there is reason to believe that these also vary according to the sport. Many of the statistics are a few years old and therefore not presented here, because there is reason to believe that they have changed. Women are underrepresented on sports governing bodies both internationally and nationally. The Scandinavian countries seem to be leading other nations in the inclusion of women, for example in Norway female representation on the executive boards of the sport districts (regional level) is more than 40% (Fasting, 1996).

Why are there so few women in sports governing bodies?

According to Kvande (1995), the development of gender research is mirrored by research about gender and organization, which started in the mid 1980s and can be divided into three phases, which she terms women's voice, women's experience and the postfeminist phase. In the first phase, which may be characterized as gender neutral, it is taken for granted that women are equal to men or like men. In the second phase, the differences between women and men are examined in detail. Women are looked upon as a resource. The male norms are criticized. Discussion focuses on female leadership and that females may be better leaders than men due to different value orientations. This perspective is criticized in the third phase because it is said to lead to essentialism, i.e. gender (sociology) became as determinant as sex (biology). The focus now is on the meaning of gender in different connections.

We now talk about many different forms of masculinity and femininity and about gender as a perspective, as a fundamental analytical category. How gender is constructed and reconstructed in the relationship between women and men becomes central. With such a perspective, how organizations construct gender and how the gender relations construct an organization become important. For example, newer research focuses on how men in an organization are often preoccupied with constructing and maintaining different forms of masculinity. The research on sports organizations, presented in the following paragraphs, to a certain extent reflects these phases, although most of the organizations can be characterized as belonging to the second phase or between the second and third phases.

Lane (1980) states that job descriptions are seldom found in sports organizations and that most organizations comprise an informal system of relationships that have their origins and present functions in the male culture and the male experience. The males within these informal systems understand and support one another and the structure: they make up the 'old-boy' network. The different aspirations and experiences that women and men have as a result of different socialization may lead to different ways of responding to typical sports management situations. This may also make it difficult for women to accept and influence the informal 'male' system. Lane (1980) also writes that the image of the female future often is sexual and sexually linked, which again is due to the fact that the people in positions of power are males. She says that:

> contrary to the stereotyped notion, females do compete, although the conditions of our culture are such that they compete in different ways, for different ends, and with different standards from the males.

According to Lane, an uneven gender distribu-

tion in an organization can also lead to women's feelings of social isolation, heightened visibility, mistaken identity and pressures to adopt stereotyped roles. This again may lead to confusion and depression.

In a study from the UK (White & Brackenridge, 1985), the low number of females in British sport is explained by some of the same factors. These authors mentioned particularly: (i) the inappropriateness of the male model of sport; (ii) women's lack of access to political systems; and (iii) recruitment mechanisms that operate in sports organizations. Raivio (1987) interviewed Finnish women in decision-making positions in sport. These women believed that there were mainly two reasons for the lack of women in these positions: (i) that men were afraid to place an equally, or more, competent woman in a leadership position; and (ii) that women did not give support to other women in elections. The respondents also thought that the sports organizations were very bureaucratic, so that they might not see their ideas carried out. Acosta and Carpenter (1985) surveyed both women and men on why there were so few women in athletic administration. The answers reflected the gender differences presented earlier. The women stressed, in order of importance: (i) perpetuation of the 'old-boy' network; (ii) weakness of the 'old-girl' network; (iii) moderate discrimination against women; and (iv) a lack of qualified women. The corresponding answers from the men were: (i) lack of qualified women; (ii) women's unwillingness to travel; (iii) women's failure to apply for openings; and (iv) family responsibilities. Bohlig (1988) discusses the fact that in the USA women disappeared from athletic administration. She suggests four main reasons: (i) the stereotypes of women in leadership roles; (ii) careers and conflicts; (iii) Title IX; and (iv) the merging of the AIAW and NCAA.

In 1985 the Norwegian Confederation of Sport established a Central Women's Committee. The work of this committee is guided by the knowledge gained from the study of gender, i.e. that women and men are different and that women have a lot to contribute to sport. Fasting and

Skou (1994) studied 43 heads of women's committees in the Norwegian Confederation of Sport and found that the most important predictors for success were:

• the knowledge and the personal characteristics of the chair of the women's committee;
• how the work was formally based and structured in the sport organization;
• the level of consciousness and the common understanding in the sport organization.

Each of these factors was also influenced by the others. The barriers for success were the opposite of those listed above:

• lack of roots in the organization: the board, the administration and the network;
• lack of common understanding concerning the work of women and sport;
• low consciousness about the female and male culture among the female chairs;
• female chairs with an unsuitable personality.

Based on this study the following conclusions were drawn. It seems to be important that someone in the organization, either an individual or a committee, has to have the responsibility for developing women-related work. This could be a man, but he needs to have knowledge about gender issues and about the difference between female and male cultures. For example, he should know that the increasing degree of professionalism, specialization and rationalization are trends that are antagonistic to traditional women's values and therefore may discourage women from taking on positions of leadership. He should also take into account that more and more women are working full-time. Also it is women who still have the main responsibility for housework and the care of children and elderly parents, which leaves them with very little time of their own. Thus the task of encouraging women to take on leadership positions has to be rooted in the organization, both formally and economically. Consciousness-raising for both female and male sports leaders seems to be important. The authors also mentioned that one cannot put into practice a plan of action to try to increase female leadership in sports without resources, both time and money. They also

stressed that the work itself has to be taken seriously and must be given status and power. This was the reason that the chair of the 'women's committee' also needed to be a member of the executive board or another decision-making body. This is exactly what the IOC has done; the chair of the Committee for Women and Sport is Anita de Franz, the only woman on the Executive Board of the IOC.

In a Canadian study (Whitson & MacIntosh, 1989) 56 senior officers in six national sports organizations were interviewed, of whom one-third were women. According to the investigators, most of the officers saw the promotion of women as a low-priority issue, even a non-issue. Having few women or no women in decision-making sports organizations was not regarded as a problem. 'Family responsibilities' was mentioned as the reason for the lack of women. As Whitson and MacIntosh state:

> The problems lay not in the practice or prejudices of the National Sports Organization, but rather with individual women, and/or with structural features of Canadian (family) life, which it was not a sport organization's task to address.

The authors focused on gender relations and the gender power structure in discussing these results. They refer to Deem (1987) who had shown that much of men's leisure is facilitated by women's services, while men affect women's leisure opportunities in their roles as policy-makers and executives.

Hall et al. (1989) focused on the processes and dynamics that structure gender in organizations. Their purpose was 'to understand and explain how organizational elites (males) work to recreate themselves in order to retain their power, and how women collude in this process'. The methods used in this study were interviews with 70 key persons in five different sports plus an analysis of documents. As in the study by Whitson and MacIntosh (1989), one of the findings was that members did not believe the organization itself was to blame for the low percentages of females. The reasons were either personal deficiencies, such as women's lack of motivation, or social factors, such as women's family situations. The solution was seen to lie not with the organization but with either society or the women themselves. This was also the opinion of many of those female officers who participated in the study. They had accepted the organizational male culture and did not want to be identified with women's issues.

In trying to understand this gender structure of sports organizations and how it could be changed in a way that could benefit the women in them, Hall *et al.* (1989) reviewed different organizational theories and feminist perspectives on organizational theory. They state that it is not enough to get more women into the organization if women are merely imitations of men. Such thinking is based on an equity model (Adler, 1986), which implies that women's and men's contributions to an organization will be identical. This model emphasizes access to management positions, with women then assimilating male norms. Progress is measured by counting the number of women and men at each hierarchical level in the organization, just as is often done in sport.

Women who enter this world must learn to play the game, which they often do. They must learn the language, symbols, myths, beliefs and values of the sporting culture (Fasting, 1994). Hall *et al.* (1989) say that the complementary model, also described by Adler (1986), recognizes, assesses and values the differing contributions that both sexes bring to the organization. Such a model can therefore have an element of change in it. In discussing feminist perspectives on organizations, the authors demonstrate how organizations construct sexuality with particular reference to the double standard that exists in relation to lesbians. Since this double standard is a mixture of the visible, the unspoken and the elusive, it also demonstrates how sexuality constructs organizations. The gender structure of organizations is characterized by power relations, which subject and control sexuality in different ways. Hall *et al.* conclude that fundamental change would be more likely if structural changes occur so that the powerful élite cannot

reproduce itself. According to the authors, more research is needed. This should focus on the intermingling of power, sexuality and structure before effective attempts for change can be suggested.

Being an officer in a sports governing body requires a heavy investment of time and energy plus a flexible home and work life. The structure of the sports organizations themselves and the way they are organized and operate are often not addressed. However, this was looked at in a Norwegian study among female coaches and administrators in the Norwegian Volleyball Federation (Hovden *et al.*, 1993). All female members of the executive board of the federation from 1982 to 1990 were surveyed plus female coaches, a total of 54 women; of these 20 were also interviewed in depth. The following factors seemed to be important in relation to recruitment and dropout among female executives and coaches in Norwegian volleyball. First, the respondents felt that they were given little support and little respect for their own resources. In addition they thought that they did not have the chance to define their own frames of action. Second, since women often had less free time than men, there were also gender differences in relation to how women and men wanted to use their free time. The women felt that their life situation was difficult to discuss within the organization. It was looked upon as something private. The organization did not take into account what is meant by gender or that women and men do not have the same starting point.

Many of the participants in this study wanted to use their knowledge and resources for the good of volleyball, but not at any cost. In spite of the fact that they were highly educated women with good resources, they found that the demands of the federation and the way the work was structured and organized made it impossible for them to work in their beloved sport. Three main reasons for this were mentioned: (i) most of them wanted to have a family and give priority to their families; (ii) they wanted to have time for friends and other types of leisure time activities; and (iii) the male-dominated culture restricted their frame of action. The respondents wished that women could have more opportunities to influence the direction of the work of the sports organization. They also believed that the coaching, as well as the executive roles, had to be practised in a less authoritarian way. A stronger female network and a stronger gender integrated network were high on the women's list of priorities. Lastly, they thought it was important to change both the league system and the activity profile of their sport, so that fewer weekends were occupied and less time was used for travelling. They also felt that the social values of the sport had to be upgraded (Hovden *et al.*, 1993).

Dorfinger and Moström (1995) surveyed 56 presidents in different sports federations in Sweden. The results showed that it was important to include more women in sports governing bodies, partly because more women would be recruited to sports practice but also because of the complementary model just mentioned. Cederberg and Olofsson (1996) comment that, in spite of this, women seem not to be recruited, which may be due to the fact that prejudice and discrimination are built into the sports system. Another study among Swedish female sports executives showed that 80% thought that women's questions had low status in the organization; 75% had also experienced that many people seemed to think it was not important to have equal gender representation, as found in the studies from Canada. The same proportion of the women thought that equity would not develop naturally by itself, but that it was necessary to have increased consciousness about the problems and a more active political approach.

In their summary of why there are so few women at the top of organizations in general, Cederberg and Olofsson (1996) stated that the construction of the gender system leads to a devaluation of women's work and an increase in the value of men's work. The structure does not often enough take into account the life situation of women, which in practice may be viewed as

an inherent type of discrimination. The studies reviewed in their survey showed that the way men experience women's situations is different to the way women describe their experiences themselves. Men believe that women are underrepresented in sports governing bodies because they do not dare, or want, to be involved, i.e. the explanation reflects the individual level. The women's explanation reflects the organizational level: they seem to focus on the structure of the organization and believe that their competence is invisible; they also lack support and encouragement. This is also in accordance with the specific studies on sports organizations presented earlier in this chapter.

Conclusion

It is essential to focus on why more women are needed in international and national sports governing bodies. First, it can be regarded as a matter of equality. Equality can be defined in different ways and I have found the following definition, taken from the Swedish Sports Confederation (1990), useful:

> Equality means that women and men have the same rights, obligations and opportunities in all the main fields of life; women and men share power, influence and responsibility in all sectors of the community.

The data presented in this chapter have shown that unfortunately this is not the case for sport. There are three arguments why it is important to change this situation.

1 Women account for more than half the population. They are underrepresented in sports organizations not only in membership but also in relation to other roles such as leadership, coaching, management and referees. Equality in decision-making assemblies is therefore a matter of democracy.

2 Women and men have different knowledge and expertise. Therefore it is important that the views of both groups are considered.

3 Women and men have different values and different interests. Therefore increased representa-

tion of women can lead to new perspectives on many issues.

In conclusion, sports organizations need the participation of women more than the women need sports organizations. The solution to recruiting more women into the leadership of sports organizations, and keeping them, is difficult. The results of the studies presented in this chapter indicate that changes in the sports organizations themselves are necessary. Emphasizing women's lives, experiences and values in the further development of sport may be one way. This can most easily be done by women themselves just because they are women. To be certain that many more women can gain access to leadership roles in practice, more knowledge, i.e. research, is needed. This should focus on the interrelationship between power, sexuality and the structure of sports governing bodies and/ or how sports organizations construct gender and how gender relations construct the sports organizations.

References

Acosta, R.V. & Carpenter, L.J. (1985) Status of women in athletics: changes and cases. *Journal of Physical Education, Recreation and Dance* **56**, 35–37.

Adler, N.J. (1986) Women in management worldwide. *International Studies of Management and Organization* **16**, 3–32.

Beamish, R. (1985) Sport executives and voluntary associations: a review of the literature and introduction to some theoretical issues. *Sociology of Sport Journal* **2**, 218–232.

Berlioux, M. (1981) Women in the promotion and administration of sport. *Federation International Education Physique Bulletin* **51**, 22–27.

Bohlig, M. (1988) Women coaches and administrators: an endangered species. *Scholastic Coach* **57**, 89–92.

Cederberg, I. & Olofsson, E. (1996) *En katt bland hermeliner: forskningsöversikt om kvinnor och ledarskap*. Umeå Universitetet, Pedagogiska Institutionen, Umeå.

Davenport, J. (1988) The role of women in the IOC and the IOA. *Journal of Physical Education, Recreation and Dance* **59**, 42–45.

Deem, R. (1987) The politics of women's leisure. *Sociological Review Monograph* **33**, 210–228.

Delforge, M. (1989) Appendix. In *Women and Sport: Taking the Lead. Synoptic Report of the National Contri-*butions by Clearing House. Proceedings from European Seminar, Bisham Abbey National Sport Center, 11–14 September. Sports Council, UK.

Dorfinger, K. & Moström, K. (1995) *Tiden hjälper til: men räcker inte! Om jämställdhet inom idrotten*. Jämställdhetsutvickling AB, Stockholm.

Dyer, K.F. (1982) *Catching up the Men. Women in Sport*. Junction Books, London.

Fasting, K. (1993) *Women and Sport. Monitoring Progress Towards Equality. A European Survey*. Norwegian Confederation of Sports, Oslo.

Fasting, K. (1994) *Sport Bodies in the 'New' Europe: Progress Towards Equality?* Norwegian Confederation of Sports/Norwegian University of Sport and Physical Education, Oslo.

Fasting, K. (1995) *European Women in Sport*. Swedish Sports Confederation, Stockholm.

Fasting, K. (1996) *Hvor går kvinneidretten?* Norges Idrettsforbund, Oslo.

Fasting, K. & Skou, G. (1994) *Developing Equity for Women in the Norwegian Confederation of Sports*. Norwegian Confederation of Sports/Norwegian University of Sport and Physical Education, Oslo.

Hall, M.A., Cullen, D. & Slack, T. (1989) Organizational elites recreating themselves: the gender structure of national sport organizations. *Quest* **41**, 28–45.

Hovden, J., Solheim, L.J. & Andreassen, S. (1993) *Er det prisen verdt? En studie av kvinnelege trenarar og tillitsvalde sine erfaringar med arbeid i Norges Volleyballforbund*. Norges Idrettsforbund, Oslo.

Hult, J.S. (1989) Women's struggle for governance in U.S. amateur athletics. *International Review for the Sociology of Sport* **24**, 249–261.

International Olympic Committee (1994) *International Olympic Congress Report*, pp. 415–419. International Olympic Committee, Lausanne.

Kvande, E. (1995) Forståelser av kjønn og organisasjon. *Sosiologisk Tidsskrift* **4**, 285–300.

Lane, K. (1980) Women as sport administrators. In S. Fraser (ed.) *The Female Athlete*, pp. 133–139. Institute for Human Performance, Burnaby, British Columbia.

Raivio, M. (1987) The life path and career of the women in leading positions in Finnish sport organizations. In J.A. Mangan & R.B. Small (eds) *Sport, Culture, Society: International Historical and Sociological Perspectives*, pp. 270–276. E. & F.N. Spon, London.

Swedish Sports Confederation (1990) *A Plan for Equality between Women and Men in Sport in the 1990s*. Swedish Sports Confederation, Stockholm.

Theberge, N. (1984) Some evidence on the existence of a sexual double standard in mobility to leadership positions in sport. *International Review for the Sociology of Sport* **19**, 169–196.

White, A. & Brackenridge, C. (1985) Who rules sport?

Gender division in the power structure of British sports organisations from 1960. *International Review for the Sociology of Sport* **20**, 95–107.

Whitson, D. & MacIntosh, D. (1989) Gender and power: explanations of gender inequalities in Canadian national sport organisations. *International Review for the Sociology of Sport* **24**, 137–150.

Women and Sport Bulletin (1999) *News about the Olympic Movement*. International Olympic Committee, Lausanne.

PART 8

SPORT-SPECIFIC INJURIES: PREVENTION AND TREATMENT

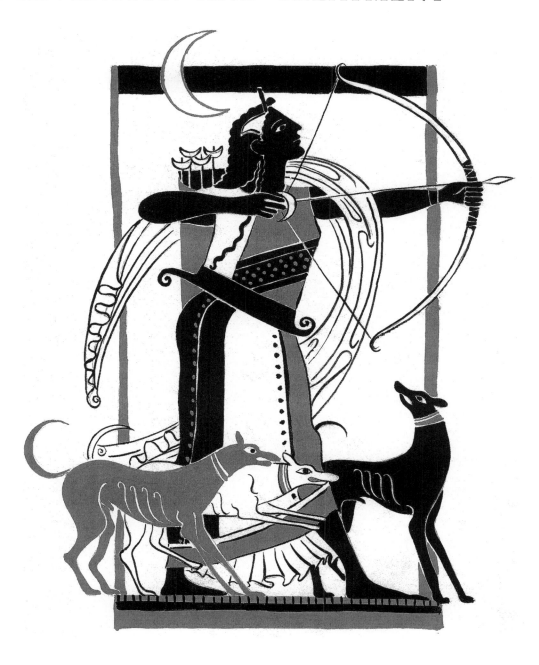

Chapter 31

Swimming

NAAMA CONSTANTINI AND MAYA CALE'-BENZOOR

Introduction

Swimming, both recreational and competitive, is one of the most popular sports and the number of females participating is continually increasing. In the 1996 Olympics Games in Atlanta, 512 females competed in the various swimming events. Female swimmers train and compete from a very young age until late adulthood as master swimmers. They participate in swimming events that previously were only performed by males, such as the 4×200m relay or the Ironman triathlon. It is not uncommon to see girls and young women training together with their male counterparts and reaching similar exercise volumes and intensities. In the past, female swimmers were believed to reach their peak performance below the age of 20 and used to be the youngest contestants in the Olympic Games except for gymnasts (Hirata, 1979). In recent years this has changed and one can find many successful female swimmers over 25 years of age. In fact, the average age of female swimmers in Atlanta was 23, almost identical to the men's average of 23.4 years.

As a training modality, swimming is beneficial for all the population, including those with various health problems such as asthma, obesity and various physical and mental handicaps. A further advantage of swimming is that injury or illness are relatively uncommon. In this chapter we discuss special issues concerning the female swimmer: physiological, medical and musculoskeletal. Emphasis is placed on aspects unique to female swimmers, although other medical aspects of swimming are discussed.

Physiological aspects

Physical characteristics

The typical female swimmer is taller and somewhat heavier than the average female. In a review on the growth and maturation of athletes, Malina (1994a) concluded that the mean stature of female swimmers from various parts of the world was generally above the 50th percentile. Nationally selected swimmers in the USA had statures at or just below the 90th percentile, while the weights of these swimmers were at or above the 50th percentile (Malina, 1994a). In the last Olympic Games in Atlanta, the average height of the female swimmers was 1.71 m and the average weight was 59 kg.

In most sports a lean body is considered an advantage as it is quicker and generally performs better than a body with a higher proportion of fat. This does not hold true for swimming, where fat provides buoyancy, thereby reducing the energy cost of staying on the surface of the water. On the other hand, excess fat can alter the body contour and increase drag. The ideal percentage of body fat for the best performance has not been established for swimmers. The percentage of body fat reported for both age-group and mature female swimmers is between 12% and 20% (Malina *et al.*, 1982a; Hergenroeder & Klish, 1990; Sinning, 1996).

Most studies on age-group female swimmers (10–17 years) suggest that skeletal age is average or advanced relative to chronological age. At an early age, female swimmers with advanced skeletal age tend to be more successful. Coaches should thus be cautious when predicting future success, since achievements of early mature females may be only temporary.

Strength

Muscular strength appears to be the second most important determinant after skill for success in competitive swimming (Costill *et al.*, 1992). Generally, males are much stronger than females; however, when expressing strength relative to lean body mass, it is interesting to note that female swimmers have similar leg strength but markedly lower arm strength compared with males (Costill *et al.*, 1992; Magnusson *et al.*, 1995). In both genders trunk extension is significantly stronger than trunk flexion, but women test significantly weaker than men in both trunk extension and flexion (Magnusson *et al.*, 1995). Swimming is a symmetrical sport, and indeed there is no significant side-to-side difference in either shoulder or thigh strength among swimmers (Magnusson *et al.*, 1995).

Anaerobic power

There is a very strong correlation between the results of anaerobic tests (especially arm tests) and swimming performance (Inbar & Bar-Or, 1977; Hawley & Williams, 1991; Hawley *et al.*, 1992; Lowensteyn *et al.*, 1992). Peak power and mean power in the Wingate anaerobic test of both arms and legs are significantly higher in male compared with female swimmers. However, when adjusted for lean body mass, Constantini and Cale-Benzoor (unpublished observations) found that leg power was greater among the female masters swimmers compared with their male counterparts. In the same study, female arm–leg anaerobic power ratios were about 55% compared with 80% in the males. Thus, it is not surprising that the difference in swimming time between females and males is generally greater when using the arms only (i.e. pulling) compared with full stroke and smaller when kicking only.

Sexual development

Data collected between the 1950s and 1970s on the age of menarche in swimmers suggested a similar (Malina, 1983) or even earlier (Astrand *et al.*, 1963) mean age of menarche compared with that of non-athletes. However, later surveys revealed a significantly later age of menarche in swimmers compared with their sedentary counterparts (Stager *et al.*, 1984; Stager & Hatler, 1988; Constantini & Warren, 1995) (Table 31.1). Malina (1994a) attributed this finding to the shift in the age of female swimmers. In earlier years female swimmers retired by 16–17 years of age, whereas nowadays they continue to train and compete into their twenties. This provides an opportunity for late-maturing swimmers, who previously retired at an early age due to relatively low success, to catch up with their early-maturing peers and to persist in the sport at an older age.

Whether early intensive training delays men-

Table 31.1 Mean age at menarche in swimmers (mean ± SD)

Reference	Swimmers (*n*)	Controls (*n*)
Constantini & Warren (1995)	13.8 ± 0.2 (SE) (69)	13.0 ± 0.1 (SE) (279)
Frisch *et al.* (1981)	13.9 (21)	12.7 (10)
Malina (1991)	14.4 ± 1.6 (43)	13.0 ± 1.4 (123)
Stager *et al.* (1984)	13.4 ± 1.4 (287)	13.0 ± 1.6 (495)
Stager & Hatler (1988)	14.3 ± 1.5 (140)	12.9 ± 1.3 (113)

arche or whether the later onset of menarche in swimmers is due to genetic factors combined with preselection is a matter of controversy (Malina, 1994b). Two studies have demonstrated that swimming training prior to menarche correlates with the age of menarche and that training delays menarche (Frisch *et al.*, 1981; Stager & Hatler, 1988). However, these observations have been challenged and may turn out to be an analytical artefact (Stager *et al.*, 1990). As in non-athletes, a high correlation ($r=0.69$) exists between age at menarche of swimmers and that of their mothers (Constantini, 1985). However, genetics is probably not the only explanation. Swimmers are older at menarche than their sisters, whereas age of menarche is similar between the control non-athletes and their sisters (Stager & Hatler, 1988).

Medical problems

Reproductive system dysfunction

The prevalence of short luteal phase and anovulation (Bonen *et al.*, 1981), oligomenorrhoea and secondary amenorrhoea (Frisch *et al.*, 1981; Sanborn *et al.*, 1982; Russell *et al.*, 1984; Fauno *et al.*, 1991) in female swimmers is about 12–40%. This is lower than the prevalence of menstrual abnormalities in ballet dancers and long-distance runners (Constantini & Warren, 1994) but significantly higher than the 5% prevalence in the non-athletic population.

In sporting disciplines that require low body weight, negative energy balance is thought to be the major cause of menstrual abnormalities and the hormonal profile shows a hypothalamic type of amenorrhoea, i.e. impaired gonadotrophin-releasing hormone secretion, altered luteinizing hormone (LH) pulsatility and low levels of gonadotrophins and oestradiol (Keizer & Rogol, 1990; Theintz, 1994). However, the case of swimmers may be different from that of ballet dancers or long-distance-runners. Swimmers are typically heavier, have a higher percentage of body fat (Malina *et al.*, 1982b; Brooks-Gunn *et al.*, 1988; Hergenroeder & Klish, 1990; Malina, 1994a) and

dieting and eating disorders are less common (Rosen *et al.*, 1986; Brooks-Gunn *et al.*, 1988; Barr, 1991; Sundgot-Borgen, 1993). Thus, it is not surprising that most studies of swimmers with either regular or irregular menses have described a different hormonal pattern: normal to high LH levels, elevated LH:FSH (follicle-stimulating hormone) ratio, normal to high oestradiol levels and increased androgen levels compared with controls (Constantini & Warren, 1995; Nichols *et al.*, 1995). It has therefore been suggested that swimmers exhibit a distinct type of menstrual dysfunction (Constantini, 1994) (Fig. 31.1), in which reproductive dysfunction is associated not with hypogonadotrophic hypo-oestrogenism but rather with mild hyperandrogenism.

Whether this specific hormonal profile (i.e. higher levels of androgens and an elevated LH:FSH ratio) is secondary to activation of the adrenal axis as a result of intensive training in the absence of energy deficit or whether it is 'primary' (genetic factors, such as polycystic ovary syndrome, precocious adrenarche, late onset of congenital adrenal hyperplasia) is unknown. Further research is needed, including follow-up studies on hormonal levels after the cessation of competitive swimming. Ultrasonic examination of the ovaries is also indicated to look for signs of polycystic ovary syndrome.

High levels of androgens can be advantageous for swimmers as they affect muscle mass positively. Since power is a major determinant in swimming performance, girls with 'naturally' elevated levels of androgens may be self-selected for this sport (Constantini & Warren, 1995). Indeed, this profile has also been demonstrated in female athletes who participate in other sports that require muscle power (Cumming *et al.*, 1987).

Bone mass

The main factor responsible for osteoporosis is reduced bone mass. The amount of bone mass is determined by the amount of bone acquired during puberty and by the rate of bone loss. Peak bone mass is determined by four major factors:

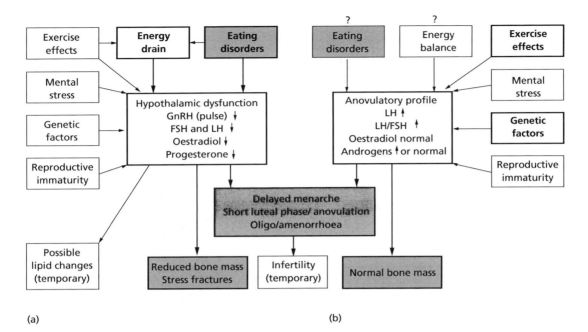

(a)   (b)

Fig. 31.1 Schematic illustration of the authors' hypothesis for the two different types of athletic menstrual dysfunction. (a) The more frequently seen 'hypothalamic amenorrhoea', which occurs in sports demanding very low body weight (e.g. dancing, long-distance running) and may result in skeletal problems secondary to hypo-oestrogenism. (b) An anovulatory hormonal profile with normal oestrogen levels in swimmers and possibly in other sports where thinness is not required. FSH, follicle-stimulating hormone; GnRH, gonadotrophin-releasing hormone; LH, luteinizing hormone; ↑, increased; ↓, decreased.

genetics, nutrition, exercise and hormonal milieu.

Physical activity increases bone mass through strain imposed on the skeleton by gravity, mechanical loading and muscle contraction. It has been claimed that since swimming is a non-weight-bearing exercise and there is no mechanical loading on the bones, bone mineral density (BMD) in swimmers is lower than that in athletes involved in high-impact, weight-bearing sports. Indeed, in several cross-sectional studies that compared BMD among different groups of athletes, female swimmers were found to have lower bone mass compared with other athletes (Heinrich *et al.*, 1990; Risser *et al.*, 1990; Lee *et al.*, 1995; Cassell *et al.*, 1996). On the other hand, higher BMD can be expected in swimmers compared with non-athletes because muscle contrac-

tion by itself affects bone mass positively (Marcus *et al.*, 1992) and because swimmers often use modalities such as zoomers and hand-paddles in their water workouts in order to increase workload on the muscles. In addition, competitive female swimmers spend many hours in the fitness room engaging in weight training.

BMD in female swimmers and non-athletes has been measured in several studies that have yielded contradictory results. Some found reduced lumbar bone density in swimmers compared with controls (Jacobson *et al.*, 1984; Risser *et al.*, 1990; Nichols *et al.*, 1995), while others found either similar (Lee *et al.*, 1995; Cassell *et al.*, 1996) or even higher (Heinrich *et al.*, 1990) densities in swimmers vs. sedentary controls. These different results are most probably due to methodological difficulties, such as small samples and different ages, training history, measurement site and measurement techniques.

Female swimmers have a later age of menarche and a higher prevalence of menstrual irregularities compared with non-athletes, but they do not suffer from low levels of oestrogens. However, high oestradiol levels have been found in young swimmers (Constantini & Warren, 1995) and androgens, which affect bone mass positively, were consistently higher in several studies. Other risk factors for reduced bone mass in dancers and long-distance runners are less prevalent among swimmers, such as low body weight, low body fat, eating disorders, insufficient caloric intake and inadequate calcium intake. Our hypothesis is that swimmers with menstrual dysfunction will not suffer from osteopenia compared with their eumenorrhoeic peers (Fig. 31.1), but this issue should be further investigated.

Swimmer's ear

OTITIS EXTERNA

The term 'swimmer's ear' refers to both acute and chronic otitis externa, which is the most common ear problem in swimmers. The cerumen (wax) that normally lubricates the external ear and prevents infection is washed away by pool water, leading to drying and cracking of the skin of the canal. In addition, swimmers often dry and 'clean'/scratch their ears, causing further local trauma. This, in conjunction with the high temperature and humid environment in the external ear canal, facilitates the invasion of endogenous or exogenous organisms.

The most common infecting organisms are *Pseudomonas aeruginosa* and fungi (Marcy, 1985). The acute infection is characterized by severe deep pain often accompanied, or preceded, by itching (especially if associated with otomycosis). There is redness, swelling and tenderness of the canal and occasionally a variable amount of discharge and lymphadenopathy. Therapy includes otic solutions and oral antimicrobial therapy in cases of severe infection.

Prevention of recurrent otitis externa includes: (i) use of water repellent prior to swimming practices; (ii) avoidance of cotton swabs for drying or cleaning since they remove the wax and can scratch the ear; (iii) drying of the canal after exposure to water with acidifying ear-drops; and (iv) use of ear-plugs while swimming if the above measures are unsuccessful.

OTITIS MEDIA

In young swimmers, middle ear infections may be a problem. Acute otitis media starts suddenly and is associated with severe pain, and often fever and hearing loss. The tympanic membrane bulges, obscuring its normal landmarks; perforation and otorrhoea may occur. The common causes are *Streptococcus pneumoniae*, *Haemophilus influenzae* and *Branhamella catarrhalis*. Treatment includes analgesics, decongestants and appropriate antibiotics. Swimming is prohibited until the acute symptoms have subsided. If the tympanic membrane ruptures, water must be kept out of the ear until the drum has healed. If healing does not occur or if tubes are inserted in cases of chronic serous otitis media, the swimmer can continue to train and compete with ear-plugs.

EXOSTOSIS

Prolonged exposure to water may cause a bony growth in the external ear called exostosis. If this becomes large it may cause ear infection by trapping water or even block the canal. Surgery is required in this case.

Nasal and sinus problems

Swimmers may suffer from vasomotor reaction of the nasal mucosa in response to stimuli such as chlorine in the pool water, bacterial pathogens or allergens in the swimming area. Sinusitis is another potential problem, especially in swimmers with pre-existing abnormalities of nasal and sinus anatomy. Nasal plugs are advised in these cases.

Eye problems

Prolonged exposure to chlorinated water can cause conjunctivitis, keratitis or corneal oedema. The eye is red and the swimmer will complain of the sensation of a foreign body in the eye as well as pain. The eye should be irrigated with ophthalmic solution. Use of swim goggles can efficiently prevent these problems. Due to chlorination of pools and use of goggles, infectious conjunctivitis, either viral or bacterial, is very rare.

Asthma

Asthma is a disease characterized by an increased responsiveness of the bronchial tree to a variety of stimuli, such as environmental irritants and allergens, resulting in widespread narrowing of the airways and decreased expiratory flow rate. With increased obstruction, there is decreased vital capacity, increased effort of breathing and mismatch of ventilation and perfusion leading to hypoxaemia and hypercarbia. In about 90% of individuals with asthma and in 35–40% of the allergic non-asthmatic population, exercise can induce bronchospasm, a phenomenon called exercise-induced asthma (EIA) (Virant, 1992). Symptoms include wheezing, chest tightness, dizziness or cough during or after exercise. A 15% decrease in peak expiratory flow rate or forced expiratory volume in 1 s during the period after exercise is diagnostic of EIA.

Swimming seems to induce less bronchoconstriction compared with land activities. The low asthmogenicity of swimming is partly explained by the high humidity of the inspired air. Other mechanisms for this protective effect have been thoroughly reviewed by Bar-Or and Inbar (1992). Whether swim training reduces the frequency and severity of EIA is not yet clear and should be further investigated. Due to the low asthmogenicity of swimming, it has long been consid-

ered a suitable sport for patients with asthma. A swim-training programme has been shown to lessen the clinical severity of asthma (Huang et al., 1989). It is also one of the sports in which these athletes can excel and even reach the top level. In a survey of 738 competitive swimmers, 13.4% reported asthma and of these 21% swam at international level (Potts, 1996).

Swimmers with clinically significant EIA should use aerosol β-adrenergic agents 15 min before exercise. Significant bronchodilatation occurs within 1 min of inhalation and continues for up to 5–6 hours. Cromolyn sodium is also effective; although it does not cause bronchodilatation, it blocks both early and late EIA and is virtually without side-effects. Another effective agent is theophylline 1–2 hours before exercise.

Other respiratory problems

Chlorine, which is often used in pool water, can cause several respiratory problems, such as sneezing, difficulty with breathing, coughing, sore throat, wheezing, chest tightness and chest congestion (Potts, 1996). The combination of chlorine gas with the ammonia and urea that comes from the sweat and urine of swimming-pool users creates inorganic compounds, which further react with amino acids to form organic molecules. These organic compounds are known to cause irritation of the respiratory tract, as well as of the eyes, skin and mucous membranes. This problem becomes worse in the winter when air is recirculated, increasing the concentration of the aforementioned factors (Bar-Or & Inbar, 1992). The problem can be minimized if fresh air is continually supplied to the indoor pool environment. Use of alternative methods of water disinfection can also reduce the concentration of the chemical irritants.

Dermatological problems

SKIN

Cutaneous problems related to swimming are uncommon and when they occur are usually relatively minor. The cause in freshwater lakes or salty sea water is usually one of various organisms, which are not discussed here. In pools they are caused mainly by chemicals that can irritate the skin. Prolonged exposure can dry the skin or cause contact urticaria.

HAIR

Prolonged contact with chlorinated water causes bleaching of the hair. This occurs especially in the summer months due to increased exposure to sunlight. Sometimes the hair of blond swimmers can become greenish due to the copper-based algicides used in swimming pools (Lampe et al., 1977).

TEETH

Prolonged contact with swimming pool water, as well as the mixture of oral flora with water, may cause yellowish-brown or dark stains on swimmers' teeth (Rose & Carey, 1995). Swimmers' calculus can be removed by routine professional dental prophylaxis (scaling and polishing).

Musculoskeletal profile characteristics

From a musculoskeletal perspective, swimming presents a number of challenges to the female swimmer. It is estimated that, on average, the competitive swimmer trains 10–11 months each year and practises 5–7 days a week, often twice daily. Swimmers may cover 8–20 km daily depending on their specialty. Richardson et al. (1980) estimated that the male swimmer takes an average of 15 strokes per 25-m lap and calculated that each shoulder undergoes about 9900 strokes per week. Since women generally have shorter limbs relative to their body length (Arendt, 1994) and are not as strong, the female swimmer might require 25 strokes to cover the same lap, thus bringing the total number of arm strokes to 16 500 per week. In addition, females are more prone to joint hyperlaxity than males and joint laxity is often associated with joint pain (Warner et al., 1990). For example, Maffuli et al. (1994)

found a strong correlation between flexibility and female gender in young swimmers.

External and internal rotation strength ratios in female swimmers were found to be lower than those in controls, being 0.6 and 0.8 respectively (Reid, 1987; Beach et al., 1992; McMaster & Troup, 1993; Fowler, 1995; Magnusson et al., 1995). The adduction–abduction ratio of the female swimmers was significantly higher than that in normal controls and higher than that reported for normals by Shklar and Dvir (1993). These torque shifts may represent a sport-specific adaptation of swimming. Assessing joint range of motion, Magnusson et al. (1995) reported external rotation values of about 116° in female swimmers, well above the standard for non-athletes. Internal rotation was also high. Fowler (1995) reported a similar incidence of posterior translation of the humerus in swimmers vs. controls and concluded that swimming does not predispose an athlete to increased posterior laxity. On the other hand, posterior and anterior excessive tightness should be considered as predisposing factors for shoulder pain. The significance and possible applications of these findings are unclear and further research is needed.

Common orthopaedic problems

Shoulder pain

The greatest orthopaedic problem that afflicts competitive swimmers is the so-called 'swimmer's shoulder'. Johnson et al. (1987) reviewed the literature and reported shoulder injury rates of 40–80%. McMaster and Troup (1993) found current shoulder complaints among 35% of élite women compared with 17.7% of men and a positive history of shoulder pain at some point in 73% of élite women swmmers. Female swimmers also complained more frequently of shoulder looseness as well as shoulder instability.

Common features of the three styles most often associated with shoulder pain (freestyle, butterfly and backstroke) are repetitive motions of progressive adduction and internal rotation of the glenohumeral joint during the power

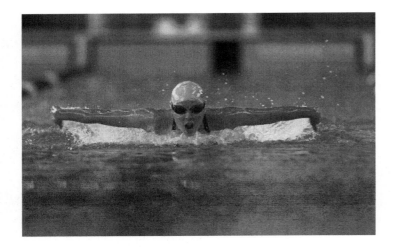

Fig. 31.2 Shoulder position during the recovery phase of the butterfly: Susan O'Neill of Australia at the 1996 Olympic Games in Atlanta.(© Allsport / Simon Bruty.)

phase and abduction and external rotation during recovery (Allegrucci *et al.*, 1994; Kenal & Knapp, 1996) (Fig. 31.2). For example, pain in the freestyle stroke was reported at either entry or first half of pull phase by 45% of swimmers (Fowler, 1995); 23% of the swimmers with shoulder pain experienced symptoms during recovery. This corresponds to a shoulder position of forward flexion, abduction and internal rotation, allowing a subacromial impingement of supraspinatus and biceps tendons. Mechanical abutment may occur as a result of degenerative changes or a hooked acromion, causing mechanical impingement of the subacromial structures. Kennedy *et al.* (1978) believed that microtears could occur in the avascular zone of the supraspinatus and biceps tendons and in turn produce an inflammatory response consisting of oedema, tendinitis and subacromial bursitis.

SIGNS AND SYMPTOMS

Primary impingement

If the supraspinatus is primarily afflicted, tenderness will be present at the greater tuberosity insertion, a painful arc in abduction may be present and a positive impingement sign will exist (Kennedy *et al.*, 1978). If the biceps tendon is involved, tenderness will be located over the

bicipital groove, resisted forward flexion will be painful and resisted supination of the forearm will occur. A more detailed review of the diagnostic steps for shoulder impingement can be found in Chapter 15 and in Kennedy *et al.* (1978) and Johnson *et al.* (1987).

Secondary impingement

Increased shoulder laxity has been shown to correlate with symptoms of impingement (Warner *et al.*, 1990). Increased capsular laxity exposes the humeral head to increased upward translation. Involuntary inferior and multidirectional instability have been recognized as causes of shoulder pain in swimmers (Johnson *et al.*, 1987). Swimmers who exhibit signs and symptoms of impingement that lessen with a relocation test may actually present with primary anterior instability (Johnson *et al.*, 1987; Kvitne *et al.*, 1995). Radiographic analysis of the shoulder should include anteroposterior views in internal and external rotation, an axillary view and a west-point prone axillary view (Johnson *et al.*, 1987).

Shoulder instability

Isolated anterior glenohumeral instability is seen primarily in backstroke swimmers (Johnson *et al.*, 1987) and is termed 'apprehension shoulder'.

The swimmer may encounter frank subluxation of the shoulder, particularly when entering the backstroke flip turn. Besides the clinical apprehension test, radiological assessment is mandatory for delineating the bony defect of the anterior glenoid in cases of recurrent subluxation (Kennedy *et al.*, 1978).

TREATMENT AND REHABILITATION

Treatment of painful shoulder conditions in the female swimmer essentially follows the guidelines for treatment of overuse injuries, consisting of relative rest and various modalities for pain and inflammation as warranted by the phase of injury (Johnson *et al.*, 1987; Fowler, 1995). The majority of swimmers with shoulder pain respond well to conservative rehabilitation measures.

The female swimmer may be more prone to fatigue. Therefore, it is of the utmost importance to address training of those muscles active throughout the stroke cycle, particularly the 'scapular pivoters' or scapular rotator muscles (Pink & Jobe, 1991; Pink *et al.*, 1991). Pink and Jobe (1991) suggest a sequence of treatment of the scapular muscles and glenohumeral protectors (rotator cuff) be carried out first. Some of these exercises are done in various weight-bearing positions and thus may be especially advantageous for female swimmers with increased shoulder laxity or instability. Closed-chain position offers an opportunity for proprioceptive and mechanoreceptor training, an area found deficient in individuals with shoulder instability (Forwell & Carnahan, 1996). Selected exercises for scapular rotators are described in Table 31.2. The later phase of strengthening of glenohumeral positioners, the deltoid, pectoralis and latissimus dorsi, requires caution during training of the supraspinatus. Worrell *et al.* (1992) found that 100° abduction and 'thumb up' position

Table 31.2 Selected exercises for scapular muscle strengthening. (Based on Pink & Jobe, 1991; Moseley *et al.*, 1992; Kenal & Knapp, 1996; Wilk *et al.*, 1996)

Exercise	Muscle emphasized	Description
Scaption With external rotation With internal rotation	Supraspinatus, upper and lower trapezius, levator scapula, rhomboids, serratus anterior, subscapularis	Elevation of arm in plane 30° anterior to coronal plane (i.e. scaption), either with thumb upwards (external rotation) or thumb downwards (internal rotation)
Rowing	Trapezius, rhomboids, levator scapula	Rowing machine in setting Prone bench with hand-held weights in simulated rowing motion
Push up with a plus	Pectoralis minor, pectoralis major, latissimus dorsi	Push-up exercise done against wall or floor, or as bench-press drill plus full scapular protraction with elbows extended
Press up	Serratus anterior	Sitting press up. May be done single-handed or sideways for additional difficulty
Supine punches		Supine (or in Trendelenberg position to minimize anterior deltoid effect) with hand-held weights for scapular protraction, or manually resisted punches, or punches with tubing

(external rotation) elicited maximal electromyographic signals from the supraspinatus. Moseley *et al.* (1992) agreed with this finding but cautioned against an inclusion of such a position in an exercise programme. Abduction alone, to a position of <90°, was not considered a core exercise by these authors.

PREVENTIVE STRATEGIES

Technical errors should be corrected. For example, dropping of the elbows in the crawl during either pull-through or recovery phases increases shoulder external rotation, which then places the muscles of propulsion at a mechanical disadvantage. Crossing the hand towards the midline causes a 'wringing out' of the hypovascular area of the supraspinatus and biceps tendons (Johnson *et al.*, 1987). Correct position of hand entry consists of shoulder internal rotation and forearm pronation. Decreased body roll may cause increased abducted flexion and extension.

Subtle changes in technique may be detected and remedied by using assistive devices such as swim fins, which reduce strain on the shoulder musculature. An upper arm band may be used (Johnson *et al.*, 1987), possibly making the biceps tendon a more effective humeral depressor and creating more space under the subacromial arch. Scapular taping has also been considered to enhance optimal scapulohumeral kinematics (Host, 1995). However, assistive devices used by swimmers may also contribute to shoulder pain. Hand paddles are used to increase the resistance through the water and also to lengthen the time spent in pull-through; thus the likelihood of impingement is also increased. The use of a kick board may also exacerbate shoulder symptoms, as the arms are essentially held in the impingement test manoeuvre position (Johnson *et al.*, 1987).

The use of paired stretching in swimming is very common and may pose special risks for the hypermobile female swimmer. Some swimmers use an isokinetic swim bench or other dry-land simulation techniques as well as various programmes for strength training. These issues should be addressed when preventive strategies are planned. Swimmers should be taught proper stretching techniques such as proprioceptive neuromuscular facilitation and careful partner selection (McMaster *et al.*, 1992; Fowler, 1995). Finally, concern has been voiced regarding the effect of weight training, particularly for the prepubescent swimmer (McMaster & Troup, 1993). A recent meta-analysis by Falk and Tenenbaum (1996) suggests guidelines for strength training of the prepubescent athlete.

Back pain

Competitive swimming is an activity that consists of many hours of training, both on land and in the water, with the spine moving into extreme positions repeatedly. As such, it withstands considerable amounts of stress (Paris, 1990). It is our observation that back pain has become a growing concern for swimmers in recent years. One study reported a 37% rate of back pain among swimmers and rated back pain as the most frequent complaint (Mutoh *et al.*, 1988). In a retrospective study we compared the prevalence of low back pain in current vs. past Israeli swimmers (Drori *et al.*, 1996): 50% of present butterfly swimmers reported back pain as opposed to 8% of past swimmers, while 47% of current breaststroke swimmers reported back pain compared with 27% of past swimmers. While taking into consideration the shortcomings of a retrospective questionnaire study, this trend warrants further consideration. Cameron *et al.* (1986) state, but without specific numbers, that the most frequent swimming-related complaint in their facility was low back pain, particularly in butterfly swimmers.

Stress to the spine in swimming is incurred in three major areas: the cervicothoracic junction, the thoracolumbar junction and the lower back (Paris, 1990). The lower cervical region is the junction of the mobile neck with the relatively inflexible thoracic spine. The breaststroke

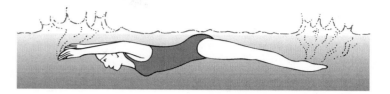

Fig. 31.3 Butterfly stroke demonstrating extension of the lumbar spine.

swimmer who forces the neck back for a quick breath is at risk of developing neck pain. An increased load is also placed on the neck during the recovery phase as the arms are thrust forward or overhead (Paris, 1990). The thoracolumbar and lumbar regions are particularly prone to compressive strain of the posterior elements due to the hyperextension motions of the lumbar spine during strenuous training using the butterfly stroke or the new breaststroke style (Kenal & Knapp, 1996) (Fig. 31.3). The same hyperextension movement has been implicated in producing a stress fracture in the pars interarticularis in gymnasts (Stinson, 1993).

DIFFERENTIAL DIAGNOSIS

The differential diagnostic procedures for the swimmer include the following, as well as consideration of metabolic, neoplastic and infectious aetiologies (Micheli, 1979).

• Musculotendinous or musculoligamentous injuries, associated with postural faults such as a hyperlordotic or roundback posture.

• Localized injuries to the growth plate. These may include Schmorl's nodes, apophyseal abnormalities (usually at the anterior part of the ring apophysis) and Scheuermann's disease (Swärd, 1992; Micheli & Wood, 1995).

• Discogenic back pain.

• Spondylolysis and spondylolisthesis may also cause low back pain in female swimmers (Fig. 31.4).

• Scoliosis has also been reported but not associated with back pain. Becker (1986) reported a 16% incidence of functional scoliosis in swimmers. With approximately 2% of the adult population

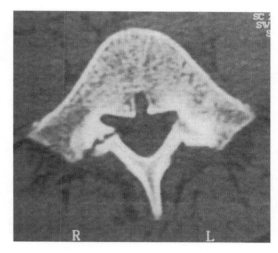

Fig. 31.4 CT scan demonstrating bilateral spondylolysis of L5 in a 13-year-old female breaststroke swimmer with a 6-month history of low back pain and a positive bone scan.

demonstrating some degree of spinal curvature (Cailliet, 1975), the higher percentage reported in swimmers may actually represent the practice of advocating swimming as a therapeutic activity for scoliosis.

DIAGNOSTIC TESTS

Plain radiographic evaluation will detect fractures and subluxations. It should be remembered that plain anteroposterior, lateral and oblique views deliver 0.11 Gy to the skin, a very high dose for an area close to the gonads (Harvey & Tanner, 1991). Bone scans may help detect early malignancy or inflammatory processes and when compared with oblique radiographs may help in identifying spondylolysis. Magnetic resonance imaging visualizes the intervertebral disc most accurately while avoiding radiation exposure. However, findings must be strictly correlated with the clinical picture because of the high rate of false-positive findings (Harvey & Tanner, 1991). Computerized tomography is also used to evaluate possible discogenic pathologies, as well as spinal fractures.

TREATMENT STRATEGIES

Treatment of the swimmer with musculotendinous pain should include stretching shortened structures (lumbodorsal fascia, hamstrings), strengthening (abdominal muscles and spinal stabilization exercises) and limitation of activities performed in painful range. Stress fractures of the pars or spondylolisthesis may require rest and protection of the area. A swimmer may respond favourably to an antilordotic brace such as the Boston brace (Micheli, 1979). While reducing stress resulting from excessive lordosis, the brace allows continued participation in swimming. Micheli (1979) also advocates the use of the Boston brace when dealing with persistent discogenic pain. The main recommendation for the swimmer presenting with Scheuermann's disease is to focus their training on the backstroke and freestyle. Training modifications should be incorporated when appropriate, for example avoidance of hand-held floats, which increase lumbosacral strain (Cameron et al., 1986). Excessive kicking and the use of a flotation device between the legs while pulling may promote excessive lordosis (Kenal & Knapp, 1996). Swimmers using a kickboard should be encouraged to keep the shoulders below the water surface on all prone strokes in order to relieve excess stress on the lumbar region.

Knee pain

Knee pain is the most frequent pain reported by breaststroke swimmers, although it is not entirely absent in other swimming styles. In a large epidemiological survey, 73% of breaststroke swimmers reported knee pain compared with 48% among other styles (Vizsolyi et al., 1987). In another study by Stulberg et al. (1980), of 18 swimmers with patellar tenderness 12 were female, lending support to the higher rates of patellofemoral pain in females reported elsewhere (Arendt, 1994).

Kennedy et al. (1978) believe that the main offender in breaststroker's knee is the tibial collateral ligament because it has been found to demonstrate dramatic increases in tension as the knee moves into extension, during valgus stress and especially with terminal external rotation. Underwater photography confirmed this sequence of events during the performance of the whip kick (Fig. 31.5). Stulberg et al. (1980) identified the medial facet of patella and the medial femoral intercondylar ridge as common sites of pain, in addition to the tibial collateral ligament. They described the mechanical fault as excessive abduction of the thighs as the knees and hips are flexed during recovery. Excessive valgus and external rotation are, again, the incriminating factors.

DIFFERENTIAL DIAGNOSIS

Pain and tenderness are typically localized to the medial aspect of the knee joint and may present as localized tenderness to the tibial collateral ligament or as diffuse tenderness around the medial aspect of the patellofemoral joint. Knee effusion and patellofemoral crepitus have also been reported (Johnson et al., 1987). Pain typically appears in the breaststroke swimmer using the whipkick and at first is present only during this activity, gradually worsening with continued participation (Stulberg et al., 1980). Clinical signs and symptoms and a physical examination are usually confirmatory. The differential diagnosis includes tibial collateral ligament stress syndrome, patellofemoral pain syndrome, medial synovitis and plica syndrome (Kenal & Knapp, 1996). Kennedy et al. (1978) suggest a diagnostic sign of pain elicited when forced

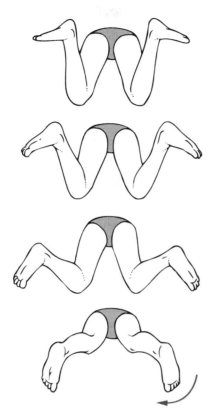

Fig. 31.5 Rear view of the breaststroke kick demonstrating the valgus position of the knee.

abduction plus external rotation with the knee in slight flexion causes pain. Plain X-rays (anterior, posterior, sunrise and tunnel view) may help in determining any bony abnormality or malalignment of the patella.

TREATMENT

In addition to regular measures aimed at reducing inflammation and restoring muscle balance around the knee, treatment should focus on eliminating the source of stress. It is the coach's task to instruct swimmers to recover with their knees together. Knees should be abducted no more than pelvic width during the recovery phase and

the middle of the kicking phase and should not achieve full extension until legs are together at the end of the kicking phase (Johnson *et al.*, 1987). Finally, the symptomatic breaststroke swimmer should minimize the use of the whipkick in practice at times of severe discomfort and attempt to find the 'critical dosage' allowing pain-free training.

Synchronized swimming

Synchronized swimming has been recognized as an official Olympic event since the 1984 Olympic Games. Synchronized swimming requires flexibility, kinaesthetic awareness and an ability to perform repeatedly under anaerobic conditions with inadequate aerobic recovery time in between. Synchronized swimming is a relatively safe sport and most problems are similar to those seen in swimmers in general.

Injuries

Most of the injuries in synchronized swimming are overuse injuries, although the prevalence of these injuries has not been adequately studied. In a study of 24 synchronized swimmers in Japan, one-third of them complained of injuries (Mutoh *et al.*, 1988). In another study of injury rates, no injuries were recorded among the 200 synchronized swimmers participating in the Junior Olympic National Championships (Rovere *et al.*, 1982).

KNEE INJURIES

These injuries, caused by the eggbeater kick, include chondromalacia, chronic patellar tendonitis, subluxation of the patella and medial collateral ligament strain (Tucker, 1980; Weinberg, 1986).

SHOULDER INJURIES

Rotator cuff impingement syndrome is seen in synchronized swimmers as in competitive swimmers (Tucker, 1980). In addition, synchronized swimmers can suffer from laxity of the anterior capsule, anterior subluxation or dislocation due to repeated support sculling. This manoeuvre stretches the anterior capsule at the point of maximal external rotation (Weinberg, 1986).

BACK PAIN

Low back pain was the most common injury reported among synchronized swimmers in a study by Mutoh *et al.* (1988). Low back pain is frequently attributed to lordosis or to the hyperextension occurring in some of the positions (split, knight, standing and walkout sequence). Other injuries described by Mutoh *et al.* (1988) are wrist and neck injuries.

MUSCLE CRAMPS

Cramping of muscles during workouts, practices and performances is common, especially in the toes, arch of the foot and calf because the ankles are extended and toes pointed for long periods of time (Weinberg, 1986). The aetiology of these cramps is not understood.

Medical problems

The medical problems associated with prolonged exposure to chlorinated water, such as skin, ear and eye problems, have been discussed earlier in this chapter. However, some specific concerns should be mentioned.

• When ear tubes are installed, the use of ear moulds becomes problematic as it prevents the synchronized swimmer from hearing the musical accompaniment.

• Near-sighted synchronized swimmers have a problem during competitions since they usually must perform without goggles. Thus, swimmers with myopia should train without corrective lenses in order to develop their confidence and to become accustomed to swimming without accurate vision.

• A problem unique to synchronized swimmers is the danger of hypoxia that may develop during competition due to the combination of breath-holding and vigorous exercise (Davies *et al.*, 1995). Symptoms include dizziness, disorientation and even momentary blackout, especially when completing the underwater component of the free programme. It has been recommended to limit the underwater sequences to 40–45 s at most.

Acknowledgements

We would like to thank Dr Bareket Falk for her thoughtful professional assistance and Professor R.J.Z. Werblowsky and Mrs Dinah Olswang for their invaluable help in editing the manuscript.

References

Allegrucci, M., Whitney, S.L. & Irrgang, J.J. (1994) Clinical implications of secondary impingement of the shoulder in freestyle swimmers. *Journal of Orthopedic Sports Physical Therapy* **20**, 307–318.

Arendt, E.A. (1994) Orthopaedic issues for active and athletic women. *Clinics in Sports Medicine* **13**, 483–503.

Astrand, P.O., Eriksson, B.O., Nylander, L. *et al.* (1963) Girl swimmers. *Acta Paediatrica* Suppl. 147, 33–38.

Bar-Or, O. & Inbar, O. (1992) Swimming and asthma: benefits and deleterious effects. *Sports Medicine* **14**, 397–405.

Barr, S. (1991) Relationship of eating attitudes to anthropometric variables and dietary intakes of female collegiate swimmers. *Journal of the American Dietetic Association* **91**, 976–977.

Beach, M.L., Whitney, S.L. & Dickoff-Hoffman, S.A. (1992) Relationship of shoulder flexibility, strength and endurance to shoulder pain in competitive swimmers. *Journal of Orthopedic Sports Physical Therapy* **16**, 262–267.

Becker, T.J. (1986) Scoliosis in swimmers. *Clinics in Sports Medicine* **5**, 149–159.

Bonen, A., Belcastro, A.N., Ling, W.Y. & Simpson, A.A. (1981) Profiles of selected hormones during menstrual cycles of teenage athletes. *Journal of Applied Physiology* **50**, 545–551.

Brooks-Gunn, J., Burrow, C. & Warren, M.P. (1988) Attitudes toward eating and body weight in different groups of female adolescent athletes. *International Journal of Eating Disorders* **7**, 749–757.

Cailliet, R. (1975) *Scoliosis: Diagnosis and Management*, 1st edn, pp. 1–2. F.A. Davis, New York.

Cameron, J.M., Goode, A.W., King, J.B. & Garrett, L.P. (1986) *Swimming Times Technical Supplement* **13**, 5–7.

Cassell, C., Benedict, M. & Specker, B. (1996) Bone mineral density in elite 7- to 9-year-old female gymnasts and swimmers. *Medicine and Science in Sports and Exercise* **28**, 1243–1246.

Constantini, N.W. (1985) *Sexual development in Israeli girl swimmers*. MD thesis, Hebrew University Medical School, Jerusalem.

Constantini, N.W. (1994) Clinical consequences of athletic amenorrhoea. *Sports Medicine* **17**, 213–223.

Constantini, N.W. & Warren, M.P. (1994) Physical activity, fitness, and reproductive health in women: clinical observations. In C. Bouchard, R. Shephard & T. Stephens (eds) *Physical Activity, Fitness and Health*, pp. 955–966. Human Kinetics Publishers, Champaign, Illinois.

Constantini, N.W. & Warren, M.P. (1995) Menstrual dysfunction in swimmers: a distinct entity. *Journal of Clinical Endocrinology and Metabolism* **80**, 2740–2744.

Costill, D.L., Maglischo, E.W. & Richardson, A.B. (eds) (1992) *Handbook of Sports Medicine and Science: Swimming*. Blackwell Scientific Publications, Oxford.

Cumming, D.C., Wall, S.R., Galbraith, M.A. & Belcastro, A.N. (1987) Reproductive hormone responses to resistance exercise. *Medicine and Science in Sports and Exercise* **19**, 234–238.

Davies, B.N., Donaldson, G.C. & Joels, N. (1995) Do the competition rules of synchronized swimming encourage undesirable levels of hypoxia? *British Journal of Sports Medicine* **29**, 16–19.

Drori, A., Mann, G. & Constantini, N. (1996) Low back pain in swimmers: is the prevalence increasing? *Program and Book of Abstracts*, p. 75. 12th International Jerusalem Symposium on Sports Injuries, Tel Aviv, Israel.

Falk, B. & Tenenbaum, G. (1996) The effectiveness of resistance training in children: a meta-analysis. *Sports Medicine* **22**, 176–186.

Fauno, P., Kalund, S. & Kanstrup, I. (1991) Menstrual patterns in Danish elite swimmers. *European Journal of Applied Physiology* **62**, 36–39.

Forwell, L.A. & Carnahan, H. (1996) Proprioception during manual aiming in individuals with shoulder instability and controls. *Journal of Orthopedic Sports Physical Therapy* **23**, 111–119.

Fowler, P.J. (1995) Upper extremity swimming injuries. In J.A. Nicholas (ed.) *The Upper Extremity in Sports Medicine*, 2nd edn, pp. 851–861. Mosby–Yearbook, St Louis.

Frisch, R.E., Gotz-Welbergen, A.V., McArthur, J.W. *et al.* (1981) Delayed menarche and amenorrhea of college athletes in relation to age of onset of training. *Journal of the American Medical Association* **246**, 1159–1163.

Harvey, J. & Tanner, S.C. (1991) Low back pain in young athletes: a practical approach. *Sports Medicine* **12**, 394–406.

Hawley, J.A. & Williams, M.M. (1991) Relationship between upper body anaerobic power and freestyle swimming performance. *International Journal of Sports Medicine* **12**, 1–5.

Hawley, J.A., Williams, M.M., Vickovic, M.M. & Handcock, P.J. (1992) Muscle power predicts freestyle swimming performance. *British Journal of Sports Medicine* **16**, 151–155.

Heinrich, C.H., Going, S.B., Pamenter, R.W., Perry, C.D., Boyden, T.W. & Lohman, T.G. (1990) Bone mineral content of cyclically menstruating female resistance and endurance trained athletes. *Medicine and Science in Sports and Exercise* **22**, 558–563.

Hergenroeder, A.C. & Klish, W.J. (1990) Body composition in adolescent athletes. *Pediatric Clinics of North America* **37**, 1057–1083.

Hirata, K. (ed.) (1979) *Selection of Olympic Champions*, Vol. 1. Institute of Environmental Stress, Santa Barbara, California.

Host, H. (1995) Scapular taping in the treatment of anterior shoulder impingement. *Physical Therapy* **75**, 803–813.

Huang, S.W., Veiga, R., Sila, U., Reed, E. & Hines, S. (1989) The effect of swimming in asthmatic children: participants in a swimming program in the city of Baltimore. *Journal of Asthma* **26**, 117–121.

Inbar, O. & Bar-Or, O. (1977) Relationship of anaerobic and aerobic arm and leg capacities to swimming performance of 8–12-year-old children. In R.J. Shephard & H. Lavallee (eds) *Frontiers of Activity and Child Health*, pp. 283–292. Pelican, Quebec.

Jacobson, P.C., Beaver, W., Grubb, S.A., Taft, T.N. & Talmage, R.V. (1984) Bone density in women: college athletes and older athletic women. *Journal of Orthopaedic Research* **2**, 328–332.

Johnson, J.E., Sim, F.H. & Scott, G.S. (1987) Musculoskeletal injuries in competitive swimmers. *Mayo Clinical Proceedings* **62**, 289–304.

Keizer, H.A. & Rogol, A.D. (1990) Physical exercise and menstrual cycle alterations: what are the mechanisms? *Sports Medicine* **10**, 218–235.

Kenal, K.A.F. & Knapp, L.D. (1996) Rehabilitation of injuries in competitive swimmers. *Sports Medicine* **22**, 337–347.

Kennedy, J.C., Hawkins, R. & Krissoff, W.B. (1978) Orthopaedic manifestations of swimming. *American Journal of Sports Medicine* **6**, 309–321.

Kvitne, R.S., Jobe, F.W. & Jobe, C.M. (1995) Shoulder instability in the overhead or throwing athlete. *Clinics in Sports Medicine* **14**, 917–935.

Lampe, R.M., Henderson, A.C. & Hansen, G.H. (1977) Green hair. *Journal of the American Medical Association* **237**, 2092.

Lee, E.J., Long, K.A., Risser, W.L., Poindexter, H.B.W., Gibbons, W.E. & Goldzieher, J. (1995) Variations in bone status of contralateral and regional sites in young athletic women. *Medicine and Science in Sports and Exercise* **27**, 1354–1361.

Lowensteyn, I., Signorile, J., Tremblay, L. & Salhanick, D. (1992) Correlation of swimming speed with various power measurements using a modified arm crank ergometer. *Medicine and Science in Sports and Exercise* **24**, S185.

McMaster, W.C. & Troup, J. (1993) A survey of interfering shoulder pain in United States competitive swimmers. *American Journal of Sports Medicine* **21**, 67–70.

McMaster, W.C., Long, S.C. & Caiozzo, V.J. (1992) Shoulder torque changes in the swimming athlete. *American Journal of Sports Medicine* **20**, 323–327.

Maffuli, N., King, J.B. & Helms, P. (1994) Training in elite young athletes (the training of young athletes (TOYA) study): injuries, flexibility and isometric strength. *British Journal of Sports Medicine* **28**, 123–136.

Magnusson, S.P., Constantini, N.W., McHugh, M.P. & Gleim, G.W. (1995) Strength profiles and performance in masters' level swimmers. *American Journal of Sports Medicine* **23**, 626–631.

Malina, R.M. (1978) Physical growth and maturity characteristics of young athletes. In R.A. Magill, M.J. Ash & F.L. Smoll (eds) *Children in Sport: A Contemporary Anthology*, pp. 79–101. Human Kinetics Publishers, Champaign, Illinois.

Malina, R.M. (1983) Menarche in athletes: a synthesis and hypothesis. *Annals of Human Biology* **10**, 1–24.

Malina, R.M. (1991) Darwinian fitness, physical fitness and physical activity. In C.G.N. Mascie-Taylor & F.W. Laskor (eds) *Application of Biological Anthropology to Human Affairs*, pp. 143–184. Cambridge University Press, Cambridge.

Malina, R.M. (1994a) Physical growth and biological maturation of young athletes. *Exercise and Sport Sciences Reviews* **22**, 389–433.

Malina, R.M. (1994b) Physical activity and training: effects on stature and the adolescent growth spurt. *Medicine and Science in Sports and Exercise* **26**, 759–766.

Malina, R.M., Meleski, B.W. & Shoup, R.F. (1982a) Anthropometric, body composition, and maturity characteristics of selected school-age athletes. *Pediatric Clinics of North America* **29**, 1305–1323.

Malina, R.M., Mueller, W.H., Bouchard, C., Shoup, R.F. & Lariviere, G. (1982b) Fatness and fat patterning among athletes at the Montreal Olympic Games, 1976. *Medicine and Science in Sports and Exercise* **14**, 445–452.

Marcus, R., Drinkwater, B. & Dalsky, G. (1992) Osteoporosis and exercise in women. *Medicine and Science in Sports and Exercise* **24**, S301–S307.

Marcy, S.M. (1985) External otitis due to infection. *Pediatric Infectious Disease* **4** (Suppl. 3), S27–S30.

Micheli, L.J. (1979) Low back pain in the adolescent:

differential diagnosis. *American Journal of Sports Medicine* **7**, 362–366.

Micheli, L.J. & Wood, R. (1995) Back pain in young athletes. *Archives of Pediatric Adolescent Medicine* **149**, 15–18.

Moseley, J.B., Jobe, F.W., Pink, M., Perry, J. & Tibone, I. (1992) EMG analysis of scapular muscles during a shoulder rehabilitation program. *American Journal of Sports Medicine* **20**, 128–137.

Mutoh, Y., Takamoto, M. & Miyashita, M. (1988) Chronic injuries of elite competitive swimmers, divers, water polo players and synchronized swimmers. In B.E. Ungerechts & K. Reichte (eds) *Swimming Sciences*, 5th edn, pp. 333–337. Human Kinetics Publishers, Champaign, Illinois.

Nichols, J.F., Spindler, A.A., LaFave, K.L. & Sartoris, D.J. (1995) A comparison of bone mineral density and hormone status of periadolescent gymnasts, swimmers, and controls. *Medicine and Exercise Nutrition and Health* **4**, 101–106.

Paris, S.V. (1990) The spine and swimming. In S.H. Hochschuler (ed.) *The Spine in Sports*, pp. 117–125. Hanley & Belfus, Philadelphia.

Pink, M. & Jobe, F.W. (1991) Shoulder injuries in athletes. *Clinical Management* **11**, 39–47.

Pink, M., Perry, J. & Browne, A. (1991) The normal shoulder during freestyle swimming. *American Journal of Sports Medicine* **19**, 569–575.

Potts, J. (1996) Factors associated with respiratory problems in swimmers. *Sports Medicine* **21**, 256–261.

Reid, D.C. (1987) Current research of selected shoulder problems. In R. Donatelli (ed.) *Physical Therapy of the Shoulder*, pp. 200–203. Churchill Livingstone, New York.

Richardson, A.B., Jobe, F.W. & Collins, H.R. (1980) The shoulder in competitive swimming. *American Journal of Sports Medicine* **8**, 159–163.

Risser, W.L., Lee, E.J., Leblanc, A., Poindexter, H.B.W., Risser, J.M.H. & Schneider, V. (1990) Bone density in eumenorrheic female college athletes. *Medicine and Science in Sports and Exercise* **22**, 570–574.

Rose, K.J. & Carey, C. (1995) Intensive swimming: can it affect your patients' smiles? *Journal of the American Dental Association* **126**, 1402–1406.

Rosen, L.W., McKeag, D.B., Hough, D.O. & Curley, V. (1986) Pathogenic weight-control behavior in female athletes. *Physician and Sportsmedicine* **14**, 79–86.

Rovere, G.D., Yates, S. & Miller, R. (1982) Junior Olympic: sport medicine health and safety recommendations. *Physician and Sportsmedicine* **10**, 120–133.

Russell, J.B., Mitchell, D., Musey, P.I. & Collins, D.C. (1984) The relationship of exercise to anovulatory cycles in female athletes: hormonal and physical characteristics. *Obstetrics and Gynecology* **63**, 452–456.

Sanborn, C.F., Martin, B.J. & Wagner, W.W. (1982) Is athletic amenorrhea specific to runners? *American Journal of Obstetrics and Gynecology* **143**, 859–861.

Shklar, A. & Dvir, Z. (1993) Isokinetics of the shoulder. In Z. Dvir (ed.) *Isokinetics: Muscle Testing, Interpretation and Clinical Applications*, 1st edn, pp. 171–191. Churchill Livingstone, New York.

Sinning, W.E. (1996) Body composition in athletes. In A.F. Roche (ed.) *Human Body Composition*, pp. 257–273. Human Kinetics Publishers, Champaign, Illinois.

Stager, J.M. & Hatler, L.K. (1988) Menarche in athletes: the influence of genetics and prepubertal training. *Medicine and Science in Sports and Exercise* **20**, 369–373.

Stager, J.M., Robertshaw, D. & Miescher, E. (1984) Delayed menarche in swimmers in relation to age and onset of training and athletic performance. *Medicine and Science in Sports and Exercise* **16**, 550–555.

Stager, J.M., Wigglesworth, J.K. & Hatler, L.K. (1990) Interpreting the relationship between age of menarche and prepubertal training. *Medicine and Science in Sports and Exercise* **22**, 54–58.

Stinson, J.T. (1993) Spondylolysis and spondylolisthesis in the athlete. *Clinics in Sports Medicine* **12**, 517–528.

Stulberg, S.D., Shulman, K., Stuart, S. & Culp, P. (1980) Breaststroker's knee. Pathology, etiology and treatment. *American Journal of Sports Medicine* **8**, 164–171.

Sundgot-Borgen, J. (1993) Prevalence of eating disorders in elite female athletes. *International Journal of Sports Nutrition* **3**, 29–40.

Swärd, L. (1992) The thoracolumbar spine in young elite athletes: current concepts on the effects of physical training. *Sports Medicine* **13**, 357–364.

Theintz, G. (1994) Endocrine adaptation to intensive physical training during growth. *Clinical Endocrinology* **41**, 267–272.

Tucker, M. (1980) Common orthopedic problems affecting synchronized swimmers. In B.J. Wenz (ed.) *Sports Medicine Meets Synchronized Swimming*, pp. 44–45. American Alliance for Health, Physical Education, Recreation and Dance, Reston, Virginia.

Virant, F.S. (1992) Exercise induced bronchospasm: epidemiology, pathophysiology and therapy. *Medicine and Science in Sports and Exercise* **24**(8), 851–855.

Vizsolyi, P., Taunton, J., Robertson, G. *et al.* (1987) Breaststroker's knee: an analysis of epidemiological and biomechanical factors. *American Journal of Sports Medicine* **15**, 63–71.

Warner, J.J.P., Micheli, L.J., Arslanian, L.E., Kennedy, J. & Kennedy, R. (1990) Patterns of flexibility, laxity, and strength in normal shoulders and shoulders with instability and impingement. *American Journal of Sports Medicine* **18**, 366–375.

Weinberg, S.K. (1986) Medical aspects of synchronized swimming. *Clinics in Sports Medicine* **5**, 159–167.

Wilk, K.E., Arrigo, C.A. & Andrews, J.R. (1996) Closed and open kinetic chain exercise for the upper extremity. *Journal of Sport Rehabilitation* **5**, 88–102.

Worrell, T.D., Corey, B.J. & York, S.L. (1992) An analysis of supraspinatus EMG activity and shoulder isometric force development. *Medicine and Science in Sports and Exercise* **24**, 744–748.

Chapter 32

Track and Field

AURELIA NATTIV

Introduction

Over the last few decades, women's participation in track and field events has received increased recognition internationally. In the early 1960s there was a growing number of girls and women interested in competing in high-level track and field events. At that time, however, women were still excluded from many Olympic events. According to many officials involved in the Olympic Movement, women were the 'weaker sex' and some of the events were felt to be too strenuous for the female athlete. Though the passage of Title IX in 1972 had a great impact on women's participation in sport in the USA, it was not until 1984 that the marathon became an Olympic event for women. During the last 20 years, women have had exposure to excellent coaching, strength and endurance training and have excelled in track and field events, breaking records and becoming stronger and faster. For the female athlete, a unique interplay exists between mechanical, hormonal and nutritional factors that in some instances may result in predisposition to bone, ligament, muscle or tendon injuries.

Medical and orthopaedic problems for the female track and field athlete

The medical problems commonly encountered in the female track and field athlete include disordered eating, amenorrhoea and premature osteoporosis (the female athlete triad), iron deficiency with or without anaemia, stress urinary incontinence while running, exercise-induced bronchospasm, heat illness, gastrointestinal problems and overtraining.

Overuse injuries of the lower extremity are by far the most common injuries seen in the female track and field athlete (Watson & DiMartino, 1987; Hoeberigs, 1992; Mechelen, 1992; Fredericson, 1996). Although there is a lack of epidemiological data on track and field injuries, the majority appear to be related to participation in the sport rather than to the gender of the athlete. However, there are some musculoskeletal problems that tend to occur more frequently in the female track and field athlete, including patellofemoral syndrome (Arendt, 1994; Ireland, 1994) and stress injury to bone (Barrow & Saha, 1988; Myburgh et al., 1990). The prevalence of these injuries, as well as other orthopaedic injuries, varies by event: stress fractures and patellofemoral syndrome are more commonly seen in the female distance runner; hamstring strains are more often seen in sprinters and hurdlers; and patellar tendonitis is common in jumpers, especially high jumpers. Although female soccer and basketball players exhibit a higher prevalence of anterior cruciate ligament (ACL) injuries compared with their male counterparts (Arendt & Dick, 1995), it is not known if this gender difference exists in female athletes competing in track and field events.

Incidence and distribution of injuries

The incidence of injuries in track and field athletes varies in the literature from 17.5% (Watson & DiMartino, 1987) to 76% (Bennell et al., 1996) and has been difficult to determine for a number of reasons. The ideal epidemiological study includes denominator-based incidence rates (Hoeberigs, 1992), where the number of new injuries observed in a defined period of time is related to the population of runners at risk. Many of the studies on track and field injuries have assessed a defined group of track and field athletes that does not necessarily reflect the entire track and field population. The definition of 'injury' and the definition of 'a runner' also vary from one study to another, as does the observation period in which the athletes are studied. In addition, there are many studies on running injuries in general that have sampled a variety of individuals, mostly recreational joggers or distance runners, often at the time of a competitive race or fun run. In contrast, there are few studies that have assessed injuries in the specific events of the track and field athlete. Exposure time is difficult to quantify in track and field because many of the training regimens are individualized. For example, the National Collegiate Athletic Association (USA) does not have injury data for track and field, mostly due to the latter problem.

In the literature the overall incidence of injury for track and field athletes does not appear to differ by gender (Macera, 1992; D'Souza, 1994; Bennell & Crossley, 1996). However, when specific injuries are assessed most studies concur that female track and field athletes are at greater risk than males for stress injury to bone (Barrow & Saha, 1988; Myburgh et al., 1990) and numerous studies of military personnel have also demonstrated a higher risk of stress fractures in female trainees (Protzman & Griffis, 1977; Kowal, 1980; Jones et al., 1989). In a recent 12-month prospective study of stress fractures in track and field athletes, Bennell et al. (1996) did not find a difference in stress fracture rates between males and females. The authors conclude that sex per se may not affect risk for stress fractures but that other factors, including diet, menstrual history and bone density, may be more important determinants of risk. Some gender differences have been noted for specific knee injuries, including a higher prevalence of patellofemoral syndrome (Clement et al., 1981; Ciullo & Jackson, 1985; Arendt, 1994; Ireland, 1994) and iliotibial band syndrome (O'Toole, 1992) in women runners. However, epidemiological studies assessing gender differences in these injuries are lacking.

The majority of injuries in female track and field athletes are overuse in nature and involve the lower extremities (Watson & DiMartino, 1987; Macera, 1992; Bennell & Crossley, 1996), with the leg (Watson & DiMartino, 1987; D'Souza, 1994; Bennell & Crossley, 1996) and the knee (Clement et al., 1981; Kutsar, 1988) being the most common site in most studies depending on the specific event. Many of the injuries in female track and field athletes are recurrent in nature (Bennell & Crossley, 1996; Bennell et al., 1996). Sprinters, hurdlers, jumpers and multi-event athletes report more acute injuries than middle-distance and distance runners (Bennell & Crossley, 1996). The greatest proportion of injuries occur during training rather than competition (D'Souza, 1994).

Risk factors for running injuries

The most frequently reported risk factors for running injuries include running distance, sudden increases in running mileage or intensity, previous running injury and lack of running experience (Hoeberigs, 1992; Brill & Macera, 1995). Running distance has been cited as the most important risk factor in running injuries (Macera et al., 1989; Hoeberigs, 1992; Brill & Macera, 1995). Higher running speed has been postulated to be a risk factor in some studies (Koplan et al., 1982; Jacobs & Berson, 1986; Lysholm & Wiklander, 1987) but not all (Blair et al., 1987; Marti et al., 1988; Walter et al., 1989). A higher performance level (Watson & DiMartino, 1987; D'Souza, 1994) has been correlated with a higher incidence of injury in male and female track and field athletes in some studies. In another study of competitive track and field athletes, increasing age, greater overall flexibility and menstrual disturbances were associated with a greater likelihood of injury (Bennell & Crossley, 1996). D'Souza (1994) has reported that more injuries occur during the beginning of the season.

Lack of proper warm-up exercise, stretching and cooling down have been proposed as risk factors for running injuries but studies are conflicting and inconclusive. The role of running shoes in shock absorbency and relationship to injury needs to be studied further. There has been little research assessing appropriate footwear for the female track and field athlete in various events.

Additional risk factors for stress fractures and stress injury to bone in the female track and field athlete include disordered eating, menstrual dysfunction and low bone density (Barrow & Saha, 1988; Myburgh et al., 1990). Intrinsic bone geometric variables such as area moments of inertia of the tibia may prove to be an important contributing variable to stress fracture risk, although most of the studies to date have been in male military recruits (Giladi et al., 1987; Milgrom et al., 1989). A narrower tibial width may provide an indicator of a biomechanically weaker structure that might be more likely to sustain a stress injury. Women have been found to have relatively narrower bones than men, which may help explain their higher incidence of stress fractures when exposed to similar training regimens.

Event-specific musculoskeletal injuries

Track and field events primarily fall into events that have explosive power requirements and those that emphasize endurance. An understanding of the mechanics of each event is essential to the understanding of the injuries that commonly occur in that event.

Sprinters and relay runners

The sprint events include the 100 m, 200 m and 400 m; the relay events include the 4×100 m and the 4×400 m. Each race event has four phases: reaction time, acceleration, maximum speed and decreasing speed (Athletics Congress, 1989). Reaction time is the time between firing of the gun and the start of the muscular reaction. Acceleration is the rate of speed increase from starting position to maximum speed, while maximum speed is the rapid repetition of neurophysiological actions and reactions. Decreasing speed includes the component of the race where neuromuscular or metabolic fatigue causes deceleration. The length of each of these phases will depend on the event as well as a number of other factors, including the competitive ability and experience of the athlete. Most injuries in the sprint and relay events occur during the acceleration and maximum speed phases.

Sprinters have a higher incidence of acute injuries (Fig. 32.1) compared with middle-distance and distance runners, who have more overuse injuries (Bennell & Crossley, 1996). The most common injuries in sprinters include hamstring strains (Lysholm & Wiklander, 1987; Kutsar, 1988; Jönhagen et al., 1994). This is most likely explained by the explosive nature of sprinting, in which the hamstring muscle group is of utmost importance. Garrett et al. (1989) used computerized tomography to show that hamstring injuries are primarily localized proximally and laterally in the hamstring group, most commonly in the long head of the biceps. Tighter hamstrings have been noted in sprinters who sustained hamstring injuries compared with non-injured sprinters (Jönhagen et al., 1994). In this same study, injured sprinters had weaker hamstrings when performing eccentric contractions at all velocities tested and weaker hamstrings and quadriceps when performing concentric contractions at slow velocities, compared with uninjured sprinters.

Yamamoto (1993) has demonstrated that a bilateral imbalence of knee extension and hip

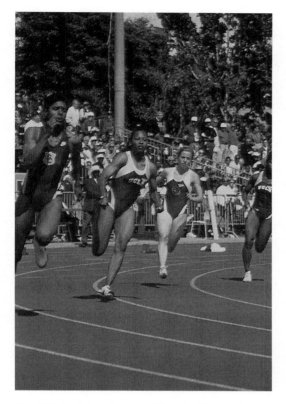

Fig. 32.1 Sprinters have a higher incidence of acute lower limb injuries, hamstring strains being the most common injury.

flexion, hamstring strength and ratio of the flexor to extensor muscle groups were parameters related to the occurrence of hamstring injury. Although it has been theorized that female athletes may have more of a discrepancy in their hamstring to quadricep ratios, this has not been consistently demonstrated. It has also not been shown that there is a gender difference in hamstring injuries.

Toe running, common in the sprinter, can predispose to musculotendinous injury of the posterior tibialis, flexor digitorum longus and flexor hallucis longus. Achilles tendonitis, plantar fasciitis and metatarsalgia may also occur in the sprinter. Appropriate stretching, softer soles, rest, and correction of biomechanical problems can be helpful in preventing and treating these problems. Stress fractures of the tibia, metatarsals and fibula can also be seen in the sprinter and are discussed in more detail in the section on middle-distance and distance runners.

Faulty running technique, sudden starting acceleration and excessive demands in weight and jumping training underlie many of the injuries seen in the sprinter (Kutsar, 1988). Avoiding block drills early in the season or on consecutive days during the season is a helpful preventive measure (Ciullo & Jackson, 1985). Hand and finger injuries can occur in relay events and can be minimized by practising coordination of baton exchange during training (Ciullo & Jackson, 1985).

Hurdlers

Hurdling is a rhythmic sprinting event and therefore the ability to perform the rhythmic pattern at speed is a critical factor for success. The techniques involved in hurdling include the start, the first strides, departure, action over the hurdle, touchdown, running between hurdles and the run-in off the last hurdle.

Hamstring injuries as well as quadricep strains are common in hurdlers. Adductor strains and pelvic avulsion fractures can also occur, especially while stretching over the hurdle (Ciullo & Jackson, 1985). Stretching exercises are important in the hurdler, as a significant stretch is required to clear the hurdle in both the lead leg and trail leg (Fig. 32.2). Heel bruises are often sustained when the hurdler lands flat footed or on her heel as opposed to the ball of the foot. If this occurs repetitively, a calcaneal fracture can occur. Heel cups can help prevent heel bruising.

Jumpers

The jumping events include the long jump, triple jump, high jump and pole vault. The jumping events are characterized by a running approach phase, a take-off phase, an aerial phase and a landing phase.

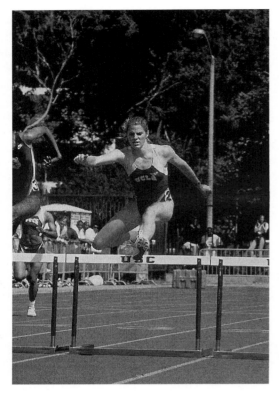

Fig. 32.2 A significant stretch of the hamstring and quadriceps muscle groups is required of the hurdler. Injuries to the myotendinous junction of these muscle groups, as well as to the adductors, are common.

LONG JUMP

The long jump is one of the original events of the ancient Olympic Games. Most long jump injuries occur during competition rather than training due to poor technique during the landing phase (Kutsar, 1988). The majority of injuries are to the knee, including meniscal injuries, ACL injuries and other ligament injuries. Ankle sprains are also common (Ciullo & Jackson, 1985; Kutsar, 1988). Preventive measures include avoidance of improper acceleration too early or too late in the jump and adherence to proper landing techniques.

TRIPLE JUMP

The triple jump is a more difficult event. The greatest injury potential exists in the landing phase (Ciullo & Jackson, 1985; Kutsar, 1988). Ankle injuries are common, as the foot can often land in plantar flexion and inversion. Lateral ankle sprains and fractures of the tibia and fibula may be seen as well as calcaneal fractures. Injuries to the knee ligaments and menisci can occur due to compressive and rotatory forces if the landing is unbalanced. Patellar tendonitis can also be commonly seen in the jumper. Muscle strains are less common.

HIGH JUMP

The high jump was introduced as an athletic event in one of the first Olympic Games. The 'Fosbury flop' was introduced in the 1968 Olympic Games and has been the most popular technique used in attaining greater heights. The 'straddle' technique is often used at the lower qualifying heights; however, ankle sprains are frequent with this approach (Ciullo & Jackson, 1985). Softer landing pits help to limit the spinal trauma that may be associated with landing on the neck or back. Proper jumping and landing techniques are very important (Fig. 32.3).

Patellar tendonitis or 'jumper's knee' is the most common injury seen in the high jumper (Ciullo & Jackson, 1985) and is often the result of repetitive braking action in conversion of linear motion. Quadriceps tendon strains, hamstring strains and patellofemoral syndrome are other problems that can be seen in the high jumper, in addition to low back strains.

POLE VAULT

Pole vaulting is one of the most complex events in track and field. The fibreglass pole was introduced in 1960 and allows greater speeds. An effective plant of the pole is the most important technique for the pole vaulter. Injuries are frequent and often due to faulty landings and falls (Kutsar, 1988). Shoulder subluxation or acromio-

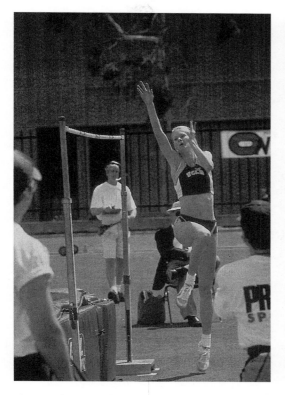

Fig. 32.3 Proper technique is important in the avoidance of injuries for the high jumper. Patellar tendonitis is the most common injury seen and can be avoided with proper jumping and landing technique.

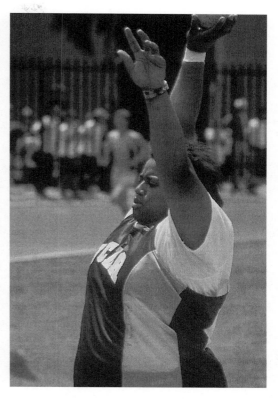

Fig. 32.4 The successful thrower must be strong and flexible as body mechanics are used maximally to produce a powerful and effective throw.

clavicular joint sprains can occur if the vaulter misses her plant. The vaulter must learn to decelerate slowly at the end of a long sprint in order to avoid injury to the ACL (Ciullo & Jackson, 1985). Abdominal and hip muscles are utilized while the athlete is crossing over the bar and falling to land on her back. Faulty technique can lead to injury. The pole vaulter should routinely check her pole before each vault, avoid training on a slippery track surface and practise single technique elements without spikes (Kutsar, 1988).

Throwers

Throwing is an event in which the athlete propels an object through the air by using the arm and involves a sequence of segmental movements of the legs, trunk, upper arm, forearm and hand. The purpose is to maximize the distance the object is thrown. The success of the throw is dependent on how effectively the thrower uses his or her body to produce the sequence of mechanical events reflective of good throwing technique (Fig. 32.4). The distance the object travels is determined by release parameters (velocity, height, angle), the force of gravity, the aerodynamic characteristics (shape) of the implement, the environment (wind and air density), temporal patterns of the feet, and the ground reaction force (Athletics Congress, 1989).

SHOTPUT

Shotputting is a power event that uses bursts of energy, since the shotput is pushed as opposed to thrown. The shotput weighs 7.25 kg at the Olympic and collegiate level, 5.45 kg in high school and 3.65 kg for the grade-school athlete (Ciullo & Jackson, 1985). The rotational motion used in the newer techniques produces tremendous torque. The common techniques in use include the Feuerbach glide, the short–long and the spin (Athletics Congress, 1989). Flexibility and strength are critical to the athlete's success. Four quick preliminary trials are necessary prior to qualification for semi-final or final events, requiring a warm-up of the muscles of the shoulder, leg and back. Sprinting, agility drills and running help develop the coordination and speed necessary for this event. The torquing techniques produce great stress on the knees, shoulder and back and repetitions should therefore be minimized during midseason.

Injury is often due to error in technique. Common injuries from faulty torquing techniques include abdominal strain (external oblique or transverse abdominus muscles), paraspinous muscle spasms and strain, and gluteus or hip capsular strain. Faulty technique leading to internal rotation on the planted non-dominant foot under the toe bar (used to stop momentum and gain balance) can cause ACL disruption. If faulty technique is used, lateral epicondylitis can also occur as the shotput is propelled forward. Proper progression of technique and form is essential to prevent injury. Wrist pain is common early in the season and can be prevented by wrist-strengthening exercises, avoidance of hyperextension techniques and taping (Ciullo & Jackson, 1985).

DISCUS

The discus is an athletic event dating back to 1300 BC. The modern discus weighs 2 kg. The technique of discus throwing involves considerable torque, and injuries of the knee, ankle and shoulder are not uncommon if the athlete becomes unbalanced. Excessive torquing can strain the cervical, thoracic and lumbar spine muscles. The most frequent injury is blistering or laceration of the fingers. Aids to increase surface friction and to secure the grip are necessary (Ciullo & Jackson, 1985). Wrist injuries and de Quervain's tenosynovitis can also be seen when faulty technique is used.

HAMMER THROW

The hammer thrower propels a shot weighing 7.25 kg forward. Strength of the back and legs is very important, as are flexibility, speed and coordination. The goal is to transfer energy from the leg and back muscles through the hips, shoulders and arms to the hammer. Paraspinous muscle strain as well as transverse process fracture is not uncommon if proper technique is not used. Hip capsular sprain, abdominal muscle strain, iliotibial band syndrome and pubic symphisitis may also occur with improper technique. Torque on the elbows may lead to medial or lateral epicondylitis; practising swings without the hammer can help prevent this from occurring. Sudden movements using faulty technique can lead to rotator cuff problems, as well as rhomboid and levator scapulae strain (Ciullo & Jackson, 1985). Chronic injuries to the knee, ankle, shoulder and back can also occur with faulty technique. Attention to equipment is also important as broken wires and wire kinking can lead to injury. Leather gloves can increase grip and decrease friction. The athlete must also be sure there are no other people within range of throws to prevent potentially devastating injury to bystanders.

JAVELIN

The javelin was the first field event in the first ancient Olympic Games. Throwing the javelin involves not only the arm but also the legs and entire body. The most crucial factor in determination of throwing distance appears to be the velocity of the javelin at the release point (Athletic Congress, 1989). The elbow leads the hand into the throw. Medial epicondylitis at the elbow is the most common injury and can be prevented by practising proper technique. The throwing motion primarily involves muscle fibre activation patterns of the deltoid, supraspinatus, infraspinatus, teres minor and subscapularis.

The most common shoulder injury in javelin throwers is impingement syndrome (Jackson, 1976). Maintaining rotator cuff strength, as well as flexibility of the shoulder and elbow, and using proper technique will prevent these common injuries. Weight training is also an integral component of training as well as a means to help prevent injuries. Strain of back muscles and triceps, as well as fingertip lacerations due to rotation of the grip cord at the release, are also common. ACL injuries can also occur while turning inward on a planted and flexed knee if faulty technique is used.

Middle-distance, distance and marathon runners

Middle-distance running includes the 800 m and 1500 m, whereas distance running typically includes the 3000 m, 5000 m and 10 000 m. The marathon is an endurance event covering 42.19 km (26 miles, 385 yards). The ideal middle-distance runner would have the speed of a sprinter and the endurance of a distance runner. In the off-season, the middle-distance runner often trains as a distance runner and injury patterns are often similar (Fig. 32.5). There are five basic components to distance training: endurance, strength, flexibility, speed and running mechanics (Athletics Congress, 1989).

Injuries to middle-distance, distance and marathon runners are primarily overuse injuries. Studies report that knee injuries comprise 30–50% of all running injuries and are generally due to overuse involving the extensor mechanism (O'Toole, 1992). Patellofemoral syndrome is more commonly seen in the female athlete with alignment abnormalities, foot pronation, tibial torsion and problems that create excessive lateral forces on the patella (Arendt, 1994; Ireland, 1994). Patella alta has been reported to be more fre-

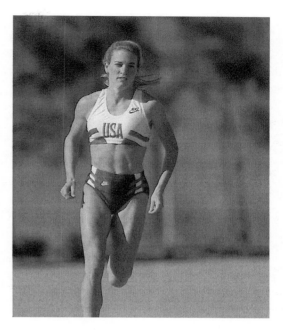

Fig. 32.5 The high-performance middle-distance runner has the speed of a sprinter and endurance of a distance runner. Overuse injuries, primarily of the lower extremity, are most frequently seen in these female runners.

quent in females and is common in those women with patellas that chronically subluxate (Insall *et al.*, 1972). Patellofemoral syndrome is best treated with quadriceps and hip abductor strengthening exercises and hamstring, gastrocnemius–soleus and iliotibial band stretching. Avoidance of full squats, stairs or hill running and correction of underlying mechanical predisposing factors, such as foot pronation or leg length discrepancies, can be helpful. Additional modification of training, such as decreasing total weekly mileage, should also be addressed.

Stress injury to bone and stress fractures have also been noted to occur more commonly in the female runner compared with the male runner in most studies (Clement *et al.*, 1981; Barrow & Saha, 1988; Myburgh *et al.*, 1990) but not all (Bennell *et al.*, 1996), especially in the presence of disordered eating, amenorrhoea and low bone density in women (Fig. 32.6a,b). Medial tibial

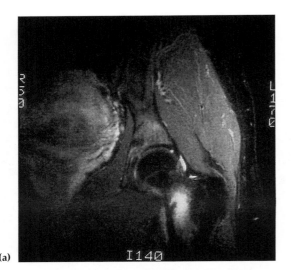

(a)

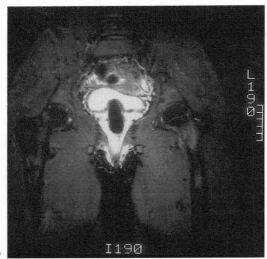

(b)

Fig. 32.6 (a) Magnetic resonance imaging (MRI) of a collegiate female distance runner with thigh pain reveals a stress fracture of the lesser trochanter of her femur. She had a history of primary amenorrhoea and low bone density (osteopenia) in her hip and spine. (b) The athlete continued to have hip pain despite rest and the MRI taken 3 months later shows a persistent stress injury. This runner had a previous stress fracture in the same region in the previous year.

stress syndrome refers to the spectrum of stress injury to bone (Detmer, 1986; Fredericson *et al.*, 1995; Fredericson, 1996). Using magnetic resonance imaging, Fredericson *et al.* (1995) have

shown that tibial periosteal inflammation and tibial stress reactions can precede frank fracture. Magnetic resonance imaging can also be useful in management and follow-up of stress fractures and stress injury to bone, including the élite athlete with repetitive stress injury (Arendt & Griffiths, 1997).

The tibia is the most common site for stress fractures in runners followed by the metatarsal bones. The most common metatarsal stress fracture in the runner is the second metatarsal. Current research in the area of stress injury to bone in the female athlete emphasizes the important interaction of mechanical, nutritional and hormonal factors on bone (Nattiv & Armsey, 1997). A nutritional and menstrual history should be assessed as part of the medical work-up of all female runners with stress injury to bone. Preventive efforts include an assessment of these factors, ideally at the time of the pre-season physical examination. If disordered eating or menstrual dysfunction is identified, the athlete should have appropriate medical tests and follow-up.

In most studies of distance runners, injuries to the foot, ankle and lower leg are the next most frequent after knee injuries (Mechelen, 1992; Rolf, 1995). In addition to stress fractures, common injuries about the leg include medial tibial stress syndrome, Achilles tendonitis and posterior tibial tendonitis (Watson & DiMartino, 1987; Kutsar, 1988; D'Souza, 1994). Plantar fasciitis is the most common cause of heel pain in runners and is often seen in conjunction with a tight Achilles tendon (Fredericson, 1996). A heel cup or heel lift can be helpful in the treatment of plantar fasciitis, in conjunction with a stretching programme and correction of biomechanical problems. A flat foot or cavus foot can predispose to excessive stress in the origin of the plantar fascia. Corrective orthotics may help in the prevention and treatment of this problem. Non-steroidal anti-inflammatory agents may be helpful in decreasing inflammation. A corticosteroid injection can give significant relief of pain in the athlete with recurrent symptoms. Low back pain and hip problems, greater trochanteric bursitis and adductor tendonitis are also commonly reported in the runner (Lysholm & Wiklander, 1987).

Achilles tendonitis is a very common overuse injury in runners. Treatment strategies include decreasing weekly running distance and cross-training, as well as local ice, non-steroidal anti-inflammatory agents, massage, mobilization techniques, electrostimulation and strengthening exercises with eccentric loading (Fredericson, 1996). A heel lift is also often helpful as well as a medial arch support if the runner pronates significantly.

Illiotibial band syndrome is common in the distance runner and commonly results from recurrent friction of the iliotibial band over the lateral femoral epicondyle (Fredericson, 1996). Messier *et al.* (1995) found that a higher total weekly distance and training on the track were predisposing factors to iliotibial band syndrome in runners. A comprehensive stretching programme for the iliotibial band and proximal hip muscles is important in treatment of iliotibial band syndrome (Fredericson, 1996).

Although chronic compartment syndrome (CCS) is not common, the physician should be familiar with this diagnosis in the runner as the presenting symptoms can be subtle. CCS has been described as an exercise-induced compartment syndrome that has been recognized in all fascial compartments of the leg but most commonly in the anterior and deep posterior compartments (Detmer, 1985; Rorabeck *et al.*, 1988). Symptoms of consistently recurring aching, tightness or weakness in the leg usually begin within 20 min of running and resolve shortly after cessation of running, although in some cases pain persists for a longer time. Numbness in the distribution of the involved nerve (often in the first web space for anterior compartment syndrome) is often noted. Symptoms may be bilateral. Compartment pressure measurements are a reliable method of assessment of CCS. Magnetic resonance imaging has also recently been used in aiding the diagnosis of CCS (Amendola *et al.*, 1990). Fasciotomy is the only treatment that provides permanent relief of symptoms in the

majority of runners. Conservative treatment, including decreased training, non-steroidal anti-inflammatory agents, stretching and rehabilitation techniques, usually provide only temporary relief.

Multi-event athletes: decathletes and heptathletes

The decathlon is the most complex track and field event. It has 10 events, with the 100 m, long jump, shotput, high jump and 400 m on the first day of competition and the hurdles, discus, pole vault, javelin and 1500 m on the second day of competition. The heptathlon has seven events. The first day of competition comprises the hurdles, high jump, shotput and 200 m, while on the second day the long jump, javelin and 800 m take place.

There is a lack of studies of injury rates and medical problems in multi-event athletes. Over-training is a concern, as are the injuries associated with each event. Psychological stamina, motivation, dedication and competitiveness to overcome obstacles are key components of success for the multi-event athlete. Studies of élite decathlon performers have shown that these athletes were outstanding young performers at many events (Freeman, 1986; Athletic Congress, 1989).

Common medical problems

Female athlete triad

The problems of the female athlete triad (disordered eating, amenorrhoea and osteoporosis) are discussed in Chapters 25–27. Distance runners have been the most frequently studied group that has demonstrated significant decreases in bone mineral density at multiple skeletal sites (Rencken *et al.*, 1996), as well as an increase in stress fracture risk (Barrow & Saha, 1988; Myburgh *et al.*, 1990). Given the repetitive mechanical forces on bone in these athletes, low bone mineral density can set the stage for a stress fracture especially if there is a history of disordered eating and amenorrhoea. A menstrual history should be obtained for any female athlete presenting with a stress fracture.

Iron-deficiency anaemia

Several studies have demonstrated chronically low serum ferritin levels in endurance athletes, especially long-distance runners (Ehn *et al.*, 1980; Clement & Asmundson, 1982; Dickson *et al.*, 1982; Colt & Heyman, 1984; Lampe *et al.*, 1986; Balaban *et al.*, 1989), although it is has not been shown that the prevalence of iron-deficiency anaemia in female runners is greater than in the general female population.

Most studies in female athletes conclude that a low ferritin level in the absence of anaemia is not associated with a decrease in performance. However, a low ferritin level with anaemia can affect athletic performance and in this situation iron supplementation is beneficial to the female athlete. Routine screening of all female athletes by assessing serum ferritin has not been found to be cost-effective. However, screening in some high-risk groups, including endurance runners with a history of nutritional deficiency, a history of anaemia or with symptoms of fatigue and decreased performance, may prove beneficial. For a complete discussion of iron-deficiency anaemia see Chapter 21.

Stress urinary incontinence

Stress urinary incontinence is experienced as involuntary loss of urine during physical activity by some athletes. It is commonly seen in female athletes in running and jumping sports, as well as in gymnastics (Nygaard *et al.*, 1990). The mechanism involves an increase in intra-abdominal pressure during exercise. Additional risk factors include multiparity and hypo-oestrogenic amenorrhoea and oligomenorrhoea.

Treatment includes avoidance of excessive fluid ingestion prior to events (tailored to sport and weather conditions to avoid dehydration), the wearing of sanitary napkins during the event and Kegel exercises to strengthen pelvic floor muscles (Nygaard *et al.*, 1990). Those with hypo-oestrogenic amenorrhoea and oligomenorrhoea should be assessed for treatment with hormone replacement. Anatomical defects, such as posterior urethrovesical angle, should be assessed if the problem persists despite treatment.

Exercise-induced bronchospasm

One of the most common medical conditions in the track and field athlete is exercise-induced bronchospasm, an attack of asthma or bronchospasm characterized by airway inflammation and hyperresponsiveness that is induced by exercise. The athlete often experiences this as shortness of breath during running, chest pain or tightness, wheezing, or coughing. The symptoms will often occur after 5–10 min of running or other form of exercise. One of the hallmarks of exercise-induced bronchospasm is that the symptoms often get worse shortly *after* exercise commences and usually resolve within 15–30 min following cessation of exercise (Cypcar & Lemanske, 1994). Athletes with a history of allergies or asthma are at higher risk for exercise-induced asthma. No gender predominance has been identified.

The fact that 11% of the 1984 USA Olympic team had exercise-induced bronchospasm yet won 41 medals illustrates that with adequate recognition and treatment exercise-induced bronchospasm can be prevented or minimized and need not impair performance (Pierson & Voy, 1988). Preventive efforts include avoidance of known allergens that may precipitate the asthma, a warm-up period approximately 30–60 min prior to prolonged running or exercise and avoidance of exercise in cold and dry environmental conditions. Schnall and Landau (1980) reported that multiple sprints of 30 s duration, 2 min apart, performed 30 min prior to prolonged running had a protective effect and may reduce the symptoms of exercise-induced bronchospasm. This strategy takes advantage of the refractory period that 40–50% of individuals with exercise-induced bronchospasm experience and is defined as the time during which less than half of the initial response is provoked by a second challenge (Cypcar & Lemanske, 1994). In other words, a mild attack of asthma makes the athlete less responsive (refractory) to an identical exercise task performed within 1 hour. The use of nasal breathing or the wearing of a scarf or surgical mask to warm and humidify the inspired air during outdoor running in the cold winter months or using an indoor track may also be helpful in the prevention of exercise-induced bronchospasm.

Pharmacological prevention and treatment includes prescription inhalers used 15–20 min prior to running. The most commonly prescribed inhalers include the β_2-adrenergic agonists, which have been effective in preventing symptoms of exercise-induced bronchospasm in 90% of patients. The β_2 agonists can also be used in acute bronchospasm. For those individuals unresponsive to the β_2 agonists, cromolyn sodium inhalers may be helpful as a preventive treatment for exercise-induced bronchospasm. Corticosteroid inhalers are not used in the sports setting acutely, unless the individual is found to have chronic asthma in addition to exercise-induced asthma or bronchospasm. In the individual with chronic asthma, inhaled corticosteroids and other medications for chronic asthma can help to treat the underlying inflammatory disorder and airway obstruction and reduce the incidence of exercise-induced bronchospasm. These inhaled agents (β_2-adrenergic agonists, cromolyn sodium and inhaled corticosteroids) are presently approved by the US Olympic Committee and the International Olympic Committee for use by athletes when accompanied by a physician note or statement of need.

Heat illness

One of the most serious conditions for the track and field athlete is heat injury. Heat injuries include heat cramps, heat exhaustion and heat stroke. Predisposing factors include previous heat injury, inadequate hydration, prolonged exercise in humid environments with a high wet bulb globe temperature (WBGT) index and lack of acclimatization. Female gender itself does not appear to be a risk factor for heat injury. Wells (1977) studied the heat response of women during different phases of the menstrual cycle and did not find differences in sweat rates or evaporative heat loss throughout the menstrual cycle. Drinkwater et al. (1977) demonstrated that there was a resistance to heat injury from physical conditioning in female marathon runners.

Prevention of heat illness in the track and field athlete includes attention to the environmental conditions prior to a track meet or race. The WBGT index is the most useful measure of heat stress. Physicians and organizers of race events should be familiar with the potential hazards of exercising in environments with a high WBGT index and be prepared to cancel events if conditions are hazardous to the athlete's well-being (Bracker, 1992; American College of Sports Medicine, 1997). Gradual acclimatization to the environmental conditions is important and avoidance of running during peak humidity is essential. In severe cases of heat exhaustion with heat stroke, intravenous fluids should be administered as well as cooling techniques and the athlete should be transferred to an emergency facility immediately.

Gastrointestinal problems

UPPER GASTROINTESTINAL PROBLEMS

Gastrointestinal problems are common in the track and field athlete, especially in distance and marathon runners. Symptoms such as heartburn, loss of appetite, nausea and vomiting appear to be more prevalent during and after intense workouts, suggesting a dose–response relationship (Keefe et al., 1984; Riddoch & Trinick, 1988). Symptoms have also been found to be more prevalent in the female runner and the inexperienced runner (Keefe et al., 1984; Riddoch & Trinick, 1988). Gastro-oesophageal reflux and decreased gastric emptying appear to be the main mechanisms responsible for the upper gastrointestinal symptoms in the runner (Green, 1992).

Measures to minimize upper gastrointestinal symptoms in the runner include reduction in the intensity of the workout and avoidance of fatty foods and high-calorie meals prior to exercise. In addition, low-osmolar cold drinks that are more readily emptied by the stomach may be helpful (Green, 1992). The use of pharmacological agents, such as histamine H_2 blockers, needs further study in the prevention of exercise-associated upper gastrointestinal problems in the runner.

LOWER GASTROINTESTINAL PROBLEMS

Lower gastrointestinal problems are also common in the runner. In fact, the term 'runner's trots' has been used to explain the well-known complaint of diarrhoea associated with running (Fogoros, 1980). Lower abdominal cramping, increased frequency of bowel movements, diarrhoea and the urge to defecate are the most common lower gastrointestinal complaints experienced while running. As is the case with upper gastrointestinal problems, symptoms are usually heightened with increased intensity of exercise.

The most likely aetiology of lower gastrointestinal problems in runners is relative ischaemia of the gastrointestinal tract during intense exercise. Preventive measures include proper hydration early in exercise to prevent cramping, preferably with cold solutions with low osmolarity, and decreasing exercise intensity if possible. Avoidance of exacerbating foods or drugs, including caffeine, is important, as is the consumption of lower residue foods before activity (Green, 1992). Pharmacological agents, such as antispasmodics, should be discouraged and have not been adequately studied in the runner.

OCCULT GASTROINTESTINAL BLEEDING

Occult gastrointestinal bleeding has been noted to be a frequent event in athletes, especially in the endurance runner (Baska et al., 1990). The intensity of exercise appears to increase the prevalence of occult gastrointestinal bleeding; non-steroidal anti-inflammatory drugs do not appear to increase the incidence (Baska et al., 1990). Strenuous exercise has been found to cause a redistribution of blood flow and reduction of visceral perfusion. Ischaemic colitis of the caecum and proximal colon have been noted in runners and may represent the main source of lower gastrointestinal bleeding in the endurance runner (Moses et al., 1988).

A complete medical history and examination is necessary to evaluate occult bleeding in the runner, especially if anaemia is associated with blood loss. Preventive measures include use of histamine H_2 blockers in those athletes without underlying disease. However, the small amount of bleeding that usually occurs in the runner has not been shown to have a detrimental effect on health or performance.

Overtraining

Overtraining can occur in the competitive female track and field athlete and is probably the most common cause of depression and fatigue in high-level athletes (Puffer & McShane, 1992). The competitive athlete, driven to excel and faced with decreased success and performance, may drive herself even harder to perform better and may become involved in a vicious cycle leading to the phenomenon of overtraining.

Studies in athletes exposed to a significant increase in training load have demonstrated increases in pressure, anger, fatigue, global mood disturbances and a reduction in a general sense of well-being as measured by the Profile of Mood States (Morgan et al., 1988). Muscle biopsies in these athletes have demonstrated markedly diminished muscle glycogen in those athletes with the greatest changes in their Profile of Mood States scores (Costill et al., 1988).

Preventive measures include adequate dietary carbohydrates and sound nutrition and psychological support for the athlete. When the diagnosis of overtraining is made, treatment should focus on a significant decrease in the intensity and frequency of training and appropriate psychological intervention. It is important to rule out other causes of depression and fatigue in the female athlete, as a number of other medical problems in addition to overtraining can contribute to these symptoms. A complete and thorough medical history and appropriate physical examination, as well as laboratory testing, may be needed prior to making the diagnosis of overtraining.

Recommendations for future research

Although there is a wealth of information on running injuries in the recreational athlete or in cross-sectional studies of athletes competing in certain events, there is a lack of sound research assessing the medical and orthopaedic problems seen in the various events of the track and field athlete. More injury surveillance research is needed in order to assess gender differences in injury patterns in male and female track and field athletes. Although it appears that there is a higher incidence of stress fractures in the female track and field athlete, there is a need for more prospective studies to assess this finding better, as well as to explore the interrelationship of mechanical, hormonal and nutritional factors on bone, ligament, muscle and tendon injury in the female athlete.

Conclusion

There are many more girls and women competing in track and field than ever before. Improvements in coaching, equipment and exercise science over the last few decades have produced female athletes who continue to improve in strength and speed. Some medical and orthopaedic problems have potentially serious health consequences for the female track and field athlete and these have been discussed in this chapter. The physician and healthcare provider need to be aware of the medical and orthopaedic problems commonly encountered in the female track and field athlete during training and competition and to work together with the athlete and her multidisciplinary team in pre-

venting these problems. Maximal performance and enjoyment from sports participation can be achieved in a safe and healthy manner for the competitive track and field athlete. Most of the problems reviewed here are preventable and can be avoided by careful screening, education and counselling during the pre-season physical examination or during other encounters with the athlete and her multidisciplinary team.

Acknowledgements

Sincere gratitude is given to Coach Dick Kampmann at Pepperdine University for his assistance.

References

Amendola, A., Rorabeck, C., Vellett, D., Vezina, W., Rutt, B. & Nott, L. (1990) The use of magnetic resonance imaging in exertional compartment syndromes. *American Journal of Sports Medicine* **18**, 29–34.

American College of Sports Medicine (1997) Position statement on prevention of thermal injuries during distance running. *Physician and Sportsmedicine* **12**, 7.

Arendt, E. (1994) Orthopaedic issues for active and athletic women. *Clinics in Sports Medicine* **13**, 483–503.

Arendt, E. & Dick, R. (1995) Knee injury patterns among men and women in collegiate basketball and soccer. NCAA data and review of literature. *American Journal of Sports Medicine* **23**, 694–701.

Arendt, E. & Griffiths, H. (1997) The use of MR imaging in the assessment and clinical management of stress reactions of bone in high-performance athletes. *Clinics in Sports Medicine* **16**, 291–306.

Athletics Congress (1989) *The Athletics Congress's Track and Field Coaching Manual*, 2nd edn. Leisure Press, Champaign, Illinois.

Balaban, E., Cox, J., Snell, P., Vaughan, R. & Frenkel, E. (1989) The frequency of anemia and iron deficiency in the runner. *Medicine and Science in Sports and Exercise* **21**, 643–648.

Barrow, G. & Saha, S. (1988) Menstrual irregularity and stress fractures in collegiate female distance runners. *American Journal of Sports Medicine* **16**, 209–216.

Baska, R., Moses, F., Graeber, G. & Kearney, G. (1990) Gastrointestinal bleeding during an ultramarathon. *Digestive Diseases and Sciences* **35**, 276–279.

Bennell, K. & Crossley, K. (1996) Musculoskeletal injuries in track and field: incidence, distribution and risk factors. *Australian Journal of Science and Medicine in Sport* **28**, 69–75.

Bennell, K., Malcolm, S., Thomas, S., Wark, J. &

Brukner, P. (1996) The incidence and distribution of stress fractures in competitive track and field athletes. A twelve-month prospective study. *American Journal of Sports Medicine* **24**, 211–217.

Blair, S., Kohl, H. & Goodyear, N. (1987) Rates and risks for running and exercise injuries: studies in three populations. *Research Quarterly for Exercise and Sport* **58**, 221–228.

Bracker, M. (1992) Environmental and thermal injury. *Clinics in Sports Medicine* **11**, 419–436.

Brill, P. & Macera, C. (1995) The influence of running patterns on running injuries. *Sports Medicine* **20**, 365–368.

Ciullo, J. & Jackson, D. (1985) Track and field. In R.C. Schneider, J.C. Kennedy & M.L. Plant (eds) *Sports Injuries: Mechanisms, Prevention and Treatment*, pp. 212–246. Williams & Wilkins, Baltimore.

Clement, B. & Asmundson, R.C. (1982) Nutritional intake and hematological parameters in endurance runners. *Physician and Sportsmedicine* **10**, 37–41.

Clement, D., Taunton, J., Smart, G. & McNicol, K. (1981) A survey of average running injuries. *Physician and Sportsmedicine* **9**, 47–58.

Colt, E. & Heyman, B. (1984) Low ferritin levels in runners. *Journal of Sports Medicine and Physical Fitness* **24**, 13–17.

Costill, D.L., Flynn, M.G., Kirwan, J.P. *et al.* (1988) Effects of repeated days of intensified training on muscle glycogen and swimming performance. *Medicine and Science in Sports and Exercise* **20**, 249–254.

Cypcar, D. & Lemanske, R. Jr (1994) Asthma and exercise. *Clinics in Chest Medicine* **15**, 351–368.

Detmer, D. (1985) Chronic compartment syndrome: diagnosis, management, and outcomes. *American Journal of Sports Medicine* **13**, 162–170.

Detmer, D. (1986) Chronic shin splints. Classification and management of medial tibial stress syndrome. *Sports Medicine* **3**, 436–446.

Dickson, D., Wilkinson, R. & Noakes, T. (1982) Effects of ultra-marathon training and racing on hematologic parameters and serum ferritin levels in well-trained athletes. *International Journal of Sports Medicine* **3**, 111–117.

Drinkwater, B., Kupprat, J., Denton, J. & Horvath, S. (1977) Heat tolerance of female distance runners. *Annals of the New York Academy of Sciences* **301**, 777–792.

D'Souza, D. (1994) Track and field athletics injuries: a one-year survey. *British Journal of Sports Medicine* **28**, 197–202.

Ehn, L., Calmark, B. & Hoglund, S. (1980) Iron status in athletes involved in intense physical activity. *Medicine and Science in Sports and Exercise* **12**, 61–64.

Fogoros, F. (1980) Runner's trots. *Journal of the American Medical Association* **243**, 1743–1744.

Fredericson, M. (1996) Common injuries in runners. Diagnosis, rehabilitation and prevention. *Sports Medicine* **21**, 49–72.

Fredericson, M., Bergman, A., Hoffman, K. & Dillingham, M. (1995) Tibial stress reaction in runners. Correlation of clinical symptoms and scintigraphy with a new magnetic resonance imaging grading system. *American Journal of Sports Medicine* **23**, 472–481.

Freeman, W. (1986) Decathlon performance success: progress and age factors. *Track Technique* **96**, 3050–3052.

Garrett, W. Jr, Rich, F., Nikolaou, P. & Vogler, J. III (1989) Computed tomography of hamstring muscle strains. *Medicine and Science in Sports and Exercise* **21**, 506–514.

Giladi, M., Milgrom, C., Simkin, A. *et al.* (1987) Stress fractures and tibial bone width. A risk factor. *Journal of Bone and Joint Surgery* **69B**, 326–329.

Green, G. (1992) Gastrointestinal disorders in the athlete. *Clinics in Sports Medicine* **11**, 453–470.

Hoeberigs, J. (1992) Factors related to the incidence of running injuries. A review. *Sports Medicine* **13**, 408–422.

Insall, J., Goldberg, V. & Salvati, E. (1972) Recurrent dislocation and the high-riding patella. *Clinical Orthopaedics and Related Research* **88**, 67–69.

Ireland, M.L. (1994) Special concerns of the female athlete. In F.H. Fu & D.A. Stone (eds) *Sports Injuries: Mechanism, Prevention, and Treatment*, 2nd edn, pp. 153–187. Williams & Wilkins, Baltimore.

Jackson, D. (1976) Chronic rotator cuff impingement in the throwing athlete. *American Journal of Sports Medicine* **4**, 231–240.

Jacobs, S. & Berson, B. (1986) Injuries to runners: a study of entrants to 10,000 meter race. *American Journal of Sports Medicine* **14**, 151–155.

Jones, B., Harris, J., Vinh, T. & Rubin, C. (1989) Exercise-induced stress fractures and stress reaction of bone: epidemiology, etiology and classification. *Exercise and Sport Sciences Reviews* **17**, 379–472.

Jönhagen, S., Németh, G. & Eriksson, E. (1994) Hamstring injuries in sprinters. The role of concentric and eccentric hamstring muscle strength and flexibility. *American Journal of Sports Medicine* **22**, 262–266.

Keeffe, E., Lowe, D., Goss, J. & Wayne, R. (1984) Gastrointestinal symptoms of marathon runners. *Western Journal of Medicine* **141**, 481–484.

Koplan, J., Rothenberg, R. & Jones, E. (1982) The natural history of exercise: a 10-yr follow-up of a cohort of runners. *Medicine and Science in Sports and Exercise* **27**, 1180–1184.

Kowal, D. (1980) Nature and causes of injuries in women resulting from an endurance training program. *American Journal of Sports Medicine* **8**, 265–269.

Kutsar, K. (1988) An overview of common injuries in track and field events. *Modern Athlete and Coach (Australia)* **26**, 3–6.

Lampe, J., Slavian, J. & Apple, F. (1986) Poor iron status of women runners training for a marathon. *International Journal of Sports Medicine* **7**, 111–114.

Lysholm, J. & Wiklander, J. (1987) Injuries in runners. *American Journal of Sports Medicine* **15**, 168–171.

Macera, C. (1992) Lower extremity injuries in runners. Advances in prediction. *Sports Medicine* **13**, 50–57.

Macera, C., Pate, R., Powell, K., Jackson, K., Kendrick, J. & Craven, T. (1989) Predicting lower-extremity injuries among habitual runners. *Archives of Internal Medicine* **149**, 2565–2568.

Marti, B., Vader, J., Minder, C. & Abelin, T. (1988) On the epidemiology of running injuries. The 1984 Bern Grand-Prix study. *American Journal of Sports Medicine* **16**, 285–294.

Mechelen, W. (1992) Running injuries: a review of the epidemiological literature. *Sports Medicine* **14**, 320–335.

Messier, S., Edwards, D., Martin, D. *et al.* (1995) Etiology of iliotibial band friction syndrome in distance runners. *Medicine and Science in Sports and Exercise* **27**, 951–960.

Milgrom, C., Giladi, M., Simkin, A. *et al.* (1989) The area moment of inertia of the tibia: a risk factor for stress fractures. *Journal of Biomechanics* **22**, 1243–1248.

Morgan, W., Costill, D., Flynn, M., Raglin, J. & O'Connor, P. (1988) Mood disturbance following increased training in swimmers. *Medicine and Science in Sports and Exercise* **20**, 408–414.

Moses, F., Brewer, T. & Peura, D. (1988) Running-associated proximal hemorrhagic colitis. *Annals of Internal Medicine* **108**, 385–386.

Myburgh, K., Hutchins, J., Fataar, A., Hough, S. & Noakes, T. (1990) Low bone density is an etiologic factor for stress fractures in athletes. *Annals of Internal Medicine* **113**, 754–759.

Nattiv, A. & Armsey, T. (1997) Stress injury to bone in the female athlete. *Clinics in Sports Medicine* **16**, 197–224.

Nygaard, I., DeLancey, J., Arnsdorf, L. & Murphy, E. (1990) Exercise and incontinence. *Obstetrics and Gynecology* **75**, 848–851.

O'Toole, M. (1992) Prevention and treatment of injuries to runners. *Medicine and Science in Sports and Exercise* **24**, S360–S363.

Pierson, W. & Voy, R. (1988) Exercise-induced bronchospasm in the XXIII Summer Olympic Games. *New England and Regional Allergy Proceedings* **9**, 209–213.

Protzman, R. & Griffis, C. (1977) Comparative stress fracture incidence in males and females in an equal training environment. *Athletic Training* **12**, 126–130.

Puffer, J. & McShane, J. (1992) Depression and chronic fatigue in athletes. *Clinics in Sports Medicine* **11**, 327–328.

Rencken, M., Chestnut, C. III & Drinkwater, B. (1996) Bone density at multiple skeletal sites in amenorrheic athletes. *Journal of the American Medical Association* **276**, 238–240.

Riddoch, C. & Trinick, T. (1988) Gastrointestinal disturbances in marathon runners. *British Journal of Sports Medicine* **22**, 71–74.

Rolf, C. (1995) Overuse injuries of the lower extremity in runners. *Scandinavian Journal of Medicine and Science in Sports* **5**, 181–190.

Rorabeck, C., Bourne, R., Fowler, P., Finlay, J. & Nott, L. (1988) The role of tissue pressure measurement in diagnosing chronic anterior compartment syndrome. *American Journal of Sports Medicine* **16**, 143–146.

Schnall, R. & Landau, L. (1980) Protective effects of repeated short sprints in exercise-induced asthma. *Thorax* **35**, 828–832.

Walter, S., Hart, L., McIntosh, J. & Sutton, J. (1989) The Ontario cohort study of running-related injuries. *Archives of Internal Medicine* **149**, 2561–2564.

Watson, M. & DiMartino, P. (1987) Incidence of injuries in high school track and field athletes and its relation to performance ability. *American Journal of Sports Medicine* **15**, 251–254.

Wells, C. (1977) Sexual differences in heat stress response. *Physician and Sportsmedicine* **5**, 78.

Yamamoto, T. (1993) Relationship between hamstring strains and leg muscle strength. *Journal of Sports Medicine and Physical Fitness* **33**, 194–199.

Chapter 33

Rowing

JO A. HANNAFIN

Introduction

Rowing was introduced as an Olympic sport for heavyweight women at the 1976 Olympic Games in Montreal and expanded to include lightweight women's rowing at the 1996 Olympic Games in Atlanta. Participation by high-school, club, élite and masters rowers has grown rapidly over the last 20 years as opportunities for participation on local, national and international levels have continued to expand.

The majority of injuries sustained in rowing are overuse injuries related to an abrupt change in training level, alteration in technique or boat, or the increasingly high volume of training seen at the national and international level. In order to understand better the injuries that occur in rowing, it will first be necessary to review the weight classes, types of boats and specifics concerning equipment and training that may affect the development of these overuse injuries.

Oarswomen are characterized by the type of boat in which they row, whether they use a single oar (sweep rowing) or two oars (sculling) and the weight class in which they compete. Figure 33.1 demonstrates the differences between sweep rowing and sculling and the variety of boats rowed in competition. The current Olympic events for women include the heavyweight single sculls (F1×), double sculls (F2×), quadruple sculls (F4×), pair (2–), eight (F8+) and the lightweight double (FPL 2×). In sweep rowing, each athlete uses a single oar that enters the water on the port or starboard side of the boat,

while in sculling each athlete uses two smaller sculls.

The phases of the rowing stroke are demonstrated in Fig. 33.2. This is the only Olympic sport in which the participating athletes do not face the start or finish line. The athletes sit on a sliding seat facing the stern of the boat with their feet anchored in shoes attached to the foot stretcher. The athlete begins at the finish, with the legs fully extended and the oar or sculls at waist height. The recovery or slide phase then begins, with coordination of trunk and arm movement as the hands extend away from the body toward the stern of the boat and the legs slowly begin to bend until a compressed position of approximately 130° is reached. During this phase, potential energy is stored in the legs, lower back and arms in preparation for the catch, when the oar enters the water, and the drive, when the legs and back extend propelling the boat through the water. In sweep rowing, considerable trunk rotation occurs at the catch and early phase of the drive in addition to the compression of the spine seen in both sweep rowing and sculling.

There are two weight classes for women in Olympic rowing. The heavyweight or open class has no height or weight restrictions for athletes. In international competition, athletes competing in the women's heavyweight events range in height from 175 to 185 cm in height and from 68 to 90 kg in weight. The coxswain of the women's eight must weigh a minimum of 50 kg. The lightweight class has been in existence in international competition since 1984 when lightweight

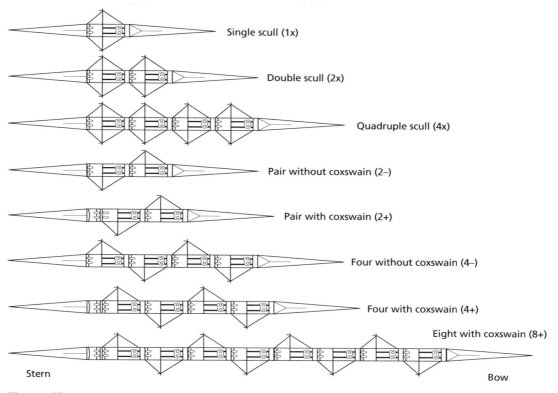

Fig. 33.1 The sweep events for women include the pair without coxswain (2–), four without coxswain (4–) and the eight (8+). Sculling events for women include the single sculls (1×), double sculls (2×) and quadruple sculls (4×).

events for women were included as exhibition events at the Lightweight World Championships in Montreal, Canada. Women participating in the lightweight class must weigh no more than 57 kg and are generally 170–180 cm in height.

Rowing injuries

Overuse injuries are seen most frequently in the knee, lower back, rib cage and upper extremity and occur with maximum frequency during periods of intense training and racing secondary to the high level of training that is perfnrmed (Hosea *et al.*, 1989; Hickey *et al.*, 1997). When an athlete presents with an injury it is critical to ascertain a description of recent training in order to determine if the injury occurred during sculling or sweep rowing and if the injury was

related to on-water training, towing ergometer training, weight lifting or land cross-training. It is also important to have a knowledge of the mechanics of the rowing stroke and to elicit symptoms that may be referable to specific phases of the rowing stroke.

The physical examination before participation should be general and should evaluate range of motion, strength and flexibility necessary for successful competition in rowing, while evaluation for an acute or overuse injury will be more specific and focused on the regional problem. Because of the complexity of the rowing stroke and the interrelationship of the arms, trunk, back and legs, the joints proximal and distal to the injury should be carefully assessed. It may also be useful to evaluate the injury via simulation of the rowing technique on an ergometer in order to

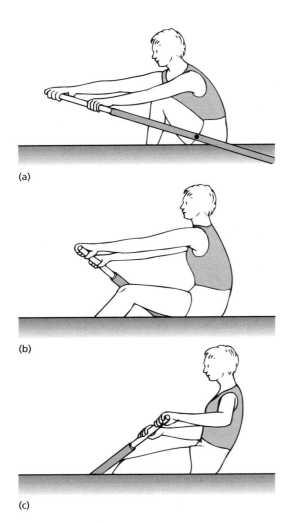

(a)

(b)

(c)

Fig. 33.2 The phases of the rowing stroke. An athlete is shown at (a) the catch, (b) the drive and (c) the finish of the rowing stroke in a sweep boat.

determine whether a correctable biomechanical abnormality may be responsible for the injury being evaluated.

The treatment of specific injuries has been outlined in previous chapters and is not discussed in detail here. However, alterations in training or technique specific to the sport of rowing are reviewed in the treatment of specific injuries. For injuries related to on-water or ergometer training it is frequently necessary to decrease the intensity

of training or to modify the type of work being performed. In mild overuse injuries it may be possible to continue to train with a decreased workload or duration of exercise while applying principles of stretching, strengthening, ice and anti-inflammatory medications. Alternatively, it is possible to alter the equipment being used by the athlete in order to diminish the load, to alter the functional range of motion or to modify the stress seen by the athlete (port vs. starboard). The load placed on the oar can be modified by changing the length or stiffness of the oar or by alteration of the inboard–outboard ratios. The height and position (toe-in vs. toe-out) of the foot stretchers can be modified to diminish rotational forces at the hip and knee. Rotational stresses on the thoracic and lumbar spine can be modified by moving an athlete from a port to a starboard position in a sweep boat. If these modifications fail, it may be necessary to discontinue on-water training if symptoms are not improving or are worsening with continued training. It may also be necessary to discontinue on-water or ergometer training at the time of diagnosis for more severe injuries, including lumbar disc disease with radiculopathy or stress fractures of the ribs. The principle of 'active rest' or cross-training must be applied in this driven and demanding group of athletes. It is virtually impossible to tell an oarswoman to stop exercising in the face of an injury. Rather it is important to educate the athlete and to provide viable alternatives to the provocative activity in order to facilitate rapid resolution of symptoms and return to sport. Bracing and physical therapy remain essential components of successful treatment.

Thoracic spine and rib

Thoracic disc herniations in oarswomen are uncommon but can nccur. The majority of thoracic injuries seen are costochondritis, costovertebral joint dysfunction and stress fractures of the ribs. Costochondritis can present with single or multiple joint involvement and is most commonly seen in the joints of the outside arm (e.g. the right costochondral junction in a starboard athlete). This syndrome is thought to result from repetitive overcompression of the costochondral junction seen with trunk torsion and outside arm cross-chest adduction in sweep rowing. Treatment is based on the principles outlined previously including ice, anti-inflammatory medication and active rest. It may be possible for the athlete to continue to train in a sculling boat, on an ergometer or on the opposite side of the boat (port vs. starboard) if symptoms allow.

Stress fractures of the ribs are an increasingly common and serious injury in the élite oarswoman. First reported by Holden and Jackson (1985) in three élite female rowers, these injuries have increased in frequency during the last decade. This increase is thought to be related to the intensity of both on-water and ergometer training and may also be related to design changes of the rowing blade from tulip to hatchet shape, which results in a heavier load at the catch. The incidence of stress fractures of the ribs was previously thought to be higher in female rowers secondary to differences in upper body strength, as described by Holden and Jackson (1985). Data collected by physicians from the Canadian Rowing Association (R. Bachus, unpublished observations) and the United States Rowing Association (Karlson, 1998) do not demonstrate any increased risk of stress fractures in sweep rowing vs. sculling or in male vs. female rowers competing at an élite level. It is estimated that 10–15% of all élite rowers will sustain a rib stress fracture at some point in their competitive careers. The roles of gender, focal strength deficits and training on the incidence of stress fractures of the ribs in the club, college or pre-élite oarswoman have not been studied. Although stress fractures of the ribs are seen with similar frequency in men and women, it is still critical to screen any female athlete presenting with a stress fracture for abnormalities in eating patterns and to assess the nutritional and menstrual status of the athlete.

Stress fractures of the ribs are often initially misdiagnosed as intercostal muscle pulls and the athlete is allowed to continue to train. A high index of suspicion must be maintained in any athlete presenting with focal chest wall pain with activity. In the early stage, pain may only be present with high-level activity but vill rapidly appear with deep inspiration, coughing or sneezing. A bone scan is diagnostic if performed after symptoms have been present for 5 days (Fig. 33.3).

The posterolateral rib at the serratus insertion is the most common site of stress fracture, although fractures at other sites have been repnrted (Brukner & Khan, 1996). Successful management of a stress fracture involves cessation of all rowing and upper body weight training for a minimum of 4 weeks, althnugh athletes should continue to cross-train in order to maintain cardiovascular fitness. A gradual transition to on-water rowing and upper body weight training is allowed at 4 weeks if the athlete is asymptomatic. Upon initial return to on-water training, mileage and speed work must be curtailed to avoid reinjury but can be gradually and steadily increased. A careful assessment of rowing technique is important with the return to on-water training in order to correct abnormal stroke mechanics and to avoid reinjury. It may be necessary to decrease the load on the nar for athletes participating in team boats so that they can train without overloading the healing rib.

Shoulder

Impingement syndrome is the most common shoulder injury in oarswomen and can be related to technique, training errors and abnormalities in the strength and flexibility of the shoulder and periscapular musculature. Impingement syndrome can also result from excessive glenohumeral laxity, which is more common in the female athlete. Over-reaching at the catch with increased glenohumeral forward flexion, coupled with excessive scapular protraction, may result in the development of impingement syndrome. Asymmetric strengthening of the deltoid without concomitant strengthening of the rotator cuff and the periscapular musculature during land-based strength training may also be provocative. Treatment of impingement syn-

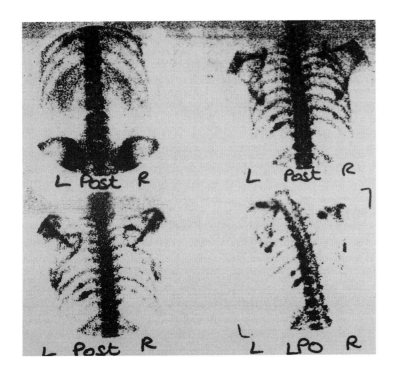

Fig. 33.3 A ^{99}Tc bone scan of an Olympic female single sculler demonstrates multiple sites of increased uptake consistent with stress fractures of the ribs.

drome includes the use of non-steroidal anti-inflammatory medications, ice and physical therapy, including a well-designed strength and flexibility programme for the rotator cuff, rhomboids, serratus and latissimus. Modification of the height of the rigger and inboard–outboard ratios may be helpful in allowing the athlete to continue to train and compete. Athletes should be monitored in order to reduce errors in technique, including over-reaching or inadequate scapular stabilization at the catch allnwing excessive transmission of load to the rotator cuff and glenohumeral joint.

Elbow and wrist

Medial and lateral epicondylitis are uncommon in the élite female rower but can be seen in club and collegiate rowers. The most common cause of these overuse injuries is a change in technique or size of the oar handle. Medial epicondylitis appears to be more common in scullers (Fig.

33.4a) and is related to a premature break in the extended elbow during the drive, resulting in compensatory hyperflexion of the wrist and overload of the flexor–pronator origin. Lateral epicondylitis is seen more commonly in sweep rowing, particularly in the inside hand, and is related to repetitive dorsiflexion of the wrist required to feather the oar at the end of each stroke (Fig. 33.4b). This injury may be related to the size of the oar handle, placing the female athlete with a smaller grip area at increased risk. Recent advances in oar handle size and grip surfaces have made this injury uncommon in the élite athlete, although it is seen frequently in the collegiate or club oarswoman secondary to training errors or equipment misfit.

Extensor tenosynovitis was first described in a group of élite oarsmen by Williams (1997) but occurs with equal frequency in male and female rowers. This extensor tenosynovitis or 'cross-over tendonitis' involves the first and second dorsal compartment of the wrist where the

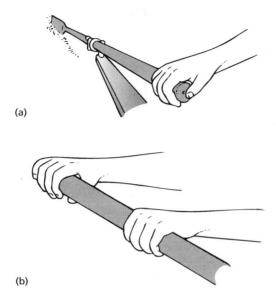

(a)

(b)

Fig. 33.4 The hand position and grip necessary for (a) sculling and (b) sweep rowing.

abductor pollicis longus and extensor pollicis brevis cross. It presents with crepitus and pain, and symptoms can be reproduced with repetitive wrist dorsiflexion. Treatment includes the use of ice, functional wrist splinting, iontophoresis or phonnphoresis, and non-steroidal anti-inflammatory medications. Adaptive splinting may be used to allow the athlete to continue to train, but must be carefully designed and padded to avoid skin breakdown. Local corticosteroid injection may be helpful in the athlete who does not respond to conservative treatment as outlined above. Surgical intervention has been described by Williams (1997) but is infrequently needed. It is not often necessary to remove the athlete from on-water training if appropriate splinting and technique modification is undertaken.

Knee

The female athlete is thought to be more prone to injuries invnlving the patellofemoral joint because of the increased Q-angle, wider pelvis

and increased incidence of ligamentous laxity. The sport of rowing places high loads on the patellofemoral joint secondary to repetitive flexion–extension during on-water and ergometer training as well as land training, which frequently involves hill running, Olympic-style lifting and plyometric training for the lower extremities. Compressive patellofemoral pain and lateral facet syndrome will often present following transition to winter land training or following the initiation of on-water speed work. Iliotibial band friction syndrome is most commonly seen during distance endurance training but can also be seen with any significant increase in the intensity of training. Genu valgum, femoral anteversion and external tibial torsion may predispose to both compressive patellofemoral pain and lateral facet syndrome, while genu varum and a tight iliotibial band may predispose to iliotibial band friction syndrome. Athletes should be carefully evaluated to determine the flexibility and strength of the hamstrings, quadriceps and hip flexors, and focal deficits should be systematically addressed. Treatment is directed to reversal of abnormal patterns of muscle weakness or inflexibility. It may also be necessary to modify training and decrease squatting, open-chain knee extension exercises, hill running and stair climbing. Patellar taping or bracing may be helpful in cases of lateral maltracking or lateral facet syndrome. It is often possible to continue on-water or ergometer training with modification of training intensity or of equipment. The foot stretcher can be altered in order to decrease knee flexion (by raising the height of the foot stretcher) or to decrease functional knee valgus or varus by increasing toe-in or toe-out of the shoes on the foot stretcher. Front or back stops can also be placed on the track of the sliding seat in order to alter the arc of knee flexion and extension.

Lumbar spine

Injuries to the lumbar spine are common in rowing secondary to the large forces transmitted from the legs through the spine to the upper

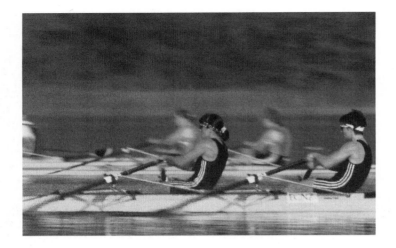

Fig. 33.5 The New Zealand double sculls team at the **Barcelona Olympics nearing the** end of the drive phase of the rowing stroke. (© Allsport / Botterill.)

extremities and the oar. In a study of lightweight élite female rowers Howell (1984) described an 82% incidence of low back pain compared with an age- and sex-matched incidence in the general population of 20–30%. Hosea *et al.* (1989) have demonstrated that significant compressive loads are placed on the lumbar spine during the drive phase of the rowing stroke (Fig. 33.5). In female rowers, these compressive forces approach 6.85 times body weight at L4 during mid-drive.

In addition, sweep rowing results in significant torsional forces across the lumbar and thoracic spine that may differentially load the disc space and facet joints. Poor technique or inequality of the strength of the leg and back musculature may predispose to lumbar spine injuries. Evaluation of the oarswoman presenting with low back pain must include a thorough examination of the spine, sacroiliac joints and hips; an assessment of the flexibility of the hip, abdominal and spine musculature; and a thorough neurological examination. The athlete presenting with pain without radicular symptoms can be treated initially with active rest (swimming), physical therapy designed to address posture, muscle strength and flexibility, and modification or discontinuation of ergometer or nn-water training. In the élite athlete, persistence of radicular symptoms for longer than 1 week or development of radiculopathy warrants more

aggressive evaluation, including a myelogram using magnetic resonance imaging or computed tomography. Central disc syndromes without radiculopathy will often benefit from conservative treatment. Addition of epidural steroid treatment may be necessary if the athlete is non-responsive to conservative treatment or if time is of the essence. It may be necessary to stop all rowing for a period of 4–6 veeks if symptoms persist in spite of appropriate conservative treatment. Disc herniation with sensory loss may worsen if the athlete is allowed to continue to train. Athletes may be allowed to compete in important events if monitored carefully and educated as to the risk of progression of the neurological symptoms. Athletes presenting with lumbar disc disease and motor loss must stop all rowing activities and must be evaluated by a physician skilled in the conservative and operative management of lumbar disc disease. Epidural steroid and physical therapy may be extremely beneficial, although surgical intervention may be warranted in specific cases. Early consultation with a spine surgeon is advisable. Élite athletes have returned to ruccessful international competition following lumbar disc surgery.

Spondylolysis or spondylolisthesis is uncommon in the skeletally mature oarswoman but can be seen in junior team candidates. This injury should be suspected when the pain is localized lateral to the midline and is exacerbated by extension rather than flexion. Lateral and oblique radiographs will confirm the diagnosis of an established spondylolysis or spondylolisthesis, while a bone scan may be required for diagnosis of an acute pars interarticularis stress fracture. Athletes with an acute stress fracture of the pars are required to stop all rowing and extension exercises until resolution of the injury.

Exercise-induced bronchospasm

Exercise-induced bronchospasm is seen in 15–20% of élite oarsmen and oarswomen. There is no known gender influence and the treatment in rowers is similar to the treatment in any athlete. Environmental factors may play an increased role in the rower as rapid changes in temperature can occur while the athlete is training on the water. In addition, these athletes may be at some distance from medical personnel during competition and must therefore be well educated in the early recognition of symptoms and the preventive use of inhaled medications. Inhaled β_2 agonists are permissible in international rowing competition but must be registered in advance of competition.

Dermatological problems

Rowers can develop a dermatological problem involving the skin of the hands, calves and buttocks. Significant callosities will develop on the palms and fingers in response to training. If these callosities are allowed to become hypertrophic they will slough, resulting in full-thickness skin loss that can significantly affect training. Athletes must be reminded to maintain optimal thickness of these calluses with the use of a pumice stone.

Gloves are not generally worn as the proprioceptive sense of oar position in the hand is critical in fine control of the position of the blade in the water.

The design of the tracks on which the seat glides, in combination with calf muscle hypertrophy, can predispose the rower to 'track bite'. Track bite presents with focal skin loss where the calves and the tip of the tracks come into direct contact. These can easily become infected and should be treated with aggressive local care and padding when needed. Skin ulceration can also occur in the gluteal crease secondary to repetitive chafing during the rowing stroke. Careful attention to personal hygiene and early treatment of focal skin irritation is successful in the management of these problems.

References

Brukner, P. & Khan, K. (1996) Stress fracture of the neck of the seventh and eighth ribs: a case report. *Clinical Journal of Sports Medicine* **6**, 204–206.

Hickey, G., Fricker, P. & McDnnald, W. (1997) Injuries to elite rowers over a 10-yr period. *Medicine and Science in Sports and Exercise* **29**, 1567–1572.

Holden, D. & Jackson, D. (1985) Stress fractures of the ribs in female rowers. *American Journal of Sports Medicine* **13**, 342–348.

Hosea, T., Boland, A., McCarthy, K. & Kennedy, J. (1989) Rowing injuries. *Postgraduate Advances in Sports Medicine* **3**, 1–16.

Howell, D. (1984) Musculoskeletal profile and incidence of musculoskeletal injuries in lightweight female rowers. *American Journal of Sports Medicine* **12**, 278–282.

Karlson, K. (1998) Rib stress fractures in elite rowers: a case series and propnsed mechanism. *American Journal of Sports Medicine* **26**(4), 516–519.

Williams, J. (1997) Surgical management of traumatic non-infective tenosynovitis of the wrist extensors. *Journal of Bone and Joint Surgery* **59B**, 408–410.

Chapter 34

Gymnastics

ANGELA D. SMITH

Introduction

Both spectators and the press exult at the athletic feats of female gymnasts. Simultaneously, however, they deplore the unhealthy behaviours apparently practised by many of the most successful gymnasts, behaviours recommended or even required by their coaches (Rosen & Hough, 1986; Roeper, 1996). The gravity-defying skills of female artistic gymnasts led to a death from a vaulting injury that occurred during competition. An eating disorder killed another élite gymnast after she barely missed qualifying for the Olympic Games. Gymnastics may give a young woman self-confidence and strength or it may stunt her growth and cause long-term health problems.

All élite sport requires particular body types, careful diet, intense training and remarkable commitment and focus. None the less, women's gymnastics has been singled out as a sport that may be particularly abusive of its élite participants (Tofler *et al.*, 1996). These young women are highly motivated and eager to please the adult coaches and judges who govern their lives. Sometimes the adults seem to fail the gymnasts in their charge. For example, many questioned the failure of coaches and officials to stop Kerri Strug's second vault after she had already sustained a serious ankle injury in the 1996 Olympic Summer Games (O'Connor & Lewis, 1997).

Both artistic and rhythmic gymnasts are judged on objective markers such as skill difficulty and excellence of skill completion. Sub-jective judging parameters include body carriage, expressiveness and music interpretation. The judges also observe and mark the gymnast's aesthetic qualities, such as body shape, leanness and overall 'look'.

Changes in recent history

BODY TYPE

Before the 1970s, élite artistic female gymnasts could usually be described as being of average height, slender, lithe and graceful. The success in 1972 of the incredibly popular gymnast Olga Korbut ushered in a new era of gymnasts with acrobatic skills, such as back flips on the balance beam, and new feats of flexibility that required excessive lumbar spine mobility. The media often described Korbut as 'pixie-ish' and lauded her girlish, pig-tailed figure that enabled her to perform such daring acrobatic stunts. In 1976, Nadia Comaneci, a prepubertal 14-year-old, increased the skills necessary to be a champion gymnast by a quantum leap, performing successive back tucks on the beam and twisting double back flips in her floor exercises. Completion of these types of rotational skills was very difficult for a woman who was 165 cm tall, so championships were increasingly won by small girls with prepubertal bodies and superb acrobatic skills. The top two medallists in the all-around competition at the 1992 Olympic Summer Games were 138 cm tall and weighed 31 kg (Ryan, 1995).

Although the gymnastics community and the

public appreciated the amazing acrobatic feats, they missed the grace and maturity generally exhibited by older gymnasts. Many female gymnasts and their coaches planned a gymnastic career to last only until age 16 years or so and tried to avoid longitudinal growth and development of the normal adult female body contours as long as possible. This was generally accomplished by long hours of training and minimal energy intake.

At the 1996 Olympic Summer Games, observers were pleased to see a few mature gymnastic champions who were over 16 years of age and had the experience, grace and artistic presence of women. In fact, five of the seven women on the gold medal team were 18 years or older (Normile, 1996). None the less, 18-year-old Kerri Strug, the final gymnast to compete for the USA team as they won the gold medal, was only 145 cm tall and weighed less than 36 kg (Roeper, 1996). Recent rule changes now require female gymnasts to be at least 16 years of age during the calendar year of a world championship or Olympic Summer Games in order to compete (Forbes, 1996). Of course, great strength, small stature and a very lean body composition are still necessary.

The body habitus of rhythmic gymnasts has perhaps been even more stereotyped than that of artistic gymnasts. Virtually all international, female, rhythmic gymnastic competitors are extremely slender, with even more aesthetic lithe body lines than artistic gymnasts. Anecdotal reports of energy consumption indicate extreme limitation of food intake. The changes in élite body type have perhaps been less obvious than for the artistic gymnasts since rhythmic gymnastics was not added to the Olympic schedule until 1984.

SKILLS

Olga Korbut's revolutionary skills at the 1972 Olympic Summer Games are now routinely accomplished by young club-level gymnasts. Somewhat less rapid change in acrobatic skills has occurred over the last decade as many moves demonstrated by Comaneci in 1976 remain the standard for world and Olympic competition. Nevertheless, in 1976 Comaneci was the only competitor to complete all the very difficult skills perfectly; now most of the top competitors expect to perform these moves successfully. In order to accomplish these feats, younger children perform increasingly difficult moves and spend a greater number of training hours working on them.

Olympic disciplines

ARTISTIC GYMNASTICS

Artistic gymnasts perform routines in four different disciplines. The floor exercise is performed to music and includes sequences of: (i) acrobatic skills, such as handsprings, flips and twisting flips; (ii) dance steps that express the music; and (iii) balance skills, such as handstands and scales (arabesques). Similar skills are performed on the 10-cm wide balance beam but without music. The uneven parallel bars require great upper body and abdominal strength: the gymnast swings around each bar, flies between them with release moves and then ends with a flying dismount. For the vault exercise, female gymnasts sprint to a springboard, punch the board for take-off, touch the vault with their hands and then land on a padded mat after performing one of several possible combinations of twisting and somersaulting manoeuvres.

RHYTHMIC GYMNASTICS

A rhythmic gymnast performs to music on a flat platform. She uses apparatus such as a ball, hoop, rope, clubs or ribbon while performing acrobatic skills and dance steps. Extreme flexibility, beautiful line and graceful interpretation of the music, along with creative and successful use of the apparatus, determine her score.

General concerns

In the last few years, both the gymnastics and medical communities have expressed increasing concern about the health of young gymnasts (Tofler *et al.*, 1996; O'Connor & Lewis, 1997). Both physical and mental health issues have been discussed. Concerns raised include possible stunting of normal growth (Theintz *et al.*, 1993; Lindholm *et al.*, 1994), unhealthy retardation of puberty with potential long-term health implications (Lindholm *et al.*, 1994), other problems related to inadequate nutrition (Lindholm *et al.*, 1994), emotional abuse by coaches and/or parents (Tofler *et al.*, 1996), inappropriate comments by officials that lead gymnasts to further malnutrition (Ryan, 1995) and eating disorders. Comments such as 'If I could, I'd take half a point off just because of that fat hanging off your butt', made by a gymnastics official to a very lean adolescent a year before she became Olympic champion (Ryan, 1995), are most unlikely to encourage healthy eating habits.

The International Gymnastics Federation has responded to these challenges by increasing the minimum age for world gymnastics competition to 16 years. USA Gymnastics has instituted the 5-Star Gym Program that rewards gymnastics clubs for providing attention to their gymnasts' nutrition, hydration, training schedules and injury prevention techniques in the hope that this strategy will allow healthy gymnasts to be adequately nourished in order to train and compete at optimal levels and develop as normally as possible. Of course, parents must also be willing to help their children follow this approach. One trainer, cautioning the mother of an undernourished young gymnast about potential bone and growth concerns, was told 'We want to keep her this way [small and undernourished]' (Ryan, 1995).

Growth and development

Nutrition

Although scientific data concerning the average energy intake and expenditure of competitive gymnasts are rare, anecdotal evidence suggests that many female gymnasts regularly consume less energy than they expend. The perceived need for extreme thinness is driven by both the perception of improved performance and the subjective component of judging. As they strive for the leanest bodies possible, gymnasts may resort to unhealthy behaviours. A study of 42 collegiate gymnasts found that two-thirds had been told to lose weight by their coach or trainer and that three-quarters of these young women resorted to dangerous methods of weight loss, such as recurrent vomiting and/or diuretic or laxative abuse (Rosen & Hough, 1986). Nutritional deficits appear to be common among rhythmic gymnasts as well as artistic gymnasts (Sundgot-Borgen, 1996).

Menarche

Until recently, élite gymnasts were thought to have delayed menarche primarily because of their severe training schedules and inadequate nutrition. Although recent studies have indicated that the most important factor determining menarche for athletes in most sports is heredity (Malina, 1994), the overriding factor determining menarche among young gymnasts may be undernourishment for extended periods of time. Virtually all studies have noted significantly delayed menarche among competitive artistic gymnasts compared with other athletes who train at similar volume and intensity. For example, in one study the average age at menarche was 14.3 years for gymnasts, 13.3 years for swimmers and 13.2 years for tennis players (Baxter-Jones *et al.*, 1994). Estimated median age at menarche for gymnasts calculated from a meta-analysis of other studies was 15.6 years compared with 13.2 years for a national sample of Flemish girls (Beunen & Malina, 1996).

Stature

At an early age successful gymnasts have shorter and lighter parents than children in other sports (Theintz *et al.*, 1989). However, when older gymnasts are examined, discrepancies between gymnasts and other groups increase. Benardot and Czerwinski (1991) studied 146 junior élite gymnasts aged 7–14 years and found a drop from the 48th percentile for height and weight among the youngest athletes to the 20th percentile among the older gymnasts. The height–weight ratio remained stable, at approximately the 50th percentile. These authors believed that the age-related decrease could be related to inadequate nutrition, sport-specific selection that favours retention of small powerful gymnasts or a combination of these factors. From age 6 years on, studies by several authors have found female gymnasts to be below the 50th percentile for both height and weight for age. Most clustered near the 10th percentile range. The gymnasts in the more recent studies were the shortest and lightest (Malina, 1994).

Although some investigators believe that the short stature of gymnasts is mainly inherited (Malina, 1994; Beunen & Malina, 1996), heredity may not account for the entire discrepancy. In a 5-year longitudinal study of 22 females involved in élite gymnastics training, Lindholm et al. (1994) found that no distinct growth spurt was seen compared with a control group who did have the normal prepubertal growth spurt as expected. All gymnasts were followed until menarche except for one athlete who still had primary amenorrhoea at age 18 years. Theintz et al. (1993) also found no discernible growth spurt among gymnasts training at least 18 h·week^{-1}; in addition, they noted 'marked' stunting of leg growth in the gymnasts.

Skeletal age correlates well with chronological age from 6 to 10 years of age, lags somewhat from 11 to 12 years and begins to fall more than a year behind chronological age by 13 years. Even by 17 years of age, female gymnasts in three studies had not reached a skeletal age of 14.5 years (Malina, 1994). The great energy demands and low nutritional intake could well be implicated as a major cause of the marked delay in maturation and the possible permanent stunting of growth. None the less, according to Beunen and Malina (1996) heredity explains 94% of the variance for skeletal maturation. Undoubtedly, most élite gymnasts are able to achieve the highest levels of competition because of their genetic attributes of short stature and great strength and speed. It seems likely that the drive to be the leanest, lightest athlete possible—by eating too little to support intense training, as well as functions such as menses and growth—markedly delays the normal prepubertal growth spurt and may permanently decrease stature from the height predicted for the athlete.

Bone mineral density

Early disquiet about the incidence of disordered eating and amenorrhoea among gymnasts raised further concerns about their bone mineral density, the third aspect of the female athlete triad. Fortunately, the bone of competitive female gymnasts seems to be preserved despite the nutritional and menstrual abnormalities (Kirchner et al., 1995; Lindholm et al., 1995; Robinson et al., 1995). Slemenda and Johnston (1993) hypothesized that the very high impact forces on both the upper and lower extremities of these athletes leads to maintenance of normal bone density for age. In support of this hypothesis, Robinson et al. (1995) found that the gymnasts they studied had greater lean body mass than either runners or the control group and that the gymnasts had greater strength of quadriceps, biceps and hip adductor muscles.

Among eumenorrhoeic collegiate gymnasts, an increase in both serum osteocalcin (a hormone associated with bone deposition) and lumbar bone mineral density was found after only a 27-week training period, even though the athletes started the study with much higher bone density values than a heavier, sedentary control group (Nichols et al., 1994).

Training

Élite gymnasts train up to 40 h·week^{-1}. Even pre-élite gymnasts may train long hours: a national team gymnast reported training 4 h·day^{-1} when she was only 4 years old (Ryan, 1995). There has been speculation about the relationship between intense gymnastics training and menarche, growth, emotional distress and injuries. Most studies find difficulty discriminating the effects of training intensity from nutritional deficits and other factors. Several authors have attempted to establish a safe threshold for the number of training hours that are unlikely to cause injury or possibly stunt growth. Absence of growth spurt and apparent stunting of leg growth was noted in gymnasts training at least 18 h·week⁻¹ (Theintz et al., 1993), but only absence of growth spurt without decreased leg growth was seen among gymnasts training less than 18 h·week⁻¹ (Lindholm et al., 1994).

Among pre-élite, élite, national and Olympic gymnasts, increased training intensity and training more than 15 h·week⁻¹ were found to correlate with spinal injury (Goldstein et al., 1991). Of 21 gymnasts with wrist pain and tenderness localized to the distal radial physis (growth plate), 17 trained at least 36 h·week⁻¹ (Roy et al., 1985). Among world-class gymnasts, there was no relationship between overgrowth of the distal ulna and weekly training volume or years of training, although gymnasts at that level would be anticipated to train extensively (Claessens et al., 1996). However, gymnasts who trained less than 10 h·week⁻¹ have been reported to exhibit osteochondritis dissecans of the elbow (Chan et al., 1991). Therefore, although it seems likely that gymnasts who train longer hours and with greater intensity are more likely to sustain injury, even those who train fewer than 10 h·week⁻¹ are not immune from serious repetitive trauma that may cause permanent problems.

Injuries

You catch your fingers on the bars, bend them back, break them, and dislocate them so you have to pull them out…you can bang up your ribs so badly that it hurts to breathe. That happens every day. You turn ankles and sprain wrists and pull muscles (Retton et al., 1986).

Gymnasts generally train while they are injured since they can often perform some of their usual activities without significantly aggravating the injury. Since some individual athletes prefer not to report their injuries (even when they partici-

pate in epidemiological studies), one Olympic champion's memoirs may provide some useful insight into the difficulties faced by epidemiological investigators. Mary Lou Retton mentions several serious injuries. She competed only a week following a concussion and sprained her wrist during the event. An injury to the wrist that appeared to be a stress fracture of the scaphoid was treated with only 4 weeks of cast immobilization instead of the 8–12 weeks recommended. 'When you're training with Bela and you have big competitions coming up, you're not going to stay out that long' (Retton et al., 1986). A cartilage injury of the knee required surgery only 6 weeks before she won the Olympic all-around title (Retton et al., 1986).

One study found female gymnasts training and competing with an injury during 71% of all exposures, training sessions or competitions (Sands, 1993). This finding makes it difficult to interpret the true incidence of injury. Few investigators have employed daily or even weekly examination, interview and/or questionnaire methods to check for injuries that do not completely preclude training or competing, so the actual incidence of injury may be greater than indicated in most of the investigations summarized below (Sands, 1993).

Incidence

Among club gymnasts, an injury rate of 3.6–3.7/1000 hours has been found (Caine et al., 1989; Backx et al., 1991). Actual injury rates are probably higher, since in one of these studies injury was defined as missing a complete practice or meet (Caine et al., 1989) and in the other study injuries were only counted if a student reported it to a teacher (Backx et al., 1991). More advanced gymnasts may sustain injuries at a higher rate. Gymnasts in a highly ranked and closely monitored collegiate programme were found to sustain a new injury during 9% of exposures (Sands, 1993). However, among 178 competitive female gymnasts monitored less rigorously the rate was only 0.52/1000 hours, with the lowest rates found among the most advanced competitors (Lindner & Caine, 1990). Similarly, at one national training centre with readily available medical coverage, artistic gymnasts sustained only two new injuries each per year on average (Dixon & Fricker, 1993). Injuries to competitive gymnasts are often serious as gauged by time lost from training and competition. A prospective study of eight Division I college teams found that more than 50% of the women could not train or compete for at least 8 days, and 17% missed more than 21 days at least once during a competitive season (Petrie, 1992).

New injury vs. reinjury

Approximately 60% of *new* injuries to collegiate gymnasts (Sands, 1993; Wadley, 1993) and club gymnasts (average age 12.6 years) were caused by a single acute traumatic event (Caine *et al.*, 1989). However, only about 40% of *all* injuries, including reinjuries, were acute (Caine *et al.*, 1989; Sands, 1993). In prospective investigations approximately 20–30% of injuries were recurrences (Caine *et al.*, 1989; Wadley, 1993). Among club gymnasts most reinjuries were to the low back, which accounted for 83% of all reinjuries; these were of the overuse or chronic type (Caine *et al.*, 1989).

Apparatus

Nearly 30% of injuries to collegiate gymnasts occurred during tumbling or during a floor exercise, while 10% occurred on the uneven bars (Sands, 1993). A similar incidence was noted for club gymnasts, with 35% of injuries occurring during a floor exercise, 23% on the balance beam and 20% on the uneven bars (Caine *et al.*, 1989).

Anatomical location

Injury to the lower back was seen most frequently, followed by injury to the shoulder, shin, ankle and wrist (Sands, 1993). Among overuse or gradual-onset repetitive motion injuries, the lower back, wrist and ankle were most commonly affected (Caine *et al.*, 1989). The ankle was the body part most frequently sustaining acute injury (Caine *et al.*, 1989). Although less attention has been given to facial injury, 7% of gymnasts in one study had experienced injury to the 'hard' tissues of the mouth during the previous year (Bayliss & Bedi, 1996).

Soft-tissue overuse

Repetitive motion and repetitive blunt trauma lead to soft-tissue overuse injury. Repetitive microtrauma may eventually cause tendinitis, muscle strain or localized tissue abnormality related to recurrent bleeding.

TENDINITIS

In gymnasts the anatomical areas prone to tendinitis include the tendons crossing the wrist and elbow and the patellar and Achilles tendons. Treatment of tendinitis in these regions is difficult since a gymnast's skills require full range of motion at these joints. A circumferential counterforce brace, made either of slightly elastic material or of inelastic strapping with a compressible air bladder against the skin, may alter the forces on an injured tendon sufficiently to allow activity. Wrist flexor tendons can be protected by a semi-flexible dorsal wrist splint that limits extension beyond the pain-free arc of motion.

The ideal treatment of tendinitis includes relative rest until symptoms completely resolve. However, a competitive gymnast may be unable or unwilling to rest from all activities that aggravate the injury for the length of time required for complete resolution. Additional methods for decreasing symptoms include local application of ice, alternating warm–cold therapy, oral anti-inflammatory medication, ultrasound or phonophoresis (with corticosteroid gel) therapy, and electrical stimulation or iontophoresis (with corticosteroid gel) therapy. Therapeutic injection of corticosteroid into the sheath of the injured tendon may be considered. However, steroid injection weakens tendon tissue, so the athlete must protect the injected area for at least 2–3 weeks following injection. Injection into the tendon itself is contraindicated because of the significant risk of tendon rupture following treatment.

REPETITIVE MICROSTRAIN

Muscle strain typically occurs at or near the musculotendinous junction, generally in the same anatomical regions as tendinitis. In addition, the rotator cuff and deltoid muscles of the shoulder and the posteromedial muscles of the lower leg may be affected by overuse muscle strain. **Delayed-onset muscle soreness** is caused typically by excessive eccentric muscle contraction. For example, a gymnast is likely to develop delayed-onset muscle soreness if she performs 15 min of plyometric exercise, repetitively jumping down from 50-cm boxes and contracting the calf muscles as they *lengthen*, without ever having done similar activity at similar intensity for a similar period of time. Overuse muscle strain injury may be treated in the same way as tendinitis, but corticosteroid injection is generally not indicated.

REPETITIVE CONTUSION

Repetitive blunt trauma can damage skin and subcutaneous fat, muscle, nerve or blood vessel. Fat necrosis occurs more often from a single episode of blunt trauma than from repetitive contusion, although the earlier traumatic injury may predispose the injured area to more significant and visible fat necrosis with subsequent contusion. Similarly, a relatively mild muscle contusion with no visible ecchymosis followed by a second contusion to the area soon after the first results in moderate pain and swelling. Subsequent reinjury may cause marked pain, discoloration and muscle fibrosis.

Meralgia paraesthetica, injury to the lateral femoral cutaneous nerve, has been reported in two gymnasts, presumably from repetitive striking against the uneven bars (Macgregor & Moncur, 1977). Similar repetitive injury is possible involving the superficial veins, mainly of the hand/wrist and foot/ankle.

Initial treatment for repetitive contusion injury is application of ice to the injured area. The area should be protected from further blunt trauma until pain and swelling have resolved. Appropriate padding may allow an injured gymnast to continue her usual training programme with minimal risk of further injury. However, if the injury is severe and padding impractical because of injury location, then she should avoid activities that could lead to further injury until pain and swelling have resolved.

Sprains and strains

ANKLE SPRAIN

Ankle sprains are probably the most frequent acute injury of female gymnasts. Gymnasts must perform with toes pointed, the least stable position of the ankle, and land on padded surfaces that are necessary to absorb landing forces but which provide a variably stable platform for the feet.

The treatment of ankle sprains is complicated by the inability of gymnasts to train with supportive shoes. The commonly used air-stirrup braces plus a supportive athletic shoe function to lock the hindfoot into place to prevent ankle inversion or eversion. A lace-up ankle brace with semi-rigid stays placed medially and laterally also has drawbacks. The heel of the brace must be covered by a soft gymnastic shoe or similar material so that the gymnast does not slip on mats. However, there are then two layers of material between the gymnast's heel and the apparatus, decreasing her sensation and jeopardizing proprioception and performance. Taping or strapping may be useful, although the efficacy of taping decreases markedly after about 20 min of activity (Greene & Hillman, 1990; Shapiro *et al.*, 1994). If the gymnast has enough plantar flexion to train or perform well in an ankle-protective device, then she probably has enough mobility to allow reinjury.

KNEE LIGAMENT RUPTURE

Anterior cruciate ligament injury is endemic among élite female artistic gymnasts (L.

Krivickas, personal communication, 1990). Gymnasts are also prone to medial collateral ligament sprains and patellar dislocations (Andrish, 1985). The combination of all three of these injuries should be considered in any female gymnast who has sustained any one of the three injuries.

Each of the three structures (anterior cruciate ligament, medial collateral ligament and/or medial patellar retinaculum) may be injured when a gymnast's foot is planted and she rotates away from the foot while flexing her knee slightly. This manoeuvre is likely to occur repeatedly whenever a gymnast is learning a twisting move. If her foot becomes stuck in the padded mat, she is likely to injure at least one of these knee structures, depending on the amount of speed and force at landing. Additional injured structures may include the meniscal cartilages, articular cartilage or bone.

SHOULDER DISLOCATION

Shoulder dislocation among gymnasts comprises two general types: the acute traumatic lesion that typically includes ligament tear or fracture; and the minimally traumatic dislocation related to joint hypermobility and muscle weakness or fatigue. Young female athletes with dislocations related to hypermobility and fatigue caused by minimal trauma, such as swinging from high to low bar in the usual manner, are often successfully treated simply with a directed strengthening programme.

MUSCLE STRAIN

Acute muscle strains most often affect muscles that cross at least two joints. For gymnasts, these include the biceps, triceps and wrist flexors and extensors in the upper extremity. Abdominal muscles may be strained, especially near the insertions on to the ilium. Paraspinous muscles are injured both in the upper back and the lumbar region. In the lower extremity, the iliopsoas, rectus femoris and hamstrings are frequently strained despite the great flexibility of these muscles in élite gymnasts.

Following acute muscle strain, ice, compression and maintaining the muscle in a lengthened position are useful. Oral anti-inflammatory medication may speed the initial resolution of pain and swelling, but probably slows the later phases of the healing process (Mishra *et al.*, 1995). Physical therapy modalities such as electrical stimulation may also decrease early pain and swelling. The injured gymnast should avoid activities that cause pain during the healing phase, while maintaining as much strength and flexibility of the muscle as possible.

Stress fractures and osteochondroses

WRIST

Among non-élite club gymnasts, 86% of females were recently reported to have wrist pain (DiFiori *et al.*, 1996). Albanese *et al.* (1989) reported three cases of apparent premature growth plate closure of the distal radius in young gymnasts. Additional stress-related changes of the distal radial physis have included widening and irregularity of the physis and cystic change. Stress-related changes were found in 10% of the skeletally immature artistic gymnasts at the world championships in 1987 (De Smet *et al.*, 1994). Among the skeletally mature gymnasts, 71% had positive and 29% neutral ulnar variance; this is significantly different from the usual situation, where the distal end of the radius is relatively longer than the distal ulna (De Smet *et al.*, 1994). Study of the skeletally immature gymnasts found that 80% of them fell within the 95% confidence limits for normal ulnar variance based on a large reference group. The taller, heavier, more muscular gymnasts were more likely to have abnormal ulnar variance. In the authors' opinion, the findings concerning possible premature distal radius growth arrest were 'less dramatic than originally stated' in previous case reports or small series (Claessens *et al.*, 1996).

A study of Chinese opera students who practised floor exercise activities for $12\,h\cdot week^{-1}$ brought to light two worrisome findings. A bony bridge suggestive of premature physeal closure was found in an asymptomatic 12-year-old girl. Also, occult injury was seen on magnetic resonance imaging (MRI) of some wrists that had normal plain radiographs (Shih *et al.*, 1995). MRI findings include horizontal metaphyseal fractures and extension of physeal cartilage into the metaphysis, suggesting that physeal widening actually occurs secondary to metaphyseal injury. Vertical fracture lines and bony bridges indicative of premature physeal closure have also been found on MRI (Shih *et al.*, 1995).

The presence of radiographic changes may predict slower resolution of symptoms. Roy *et al.* (1985) found that gymnasts (19 of 21 were female) with wrist pain and distal radial changes on plain X-ray took at least 3 months to recover; five actually took more than 6 months to return to gymnastics. Those without radiographic changes recovered within an average of 4 weeks.

A single case of osteonecrosis of the capitate bone of a 19-year-old collegiate gymnast has been reported (Murakami & Nakajima, 1984). Since this athlete began having pain when she was not doing any active athletic training and this is the only case apparently reported in the English literature, the relationship between gymnastics and the pathology remains unclear (Murakami & Nakajima, 1984).

ELBOW

Osteochondritis dissecans, usually of the capitellum or the radial head, may limit a gymnast's ability to compete. Surgical removal or internal fixation of loose fragments may be necessary. Although relatively rare, osteochondritis dissecans of the elbow represented nearly 1% of all gymnastics injuries seen over a 12-year period by Maffulli *et al.* (1992a). Six of the injured were girls, all but one 14 or 15 years old. All had limited elbow extension and only one of the 12 (including the boys) was able to continue competing at the same level. In another study similar problems were found among seven high-performance female gymnasts, three of whom had both elbows affected by osteochondritis dissecans of the capitellum. These athletes trained 20–25 h·week^{-1} and all had trained for at least 5 years. Despite conservative physical therapy in all, and surgical

treatment of all but one elbow, the average extension lost was 10°. Only one gymnast was able to continue competing (Jackson *et al.*, 1989). The inability of athletes with osteochondritis dissecans of the capitellum or radial head to continue competitive gymnastics has been found by others who studied groups consisting of both male and female gymnasts (Chan *et al.*, 1991). At least one study has found that radiographically visible osteochondritis dissecans is unlikely to be found among asymptomatic high-performance female gymnasts training 20–25 h·week^{-1}, with no cases found among 43 asymptomatic athletes (Jackson *et al.*, 1989).

Traction apophysitis of the olecranon may also occur, with fragmentation of the epiphysis and widening of the growth plate. Gymnasts with this problem are able to return to their previous level of competition (Maffulli *et al.*, 1992b).

OSTEOCHONDRITIS DISSECANS OF THE KNEE

Osteochondritis dissecans may affect the femoral condyles of young gymnasts. Although heredity seems to be a factor in this disorder, repetitive high-impact trauma is thought to play a significant role (Mubarak & Carroll, 1981). Rest from high-impact activities or surgical drilling of the lesion may allow healing to occur, although internal fixation of the lesion may be preferred treatment for the high-performance gymnast. Internal fixation is generally indicated for unstable lesions as well.

SPONDYLOLYSIS

At one élite national training centre, where the average duration of scholarship for female gymnasts was 2.2 years, the incidence of symptomatic spondylolysis was 9.5% during the period of scholarship (Dixon & Fricker, 1993). The true incidence remains unknown as an MRI study found one asymptomatic case of spondylolysis among 17 female gymnasts of wide-ranging competitive levels who used many different training regimens (Tertti *et al.*, 1990). Another

MRI study of 33 female gymnasts, from pre-élite to world-class athletes, found spinal abnormalities consisting of spondylolysis in five gymnasts and disc abnormalities in seven additional gymnasts, with the incidence related to competitive level and weekly training hours; 80% of the gymnasts with abnormalities on MRI trained at least 15 h·week^{-1}, while 87% of the gymnasts who trained less than 15 h·week^{-1} had normal MRI scans (Goldstein *et al.*, 1991).

Gymnasts with spondylolysis (Fig. 34.1) have

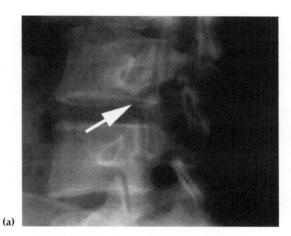

(a)

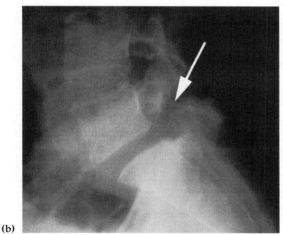

(b)

Fig. 34.1 (a) Spondylolysis, a defect in the pars interarticularis of the vertebra (arrow), related to repetitive lumbar flexion and extension. (b) This athlete had bilateral pars interarticularis defects, as seen on the lateral view (arrow tip is in the defect).

been treated successfully with an anti-lordotic Boston brace (Micheli *et al.*, 1980; Steiner & Micheli, 1985). They can even train in the brace, although it limits their ability to perform certain activities such as back tucks and back handsprings (L.J. Micheli, personal communication, 1984).

ILIAC APOPHYSITIS

The growth plate of the iliac crest may become inflamed from blunt trauma or from repeated traction injuries. Gymnasts sustain both types of trauma frequently. Treatment is rest from aggravating activities and consideration of physical therapy modalities such as ultrasound or phonophoresis.

Acute fractures and dislocations

The most devastating injuries in gymnastics are catastrophic injuries to the head and spine, possibly resulting in paralysis or even death. According to statistics from the National Centre for Catastrophic Sports Injury Research, the highest risk of head and spine injury among common school sports is found in American football, gymnastics, ice hockey and wrestling (Cantu, 1995). Although 18 acute head and neck injuries occurred during a 10-year period (0.11 per athlete per year) at a national élite gymnastics training centre, none were catastrophic (Dixon & Fricker, 1993).

The most frequently occurring fractures and dislocations among gymnasts involve the fingers and toes. However, other upper and lower extremity fractures are not uncommon, particularly due to missed moves from the uneven bars. Figures 34.2 and 34.3 illustrate injuries in two female gymnasts seen by the author within a 2-week period, both caused by missed moves; the pre-élite 7-year-old sustained bilateral elbow fractures after missing her hold on the high bar.

Long-term sequelae

A study of 24 national-team artistic gymnasts

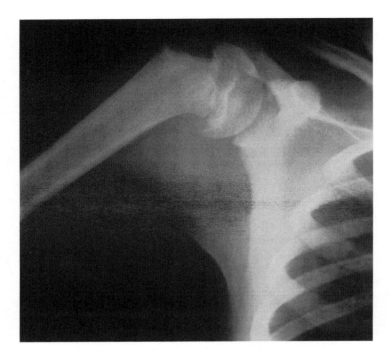

Fig. 34.2 Injury to a female gymnast caused by a missed move: severely displaced growth plate fracture of the proximal humerus.

who had completed their competitive careers found that seven continued to have the low back pain that had been present while they competed. Lumbar radiographs of many of the gymnasts showed significant abnormalities at the lumbosacral junction: bilateral L5 spondylolysis in six gymnasts, unilateral L5 spondylolysis in one and L5–S1 spondylolisthesis in three (Konermann & Sell, 1992). However, a comparison of former élite gymnasts with an age-matched control group found no difference in subjective rating of back pain between the two groups and no difference in posture (Tsai & Wredmark, 1993).

Of 12 gymnasts (six female and six male) who sought medical attention for osteochondritis dissecans of the elbow, only one was able to continue competing. At follow-up 6 months to 11 years later, the elbow symptoms of two former gymnasts interfered with their work, and three had been counselled not to follow their planned careers in physical education because of their elbow disability. The loss of elbow extension became even worse between the initial and follow-up examinations (Maffulli *et al.*, 1992a).

Inability to continue competing was confirmed in another group of seven high-performance female gymnasts, who lost an average of 10° of elbow extension (Jackson *et al.*, 1989).

A prospective study of gymnasts through their 4 years of college, with follow-up interviews 10–70 months after they retired from competition, presented a relatively bleak prognosis for female gymnasts in the first few years after retirement. These women were still bothered by 45% of the injuries that they had reported during their competitive years. The anatomical areas that hampered them most frequently were the lower back, ankle, great toe, shoulder and knee. In 29% of the women, sport activity was limited by their previous injuries. Only one of the 22 gymnasts available for follow-up reported no residual problems (Wadley, 1993).

Prevention

DECREASED TRAINING HOURS

It is difficult to establish a safe threshold for the number of training hours unlikely to cause injury

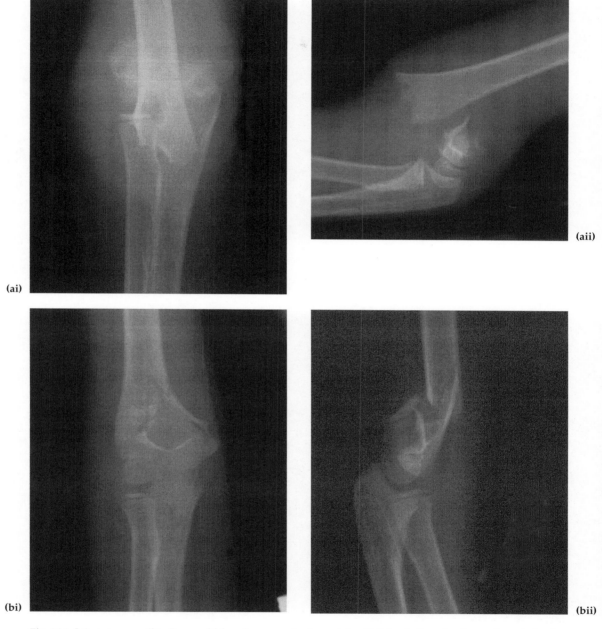

Fig. 34.3 Injury to a pre-élite 7-year-old female gymnast who sustained bilateral elbow fractures after missing her hold on the high bar: (ai) anteroposterior and (aii) lateral views of severely displaced left supracondylar humerus fracture, with vascular injury that caused loss of the radial and ulnar pulses; (bi) anteroposterior and (bii) lateral views of right supracondylar humerus fracture.

or possibly to stunt growth. Micheli, commenting on a study of spinal injuries in female gymnasts, stated that '15 h·week^{-1} may be an upper level for safe training for female gymnasts before incurring spinal injury' (Goldstein *et al.*, 1991). However, studies of other injuries have found problems related to overuse in gymnasts training as little as 4.5 h·week^{-1} (Chan *et al.*, 1991). Theintz *et al.* (1993) suggested 15–18 h·week^{-1} as a training threshold when there are concerns about growth restriction. However, Lindholm *et al.* (1994) found evidence of growth abnormality among gymnasts who trained on average only 10 h·week^{-1}. Therefore, it seems most likely that training hours are only one variable in the aetiology of injury and growth anomaly. Other factors, such as intensity of training and nutrition, must be considered.

DECREASED TRAINING WHEN GROWING RAPIDLY

Rapidly growing gymnasts have approximately twice the injury rate of gymnasts in a stable phase of growth as determined by Tanner staging and menarcheal status (Caine *et al.*, 1989). Among non-élite club gymnasts of average age 12.3 years (SD=2.0), the most important factors related to wrist pain were found to be intensity of training as related to age and later age of starting training, perhaps due to the gymnast's attempt to attain the skill level of her same-age peers (DiFiori *et al.*, 1996). This study also suggests that training should be less intense during times of rapid growth.

DECREASED TRAINING WHEN INJURED

A gymnast who trains before a significant injury has healed risks sustaining overuse injuries, as other structures must compensate for the weakened part. In addition, if she misses a move because the injured part gives way or because she buckles due to pain, she is likely to sustain a new acute injury. Although it is reasonable to practise moves that do not use the injured part,

most gymnastic moves use all parts of the body. Therefore, the safest course would often be simply to perform conditioning and flexibility work that would not aggravate the injury. Highly competitive gymnasts do not seem to heed such recommendations judging by the studies and memoirs discussed above.

COMPLETE REHABILITATION

In other sports, reinjury has been reported as a major source of time lost from training or competition. Among female gymnasts, a reinjury rate of 33% has been reported (Caine *et al.*, 1989). Both complete healing of the injury and complete rehabilitation of the injured region are important in preventing reinjury.

POSITIVE EMOTIONAL OUTLOOK

A retrospective study of 83 female club gymnasts found that the athletes who reported more injuries scored higher on measures of anxiety and tiredness, lower on composure and feeling energetic, and higher on cognitive anxiety. The question of whether these mood variables were the cause or the result of the injuries was not determined in this survey (Kolt & Kirkby, 1994). A prospective study of female competitive club gymnasts found an increased incidence of injury after an athlete had been practising a discipline for an extended time and the authors surmised that loss of focus or concentration might be a cause for these injuries (Lindner & Caine, 1990). Of course, muscle fatigue could be implicated at least equally with mental fatigue.

A prospective study of collegiate gymnasts did find that life stress in the preceding year, when coupled with poor current social support, predicted incidence of injury (Petrie, 1992). Since injury in a previous year would undoubtedly contribute to life stress, it may be impossible to sort out the contributions of previous injury, inadequate rehabilitation and poor focus from depression or anxiety not related to these other factors predisposing to injury.

Conclusion

Although research in the past 15 years has contributed to our understanding of the potential nutritional, developmental and musculoskeletal problems among competitive artistic gymnasts, very few investigators have published work concerning rhythmic gymnasts. Although the nutritional and developmental issues may be similar, injury patterns may be quite different.

Despite a high incidence of menstrual abnormalities among gymnasts during their competitive years, anecdotal evidence suggests that menarche is eventually attained and fertility unlikely to be impaired permanently. Growth may be permanently stunted among those gymnasts who train long hours and consume inadequate diets. However, additional investigation is needed to confirm both the findings and the possible causes of growth abnormalities.

Gymnastics is clearly one of the most dangerous sports practised by large numbers of girls and young women. Fortunately, there have been few cases of paralysis or death. However, the studies cited suggest that most competitive gymnasts can expect years of musculoskeletal problems related to injuries sustained during their gymnastics careers. Long-term follow-up of these athletes is needed to determine the severity and extent of these disabilities.

References

Albanese, S.A., Palmer, A.K., Kerr, D.R., Carpenter, C.W., Lisi, D. & Levinsohn, E.M. (1989) Wrist pain and distal growth plate closure of the radius in gymnasts. *Journal of Pediatric Orthopedics* **9**, 23–28.

Andrish, J.T. (1985) Knee injuries in gymnastics. *Clinics in Sports Medicine* **4**, 111–121.

Backx, F.J.G., Beijer, H.J.M., Bol, E. & Erich, W.B. (1991) Injuries in persons in high-risk sports: a longitudinal study of 1818 school children. *American Journal of Sports Medicine* **19**, 124–130.

Baxter-Jones, A.D., Helms, P., Baines-Preece, J. & Preece, M. (1994) Menarche in intensively trained gymnasts, swimmers and tennis players. *Annals of Human Biology* **21**, 407–415.

Bayliss, T. & Bedi, R. (1996) Oral, maxillofacial and general injuries in gymnasts. *Injury* **27**, 353–354.

Benardot, D. & Czerwinski, C. (1991) Selected body composition and growth measures of junior elite gymnasts. *Journal of the American Dietetic Association* **91**, 29–33.

Beunen, G. & Malina, R.M. (1996) Growth and biological maturation: relevance to athletic performance. In G. Beunen & R.M. Malina (eds) *The Child and Adolescent Athlete*, pp. 3–24. Blackwell Science, Oxford.

Caine, D., Cochrane, B., Cain, C. & Zemper, E. (1989) An epidemiologic investigation of injuries affecting young competitive female gymnasts. *American Journal of Sports Medicine* **17**, 811–820.

Cantu, R.C. (1995) Head and spine injuries in youth sports. *Clinics in Sports Medicine* **14**, 517–532.

Chan, D., Aldridge, M.J., Maffulli, N. & Davies, A.M. (1991) Chronic stress injuries of the elbow in young gymnasts. *British Journal of Radiology* **64**, 1113–1118.

Claessens, A.L., LeFevre, J., Beunen, G., De Smet, L. & Veer, A.M. (1996) Physique as a risk factor for ulnar variance in elite female gymnasts. *Medicine and Science in Sports and Exercise* **28**, 560–569.

De Smet, L., Claessens, A., Lefevre, J. & Beunen, G. (1994) Gymnast wrist: an epidemiologic survey of ulnar variance and stress changes of the radial physis in elite female gymnasts. *American Journal of Sports Medicine* **22**, 846–850.

DiFiori, J.P., Puffer, J.C., Mandelbaum, B.R. & Mar, S. (1996) Factors associated with wrist pain in the young gymnast. *American Journal of Sports Medicine* **24**, 9–14.

Dixon, M. & Fricker, P. (1993) Injuries to elite gymnasts over 10 yr. *Medicine and Science in Sports and Exercise* **25**, 1322–1329.

Forbes, L. (1996) Physical and emotional problems of elite female gymnasts (letter). *New England Journal of Medicine* **336**, 140–141.

Goldstein, J.D., Berger, P.E., Windler, G.E. & Jackson, D.W. (1991) Spine injuries in gymnasts and swimmers. An epidemiologic investigation. *American Journal of Sports Medicine* **19**, 463–468.

Greene, T.A. & Hillman, S.K. (1990) Comparison of support provided by a semirigid orthosis and adhesive ankle taping before, during, and after exercise. *American Journal of Sports Medicine* **18**, 498–506.

Jackson, D.W., Silvino, N. & Reiman, P. (1989) Osteochondritis in the female gymnast's elbow. *Arthroscopy* **5**, 129–136.

Kirchner, E.M., Lewis, R.D. & O'Connor, P.J. (1995) Bone mineral density and dietary intake of female college gymnasts. *Medicine and Science in Sports and Exercise* **27**, 543–549.

Kolt, G.S. & Kirkby, R.J. (1994) Injury, anxiety, and

mood in competitive gymnasts. *Perceptual and Motor Skills* **78**, 955–962.

Konermann, W. & Sell, S. (1992) The spine: a problem area in high performance artistic gymnastics. A retrospective analysis of 24 former artistic gymnasts of the German A team. *Sportverletz Sportschaden* **6**, 156–160.

Lindholm, C., Hagenfeldt, K. & Ringertz, B.M. (1994) Pubertal development in elite juvenile gymnasts. Effects of physical training. *Acta Obstetricia et Gynecologica Scandinavica* **73**, 269–273.

Lindholm, C., Hagenfeldt, K. & Ringertz, H. (1995) Bone mineral content of young female former gymnasts. *Acta Paediatrica* **84**, 1109–1112.

Lindner, K.J. & Caine, D.J. (1990) **Injury patterns of female competitive club gymnasts.** *Canadian Journal of Sport Science* **15**, 254–261.

Macgregor, J. & Moncur, J.A. (1977) Meralgia paraesthetica: a sports lesion in girl gymnasts. *British Journal of Sports Medicine* **11**, 16–19.

Maffulli, N., Chan, D. & Aldridge, M.J. (1992a) Derangement of the articular surfaces of the elbow in young gymnasts. *Journal of Pediatric Orthopedics* **12**, 344–350.

Maffulli, N., Chan, D. & Aldridge, M.J. (1992b) Overuse injuries of the olecranon in young gymnasts. *Journal of Bone and Joint Surgery* **74B**, 305–358.

Malina, R.M. (ed.) (1994) Physical growth and biological maturation of young athletes. *Exercise and Sport Sciences Reviews* **22**, 389–434.

Micheli, L.J., Hall, J.E. & Miller, M.E. (1980) Use of modified Boston brace for back injuries in athletes. *American Journal of Sports Medicine* **8**, 351–356.

Mishra, D.K., Friden, J., Schmitz, M.C. & Lieber, R.L. (1995) Anti-inflammatory medication after muscle injury: a treatment resulting in short-term improvement but subsequent loss of muscle function. *Journal of Bone and Joint Surgery* **77A**, 1510–1519.

Mubarak, S.J. & Carroll, N.C. (1981) Juvenile osteochondritis dissecans of the knee: etiology. *Clinical Orthopaedics and Related Research* **157**, 200.

Murakami, S. & Nakajima, H. (1984) Aseptic necrosis of the capitate bone in two gymnasts. *American Journal of Sports Medicine* **12**, 170–173.

Nichols, D.L., Sanborn, C.F., Bonnick, S.L., Ben-Ezra, V., Gench, B. & DiMarco, N.M. (1994) The effects of gymnastics training on bone mineral density. *Medicine and Science in Sports and Exercise* **26**, 1220–1225.

Normile, D. (1996) Where is women's gymnastics going? *International Gymnastics* **38**, 46–47.

O'Connor, P.J. & Lewis, R.D. (1997) Physical and emotional problems of elite female gymnasts (letter). *New England Journal of Medicine* **336**, 140–141.

Petrie, T.A. (1992) Psychosocial antecedents of athletic injury: the effects of life stress and social support on female collegiate gymnasts. *Behavioral Medicine* **18**, 127–138.

Retton, M.L., Karolyi, B. & Powers, J. (1986) *Mary Lou: Creating an Olympic Champion.* McGraw-Hill, New York.

Robinson, T.L., Snow-Harter, C., Taaffe, D.R., Gillis, D., Shaw, J. & Marcus, R. (1995) Gymnasts exhibit higher bone mass than runners despite similar prevalence of amenorrhea and oligomenorrhea. *Journal of Bone and Mineral Research* **10**, 26–35.

Roeper, R. (1996) Gymnastics: triumph or tragedy? *Chicago Sun-Times.*

Rosen, L.W. & Hough, D.O. (1986) Pathogenic weight-control behaviors of female college gymnasts. *Physician and Sportsmedicine* **16**, 140–146.

Roy, S., Caine, D. & Singer, K.M. (1985) **Stress changes of the distal radial epiphysis in young gymnasts.** A report of twenty-one cases and a review of the literature. *American Journal of Sports Medicine* **13**, 301–308.

Ryan, J. (1995) *Little Girls in Pretty Boxes: The Making and Breaking of Elite Gymnasts and Figure Skaters.* Doubleday, New York.

Sands, W.A. (1993) Women's gymnastics injuries: a 5-year study. *American Journal of Sports Medicine* **21**, 271–276.

Shapiro, M.S., Kabo, J.M., Mitchell, P.W., Loren, G. & Tsenter, M. (1994) Ankle sprain prophylaxis: an analysis of the stabilizing effects of braces and tape. *American Journal of Sports Medicine* **22**, 78–82.

Shih, C., Chang, C.Y., Penn, I.W., Tiu, C.M., Chang, T. & Wu, J.J. (1995) Chronically stressed wrists in adolescent gymnasts: MR imaging appearance. *Radiology* **195**, 855–859. [Published erratum appears in *Radiology* 1995, **197**, 319.]

Slemenda, C.W. & Johnston, C.C. (1993) High intensity activities in young women: site specific bone mass effects among female figure skaters. *Bone and Mineral* **20**, 125–132.

Steiner, M.E. & Micheli, L.J. (1985) Treatment of symptomatic spondylolysis and spondylolisthesis with the modified Boston brace. *Spine* **10**, 937–943.

Sundgot-Borgen, J. (1996) Eating disorders, energy intake, training volume, and menstrual function in high-level modern rhythmic gymnasts. *International Journal of Sports Nutrition* **6**, 100–109.

Tertti, M., Paajanen, H., Kujala, U.M., Alanen, A., Salmi, T.T. & Kormano, M. (1990) Disc degeneration in young gymnasts. A magnetic resonance imaging study. *American Journal of Sports Medicine* **18**, 206–208.

Theintz, G.E., Howald, H., Allemann, Y. & Sizonenko, P.C. (1989) Growth and pubertal development of young female gymnasts and swimmers: a correlation with parental data. *International Journal of Sports Medicine* **10**, 87–91.

Theintz, G.E., Howald, H., Weiss, U. & Sizonenko, P.C. (1993) Evidence for a reduction of growth potential in adolescent female gymnasts. *Journal of Pediatrics* **122**, 306–313.

Tofler, I.R., Stryer, B.K., Micheli, L.J. & Herman, L.R. (1996) Physical and emotional problems of elite female gymnasts. *New England Journal of Medicine* **335**, 281–283.

Tsai, L. & Wredmark., T. (1993) Spinal posture, sagittal mobility, and subjective rating of back problems in former female elite gymnasts. *Spine* **18**, 872–875.

Wadley, G.H. (1993) Women's intercollegiate gymnastics: injury patterns and 'permanent' medical disability. *American Journal of Sports Medicine* **21**, 314–320.

Chapter 35

Figure Skating

JANE M. MORAN

Introduction

Ice skating originated in northern Europe as an important means of transportation on frozen rivers, canals, lakes and ponds, and secondarily became an activity of recreational and social importance. As a sport, figure skating was recognized as a unique combination of art and athleticism. It was also one of the few sports considered 'lady-like' and so could be enjoyed by both women and men. Figure skating emerged as a form of entertainment for the European nobility and royalty during the 18th century. The International Skating Union (ISU) was founded in July 1892 at Scheveningen, The Netherlands. Today figure skating is recognized, practised and regulated in 55 nations around the world.

In this century, figure skating has enjoyed ever-increasing popularity in the recreational, competitive and professional arenas. The associated proliferation of indoor skating facilities has provided year-round access to high-quality ice surfaces. There are increasing demands on athletes at the competitive and professional levels to perform more and more difficult elements. This steady expansion of the 'performance envelope' has placed greater demands on those who assist athletes in gaining and maintaining the competitive edge: the coaches, who manage the complex process of performance enhancement, and the health professionals, who prevent and manage performance-threatening injury. Increased performance demands, increased training complexity and a broadening spectrum of injury point to

a need in modern figure skating for well-coordinated and focused research programmes to identify optimal methods of training and injury management.

The sport

The sport of figure skating includes five disciplines: compulsory figures, free (singles) skating, pairs, dance and precision (team skating). The ability to care for figure skaters properly requires at least a basic understanding of the unique skills, demands and risks of each of the five disciplines.

Compulsory figures

Each compulsory figure requires the skater to perform, or 'trace', two or three superimposed circles that form a variation of the figure 8. There are a total of 41 figures of increasing degrees of difficulty. In each figure, the skater must demonstrate control of the edge of the skate blade by tracing, with a bent knee, each circle of the figure as exactly as possible over the initial tracing. The skater traces each figure twice on each foot. This exercise demonstrates a skater's mastery of skate blade edges in controlling motion, speed, balance and precision of movement.

Free skating

In this discipline, a single skater performs jumps, spins and stroking (footwork) depending on the skater's level of technical ability. It is particularly important to understand the physical demands of jumps in order to advise the skater which elements he or she is ready to return to after injury. Figures 35.1 and 35.2 illustrate the various jumps and identify the approach, take-off and landing phases.

When 'approaching' a jump, a skater will be on an inside or outside edge of one skate. The take-off is from the blade of one skate (inside or outside edge) or from the blade with an assist from the toe-piece of the other skate blade. Single jumps or jumps of one and a half rotations do not produce significant torque on the take-off or landing leg. As the level of skill increases and

the skater begins to perform double, triple or quadruple jumps, increasingly greater rotational stresses are placed on the landing leg. When landing a jump, the skater must control the rotational component as well as absorbing the impact force when the blade contacts the ice. In controlling the rotational component during a spin or jump, the skater pushes both arms and free leg away from the axis of rotation. This increases the moment of inertia and reduces rotational speed. In this manner most of the rotational force is eliminated before the skater lands or changes feet and exits from the spin. In jumps, this manoeuvre must be timed perfectly so that the arms and legs open immediately before landing. If the

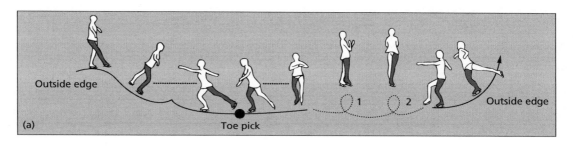

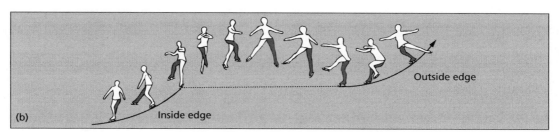

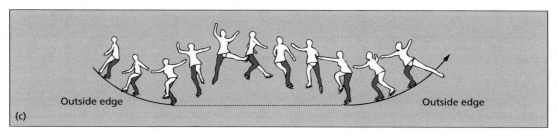

Fig. 35.1 Technique of figure skating jumps: approach, flight and landing for (a) the toe loop, (b) the salchow and (c) the loop. (From *Official Guide Book, Nagano*, 1998.)

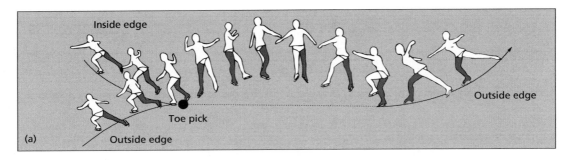

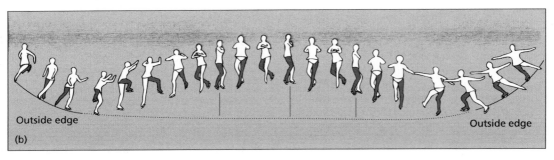

Fig. 35.2 Technique of figure skating jumps: approach, flight and landing for (a) the flip or Lutz and (b) the triple axel. (From *Official Guide Book, Nagano*, 1998.)

rotational forces are not controlled and dissipated just before landing, the rotational force is transmitted to the landing leg. When learning a multi-revolution jump, the skater will quite often over-rotate or under-rotate. This subjects the skater's landing leg to repeated impact and rotational forces and can lead to overuse injury.

During spins, rotation speeds are faster than during jumps but there is no landing impact for the skater to absorb. Spin direction is determined by the 'footedness' of the skater: right-footed skaters rotate anticlockwise; left-footed skaters clockwise. The skater rotates with arms and legs close to the body, usually in a tighter position while spinning than during a jump.

Pairs

Pairs skating combines free skating elements performed in unison by a pair of skaters, with other elements performed together such as lifts, throw jumps and coordinated and 'common-axis' spins. Whether the partners are together or apart, their movements should be synchronized. During spins about a common axis or side by side in unison, the skaters are vulnerable to lacerations from the blade of the partner's skate.

The lifts in pairs skating are becoming ever more daring and are increasingly the cause of fall-related injury. There are two kinds of lifts: the overhead lift and the twist lift. In the overhead lift, the male partner maintains physical contact with the female except momentarily during change in her position or during dismount. The male performs a one- or two-handed lift, raising the female partner overhead by her hips, axillae or hands. He supports her overhead with one or both of his hands with his arms fully extended while he skates forward, backward or rotates on the ice. The female must maintain her balance and centre of gravity once in the lifted position. The position of the female partner during the lift can be upright, horizontal or head down. The male partner must then check his position or rotation before lowering her smoothly to the ice.

In twist lifts (Fig. 35.3), the male lifts the female

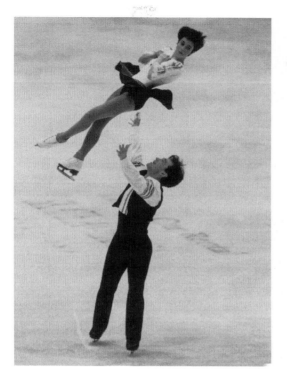

Fig. 35.3 Pair's twist lift: Shelby Lyons and Brian Wells of the USA at Skate America 1996. (Photo courtesy of ISU Media and Allsport.)

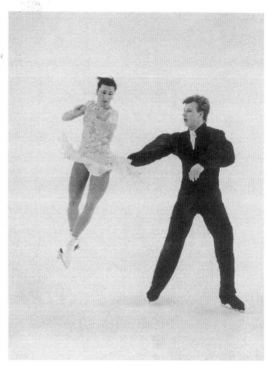

Fig. 35.4 Pairs throw jump: Marina Elstova and Andrei Bushkov of Russia at Skate Canada 1996. (Photo courtesy of ISU Media and Allsport.)

partner overhead and tosses her in the air. While airborne, she performs a half or full rotation before he catches her and lowers her to the ice. The couple may fall at any time during the execution of these lifts because of tripping, mistiming or fatigue. There is potential for serious injury if the female partner falls from the height of the lift or the male partner fails to catch her during the twist lift. Fortunately, in the majority of lifts, the male partner is often able to offer some assistance partially to break the force of the female partner's fall.

Throw jumps (Fig. 35.4) are another very exciting aspect of pairs skating that have an associated risk of injury to the female partner. In throw jumps, the male partner throws the female into the air and across the ice while she completes two or three revolutions in the air. Her height and dis-tance covered is far greater than any jump she could perform individually. The forces of impact on landing are consequently magnified, as are any errors in correcting the rotational forces discussed in the previous section.

Ice dancing

Ice dancing is based on the various aspects of dance and emphasizes rhythm, interpretation of music, precise steps, speed and carriage. It includes varied dance holds, intricate footwork, deep edges, and small lifts and spins. The ice dancer's skate blades have shorter tails in order to avoid becoming entangled with a partner's skates during the close footwork (Fig. 35.5). However, because of the intricate and at times rapid and entwined footwork, falls still occur,

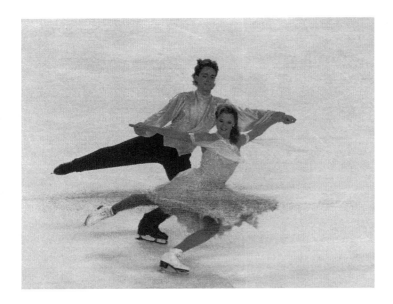

Fig. 35.5 Ice dancing: Shae Lynn Bourne and Victor Kraatz of Canada at Skate Canada 1996. (Photo courtesy of ISU Media and Allsport.)

often at high skating speeds, causing lacerations and other injuries.

Precision skating

Precision skating, also known as team skating, is characterized by complex formations and intricate transitions performed by teams of 12–24 skaters. The precision teams perform manoeuvres such as circles, lines, wheels, intersections and blocks (skaters lined up in more than two lines) (Fig. 35.6). The emphasis is on unison, accuracy of formations and synchronization of the team. Skaters are in close proximity to each other and one fall frequently causes a domino effect, resulting in more than one injury.

Physiological profile of skaters

Figure skating is a physically demanding sport that requires a unique combination of artistic ability and speed, agility, flexibility and power (Fig. 35.7). The increasing technical difficulty of figure skating has resulted in heightened demands on physical fitness. International study of figure skaters has helped to develop a physiological profile of these athletes. Gledhill (1997),

for example, reported that muscular power, flexibility, aerobic and anaerobic fitness all increase over the course of an individual skater's development, but body composition remains essentially unchanged. The developing physiological profile of the competitive figure skater has in turn formed the basis for monitoring and training programmes for skaters that address aerobic power, anaerobic power, muscular power, flexibility and body composition.

Competitive figure skaters train for approximately 10–11 months per year. Training frequency, duration and intensity of on-ice and off-ice training time parallels an increase in the technical calibre of the skater. Kjaer and Larsson (1992) showed that figure skaters have oxygen requirements comparable with those athletes whose sports are endurance related. When monitoring heart rates during the long programme it was demonstrated that skaters are at their maximal heart rates within the first minute of the programme. While skaters have above-average maximal oxygen consumption, their aerobic capacity is generally lower than many competitive athletes (Provost-Craig, 1997). The skater must therefore be maximally conditioned, both aerobically and anaerobically, in order to

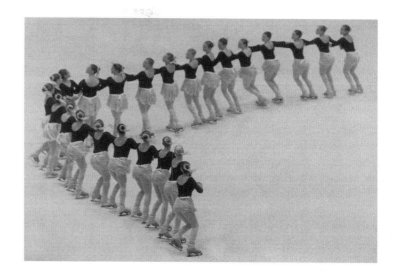

Fig. 35.6 Line formation in synchronized skating. (Photo courtesy of ISU Media and Allsport.)

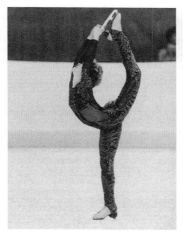
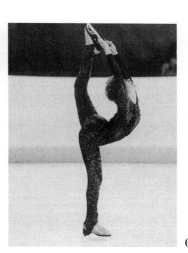

Fig. 35.7 Denize Biellman of Switzerland performing her famous spin, shown from two different sides. (Photo courtesy of Michel Perret, Foulis 4, CH-1260 Nyon.)

(a)   **(b)**

perform continuously at a high level throughout a modern free skating programme, maintaining sufficient strength and cardiovascular fitness to perform difficult jumps and maintain speed to the end. Now that the competitive season extends throughout the year, it is particularly important that skaters plateau at the peak of physical fitness.

Ross *et al.* (1976) demonstrated that both male and female figure skaters matured later than the average population. This corresponds with the study by Lockwood (1997) who reported that

the mean age at puberty of male and female skaters (Tanner stage 3) was 14±1.73 years. Lockwood (1997) and Niinima *et al.* (1979) reported that the mean starting age of competitive training has become significantly younger. Whereas senior skaters began training at a mean age of 7.7 years, juvenile skaters today begin training at an average age of 5.85 years. Not only are athletes training and competing at a younger age, but the physical demands of the sport have also changed dramatically, particularly jumping. Current figure skaters are generally shorter and leaner than skaters in the past. The increased and earlier emphasis on the performance of triple jumps has given younger, leaner skaters a competitive advantage and allowed them to surpass the jumping performance of the more physically mature senior skaters. In these young skaters, the vigorous physical demands of training and of impact loading are being superimposed on the biological demands of normal growth and development. There are few research studies that document the ability of the developing human body, and specifically the musculoskeletal system, to respond to these increased forces and stresses. Slemenda and Johnston (1993) and Lockwood (1997) have reported that high-impact, repetitive load-type training affects bone mineral density at the specific loaded sites. Lockwood (1997) reported a significant difference in bone mineral density between the dominant and non-dominant lower extremity of figure skaters in the prepubertal, pubertal and postpubertal populations. However, there are no longitudinal studies that document what effects training at this young age will have on the musculoskeletal system in the years to come.

Equipment

As in any sport, the equipment necessary to participate plays an integral part in safety, enjoyment and performance. In the case of figure skating, equipment issues focus on the skate. The components of a modern skate are illustrated in Fig. 35.8. Injuries to the figure skater can be related to both boot components and blade placement.

Boots

The skate boot is made of leather and is constructed around a steel shank that runs down the centre of the boot sole. This steel shank forms the compound curve of the sole and holds the other boot components in place. The top portion of the

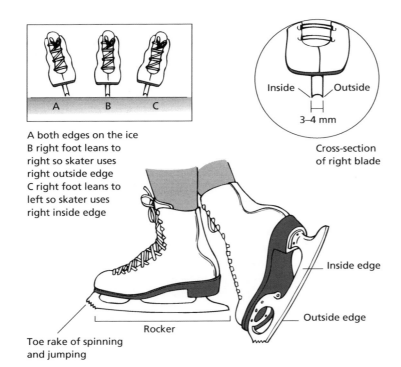

A both edges on the ice
B right foot leans to right so skater uses right outside edge
C right foot leans to left so skater uses right inside edge

Cross-section of right blade

Fig. 35.8 Parts of a skate.

boot surrounding the leg is lower at the back to allow some degree of plantar flexion. A dancer's boot may be modified by a 'danceback stay': a notch is cut in the rear of the boot and the lining extended and rolled over for softness, thus allowing for greater knee bends and toe points. Boots can be obtained from stock or custom made. Boots purchased off the shelf are generally made of thinner leather and vary greatly in quality and price. Custom boots, while generally more expensive, are available for skaters who require a closer fit and increased support. There is a spectrum of boot strength or stiffness, and it is important to match the boot to the skater's age, weight, technical level and frequency of skating. All skaters require a boot that fits well and offers adequate support. Overly stiff boots require excessive breaking-in times and also place the skater at risk for injury. Conversely, if the boot is not stiff enough, the skater does not have the required support to perform the more demanding jumps, and the boot breaks down quickly. This also places the skater at risk for injury. The boot strength equation is therefore modified by the uniqueness of each skater. For example, the beginner, who is younger with less weight and muscular force, requires a boot pliable enough to allow for ankle and knee bends, while the skater performing triple jumps requires a heavily re-inforced boot for increased support on landing. Because the shape of the foot is unique to every skater and in order to avoid injuries to the feet and ankles, the boot must be constructed to afford enough space for the foot and yet fit snugly so as not to cause any movement of the foot in the boot. In order to avoid soft tissue injuries as well as stress fractures, the boot must be adaptable in order to allow corrections to accommodate irregular feet or to allow the use of orthotics.

There are a variety of methods for softening the leather of new boots. Some time should be spent with the feet in new boots before wearing the skates on the ice. Wearing boots around the house (e.g. while watching TV and doing homework) with blades mounted and guards in place is a common method. Wearing boots without the blades mounted is not recommended as it allows flexion of the forefoot, a movement that does not normally occur during skating. Also, this could predispose the midsole and outsole of the boot to separate from the central shank. Feet should be regularly checked for any pressure areas and the corresponding part of the boot padded or punched out. Manoeuvres such as stroking, back crossovers and knee bends allow the skater to adjust to the feel of the boot and allow proper boot motion to be obtained. New boots should not be laced too tightly; instead, the skater should unlace and lace the boots frequently as they soften.

A consensus statement developed at the 1997 International Congress in Medicine and Science of Figure Skating (sponsored by the ISU) recommends that a boot should:

- be lightweight;
- be aesthetically pleasing;
- allow plantar flexion and dorsiflexion;
- limit inversion and eversion;
- fit well and adapt to the shape of the skater's foot easily;
- accommodate a device to balance the foot within the boot such as an orthotic;
- be dry inside;
- be made of materials with characteristics as good as or better than leather.

Further research to develop a boot that meets these criteria will hopefully aid in the prevention of boot-related injuries.

Blades

The skate blade is purchased separately and selected according to intended use (e.g. free skate or dance). In coronal section the blade is approximately 3–4 mm in width, with the contact surface grooved convexly upward so that there is a hollow between the medial or inside edge and lateral or outside edge. The blade is also curved along its length, referred to as the rocker (see Fig. 35.8). Therefore at any time the skater should be balanced on either an outside or inside edge, with only a small portion of the total blade in contact with the ice. In the figure skating disciplines the blades vary in the degree of rocker or curvature of the blade, the depth of the hollow, and the number, size and distribution of toe-picks. Figures blades have a greater rocker, while dance blades usually have a shorter tail to permit close footwork with a partner.

The blade is either riveted or screwed to the sole of the boot. The skater is very sensitive to placement of the blade: small adjustments can have an inordinate effect on balance when performing complex elements. Inappropriate blade placement can also lead to overuse injuries in the lower extremities as a result of overcorrecting an edge on landing jumps. As a rule, the skate blade should line up just medial to the front toe seam and directly midline on the heel. The skater should make frequent checks to ensure that the blade is securely fixed to the sole in order to prevent injury when landing with an unstable blade mount.

Skate fit

When the boot is laced, the foot should fit snugly in the heel, arch and ball areas in order to provide optimal support. The toes should be able to wiggle freely, but not slide from side to side. The heel should not move out of the back cup of the boot when bending the knees. The foot should fit in the boot locked in a neutral position (Podhajsky, 1997).

Because figure skaters begin skating at an early age, boot fit is critically important. Young skaters spend long hours on the ice perfecting both free skating and compulsory figures. Boots are selected to fit snugly, with only a skating leotard over the foot. This fit may be perfect at first, but as the young skater's foot grows the boot remains the same size. The average skater changes boots about once per year and perhaps less frequently than ideal (often due to the cost of new boots). If not closely monitored in the young skater, the feet may become increasingly cramped leading to the development of hammer-toes, corns, calluses and other pressure-related injuries.

Injuries

Documentation of trends in the type and frequency of injury encountered in figure skating will require marked improvements in, and standardization of, reporting. The following section is intended as a summary of the available information on figure skating injuries.

The frequency and spectrum of injury in figure skating appear to be increasing. There are many aspects of the sport contributing to this increase: (i) figure skating has experienced a rapid growth in popularity; (ii) the number of participants and the hours of training have increased; (iii) since figures were dropped from the competitive aspect of skating in 1991, skaters spend more time training in free skating than compulsory figures; (iv) there has also been rapid growth in the technical and physiological demands of the free skating programmes; and (v) there has been a trend for children to begin training seriously at younger ages (Niinima et al., 1979; Zauner et al., 1989; Lockwood, 1997).

Notwithstanding the above, there are a number of reasons why it is difficult to document the incidence, severity and aetiology of figure skating injuries. To begin with, there are few acceptable studies that address this issue. Those studies that are available may not reflect the true incidence of injuries due to under-reporting. Like other athletes, skaters may not report an injury if they feel it will affect their chances of selection for competitions. Athletes may also perceive that they would appear weak or disadvantaged to their competitors or to the judges. Figure skaters who do continue to train and compete with overuse-type injuries may be excluded from a study if the injury is of insufficient severity to curtail practice or competition. Finally, as illustrated by Kjaer and Larsson (1992), athletes may simply forget an injury. The subjects in their prospective study only recalled 83% of their injuries at the end of a 1-year period. This is particularly relevant when reviewing the literature on figure skating injuries as the majority of published information is derived from questionnaires administered retrospectively to skaters.

The injury rate in figure skating relative to other sports is largely unknown. Studies by Brock and Striowski (1986), Smith and Ludington (1989) and Kjaer and Larsson (1992) report a lower injury rate in figure skaters compared with that reported in a study by Lowry and Leveau (1982) on gymnasts, athletes who spend similar amounts of time in practice and performance.

Figure skating injuries can be classified into acute (due to episodic macrotrauma) and overuse (due to repetitive microtrauma) injuries. Several studies have reported the proportion of acute and overuse injuries and the predominance of lower extremity injuries in figure skaters. Table 35.1 shows the number of injuries compared with the number of participating skaters, Table 35.2 the types of injuries sustained and Table 35.3 the anatomical location of the reported injuries. In a retrospective study by Brock and Striowski (1986), 50% of reported injuries were acute, including fractures, sprains and cartilage tears, while 43% were overuse injuries, including tendonitis, shin splints and chondromalacia patellae. A retrospective study of 14 skaters by Brown and McKeag (1987) showed that acute injuries (muscular strains, ligamentous sprains, fractures, haematomas) accounted for the largest proportion of injuries in singles skating, and that the lower extremities were the site of two-thirds of all injuries.

Smith and Ludington (1989) reported a 9-month prospective study that examined the incidence, severity and cause of injuries sustained by 48 skaters, of whom 32 were élite pairs skaters

and 16 élite ice dancers. The élite senior female pairs skaters and female ice dancers sustained the highest injury rate. Of the 49 injuries reported, 33 were serious enough significantly to alter or interrupt training for at least 7 days. The types of injury were similar to those seen in the study by Brown and McKeag (1987), and included concussions, lacerations, fractures, dislocations, haematomas and muscle strains. Smith and Ludington (1989) also showed that lower extremity injuries predominated in both pairs and ice dancing, and that the number of acute injuries (mostly lift-related) outnumbered overuse injuries. A smaller sample of 14 pairs skaters studied by Brown and McKeag (1987) showed less involvement of the lower extremity and a higher prevalence of injuries in the upper extremities and axial region.

In a retrospective study by Garrick (1982), females had more overuse than acute injuries; again, the lower extremity predominated, the knee, foot and ankle being the common sites of injury. The predominance of injury to the lower extremity is a recurrent theme in the studies by Smith and Micheli (1982), Brock and Striowski (1986), Brown and McKeag (1987), Smith and Ludington (1989) and Kjaer and Larsson (1992). The commonest injuries in these studies include joint sprains, muscle strains, patellofemoral pain, tendonitis, tibial periostitis, haematomas, lacerations and fractures.

Tight, unyielding boots have been implicated in the aetiology of many lower extremity injuries. Jumping sports depend not only on the knee, hip and thigh but also on the ankle and calf to generate the forces and counter-forces necessary to

Table 35.1 Number of figure skating injuries compared with the number of participating skaters

	Smith & Micheli (1982)	Brock & Striowski (1986)	Brown & McKeag (1987)	Smith & Ludington (1989)	Kjaer & Larsson (1992)
No. of skaters	19	60	14	48	8
No. of injuries	52	28	39 singles 9 pairs	49	18

Table 35.2 Types of figure skating injuries

	Smith & Micheli (1982)	Brock & Striowski (1986)	Brown & McKeag (1987)	Smith & Ludington (1989)	Kjaer & Larsson (1992)
Concussion	3 (5.8%)		Singles, 3 (8%) Pairs, 3 (33%)	2 (4%)	
Fracture	3 (8%)	1 (3.6%)	Singles, 8 (21%) Pairs, 2 (22%)	4 (8%)	
Lacerations	2 (3.8%)		Singles, 2 (5%) Pairs, 1 (11%)	5 (10%)	
Periostitis	5 (9.6%)			1 (2%)	2 (11%)
Joint strain	9 (17.3%)	6 (21%)	Singles, 3 (8%) Pairs, 1 (11%)	8 (16%)	9 (50%)
Muscle sprain	9 (17.3%)		Singles, 12 (31%)	13 (28%)	2 (11%)
Soft tissue, non-specific	8 (15.3%)	8 (28.5%)	Singles, 3 (8%)		1 (5.6%)
Haematoma/ contusion	2 (3.8%)		Singles, 6 (15%) Pairs, 2 (22%)	5 (10%)	
Bursitis	6 (11.5%)			4 (8%)	
Tendon	5 (9.6%)	10 (37.5%)	Singles, 1 (3%)	7 (14%)	4 (22.2%)
Nerve			Singles, 1 (3%)		
Teeth		1 (3.6%)			
Non-skating		2 (7.1%)			

Table 35.3 Anatomical location of figure skating injuries*

	Smith & Micheli (1982)	Brown & McKeag (1987)	Smith & Ludington (1989)	Kjaer & Larsson (1992)
Foot	6 (12%)	3 (6%)	6 (12%)	1 (6%)
Ankle	10 (19%)	3 (6%)	7 (14%)	7 (39%)
Leg	9 (17%)	3 (6%)	3 (6%)	2 (11%)
Knee	6 (12%)	11 (23%)	10 (20%)	5 (28%)
Thigh	1 (2%)		4 (8%)	
Hip/buttock	6 (12%)	9 (19%)	5 (10%)	
Low back	6 (12%)	4 (8%)	4 (8%)	2 (11%)
Upper back		2 (4%)	2 (4%)	
Chest/rib	1 (2%)	1 (2%)	1 (2%)	
Head	4 (8%)	6 (13%)	2 (4%)	
Shoulder/arm	1 (2%)	4 (8%)	1 (2%)	
Elbow/forearm		1 (2%)		
Wrist		1 (2%)	1 (2%)	
Hand	2 (4%)		3 (6%)	1 (6%)
Total	52	48	49	18

*The studies reviewed did not use standardized inclusion criteria; therefore, although it is possible to obtain a general impression of the relative frequency of injury to various anatomical areas, these proportions should be interpreted with caution. Figures are number of reported injuries to that anatomical area. Figures in parentheses represent percentage of total reported injuries; total may exceed 100% due to multiple areas of injury in a particular skater.

obtain maximum jump height and to absorb the impact of landing. Figure skating is the only jumping sport that limits the ankle joint and calf muscles by the use of rigid boot support. The high heel and inflexible ankle portion of the boot do not allow skaters to use their ankles effectively in plantar flexion during jump take-offs or to cushion their landings. Lockwood (1996) performed a kinematics analysis of the landing phase of two technically different types of single, double and triple jumps performed on ice. The results indicated that both knee and hip flexion increased with additional revolutions but that only minimal ankle flexion occurred. This was attributed to the stability of the boot, which provided a mechanical block to increased ankle flexion. The lack of dorsiflexion flexibility in the skating boot may cause increased forces to be transmitted higher up the leg on landing. The force absorbed by the knee extensor mechanism during landing contributes to the development of anterior knee pain and overuse injury. Smith et al. (1991) reported on anterior knee pain in adolescent figure skaters. They examined 46 skaters, 14 (30%) of whom had anterior knee pain syndromes, including patellar tendonitis, Osgood–Schlatter disease and patellofemoral pain syndrome. The female-to-male ratio of anterior knee pain was 2:1. In the study by Brown and McKeag (1987) more than half the skaters reported knee pain. Richards and Henley (1996) stated that the ankle plays an important role in jumping and landing, and that a significant portion (>30%) of the impact at landing is attenuated by the ankle. Richards et al. studied ground reaction forces, limb kinematics and limb kinetics for backward drop jumps from a height of 30 cm in skaters wearing a rigid boot and those wearing a boot with an articulation to allow free motion of the ankle in the sagittal plane. They found that ground reaction forces were 23% less, ankle range of movement in the sagittal plane was about 25% greater and the knee angle was significantly straighter at impact in the articulated boot. Considering these findings it was concluded that the increased mobility afforded the ankle in the sagittal plane enabled the skaters

more effectively to attenuate the forces generated at impact on landing. Smith and Ludington (1989) identified 21.2% of injuries as related to the boot, while Brock and Striowski (1986) noted a comparable incidence of 14.3%. Davis and Litman (1979) noted the foot as a primary site of lower extremity discomfort and injury among 45 female skaters aged 9–18 years. Figure 35.9 illustrates the primary areas of the foot affected by the boot but does not include all the possible secondary overuse-type injuries incurred as a result of altered ankle biomechanics.

Rapid growth may contribute to injuries related to muscle flexibility or boot fit. Achilles tendonitis is a very common boot-related problem. The boot has a slight heel raise so that the foot is slightly plantar flexed, which leads to relative shortening of the gastrosoleus muscle and the Achilles tendon. This lack of flexibility seems to have a strong relationship with development of Achilles tendonitis. The Achilles tendon is also subject to pressure from the proximal rim of the boot and may be injured during repeated toe jumps where the foot is maximally plantar flexed in the boot.

Ankle sprains are a common injury reported in the majority of articles on skating injuries. Authorsen et al. (1997) and Danowski (1997) found that the foot and ankle incur the largest number of injuries in the figure skater. Danowski (1997) described a foot instability syndrome in which skaters spend so much time (several hours per day since childhood) in a reinforced boot that they lose strength and proprioception about the ankle joint. The skater's conditioning programme should therefore incorporate exercises to maintain and improve on the ankle joint's inherent proprioception and stability. Although less directly related to the boot, groin strain and plantar fasciitis are common, especially in skaters with high arches and tight calf muscles.

Of the overuse injuries reported by Smith and Micheli (1982) in 19 competitive skaters, low back pain was the most frequent complaint. Lumbar strain was also reported by Smith and Ludington (1989) and Kjaer and Larsson (1992) and is associated with the repeated hyperexten-

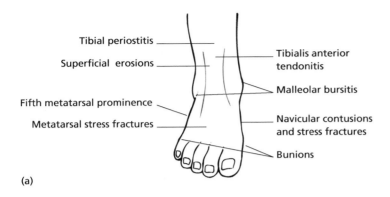

(a)

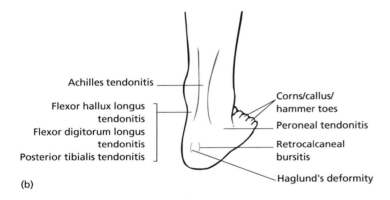

(b)

Fig. 35.9 Principal areas of the skater's foot affected by the boot fit: (a) front and (b) back of the foot.

sion and disc-loading of the low back during frequent jumping and landing.

Precision team skating is just developing into a recognized competitive sport and there are no published data available with regard to injuries. However, the potential for injury during competition or practice is great because of the number of skaters in close proximity on a limited ice surface. A review of injuries sustained at the ISU World Challenge Cup in 1996 (374 skaters participating in 14 teams) revealed 109 reported injuries (C.F. McCarthy, personal communication, 1996) (Table 35.4).

Injury prevention

Figure skating injuries occur as a result of episodic macrotrauma (acute) or recurrent microtrauma (overuse), or a combination of these, to the musculoskeletal structure of the skater. In the case of acute injury, it is difficult to decrease the numbers of lacerations, contusions, fractures and concussions that occur in a sport with some inherent risk. However, microtrauma or overuse syndromes, unlike acute injuries, are largely preventable through effective training programmes and education. Brock and Striowski (1986) documented the time lost due to acute and overuse injuries and found that the potentially preventable overuse injuries kept skaters off the ice longer than acute injuries.

Figure skating has drawn on the experience of other sports that suggest proper conditioning reduces overuse injuries and thereby decreases training time lost due to these injuries. Aleshinsky et al. (1988) state that strengthening and conditioning programmes are essential to continued success in figure skating because they maximize performance and reduce injury. Smith et al. (1991) showed a direct relationship between

Table 35.4 ISU World Challenge Cup 1996: injuries by anatomical location. (Data from C.F. McCarthy, personal communication, 1996)

	Concussion	Fracture/ dislocation	Soft-tissue injury
Head	5		
Nasal		2	
Coccyx		2	
Vertebrae		3	
Clavicle		4	
Finger		7	6
Wrist		9	1
Forearm/arm		4	
Elbow		2	
Shoulder		2	2
Toe/foot		2	1
Ankle		6	20
Patella		1	
Knee		2	8
Lower leg		3	2
Neck			2
Low back			5
Other			
Muscle tear			2
Tendonitis			4
Tendon laceration			2
Total	5	49	55

hamstring and quadriceps muscle tightness and knee pain. Lack of flexibility in the quadriceps causes an increased load to be placed on the quadriceps mechanism, leading to overuse syndromes such as traction apophysitis, patellofemoral symptoms and patellar tendonitis. Lack of quadriceps strength results in decreased ability to absorb forces through the knees, which in turn leads to lateral patellar compression. Ferstle (1979) described the use of off-ice training for the prevention of injuries. McMaster et al. (1979) published a 3-month programme which showed that graduated on-ice interval training and off-ice weight training and flexibility improved cardiovascular fitness and enhanced performance. Smith (1996) conducted a 4-year longitudinal study of 48–52 skaters aged 11–29 years. Over the 4-year period various training adjuncts and recommendations were introduced to the skaters at the training camps, including advice about weight training, preseason medical advice and examinations, boot checks, ballet and sports psychology. Over this time there was a marked reduction in injuries. The decreased injury rate was attributed to increased strength, flexibility and knowledge, which led to earlier intervention and decreased emotional stress in the course of injury. Yu (1996) supports the concept that the incidence of injury decreases dramatically with increased flexibility and routine stretching regimes.

Good postural alignment, adequate flexibility and sufficient strength are basic requirements for the athletic and artistic components of figure skating. Correct biomechanics, graduated training time and intensity, and progression of muscle strength and flexibility are the keys to avoiding overuse injuries. The areas that predominantly require increased flexibility are the lower extremity (quadriceps, gastrosoleus complex, hamstrings, hips), trunk (extension, flexion and lumbodorsal fascia) and upper extremity (shoulders). The areas that require strengthening include the primary muscles for jumping (gluteus maximus, gluteus medius, hamstrings, quadriceps, gastrosoleus, tibialis anterior). Trunk stability, including stabilization of the spine through abdominal strengthening, is very important in jumping. Better jumpers have larger differences between their moments of inertia (degree of 'openness') at the instant of take-off and the most closed position during flight. This **requires good upper body strength, particularly** all the shoulder girdle muscles (abductors, adductors and internal rotators) (Aleshinsky *et al.*, 1988). Upper body strength is particularly important in pairs skaters in order to prevent injuries during lifts. In the male partner, upper body and trunk strengthening should include a weight programme that incorporates the manner in which the lifts are performed on the ice. Improved strength of the arm and leg adductor muscles improves the quality of a skater's spin.

Acute injuries such as contusions and haematomas can be decreased by wearing touchdown pants, which have padding over the buttock and lateral thigh to cushion bony prominences during falls. Acute ankle injuries can be prevented by incorporating strengthening and proprioception exercises into off-ice conditioning programmes. Authorsen *et al.* (1997) reported that off-ice testing of the ankles of élite skaters indicated poorly developed strength of the ligaments and peroneal muscles stabilizing the ankle. Figure skaters should therefore increase strength and proprioception training of the ankle in order to develop and maintain the active muscular stability and response time of the ankle. Not only will this help to prevent inadvertent ankle injuries away from the ice, which affect the ability to return to skating, but will also protect the skater from ankle injury on the ice as the passive stability inherent in new boots progressively lessens throughout the season.

Some of the acute injuries that occur in pairs skating because of the risks inherent in the lifts, throws and jumps can be avoided by off-ice training. Moskvina (1997) advocates practising these techniques in a gym in order to develop strength, timing, height and lean in the air, and recommends that acrobatic manoeuvres be performed using a rubber or foam mat in order to decrease the impact on landing. This allows skaters to learn increasing control of the lift, the number of revolutions in the twist lift and to correct landing technique before attempting the same elements on the ice. Injuries due to falls from heights can be avoided if the **female partner practises the necessary movements of a lift on the** floor or gymnastics bar. Practising the motor components of a lift with the male lying on the floor or sitting in a chair eliminates both the risk of falls for the female partner and the risk of back injury for the male partner. Practising lifts as a pair off the ice improves strength and technique and improves confidence when the manoeuvres are transferred to the ice.

Although figure skaters invest many hours of daily training, only a small portion of this time incorporates activities that enhance conditioning. Skating is a highly anaerobic and moderately aerobic activity in which the skater performs with a maximal heart rate for 2–5 min. Off-ice training allows the skater to train at the supramaximal cardiovascular levels reached while doing difficult jumps. A high $\dot{V}_{O_{2max}}$ in conjunction with an ability to tolerate high levels of lactic acid is recognized as a competitive advantage in figure skating.

In response to the gradually emerging body of research specific to their sport, figure skaters have gradually expanded off-ice training in order to enhance overall conditioning and performance and to decrease training time lost to injury. Off-ice conditioning must be incorporated into the training programme so that it does not interfere with the on-ice component but rather supplements it. A comprehensive training programme must be focused as closely as possible on the skater's stated goals and should be based on the results of physiological testing, biomechanical alignment and present level of technical ability.

Medical concerns

Exercise-induced bronchospasm

Exercised-induced bronchospasm (EIB) results in airflow obstruction that typically occurs 5–15 min after strenuous exercise. Symptoms may include shortness of breath or wheezing, although occasionally the only symptom may be coughing after exercise. EIB has been documented in 70–80% of athletes with asthma and 40% of people who have allergies (Schroeckenstein & Busse, 1988; McCarthy, 1989). Athletes at risk for EIB include those with a past history of asthma or environmental allergies and those with a history of coughing or wheezing after strenuous exercise. EIB can be exacerbated when competing in a cold, dry environment. Conversely, the severity of the bronchospasm associated with exercise can be decreased by a long warm-up prior to the event.

Provost-Craig *et al.* (1996) studied 100 competitive skaters to determine the incidence of EIB in competitive skating. In this study, pulmonary function tests completed at rink-side showed an overall incidence of EIB of 30–38%. Screening for EIB in youths participating in physically demanding, cold-weather sports such as figure skating is necessary for proper identification and treatment. With appropriate treatment, athletes can improve their performance as well as their enjoyment of the sport. Education is important in both identification and treatment. Early identification depends on education of athletes, parents and coaches. An effective treatment programme should communicate the knowledge that EIB is an exaggerated, reversible airway response to exercise that occurs in many athletes and that can be successfully managed in most cases. Athletes must be aware that using an inhaler for EIB does not necessarily mean that they have asthma. Treatment compliance with non-pharmacological and pharmacological interventions is improved through education. Athletes who exhibit a reduction in peak expiratory flow rates of >10% after exercise are candidates for treatment (Pierson, 1988).

Nutrition

Competitive success in figure skating demands grace, strength, flexibility and endurance, as skaters are judged on both technical and artistic performance. It is extremely important for the skater to satisfy the energy requirements for training and competition while maintaining optimum weight and body composition for the artistic aspect of the sport, and nutrition is therefore a vital component of performance enhancement and injury avoidance.

The aesthetic quality a skater presents to the judges often adds to the artistic merit of the performance, although this aspect should not overshadow other factors in achieving success (technical ability, training, mental preparedness). It is imperative that a skater does not succumb to pursuing a set weight for aesthetic reasons that, in the long run, adversely affects her health and performance. Nutritional deficiencies result in reduced exercise capacity, increased heart rate, decreased oxygen uptake, decreased work tolerance, a weakened immune system and an increased risk of overuse injury. Coaches, families, skaters and the medical profession all have a part to play in preventing eating disorders in athletes.

Generally, most trained athletes have a lower body fat content than non-athletic subjects of similar age and maturity. Several nutritional studies have been conducted on competitive female figure skaters. Ziegler (1996) noted that in both males and females aged 11–18 years caloric intakes were below the recommended daily allowance for age and energy output, especially for females. He also reported that the iron and folic acid status, as well as the endurance, of figure skaters varied with the seasons and were significantly lower during the competitive season.

It is often difficult for competitive skaters and coaches to eat properly. At rink-side, in hotel restaurants and at competitions in foreign countries, healthy nutritional choices are sometimes limited. Proper nutrition promotes effective weight control, allows the individual to be comfortable with her appearance, improves physical and mental performance, and improves the perception of health and well-being. All of this helps to improve self-esteem. Skaters who are well nourished can train effectively, with increased concentration and decreased stress, in order to perform more consistently to their full potential.

Psychological stress

Some skaters experience significant psychosocial stresses at very young ages compared with non-skating, non-competitive counterparts. Stress can be increased if the skater lives away from home and lacks the support of the family environment. Parents and other family members may sacrifice time and money, which sometimes increases the pressures on the skater to attain unrealistic goals. In addition to these sources of stress, there is also the social isolation from non-skating peer groups imposed by the time requirements of rigorous training schedules.

A supportive family and a good working relationship with a sensitive coach are two elements necessary for success in competitive figure skating. Success for a particular skater is represented by the achievement of a common goal arrived at through discussions with the skater, other family members and the coach. In pursuit of this goal, competitive skaters can benefit from effective stress management training, psychosocial skills enhancement and motivational interventions.

Injury management (rehabilitation)

Rehabilitation of musculoskeletal injury is most effective when conducted in a multidisciplinary environment. Depending on the nature and severity of the injury and the anticipated time away from competition, the rehabilitation team may include a sports medicine physician, physiotherapist (manual therapist), physiologist, sports psychologist and nutritionist. The degree of involvement of various members of the team with the athlete, coach and parent depends

on the injury and the goals of rehabilitation. Throughout the rehabilitation programme, constant re-evaluation and modification are necessary to accommodate the athlete's progress and graduated return to full participation. Overall, the goal is safely to return the athlete to her previous level of participation as soon as possible by maximizing function and minimizing reinjury. The general sports medicine rehabilitation approach and the treatment of soft-tissue injuries has been well delineated in other sports medicine texts. The following therefore only outlines those techniques of specific use in the recovery of figure skaters.

Like all athletes, injured skaters are reluctant to give up their sport for any period of time. Even if the skater is following an off-ice conditioning and rehabilitation programme, she will become isolated. The medical personnel responsible for the rehabilitation of a skater should make every attempt to keep the skater on the ice in some capacity. In this regard it is important that physicians and therapists treating an injured skater have an understanding of the various aspects of skating so that they can advise the skater about 'relative rest' and protection of the injured body part while maintaining some on-ice training. Assuming this knowledge of the sport, the medical team can provide guidance to the skater, coach and often the parent as to the ability of the injured area to tolerate the stresses of the various skating elements. Uninterrupted association with the arena of competitive endeavour maintains the psychological health and commitment of the serious or competitive skater.

Almost all overuse injuries are treated non-operatively. Treatment involves settling the body's inflammatory response in order to allow healing to occur, while investigating the likely cause of repetitive localized microtrauma, which usually involves altering the skater's boot, technique, training programme, muscle strength, flexibility or biomechanics. This applies to the majority of knee and lower leg injuries excluding the specific boot-related injuries discussed below.

Boot-related injuries

STRESS FRACTURES

All stress fractures require review of the skater's nutritional, training and menstrual history. Stress fractures of the fibula are caused by pressure from the hard rim of the boot and can be prevented by padding the proximal portion of the boot with orthopaedic felt or lamb's-wool, ensuring correct placement of the skate blade, and improving strength and flexibility of the lower extremity. Navicular stress fractures should bear no weight during the healing period. Rarely, surgery is required for ununited or displaced fractures. Biomechanical stresses must be identified and relieved. Metatarsal stress fractures are caused by the repetitive localized trauma of landing from jumps. The skate itself provides no shock absorption and in addition limits ankle dorsiflexion, which would normally attenuate the impact force. In this situation, skaters must eliminate all moves that aggravate their symptoms both on and off the ice. Most skaters can continue stroking and compulsory figures but may require increased support for walking activities off the ice. To prevent recurrence of metatarsal stress fractures, a shock-absorbing insole is placed in the skate and any abnormal weight distribution across the foot corrected by use of an orthotic.

PAINFUL BUMPS

Painful accessory navicular bones are very common. These accessory navicular bones can cause a medial mid-foot prominence that can be exacerbated by overpronation. Correction of overpronation is helpful, although the boot-maker should also punch out the appropriate part of the boot in order to avoid pressure on these areas. Similar pressure areas occur over the base of the fifth metatarsal. Calluses and corns over the dorsal aspect of the toes are very common. The dorsal portions of the digits rub against the toe box of the boot while trying to grip the insole to achieve better control of the

skate. These are rarely painful but at times require doughnut-shaped padding.

Large bursae can develop over the bony prominences of the foot and ankle due to excessive pressure of the boot against these areas. These bursae occur over the malleolli, calcaneal tuberosity, navicular bone and anterior tibial tendon (Fig. 35.10). In most cases malleollar bursae do not interfere with training but are more of a nuisance in getting the boot to fit. Once the skate is on, the skater adjusts the laces repeatedly as fluid is extruded from the bursae due to increasing pressure from the tightened boot. However, the fluid tends to reaccumulate once the skate is removed. Although the bursae can be aspirated and injected with corticosteroid in an attempt to prevent reaccumulation, this is not particularly successful. The skater can also pad

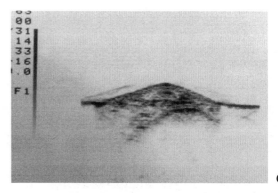

(a)

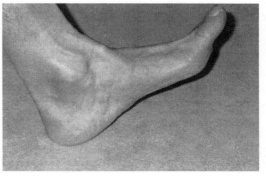

(b)

Fig. 35.10 (a) Cyst development on the anterior tibial tendon with (b) corresponding ultrasound confirming fluid collection. (Photo courtesy of Dr R.G. Danowski.)

the area in order to prevent further pressure prior to correction of the boot. Treatment involves altering the boot either by punching out the appropriate spots to avoid pressure over these bony prominences or by decreasing the padding over the pressure area and increasing the padding around the prominence. Some skaters have the bursa excised, although care must be taken not to replace a non-painful bursa with an irritating and painful scar that continues to be a pressure area inside the boot.

Haglund's deformity of the calcaneal tuberosity is caused by the heel slipping within the boot during knee and ankle flexion because of excessive movement of a narrow heel in a wide heel cup. This is treated by improving the fit of the boot by adding padding over the medial and lateral aspects of the Achilles tendon and by increasing the flexibility of the boot to allow more ankle dorsiflexion. The back stay can also be punched out to relieve pressure over the calcaneal prominence. Alternatively, the skater can replace the skate with a make that has an appropriately narrow heel counter.

TENOSYNOVITIS

Tenosynovitis of the anterior ankle is caused by the pressure of boot laces and tongue crease on the dorsum of the ankle during ankle flexion. This can be relieved by adding padding, such as orthopaedic felt or sheepskin, to the tongue of the skate. Smith (1990) suggests using Plastazote or other malleable plastic insert between the leather of the boot and the padding of the tongue. The plastic insert is heated and placed between the leather and padding of the tongue and the skate is then laced up loosely. This allows grooves to form in the hardening plastic that form a firmer area over the tendon and distribute the forces over a wider area, alleviating the pressure of the laces and leather over the tendon.

Achilles tendonitis may result from pressure of the proximal rim of the boot when performing toe jumps repeatedly. In this case, toe jumps should be limited until symptoms subside. The upper rim of the boot should be padded to decrease the pressure and limit forceful plantar flexion. This should alleviate the problem. It should be noted that skating boots have an elevated heel, which tends to maintain the ankle in slight plantar flexion. This leads to relatively shortened Achilles tendons and predisposes skaters to Achilles tendonitis. Skaters should stretch their Achilles tendon both before wearing their boots and when they have their boots on. Occasionally, the boot padding in this area also causes irritation to the tendon as the ankle is moved through plantar flexion and dorsiflexion. In this case, the padding should be compressed or removed in order to alleviate the pressure adjacent to both sides of the tendon.

ANKLE INJURY

Ankle injuries constitute a large proportion of figure skating injuries. Retraining of proprioception is a critical element in the off-ice training programme, and should include walking on even and uneven surfaces and running in straight lines and zigzag patterns. Balance and proprioception can be enhanced by hopping and jumping or by the use of a trampoline or balance board (Fig. 35.11a). Varying the free leg and arm position on the balance board can enhance balance. Resistance exercises are important in the restoration of ankle strength (Fig. 35.11b,c) and are important in the prevention of recurrent injury. The skater may begin stroking as soon as the foot can fit into the skating boot but should avoid double or triple jumps, especially those that land on an outside edge, until normal peroneal strength and proprioception have been restored. Normal strength and proprioception can be judged to have been restored when the skater can maintain balance on the injured limb alone during continuous independent movement of one or more of the unaffected extremities.

General aspects of injury management

All muscle groups that provide support and balance are important for figure skating. All

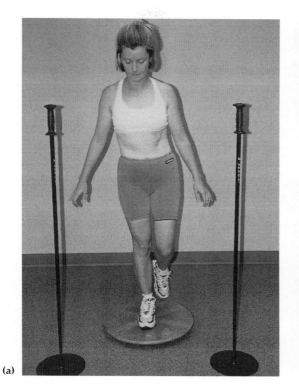

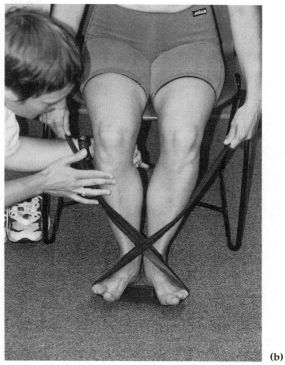

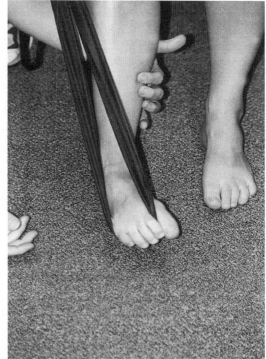

Fig. 35.11 (a) Balance board exercises to increase proprioception and strengthening of the ankle. (b, c) Two ankle strengthening exercises using resistant elastic bands. (Photos courtesy of Dr Kelly Flannigan.)

skating disciplines require adequate strength of the muscle groups stabilizing the ankle, knee and hip joints, as well as those muscle groups responsible for maintenance of body posture, especially arm position. If an injury has limited on-ice training, effective injury management must provide for maintenance of all these components during the rehabilitation period.

One particularly effective off-ice conditioning activity that can be incorporated into a rehabilitation programme is the slide board, which offers sport-specific cardiovascular fitness and strengthening of the lower extremity without impact forces. Provost-Craig and Pies (1997) reported that heart rate response to 70–80 slides per minute did not differ from the mean heart rate response during the 4-min programme on the ice. Correct use of the slide board increases back stabilization, promotes good body alignment and balance, and simulates skating movement patterns. In addition to its usefulness in rehabilitation, it is an effective non-impact, off-ice conditioning device for preseason training programmes. Depending on the injury, other appropriate activities, such as swimming, cycling, rowing and treadmill, could be used to maintain cardiovascular fitness and ideal body weight during the rehabilitation phase.

A harness device (Fig. 35.12) can be used to limit weight-bearing during practice sessions for skaters recovering from injury. This device decreases the impact load by 10–30% during landing from jumps and prevents skaters from falling as they gradually recover their training programme (Gross, 1997). It allows skaters to return to training without the fear of falling and reinjury, thus improving confidence and helping to overcome any psychological barriers. Skaters with upper extremity injuries, including hand and wrist fractures, can continue skating as long as immobilization is sufficient to prevent symptoms during practice. The skater may need to decrease lifts if involved in pairs or dance. If involved in precision skating, the athlete will need an adequate grip required for precision elements.

Trunk stability in relationship to the pelvis is

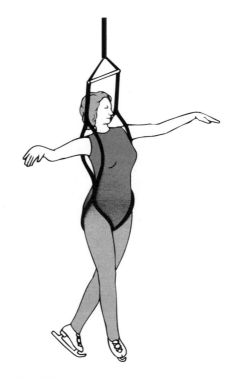

Fig. 35.12 Harness support used as a training or rehabilitation device.

very important for balance on the ice and for jumping. Neuromuscular stability of the lumbar–pelvic region requires both the neurological control to attain the proper lumbar–pelvic position via proprioception and the muscular control to maintain this position. This trunk stability is maintained by the coordinated action of the back extensor, abdominal flexor and gluteus muscle groups. Weakness of the gluteus medius and poor trunk stability allows unwanted lateral movement of the pelvis. Conversely, strengthening of these muscle groups and increasing their endurance increases core trunk stability. This in turn increases the skater's ability to absorb multiaxial loading through the trunk of the body, rather than through the vertebral joints and the lower extremity. In addition to the obvious role in enhancement of performance, core trunk stability and balance are therefore also an integral

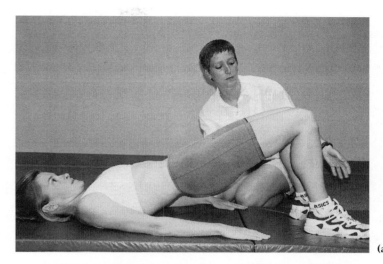

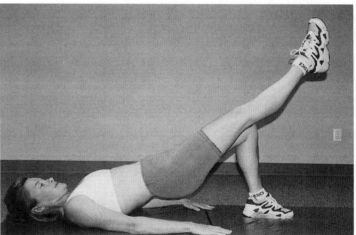

Fig. 35.13 Examples of two spine stabilization exercises where a level pelvis is maintained in order to increase core stability. (Photos courtesy of Dr Kelly Flannigan.)

(a)

(b)

part of injury prevention. Specific spine stabilization exercises (Fig. 35.13) are used to improve trunk strength and core stability selectively. Weakness of the hip and trunk stabilizers can present as knee pain because of inability to control the pelvis on landing. This causes more rotation, overcorrection and consequently more shock absorption at the knee.

Groin strains involving hip flexors and adductors are not uncommon in figure skaters, although fortunately they respond to flexibility and strengthening exercises. Low back pain is a common complaint and usually involves musculoligamentous strains. However, because of skating's emphasis on lumbar lordosis and holding the free leg extended at all times, skaters are at increased risk of spondylolysis. If skaters lack flexibility in the hip joint, they attempt to achieve further leg extension through the lumbosacral area, thus increasing strain and the possibility of injury to the structures of the low back. It is also important that the skater has full physiological movements at the uncovertebral joints of the lumbar spine, as stresses that result from inadequate joint ranges will present as overuse injuries. Tight lumbodorsal fascia is also a cause of back pain in figure skaters. Stretching of the lumbodorsal fascia is important in maintaining muscle balance and proper lumbar mobility (Fig. 35.14). Spine stabilization exercises are used in rehabilitation of back injury and for prevention of recurrent injury.

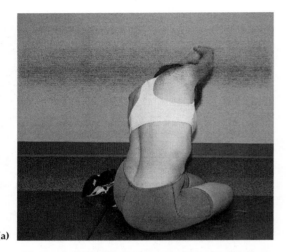

(a)

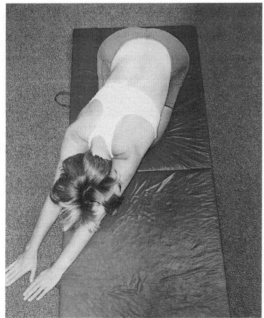

(b)

Fig. 35.14 Two different methods to stretch the lumbodorsal fascia. (Photos courtesy of Dr Kelly Flannigan.)

With the increased popularity of figure skating, there are more skaters seeking advice from their physicians with respect to the more common problems encountered. Physicians who understand the basics of the sport will be able to provide more effective injury prevention and management services to this group of recreational and competitive athletes.

Recommendations for future research

Because of the increased demands in the training of competitive figure skaters and in recognition of the lack of research delineating the effects of high-impact, repetitive loading on the growth and development patterns of young athletes, the ISU has recently reviewed and raised the age limits for competing at international and Olympic events. Further prospective and longitudinal studies are necessary in order properly to advise skaters and coaches on the content of figure skating training programmes. In this highly technical world, the skating boot (the source of most injuries in figure skating) has not changed significantly in the last century. A hinged plastic boot is currently undergoing evaluation, although much further study will be required to develop a skate that can match the abilities of the athletes who wear them.

In the last few years, several international meetings specific to figure skating have been held in America and Europe. These events have provided skaters, coaches, therapists, scientists and physicians the opportunity to expand their knowledge and to plan future research for the benefit of all figure skaters and those who help them reach their goals.

Acknowledgements

I would like to thank the following who assisted in creating this chapter: Penny Dain, International Skating Union Media Relations, Sue Pavlicic and Kim Ward for their time and energy devoted to the clinical photographs; Audiovisual Services of the Capital Health Region of Victoria, BC for the reproduction of slides and photographs; and Dr Kelly Flannigan for his professional photography, valued insight and computer mastery.

References

Aleshinsky, S., Podolsky, A., McQueen, C., Smith, A. & Van Handel, P. (1988) Strength and conditioning program for figure skating. *National Strength and Conditioning Association Journal* **10**, 26–30.

Authorsen, S., Wingendorf, M. & Weyer, R. (1997) Boot related injuries as seen at the Olympic Training Center, Dortmund, Germany. In *ISU International Congress on Medicine and Science in Figure Skating*, p. 15. International Skating Union, Lausanne, Switzerland.

Brock, R. & Striowski, C. (1986) Injuries in elite figure skaters. *Physician and Sportsmedicine* **14**, 111–115.

Brown, E. & McKeag, D. (1987) Training, experience, and medical history of pairs skaters. *Physician and Sportsmedicine* **15**, 100–114.

Danowski, R.G. (1997) The foot instability syndrome of the ice skater. In *ISU International Congress on Medicine and Science in Figure Skating*, p. 9. International Skating Union, Lausanne, Switzerland.

Davis, M.W. & Litman, T. (1979) Figure skater's foot. *Minnesota Medicine* **62**, 647–648.

Ferstle, J. (1979) Figure skating: in search of the winning edge. *Physician and Sportsmedicine* **7**, 129–136.

Garrick, J. (1982) Figure skating injuries. *Medicine and Science in Sports and Exercise* **14**, 141.

Gledhill, N. (1997) Physiological changes in figure skaters over the years. In *ISU International Congress on Medicine and Science in Figure Skating*, p. 12. International Skating Union, Lausanne, Switzerland.

Gross, J. (1997) Automatic harness. In *ISU International Congress on Medicine and Science in Figure Skating*, p. 14. International Skating Union, Lausanne, Switzerland.

Kjaer, M. & Larsson, B. (1992) Physiological profile and incidence of injuries among elite figure skaters. *Journal of Sports Sciences* **10**, 29–36.

Lockwood, K. (1996) Kinetic and kinematic characteristics of impact upon landing single, double, and triple revolution jumps in figure skating. In *First Congress on the Sports Medicine and Sports Science of Skating*, pp. 5–7. US Figure Skating Association, San Jose, California.

Lockwood, K. (1997) *The effects of repetitive impact load-type training on skeletal health and integrity in competitive figure skaters*. PhD thesis, Faculty of Physical Education and Recreation, Edmonton, Alberta.

Lowry, C.B. & Leveau, B.F. (1982) A retrospective study of gymnastics injuries to competitors and non-competitors in private clubs. *American Journal of Sports Medicine* **10**, 237–239.

McCarthy, P. (1989) Wheezing or breezing through exercise-induced asthma. *Physician and Sportsmedicine* **17**, 125–130.

McMaster, W., Liddle, S. & Walsh, J. (1979) Conditioning program for competitive figure skating. *American Journal of Sports Medicine* **7**, 43–47.

Moskvina, T. (1997) Preventing injuries with off ice training. In *ISU International Congress on Medicine and Science in Figure Skating*, p. 20. International Skating Union, Lausanne, Switzerland.

Niinimaa, V., Woch, Z. & Shephard, R. (1979) Intensity of physical effort during a free figure skating program. In *Science in Skiing, Skating and Hockey*, pp. 74–81. Academic Publishers, Edmonton, Canada.

Pierson, W.E. (1988) Exercise induced bronchospasm in children and adolescents. *Pediatric Clinics of North America* **35**, 1031–1040.

Podhajsky, H. (1997) Foot alignment and the skating boot fit. In *ISU International Congress on Medicine and Science in Figure Skating*. International Skating Union, Lausanne, Switzerland.

Provost-Craig, M.A. (1997) Off ice training of the specific parameters. In *ISU International Congress on Medicine and Science in Figure Skating*, p. 27. International Skating Union, Lausanne, Switzerland.

Provost-Craig, M.A. & Pies, N. (1997) Heart rate response of the long program and guides for improvement. In *ISU International Congress on Medicine and Science in Figure Skating*, p. 26. International Skating Union, Lausanne, Switzerland.

Provost-Craig, M.A., Whaler-Beck, P., Arbour, K., Sestili, D., Chabalko, J. & Ekinci, D. (1996) The incidence of exercise induced bronchospasm in competitive figure skaters. In *First Congress on the Sports Medicine and Sports Science of Skating*, p. 20. US Figure Skating Association, San Jose, California.

Richards, J. & Henley, M.S. (1996) Effects of ankle mobility on landing forces in skating. In *First Congress on the Sports Medicine and Sports Science of Skating*. US Figure Skating Association, San Jose, California.

Ross, W.D., Brown, S.R., Faulkner, R.A., Vajda, A. & Savage, M.V. (1976) Monitoring growth in young skaters. *Canadian Journal of Applied Science* **1**, 163–167.

Schroeckenstein, D.C. & Busse, W. (1988) Exercise and asthma: not incompatible. *Journal of Respiratory Disease* **9**, 29–45.

Slemenda, C.W. & Johnston, C.C. (1993) High intensity activities in young women: site specific bone mass effects among female figure skaters. *Bone and Mineral* **20**, 125–132.

Smith, A. (1990) Foot and ankle injuries in figure skaters. *Physician and Sportsmedicine* **18**, 73–86.

Smith, A. (1996) Reduction of injuries among elite figure skaters: a 4-year longitudinal study. In *First Congress on the Sports Medicine and Sports Science of Skating*, p. 18. US Figure Skating Association, San Jose, California.

Smith, A. & Ludington, R. (1989) Injuries in elite pair skaters and ice dancers. *American Journal of Sports Medicine* **17**, 482–488.

Smith, A. & Micheli, L. (1982) Injuries in competitive figure skaters. *Physician and Sportsmedicine* **10**, 36–47.

Smith, A., Stroud, L. & McQueen, C. (1991) Flexibility and anterior knee pain in adolescent elite figure skaters. *Journal of Pediatric Orthopedics* **11**, 77–82.

Yu, L. (1996) Injuries of national and international competitive skaters. In *First Congress on the Sports Medicine and Sports Science of Skating*, p. 17. US Figure Skating Association, San Jose, California.

Zauner, C., Maksud, M. & Melichna, J. (1989) Physiological considerations in training young athletes. *Sports Medicine* **8**, 15–31.

Ziegler, P. (1996) The nutritional status of teenage female competitive ice skaters. In *First Congress on the Sports Medicine and Sports Science of Skating*, p. 9. US Figure Skating Association, San Jose, California.

Chapter 36

Cycling

LISA LAMOREAUX

Introduction

The sport of cycling takes many forms: road, track, mountain and BMX to name a few. Women are quite active in the sport of cycling. In 1995 and 1996, the number of women competing in the National Off Road Biking Association (NORBA) National Series rose by 60% and 75% respectively. These statistics also reveal that the median age of the female NORBA rider is 32. This is an interesting statistic and may, in part, reflect the fact that many women enter the sport as a method of rehabilitation from injuries in other sports. Cycling offers a wide range of aerobic and anaerobic exercise without the high price of repetitive impact.

Cycling injuries fall into two broad categories: traumatic and overuse. An understanding of the mechanics of cycling aids in the prevention and treatment of both types of injuries. This chapter attempts to compile the current scientific literature on the biomechanics of cycling and places it alongside the experience gained by the author as both an orthopaedic surgeon and professional cyclist. Though professional cycling is still a male-dominated sport, women are receiving increasing support and interest. An understanding of the specific cycling problems of women will aid in keeping them active in their sport.

Bike fit: the foundation for prevention of overuse injury

Cycling is a concentric form of exercise and is therefore less likely to cause muscle strain type injuries. However, due to the repetitive nature of cycling any mechanical malalignment that produces undue strain on a tendon or a joint can eventually lead to injury. Overuse injuries generally are attributable to one of three factors: poor fit of rider and bike, training error or increased stress. These three factors are relevant not only when evaluating a cyclist with an overuse injury but also for the athlete using cycling for rehabilitation or entering the sport for the first time.

What is proper bike fit and how does this apply to the female cyclist? Traditional bike fit has been based upon the proportions of the average male, thus leaving most women and many men struggling with back, shoulder or knee pain. Most traditional fit systems are based on standover clearance or inseam length (Burke, 1994). However, women tend to be proportionately longer in the legs than the torso compared with a male of the same height. Additionally, most women have shorter arms than a male of comparable height. What constitutes proper fit is influenced not only by body configuration but also by riding style, flexibility and goals. Proper fit can mean upright and comfortable for a recreational rider with neck pain, while it can mean the most aerodynamic and metabolically efficient position for an élite time triallist. Proper fit is as dependent upon riding style and goals as it is upon body size.

The frame

Frame geometry fits into several general categories: road racing, touring, mountain and BMX. The traditional 'double diamond' frame configuration is still the most prevalent but many monocoque designs and alternative geometries are becoming more common (Fig. 36.1).

Frame size is best determined by the cyclist's total **height** and **riding** style. The **reach** and height of the cyclist determines the position of the top of the head tube and the handle bar and therefore frame size. This is because, unlike the saddle, there is not very much useful adjustment in the handlebar and stem. There is one factor common in comfortable fit and that is centre of gravity. For most riders, having the centre of gravity just in front of the bottom bracket spindle results in a comfortable fit. Again this is not a fixed rule. For an élite time triallist in an aero position, the centre of gravity will be pushed further forward. For the 'average' rider with 'average' body proportions, a comfortable seat position will be achieved using the knee-over-spindle rule. This is accomplished by positioning the seat so that a plumb-line dropped from the tibial tuberosity bisects the pedal spindle of the forward leg when the crank is parallel to the floor (Fig. 36.2). This will not be optimal for many riders, but provides a good starting point. For example, a rider with proportionately greater femoral length will find that her centre of gravity is placed too far back with this positioning. When pedalling, it is best if the cyclist supports most of her weight through her legs, which are generally pushing down on the pedals. Some weight should be supported on the saddle and some on the hands; however, the hands are least tolerant of load-bearing.

Good fit is not only important for achieving comfort but is also a key element in the maximization of transfer of power from the body to the cycle drive train (Gonzalez & Hull, 1989). The transfer of power depends primarily upon five variables: seat-tube angle, seat height, crank length, longitudinal foot position on the pedal and pedal cadence.

The seat-tube angle (STA) determines the position of the seat and thus the hip axis relative to the crank axis. There are varying opinions as to the 'optimal' STA. Traditionally, competitive road cyclists ride with STAs of 72–76°, while triathletes ride with steeper STAs, sometimes as much as 80–90°. The STA tends to decrease with increasing frame size as it mostly reflects the length of the femur. This allows the taller cyclist with a longer femur to shift her position

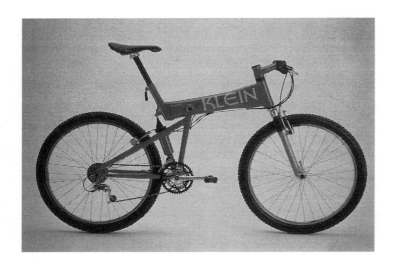

Fig. 36.1 Although the traditional double-diamond frame configuration is still most prevalent, alternative geometries are becoming more common.

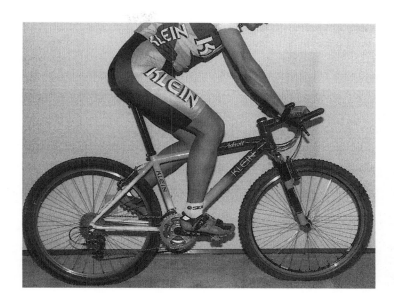

Fig. 36.2 Saddle fore–aft positioning: with the cranks parallel to the floor the 'average' rider will find that a good starting position is with the tibial tuberosity over the pedal spindle.

rearward, maintaining the body's centre of gravity. STA may also be altered effectively by sliding the seat forward or backwards. Different riding styles and events are reflected by different geometries. This is seen in mountain and touring bikes, which have shallower STAs (more laid back) to aid in seated climbing. The effect of varying STA on cardiorespiratory responses during steady-state cycling has been studied by Heil *et al.* (1995). Trend analysis suggested that cardiorespiratory responses minimize around STAs in the range of 83–90°. This study reflects conditions similar to time trialling and thus may not reflect other forms of cycling. The observed responses may be largely due to increased hip angle, as mean hip angle increases with increased STA thus affecting muscle forces. Although the cardiorespiratory responses were small, it was calculated that the 2.5% reduction in $\dot{V}_{O_2}$ between an STA of 83° and an STA of 69° would result in a difference of 54 s over a 40-km time trial.

Optimal seat height has been evaluated with respect to oxygen consumption and lower limb kinematics (Asmussen, 1953; Shennum & deVries, 1976; Nordeen-Snyder, 1977). Oxygen consumption is minimized at approximately 100% of trochanteric height or 106–109% of symphysis pubis height. These studies, when corrected for the different methods of measuring leg length, correlated well. Leg length should be measured with the subject wearing cycling footwear, the feet spread 30 cm, body erect and back flush with the wall. Saddle height is measured from the pedal, at its most distal position from the seat, to the top of the seat at a point directly through the pedal axis. A simpler, less scientific method of adjusting seat height is to sit comfortably on the bike with heels on the pedals and pedal backwards. The leg should come to full extension with the foot flat. Now clip in and pedal. At the bottom of the stroke the knee should have a slight flexion angle; recommendations range from 15 to 30° (Fig. 36.3). Observing the rider from behind, the hips should not be rocking back and forth to gain extension as this indicates that the seat is too high. A second indicator of excessive seat height is 'ankling', excessive ankle flexion in an attempt to reach the bottom of the pedal stroke. Additionally, a seat that is too low results in excessive patellofemoral loading, as the knee experiences increased flexion with each revolution.

With limb length discrepancy, it is easiest to fit

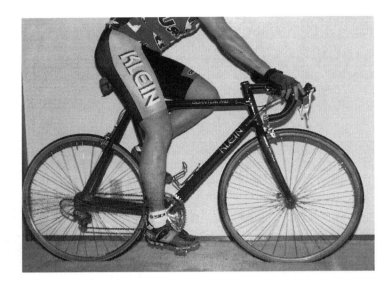

Fig. 36.3 Seat height: at the bottom of the pedal stroke the knee should have a slight flexion angle.

the bike to the longer leg. The shorter leg should be evaluated to determine if the discrepancy is primarily tibial or femoral. If it is tibial, adding a lift or shim of slightly less than the total discrepancy between the cleat and shoe solves the problem. If it is femoral, a lift of approximately half the discrepancy should be combined with moving the shorter leg back slightly on the pedal. Limb length discrepancy may also be adressed by using a shorter crank for the shorter leg.

Crank length is another important variable in the transfer of power from the body to the bike (Hull & Gonzalez, 1988). Optimum crank arm length depends on several factors, particularly riding style, whether sprinting, touring, time trialling or hill climbing. For every style there is an optimum crank arm length, for example a longer crank arm increases the leverage and decreases the revolutions and is good for pushing big gears. In general the minimum cost function occurs at longer crank arm lengths and lower pedalling rates in tall people compared with short people (Faria, 1992). It is not uncommon to see a short woman using a long crank arm that will result in excess hip and knee flexion at the top of the pedal stroke. Mechanical power output tends to be greatest with a ratio of leg length (trochanter to floor in centimetres) to crank

length of 6.3:1 (Inbar *et al.*, 1983). General guidelines are that shorter cyclists use crank arm lengths of 165–166.5 mm, with 160 mm being a consideration for those under 1.5 m tall. Cyclists 1.6–1.8 m tall use a crank arm length of 175 mm; in mountain biking 177.5 mm should be considered.

The pedal provides the platform through which the cyclist transfers energy to the bike. A variety of pedal styles are currently available. The traditional platform pedal is still commonly used for recreational and children's bikes, BMX, slalom and stationary bikes. This allows the rider to use any type of shoe. Toe-clips and cleated cycling shoes have been found to improve cycling efficiency (Davis & Hull, 1981). When cleating the shoe to the pedal, proper placement becomes an important issue. Several studies have evaluated cycling parameters in relation to changes in foot position (Ericson *et al.*, 1985, 1988; Ericson & Nisell, 1986; Gonzalez & Hull, 1989; Mandroukas, 1990). Longitudinal position of the foot on the pedal plays an important role in knee and ankle kinematics, as well as in perceived exertion and transfer of power to the pedal. Ericson *et al.* defined the anterior foot position as the second metatarsal head in contact with the centre of the pedal (Ericson *et al.*, 1985, 1988;

Ericson & Nisell, 1986, 1987). This position was shown to result in a 5° increase in ankle joint dorsiflexion, increased ankle load moment and increased mean force efficiency ratio with increased soleus electromyographic activity. The posterior position (foot moved distally 10 cm from the anterior position so that the midfoot is in contact with the centre of the pedal) increased hip joint motion by 7°, knee joint motion by 3° and increased stress on the anterior cruciate ligament. Mandroukas (1990) analysed foot placement and seat height and also found that the anterior foot position with the seat height allowing near full knee extension was more effective and perceived as easier.

The position of the foot on the pedal is also influenced by anatomical alignment. Many women tend to have slight valgus knee alignment or increased external tibial torsion. With this type of alignment, if the foot is locked to the pedal in a straight-ahead position tendon strain will probably result. This is well demonstrated in a study by Ruby and Hull (1993) that evaluated the response of intersegmental knee loads to foot pedal platform degrees of freedom. With a platform that allowed rotation, there was significant reduction in axial and varus/valgus knee moments. For the average cyclist this means using a clipless pedal with a few degrees of float to allow this rotational degree of freedom. There are cases of extreme alignment anomalies that may not be so easily adapted to the standard bicycle. Excessive varus or valgus alignments can produce increased stress on the medial or lateral knee. Spacers can be used to widen stance width and improve alignment from hip to knee. Lifts or cants can often be used to aid the valgus knee, placing these between the pedal and the shoe. The structure of the foot also influences low-level load transmission to the knee. Extreme inversion of the forefoot relative to the transverse plane causes significantly greater average posterior knee forces and extensive knee moments (Ruby et al., 1992). This suggests that corrective orthotics may play a role in preventing overuse injury. However, there is some debate as to whether using inserts to optimize alignment and support foot structures has a significant effect on the energy cost of cycling. Anderson and Sockler (1990) found no benefit from orthotics in the energy cost of submaximal cycling. However, Hice et al. (1988) found reduced oxygen consumption and heart rate when orthoses were used to place the rear foot at its neutral calcaneal stance position.

Although technically not an aspect of bike 'fit', cadence is one of the elements significant in the transfer of power from the cyclist to the bike. Cadence is also one of the most frequently implicated culprits in cycling overuse injuries. The optimal cadence for gross work efficiency is 60–91 r.p.m. for moderate to high workloads (Seabury et al., 1977; Faria et al., 1982; Boning et al., 1984). Coast et al. (1986) demonstrated a trend for the most economical cadence to rise from 50 to 78 r.p.m. as power output increased from 100 to 800 W, or approximately 80% $\dot{V}_{O_{2max}}$. Both force at the pedal and muscle stress are minimized at cadences between 90 and 100 r.p.m. This suggests that a pedalling rate of 90–110 r.p.m. may minimize peripheral muscle fatigue, even though this rate may result in higher oxygen uptake (Patterson & Moreno, 1990; Widrick et al., 1991). Even when climbing, a high cadence is more economical than a low cadence (although standing to climb has other advantages, such as recruiting other muscle patterns and relieving fatigue, or enhancing power production) (Swain & Wilcox, 1992).

For most cyclists bike fit is a very haphazard process. Most riders, whether entering the sport for the first time, being prepared for a team or even riding a bike in a health club, depend on peers and friends to make these important adjustments. It is unlikely that even most élite athletes have analysed these studies, and most cyclists probably set up their bikes by trial and error. Women quite commonly enter the sport for the first time riding a second-hand bike from a boyfriend or spouse. By aiding the understanding of good fit, not only can the rider's enjoyment be improved but additionally a significant impact can be made in prevention of injury.

Traumatic injuries

There is very little in the literature that differentiates cycling injury patterns by gender. Pfeifer (1994) used a self-administered questionnaire to evaluate injury in NORBA Pro/Elite racers. Although the numbers were small (47 males and 14 females), this is one of the few studies that investigated gender-specific injury differences. Of the female cyclists who responded, bruises and wounds accounted for 68% of injuries, strains and tendinitis 21% and fractures 4.4%. This was not much different from the male distribution of injury. When analysed by region, the knee was most commonly injured in males, accounting for more than half of reported injuries. In female riders lower extremity injury was also quite high (39%); however, the low back accounted for the greatest number of injuries. It would be interesting to evaluate this discrepancy further. Is it secondary to training error, representing possibly poor upper body and trunk strength or flexibility, or is it the result of difficulties with bike fit? Mountain biking also represents a 'young' sport and there are few data regarding specific injuries.

Road cycling has been popular for quite some time, so it would seem more likely that a database on injuries would be available. However, there is very little information with respect to gender-specific injury. Wilber et al. (1995) evaluated 294 male and 224 female recreational cyclists selected at random. Significant differences were noted between male and female training characteristics. Overall, 85% reported one or more overuse injury with 36% requiring medical treatment. The odds of female cyclists developing neck and shoulder overuse injury were 1.5–2 times greater than their male counterparts. This brings up the recurring issue of bike fit. Traditional methods of bike fit would leave many women in a stretched-out position, contributing to neck and shoulder problems. In the paediatric population, several studies have observed higher traumatic injury rates in boys than girls (Gerbesich et al., 1994; Noakes, 1995), while in a survey evaluating BMX racers it was noted that women were injured twice as frequently as men (Brogger et al., 1990).

Estimates of overall accidental injury rates vary (Thompson et al., 1990a). Estimates of a 2–3% incidence of injury in competitive criterium, road, and track and circuit races have been reported (Kiburz et al., 1986; Mclennan et al., 1988), while Kronisch et al. (1996) reported an overall injury rate of 0.4% at a mountain bike national series event in 1994 that encompassed 4027 individual starts in five events. For the entire 1995 NORBA national series season, the rate of injuries for all entries was 0.1% (National Off Road Biking Association, 1996). In BMX racing, an injury rate of 6.3% was reported at the 1983 BMX European Championship (Brogger et al., 1990).

Although traumatic injuries are an inherent risk of cycling, the severity and incidence can be greatly influenced. Head injuries account for most fatal accidents in cyclists and helmets can have a significant effect on lessening the severity of injury (Sacks et al., 1991; Spaite et al., 1991; Ashbaugh et al., 1995; Noakes, 1995). Many helmet manufacturers have designed helmets specifically for women, taking into account head size and shape and even hair. Newer helmet designs have also focused on improving weight, ventilation and aerodynamics, leaving very few excuses for not wearing them. Helmets not only influence the severity of head injury, but also have a significant effect on decreasing facial injury (Thompson et al., 1990b). In downhill mountain bike racing helmets now even offer full-face protection (Fig. 36.4). All cycling governing bodies in the USA require helmet use at sanctioned events.

Road rash is probably the most common cycling injury (Coyle et al., 1991; Mellion, 1991; Chan et al., 1993; Pfeifer, 1994). Although protective clothing can be of some aid, the frictional abrasion that results in road rash occurs even beneath clothing. The padded armour of the downhill mountain bike racer offers significant protection to direct contact, but is impractical in most other events where heat dissipation and aerodynamics are an issue. The care of road rash

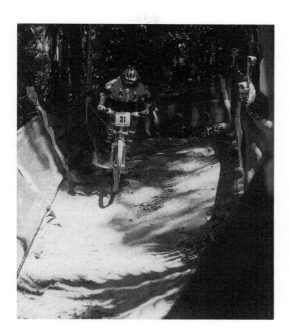

Fig. 36.4 Padded body wear and full-face helmets add extra protection for the downhill mountain bike racer.

is directed first at preventing infection and second at maximizing cosmesis. The first priority is complete cleansing and removal of any foreign body, which can result in infection or tattooing. Non-viable skin is also débrided. Scrubbing should be thorough and can be aided by the use of chlorhexidine or an iodophor scrub. The use of viscous lignocaine or a slush of ice and lignocaine may make it easier for the rider to tolerate. Allergic sensitivity, although very rare, may occur in association with the preservatives (methylparaben) used in multidose vials of lignocaine. Using lignocaine from a crash cart or for intravenous use avoids this problem. Lignocaine toxicity is probably more common than allergic sensitivity and manifests as seizure; doses of lignocaine should be limited to $5\,mg\cdot kg^{-1}$ to avoid this. Daily care should include keeping the newly forming dermis clean and lubricated, whether by antibiotic ointment or hydrocolloid dressing (Mellion *et al.*, 1988; Hermans, 1991). Pigmentation may be decreased by using sun-

block for 6 months to a year to protect the affected area.

Upper extremity trauma is a significant issue in cycling. Tucci and Barone (1988) evaluated urban cycling injuries and reported that 41.9% of subjects had injuries to the upper extremity; this was nearly twice that of the lower extremity. If there is time, a common reaction is to try to break the fall with an outstretched hand, commonly resulting in fracture of the wrist or forearm. Frequently, however, the rider is still gripping the bars or is thrown over the bars to land on the point of the shoulder. This results in shoulder girdle injury, such as fracture of the clavicle and injury to the acromioclavicular joint (Davis *et al.*, 1980). Clavicle fractures and acromioclavicular joint injuries are most commonly treated conservatively. For the competitive rider a stationary trainer may be tolerated within a few days of injury. Return to the road or dirt will be as tolerated, frequently by 3 weeks. Fracture union requires approximately 6 weeks. Return to riding must be based on clinical findings and risk of non-union. Fractures at highest risk for non-union are those involving the distal end with the coracoclavicular ligaments detached from the proximal fragment. This allows the proximal fragment to retract upwards and into the trapezius while the distal fragment drops downwards. Competitive cyclists may opt for surgical stabilization to speed their return to competition. This must be approached with caution, as the stresses induced by cycling may cause the orthopaedic hardware to fail with potential for migration (potentially into the chest).

Injury may occur at any level of the upper extremity. Injury to the hand may result in abrasion, contusion or fracture. One injury of interest has become more common since the advent of twist-shifters, particularly in mountain biking. As with skiing, the 'grip', or position of the hand at impact, may predispose the thumb to an abduction force, resulting in tear of the ulnar collateral ligament of the thumb. With twist-shifters the grip is around the shifter with the thumb under the bar and a fall such as an 'endo' (rider launched over the bars, either from locking up the front brake or the bike coming to a dead stop as the front tyre hits an obstacle) can easily result in tear of the ulnar collateral ligament. Prevention is readily addressed by consciously remembering to keep the thumb over the top of the bar. Treatment depends upon the degree of disruption of the ligament. In my experience with mountain bike riders, a fairly circumferential dislocation with volar plate injury frequently occurs; this requires surgical repair. Return to riding can be quite rapid. The surgical repair or sprain can be protected with a hand–thumb spica cast or heat-moulded plastic spica splint, custom moulded to the cyclist's grips.

Overuse injuries

Overuse injuries account for the majority of injuries in cycling and most commonly result from training errors, poor position or excessive stress, which need to be specifically evaluated and addressed.

Neck and back pain

Neck and back pain are extremely common problems with cyclists, particularly women (Weiss, 1985; Pfeifer, 1994). Most neck and back pain in road cyclists is caused by load-bearing through the arms and shoulders and hyperextension of the neck, particularly in the horizontal and dropped riding position (Fig. 36.5). The more upright position assumed for mountain biking and BMX produces less positional strain. However, the trade-off is increased impact in off-road conditions and jumps. Trigger points about the neck and shoulder girdle occur most commonly in the levator scapula, trapezius, rhomboid and sternocleidomastoid muscles (trigger points are irritable foci arising in muscle or fascia due to trauma). Overuse, repetitive motion and strained or abnormal postures can all contribute to the trigger point pain–spasm–pain cycle.

Wilbur *et al.* (1995) used a mailed questionnaire to survey randomly 294 male and 224 female recreational cyclists. The odds of the female cyclists developing neck overuse

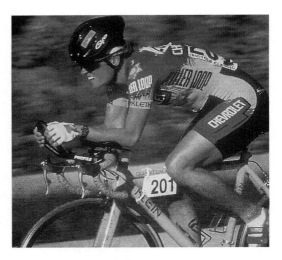

Fig. 36.5 Most neck and back pain in cyclists is caused by load-bearing through the arms and shoulders and by hyperextension of the neck.

injury/complaint was 1.5 times that of the males; shoulder overuse injury/complaint was 2.12 times more frequent in the females than the males. In evaluating the female cyclist with neck, shoulder or back pain, bike fit should be reviewed. Many women are matched to a bike with too long a top tube, the fit being based on their leg length. There is some room for modification by using a shorter stem, although this will be limited and also alters the handling characteristics of the bike. In mountain biking, a bike that is too small can also be a culprit. This may result in the rider being in an excessively dropped position and bearing increased load through the arms and shoulders. Changing the stem to one with increased rise may be sufficient to resolve this. Stems for mountain bikes are commonly marketed with 0, 10 and 20° rise; 15 and 30° rise are also available or a custom stem can be designed.

Riding technique is also an important element. A rigid riding position transmits force directly to the neck and shoulder girdle, while a stiff inflexible back increases low back strain. Changing position frequently, absorbing shock through a flexed elbow position, stretching and standing are all important in preventing or resolving the pain. Strength and flexibility exercises are an important element of the medical management of these problems. Additionally, women should not ignore upper body strengthening and conditioning. All too frequently the emphasis of the competitive female cyclist is so focused on developing leg power and endurance that upper body conditioning is ignored. Good upper body and trunk strength and flexibility are an important factor in bike handling and are very necessary to add power to sprinting and hill climbing.

Hand and wrist

Ulnar neuropathy is an extremely common problem in cyclists at all levels (Noth *et al.*, 1980; Burke, 1981; Hankey & Gubbay, 1988). This is the result of compression of the ulnar nerve at or adjacent to Guyon's canal or from traction on the nerve secondary to wrist hyperextension (Eckman *et al.*, 1975; Wilmarth & Nelson, 1988). The ulnar nerve in Guyon's canal is more superficial than the median nerve in the carpal tunnel, making it potentially more prone to external compression. The ulnar nerve as it enters the hand contains both sensory and motor fibres, and in cyclist's palsy both the superficial sensory and deep motor branch are involved (Munnings, 1991). The symptoms of ulnar neuropathy in the cyclist may be mild, with intermittent paraesthesias relieved by positional change, or severe, with significant neuropraxia lasting for several months after all pressure is relieved.

Ulnar neuropathy is markedly influence by bike fit. Compression and traction are both induced by increased weight-bearing through the hands, especially with the wrists in a hyperextended position. The reach and drop to the bars should be evaluated, reach being shortened and drop being raised as necessary. Less than one-third of the rider's weight should be borne on the bars (Gardner, 1975). Padded cycling gloves and handlebar padding are also important.

Tenosynovitis and tendinitis about the hand and wrist are problems that may be more inher-

ent to mountain biking than road cycling. These are poorly documented in the literature. Mountain bike riding is associated with greatly increased repetitive impact and vibratory trauma, which are borne by the hands. Beginners in particular may grip the bars or brakes with undue ferocity during long or technical descents, resulting in tenosynovitis. Triggering of the flexor tendons tends to be more common in the little and ring fingers, suggesting that this is primarily associated with increased braking strain. This deserves further evaluation, particularly as it appears to be more common in female cyclists. It may be due to smaller hand size and component mismatch or may simply be secondary to overgripping. Getting the rider to relax her grip is an important element in addressing the problem. This should be coupled with stretching, anti-inflammatory drugs and padded gloves. In mountain biking a front shock absorber does much to resolve the vibration and trauma transmitted to the hands, different shocks having differing characteristics. Triggering that does not resolve with conservative management may benefit from steroid injection into the A1 pulley of the flexor sheath or surgical release of the A1 pulley (Green, 1993).

Tendinitis may also occur from repetitive gripping and shifting, resulting in either de Quervain's tenosynovitis or crossover syndrome (Green, 1993). De Quervain's tenosynovitis involves the extensors and abductors of the thumb in the first extensor compartment of the wrist and may result from a long hilly ride requiring frequent shifting, particularly early in the season. Intersection syndrome is more often the result of twist-shifting, particularly if the shifters are slippery or muddy. Stretching the involved tendons, along with anti-inflammatory medication or injection, may be sufficient to resolve this. The competitive cyclist may require a moulded orthoplast splint in order to allow continued racing and training. The tension in the shifters may also be altered to decrease the resistance; this may be an important factor in a woman with small hands or poor hand strength.

Saddle problems

Although buttock and saddle problems are well documented in the cycling literature, most of this is empirical evidence rather than scientific research. Women's issues are particularly poorly addressed. Recently, saddles designed specifically for women have become more widely marketed. Whereas previously women's saddles were essentially something wide, bulky and heavily padded, they are now available in lightweight aero designs. These designs commonly have a slightly wider seat to accommodate the increased distance between the ischial tuberosities while still tapering to a narrow nose. Frequently, cutouts are incorporated to decrease perineal and labial pressure. As to what factors are associated with seat symptoms there is very little in the medical literature. Weiss (1985) evaluated the relationship between seat symptoms and seat height, seat tilt, handlebar height, relative height of handlebars and seat, and seat construction in a group of recreational cyclists on a week-long bike tour. The only significant association was that riders who used a padded seat were more likely to experience buttock problems.

Chafing of the skin of the medial thigh and groin can be a painful problem. This is thought to be more common in women, although again this is based on speculation (Weiss, 1994). The saddle may very well be the culprit here, as a wider nose with increased padding will result in increased chafe. An important element in preventing saddle sores, whether on the thigh, groin or buttocks, is keeping the skin clean and dry. Padded cycling shorts with an absorbent lining help in wicking moisture away, as well as adding padding without increasing friction. It is very important that these shorts are cleaned and dried between each ride. Additionally, after a strenuous race or training ride it is helpful to change into dry clean shorts as soon as possible, decreasing the risk of furunculitis.

Saddle position may play a role in saddle sores and chafe. A seat that is too high results in increased rocking in the saddle in order to gain extension at the bottom of the pedal stroke, thus increasing chafe. Additionally, a saddle that is too far forward or backward does not support the weight of the rider as it is meant to. Tilt is a matter of personal preference; neutral to slightly downward tilt is most commonly recommended to decrease perineal and labial pressure.

Knee

Cycling kinematics reveals that the knee flexes and internally rotates from bottom dead centre to just past top dead centre, and then extends and externally rotates until bottom dead centre. During gait, when the knee flexes and internally rotates there is associated subtalar joint pronation; when the knee extends and externally rotates there is subtalar joint supination. However, in cycling the foot is fixed, preventing this compensatory subtalar joint motion and referring it proximally, primarily to the knee (Ericsson & Nisell, 1987; Ericson et al., 1988). Although there is no impact in steady-state cycling, it is highly repetitive and thus any malalignment of the rider or cycle will be accentuated over time. The knee was the second most commonly reported site of overuse injury/complaint in recreational cyclists (Wilber et al., 1995). It is easy to see how mechanically the knee is at risk for overuse injury in the cyclist; however, cycling is also one of the most widely prescribed forms of rehabilitation for the injured knee.

PATELLOFEMORAL PAIN

Patellofemoral pain is not uncommon in cyclists and can generally be traced to errors in training technique or bike fit. Patellofemoral disorders and valgus knee problems are quite common in women so this is an important issue (Zelisko et al., 1982; Ireland & Wall, 1990; National Collegiate Athletic Association, 1991). Training errors to look for are too many miles too fast, addition of hill or interval work, pushing too big a gear (riding at a relatively low cadence with high pedal resistance) or standing to climb. Training errors must also be sought outside the cycling routine, such as extension weight training. Errors of bike fit include positioning the seat too low or too far forward; this increases knee flexion angle and increases strain. Pedal alignment and float are also important. A cleat that is set toe-out increases valgus strain, while a pedal with no float locks the foot in and increases knee strain (Ruby & Hull, 1993).

Treatment must be aimed at altering the training or fitting error. This takes patience, particularly in the competitive cyclist who is worried about losing fitness. Maintaining a high cadence and avoiding hills, along with appropriate adjustments to the bike, are the first steps. Stretching should be aimed at not only the quadriceps patellofemoral mechanism but also the iliotibial band (ITB) and hamstrings, as tightness in these structures has been shown to be a significant factor in patellofemoral pain (Zappala et al., 1992). Ice massage is useful for patellar tendinitis and a short course of anti-inflammatory medication may be beneficial. Generally patellar bracing or taping is poorly tolerated in cycling, although a simple patellar strap may be beneficial in patellar tendinitis. Cyclists with marked hyperpronation may benefit from orthotics, use of a medial heel wedge or use of a medial washer on the pedal. Cleat alignment should be checked. Patellofemoral problems are best managed with rehabilitation and very rarely require surgical intervention (Fulkerson, 1994).

QUADRICEPS TENDINITIS

A less common but similar problem about the knee is quadriceps tendinitis. This may occur at the superior pole of the patella and be confused with chondromalacia; more commonly in cyclists, it may present laterally and be confused with ITB syndrome. Inciting factors for quadriceps tendinitis are the same as those for patellofemoral problems and thus diagnosis and treatment follow the same process. Ultrasound may be a useful adjunctive modality.

ILIOTIBIAL BAND SYNDROME

ITB syndrome presents as sharp pain along the lateral aspect of the knee. The ITB is a thickening of the fascia lata that commences at the level of the greater trochanter, where three-quarters of the gluteus maximus and tensor fasciae latae are inserted into it. It passes down the posterolateral aspect of the thigh, crossing the lateral epicondyle of the femur. With knee flexion the ITB passes anterior to the lateral epicondyle and with extension posterior to the lateral epicondyle (Last, 1984). Thus with cycling the ITB can become inflamed with repetitive friction across the lateral epicondyle. The pain of ITB syndrome can begin quite suddenly, possibly during a ride, making it very difficult for the rider to complete. Evaluation should look for point tenderness at the lateral epicondyle, along with pain with compression of the ITB as the knee is flexed and extended. Tightness of the ITB is evaluated with Ober's test (Magee, 1987). Increased pronation, internal tibial rotation or varus alignment increase tension in the ITB, as does limb length discrepancy and a foot too far forward on the pedal. It is important to check that the cleat position is not internally rotated and that saddle height is not too high. Excessive hill work is a common training error in the cyclist with ITB syndrome. Treatment is aimed at stretching (Ober's stretch and lateral hip drop stretch), training modifications and decreasing inflammation with ice and modalities. In extremely recalcitrant cases that fail to respond to prolonged conservative management, surgical intervention has been shown to have effective results (Noble, 1980). This is accomplished by resecting a portion of the distal posterior fibres of the ITB over the lateral femoral epicondyle (Martins et al., 1989; Holmes et al., 1993).

MEDIAL KNEE PAIN

Medial knee pain may be the result of several different problems. In mountain bikers, climbing, particularly steep, loose or prolonged climbs, or grinding through loose sand may result in pes anserinus bursitis or semimembranosus tendinitis/bursitis. The pes anserinus is the tendinous insertion of the sartorius, gracilis and semitendinosus muscles on the anteromedial aspect of the proximal tibia. A bursa lies between the aponeurosis of these tendons and the medial collateral ligament, about 5 cm below the anteromedial joint line. Pes anserinus bursitis and tendinitis of the pes tendons are caused by overuse friction or direct contusion (O'Donoghue, 1987). Semimembranosus tendinitis presents as persistent aching pain located on the posterior medial aspect of the knee, just below the joint line (Ray & Clancy, 1988). Semimembranosus tendinitis occurs in the endurance athlete as a result of repetitive loading or overloading. Both of these injuries must be differentiated from the joint line pain of a meniscal tear; bursal swelling may help in this differentiation (Henningan et al., 1994). A history of the sensation of locking or catching must not be assumed to be meniscal, as semimembranosus tendinitis with an enlarged bursa may cause the sensation of catching, particularly when the cyclist stands to climb. Both conditions significantly inhibit hamstring power. Again, both these tendon injuries are due to overuse and inflammation, rather than the eccentric muscle–tendon junction injury that occurs in runners (Garrett, 1990). Treatment must first be aimed at altering training. Hill work should be avoided and hamstring weight training discontinued. Stretching and modalities to fight inflammation are beneficial. The bursa may be aspirated and injected with a small amount of cortisone. If the bursal inflammation becomes chronic, surgical resection may be indicated (Ray & Clancy, 1988).

Foot and ankle

In cycling the foot functions mainly as a rigid platform through which force is applied to the pedal (O'Brien, 1991). Foot and ankle problems in cycling tend to be less debilitating than in impact sports. Foot paraesthesias are one of the more common problems, particularly when associated with long-distance rides. Fortunately this is usually a self-limiting problem. Paraesthesias most commonly arise secondary to pressure from straps, whether on shoes or clips (the cages some cyclists use for securing the foot to the pedal). Using clipless pedals relieves this source of pressure and also allows a small amount of float (rotation about the cleat) that allows the cyclist to alter position occasionally and relieve fatigue. Cleat position can be the source of irritation and needs to be evaluated both for rotational and fore–aft positioning. Cycling shoes are designed for rigidity in order to improve transfer of pressure to the pedal. A good cycling shoe is essentially the most comfortable shoe for that particular rider's foot, generating no pressure points or sites of friction. There are no cycling shoes designed specifically for women.

Achilles tendinitis, although far less common than in impact sports, may cause significant disability in the cyclist. This most commonly results from problems of bike fit or technique. A seat that is too low or a foot that is placed too far behind the pedal spindle may produce ankling (excessive flexion extension at the ankle). Leg length discrepancies should also be sought, as many cyclists adapt by ankling on the short side. Ankling may also be simply an error of technique and can be sought by watching the athlete ride. Treatment is aimed at correcting bike fit and technique. The fit can even be modified temporarily by placing the foot a few millimetres forward of the pedal axis in order to decrease motion. Conservative measures aimed at stretching, decreasing inflammation and then strengthening aids return to sport.

Rehabilitation

In rehabilitating the knee after injury or surgery, the bicycle can be a very useful tool. This also seems to be a frequent entry point into the sport of cycling for women. Many women have significant disorders of the patellofemoral joint and cycling for rehabilitation is commonly recommended (Hungerford & Lennox, 1983; Zappala et *al.*, 1992). Cycling is a closed-chain exercise and allows neuromuscular development without significant patellofemoral joint reaction forces. As a closed-chain exercise, cycling is also commonly used for rehabilitation after anterior cruciate ligament reconstruction. After injury or surgery the bicycle or ergometer can be used to work on range of motion and strength, as well as cardiovascular fitness. Cycling can frequently be started before full weight-bearing. Approximately 100° of flexion is needed before a complete crank cycle can be performed.

The electromyographic activity of various muscles during cycling has been evaluated by Mcleod and Blackburn (1980). Activity in the quadriceps and gastrocnemius was well documented, although, interestingly, under normal conditions the hamstrings were relatively inactive. With instruction, hamstring activity could be enhanced. In trained cyclists electromyographic recordings show significant hamstring activity during the crank stroke from 90 to 270° (Faria, 1992). Thus with training, cycling can be used to build strength and endurance in multiple muscle groups.

Conclusion

Although cycling, particularly in professional circles, is still a male-dominated sport, women are participating in increasing numbers. There is very little in the way of gender-specific information regarding women in cycling. It seems sensible to suggest that traumatic injuries in cycling will not be greatly influenced by gender. On the other hand, overuse injuries have great potential to be influenced by gender. Women may have more frequent problems with bike fit due to gender-influenced guidelines. Another issue may be differences in training techniques. This is an area wide open for further investigation.

References

Anderson, J.C. & Sockler, J.M. (1990) Effects of orthoses on selected physiologic parameters in cycling. *Journal of the American Podiatric Medical Association* **80**, 161–166.

Ashbaugh, S.J., Macknin, M.L. & VanderBrug M.S. (1995) The Ohio bicycle injury study. *Clinical Pediatrics* **34**, 256–260.

Asmussen, E. (1953) Positive and negative muscular work. *Acta Physiologica Scandinavica* **28**, 364–382.

Boning, D., Gonen, Y. & Massen, N. (1984) Relationship between work load, pedal frequency, and physical fitness. *International Journal of Sports Medicine* **5**, 92–97.

Brogger, J.T., Hvass, I. & Bugge, S. (1990) Injuries at the BMX cycling European championship, 1989. *British Journal of Sports Medicine* **24**, 269–270.

Burke, E.R. (1981) Ulnar neuropathy in bicyclists. *Physician and Sportsmedicine* **9**, 53–56.

Burke, E.R. (1994) Proper fit of the bicycle. *Clinics in Sports Medicine* **13**, 1–14.

Chan, K.M., Yuen, Y., Li, C.K., Chien, P. & Tsang, G. (1993) Sports causing most injuries in Hong Kong. *British Journal of Sports Medicine* **27**, 263–267.

Coast, J.R., Cos, R.H. & Welch, H.G. (1986) Optimal pedalling rate in prolonged bouts of cycle ergometry. *Medicine and Science in Sports and Exercise* **18**, 225–230.

Coyle, E.F., Fletner, M.E., Kautz, S.A. *et al.* (1991) Physiological and biomechanical factors associated with elite endurance cycling performance. *Medicine and Science in Sports and Exercise* **23**, 93–107.

Davis, M.W., Litman, T., Crenshaw, R.W. & Mueller, J.K. (1980) Bicycling injuries. *Physician and Sportsmedicine* **8**, 88–96.

Davis, R. & Hull, M. (1981) Measurement of pedal loading in bicycling. II. Analysis and results. *Journal of Biomechanics* **14**, 857–872.

Eckman, P.B., Perlstein, G. & Altrocchi, P.H. (1975) Ulnar neuropathy in bicycle riders. *Archives of Neurology* **32**, 130–131.

Ericson, M.O. & Nisell, R. (1986) Tibiofemoral joint forces during ergometer cycling. *American Journal of Sports Medicine* **14**, 285–290.

Ericson, M.O. & Nisell, R. (1987) Patellofemoral joint forces during ergometer cycling. *Physical Therapy* **67**, 1365–1371.

Ericson, M.O., Ekholm, J., Svensson, O. & Nisell, R. (1985) The forces of ankle joint structures during ergometer cycling. *Foot and Ankle* **6**, 135–142.

Ericson, M.O., Nisell, R. & Nemeth, G. (1988) Joint motions of the lower limb during ergometer cycling. *Journal of Orthopedic Sports Physical Therapy* **9**, 273–279.

Faria, I.E. (1992) Energy expenditure, aerodynamics and medical problems in cycling, an update. *Sports Medicine* **13**, 43–63.

Faria, I.E., Sjogaard, G. & Bonde-Petersen, F. (1982) Oxygen cost during different pedalling speeds for constant power outputs. *Journal of Sports Medicine and Physical Fitness* **22**, 295–299.

Fulkerson, J.P. (1994) Patellofemoral pain disorder:

evaluation and management. *Journal of the American Academy of Orthopedic Surgery* **2**, 124–132.

Gardner, K.M. (1975) More on bicycle neuropathies. *New England Journal of Medicine* **292**, 1245.

Garrett, W.E. (1990) Muscle strain injuries: clinical and basic aspects. *Medicine and Science in Sports and Exercise* **22**, 436–442.

Gerbesich, S.G., Parker, D. & Dudzik, M. (1994) Bicycle–motor vehicle collisions. Epidemiology of related injury incidence and consequences. *Minnesota Medicine* **77**, 27–31.

Gonzalez, H. & Hull, M.L. (1989) Multivariate optimization of cycling biomechanics. *Journal of Biomechanics* **22**, 1151–1161.

Green, D.P. (1993) In D.P. Green (ed.) *Operative Hand Surgery*, 3rd edn, pp. 1988–1998. Churchill Livingstone, New York.

Hankey, G.J. & Gubbay, S.S. (1988) Compressive mononeuropathy of the deep palmar branch of the ulnar nerve in cyclists. *Journal of Neurology, Neurosurgery and Psychiatry* **51**, 1588–1590.

Heil, D.P.W., Ilcox, A.R. & Quinn, C.M. (1995) Cardiorespiratory responses to seat-tube angle variation during steady-state cycling. *Medicine and Science in Sports and Exercise* **27**, 730–735.

Henningan, S.P., Schneck, C.D., Mesgarzadeh, M. & Clancy, M. (1994) The semimenbranosus–tibial collateral ligament bursa. *Journal of Bone and Joint Surgery* **76A**, 1322–1327.

Hermans, M.H.E. (1991) Hydrocolloid dressing versus tulle gauze in the treatment of abrasions in cyclists. *International Journal of Sports Medicine* **12**, 581–584.

Hice, G.A., Kendrick, A. & Weber, K. (1988) The effect of foot orthoses on oxygen consumption while cycling. *Journal of the American Podiatric Medical Association* **75**, 513–521.

Holmes, J.C., Pruitt, A.L. & Whalen, N.J. (1993) Iliotibial band syndrome in cyclists. *American Journal of Sports Medicine* **21**, 419–424.

Hull, M.L. & Gonzalez, H. (1988) Bivariate optimization of pedalling rate and crank arm length in cycling. *Journal of Biomechanics* **21**, 839–849.

Hungerford, D.S. & Lennox, D.W. (1983) Rehabilitation of the knee in disorders of the patellofemoral joint: relevant biomechanics. *Orthopedic Clinics of North America* **14**, 397–402.

Inbar, O., Dotan, R., Trousil, T. & Dvir, Z. (1983) The effect of bicycle crank-length variation upon power performance. *Ergonomics* **26**, 1139–1146.

Ireland, M.L. & Wall, C. (1990) Epidemiology and comparison of knee injuries in elite male and female United States basketball athletes. *Medicine and Science in Sports and Exercise* **22**, 582.

Kiburz, D., Jacobs, R. & Reckling, F. (1986) Bicycling accidents and injuries among adult cyclists. *American Journal of Sports Medicine* **14**, 416–419.

Kronisch, R.L., Chow, T.K., Simon, L.M. & Wong, P.F. (1996) Acute injuries in off road bicycle racing. *American Journal of Sports Medicine* **24**, 88–93.

Last, R.J. (1984) *Anatomy, Regional and Applied*, 7th edn. Churchill Livingstone, London.

Mclennan, J.G., Mclennan, J.C. & Ungersma, J. (1988) Accident prevention in competitive cycling. *American Journal of Sports Medicine* **16**, 266–268.

Mcleod, W.D. & Blackburn, T.A. (1980) Biomechanics of knee rehabilitation with cycling. *American Journal of Sports Medicine* **8**, 175–180.

Magee, D.J. (1987) *Orthopedic Physical Assessment*. W.B. Saunders, Philadelphia.

Mandroukas, K. (1990) Some effects of knee angle and **foot placement in bicycle ergometer.** *Journal of Sports Medicine and Physical Fitness* **30**, 155–160.

Martins, M., Librecht, P. & Burssens, A. (1989) A surgical treatment of the iliotibial band friction syndrome. *American Journal of Sports Medicine* **17**, 651–654.

Mellion, M.B. (1991) Common cycling injuries. *Sports Medicine* **11**, 52–70.

Mellion, M.B., Fandel, C.M. & Wagner, W.F. (1988) Hydrocolloid dressings in the treatment of turf burns and other athletic abrasions. *Athletic Training* **23**, 341–346.

Munnings, F. (1991) Cyclist's palsy. *Physician and Sportsmedicine* **19**, 113–119.

National Collegiate Athletic Association (1991) *NCAA Injury Surveillance System*. NCAA, Overland Park, Kansas.

National Off Road Biking Association (1996) *Jeep Series Information*. NORBA, Colorado Springs.

Noakes, T.D. (1995) Fatal cycling injuries. *Sports Medicine* **20**, 348–362.

Noble, C.A. (1980) Iliotibial band friction in runners. *American Journal of Sports Medicine* **8**, 232–234.

Nordeen- Snyder, K.S. (1977) The effect of bicycle seat height variation upon oxygen consumption and lower limb kinematics. *Medicine and Science in Sports* **9**, 113–117.

Noth, J., Dietz, V. & Mauritz, K.H. (1980) Cyclist's palsy: neurological and EMG study in 4 cases with distal ulnar lesions. *Journal of the Neurological Sciences* **47**, 111–116.

O'Brien, T. (1991) Lower extremity cycling biomechanics: a review and theoretical discussion. *Journal of the American Podiatric Medical Association* **81**, 585–592.

O'Donoghue, D.H. (1987) Injuries of the knee. In D.H. O'Donoghue (ed.) *Treatment of Injuries to Athletes*, 4th edn, pp. 470–471. W.B. Saunders, Philadelphia.

Patterson, R.P. & Moreno, M.I. (1990) Bicycle pedalling forces as a function of pedalling rate and power output. *Medicine and Science in Sports and Exercise* **22**, 512–516.

Pfeifer, R.P. (1994) Off road bicycle racing injuries: the

NORBA pro/elite category. *Clinics in Sports Medicine* **13**, 207–218.

Ray, J.M. & Clancy, W.G. (1988) Semimembranosus tendinitis: an overlooked cause of medial knee pain. *American Journal of Sports Medicine* **16**, 347–351.

Ruby, P. & Hull, M.L. (1993) Response of intersegmental knee loads to foot/pedal platform degrees of freedom in cycling. *Journal of Biomechanics* **26**, 1327–1340.

Ruby, P., Hull, M.L., Kirby, K. & Jenkins, D.W. (1992) The effect of lower-limb anatomy on knee loads during seated cycling. *Journal of Biomechanics* **25**, 1195–1207.

Sacks, J.J., Homgren, P., Smith, S.M. & Sosin, D.M. (1991) Bicycle-associated head injuries and deaths in the United States from 1984 to 1988: how many are preventable? *Journal of the American Medical Association* **266**, 3016–3018.

Seabury, J.J., Adams, W.C. & Ramey, M.R. (1977) Influence of pedalling rate and power output on the energy expenditure during bicycle ergometry. *Ergonomics* **20**, 491–498.

Shennum, P.L. & deVries, H.A. (1976) The effect of saddle height on oxygen consumption during bicycle ergometer work. *Medicine and Science in Sports* **8**, 119–121.

Spaite, D.W., Murphy, M., Criss, E.A., Valenzuela, T.D. & Meslin, H.W. (1991) A prospective analysis of injury severity among helmeted and nonhelmeted bicyclists involved in collisions with motor vehicles. *Journal of Trauma* **31**, 1510–1516.

Swain, D.P. & Wilcox, J.P. (1992) Effect of cadence on economy of uphill cycling. *Medicine and Science in Sports and Exercise* **24**, 1123–1127.

Thompson, D.C., Thompson, R.S. & Rivara, F.P. (1990a) Incidence of bicycle related injuries in a defined population. *American Journal of Public Health* **80**, 1388–1390.

Thompson, D.C., Thompson, R.S., Rivara, F.P. & Wolf, M.E. (1990b) A case control study of the effectiveness of bicycle safety helmets in preventing facial injury. *American Journal of Public Health* **80**, 1471–1474.

Tucci, J.J. & Barone, J.E. (1988) A study of urban bicycling acccidents. *American Journal of Sports Medicine* **16**, 181–184.

Weiss, B.D. (1985) Nontraumatic injuries in amateur long distance bicyclists. *American Journal of Sports Medicine* **13**, 187–191.

Weiss, B.D. (1994) Clinical syndromes associated with bicycle seats. *Clinics in Sports Medicine* **13**, 175–186.

Widrick, J.J., Freedson, P.S. & Hamill, J. (1991) Effect of internal work on the calculation of optimal pedalling rate. *Medicine and Science in Sports and Exercise* **24**, 376–382.

Wilber, C.A., Holland, G.J., Madison, R.E. & Loy, S.F. (1995) An epidemiological analysis of overuse injuries among recreational cyclists. *International Journal of Sports Medicine* **16**, 201–206.

Wilmarth, M.A. & Nelson, S.G. (1988) Distal sensory latencies of the ulnar nerve in long distance bicyclists. *Journal of Orthopedic Sports Physical Therapy* **9**, 370–374.

Zappala, F.G., Taffel, C.B. & Scuderi, G.R. (1992) Rehabilitation of patellofemoral joint disorders. *Orthopedic Clinics of North America* **23**, 555–566.

Zelisko, J.A., Noble, H.B. & Porter, M.A. (1982) A comparison of men's and women's professional basketball injuries. *American Journal of Sports Medicine* **10**, 297–299.

Chapter 37

Tennis

CAROL L. OTIS

Introduction

Tennis is one of the most popular and widely played of all Olympic sports. An estimated 40–50 million children and adults worldwide play tennis each year on more than 1 million tennis courts (B. Patterson, personal communication, 1997). They play on different types of court surface and at different levels of competition, from the beginner hitting against a wall to professionals competing before thousands of spectators for hundreds of thousands of dollars. In the USA, the Tennis Industry Association estimates that 19.4 million people played tennis in 1996, comprising 60% men and 40% women (Tennis Industry Association, 1997). Approximately 1 million players are aged over 50. Called 'the sport for a lifetime' by the United States Tennis Association, tennis can be played and enjoyed by people aged 6 to 96.

History

The game of tennis as we recognize it today was 'invented' in 1874 when an Englishman, Major Walter Clopton Wingfield, patented a set of equipment and instructions for the game called lawn tennis (Collins & Hollander, 1994). Lawn tennis was first played on hourglass-shaped croquet lawns. Grass was the first court surface and the most traditional one. James Dwight brought tennis to the USA in 1876 and the rectangular court outline was codified in 1882 (Yeomans, 1987; Collins & Hollander, 1994).

Tennis was an Olympic sport in the first revival of the modern games in Athens in 1896 and continued in the Olympics until 1924. Tennis returned as a demonstration sport in the 1968 Olympics in Mexico City and in Los Angeles in 1984, and has been a full Olympic sport since the 1988 Olympics in Seoul.

Women first played Olympic tennis in the 1900 Paris Olympics, where Charlotte Cooper of Great Britain defeated Helene Prevost of France in the final. Women played mixed doubles in 1900, 1906 and 1912. Women's doubles were not played at the Olympics until 1920 in Antwerp. In the 1924 Paris Olympics, 28 countries sent a total of 113 tennis players, 82 men and 31 women (Collins & Hollander, 1994).

Women have represented their countries in international tennis competitions. Hazel Hotchkiss Wightman, an American tennis champion, founded the Wightman Cup, a competition modelled on the men's Davis Cup. The first Wightman Cup competition was contested between American and British teams in 1923. It continued between these two countries until 1989. In 1963, the International Tennis Federation (ITF) approved an international competition among women playing in teams representing their countries. Modelled on the Davis Cup competition and called the Federation Cup (Fed Cup), the first competition was played in London in 1963. It was won by the American team of Billie Jean Moffitt, Darlene Hard and Carole Caldwell. Today the Fed Cup is played yearly by teams of professional and amateur women representing their countries.

Tennis was traditionally an amateur sport but in 1968 the era of 'open tennis' and payment to players began. In 1971, 12 women's tournaments were designated as 'open' to both amateurs and professionals, with prize money going to the players who declared themselves as professionals (Collins & Hollander, 1994). The women's professional tour was formed in 1970 by eight players, who included Billie Jean King, Rosie Casals, Peaches Bartkowicz and Nancy Richey. Dubbed the 'Houston Eight', they played for US$7500 in prize money at a tournament in Houston, Texas (Collins & Hollander, 1994). In 1971, 14 tournaments sponsored by Virginia Slims were held, with total prize money of US$309 000. That year, Billie Jean King won US$117 000, becoming the first woman athlete to break the milestone of US$100 000 a year in winnings.

Physiological demands of the sport

Tennis has been called 'a game of continual emergencies' (Groppel & Roetert, 1992), featuring long rallies interspersed with short bursts of activity. Playing the game takes all of an individual's skill, agility, strength, speed, coordination, endurance, flexibility and mental toughness. It requires both anaerobic bursts of speed and intervals of submaximal effort during rallies. Women's matches can last as long as 2–3 hours with 90 s between change-overs every two games. The physical demands of the sport involve both the aerobic and anaerobic cardiorespiratory systems and the entire kinetic chain of the musculoskeletal system. Mastery of the game requires a progression from learning stroke technique to achieving ball control and placement with consistency, depth and power. These skills are then used with court sense, concentration and mental toughness (Fig. 37.1). Movement on the court is forward, back, diagonal and lateral.

Training for the sport

Professional and amateur tennis is played the entire year. Successful training involves a preparation phase, followed by precompetition, competition and transition (active rest) phases. Since tennis can be played all year, periodization of training cycles with a build-up to the competitive phase and a period of recovery and rest are important in minimizing burnout, overtraining and injuries (Groppel & Roetert, 1992; Gould *et al.*, 1996). Training should emphasize: (i) muscular strength and endurance; (ii) cardiovascular training for both aerobic and anaerobic conditioning; and (iii) flexibility, i.e. full range of

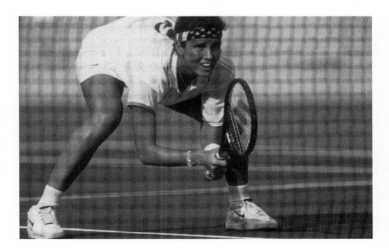

Fig. 37.1 Mary Joe Fernandez (USA) in a doubles match, Atlanta 1996. (© Allsport / S. Dunn.)

motion of the upper and lower extremities and trunk (Kibler *et al.*, 1988; Chandler, 1995). Sport-specific strengthening for tennis emphasizes abdominal, low back, shoulder, trunk, wrist, scapular and forearm muscles (Groppel & Roetert, 1992).

Equipment

Racquet

The most significant changes in tennis equipment are the modifications in racquet design. The original racquets were made of laminated wood. Racquets have been made from aluminium, steel, graphite, ceramic, magnesium, titanium, composites, fibreglass and boron. The head size and shape have also varied. A larger head allows greater surface area for ball contact. In 1981, the ITF proclaimed formal rules regarding racquet size for competition play (Collins & Hollander, 1994). The frame of the racquet cannot exceed 81.28 cm in length from the bottom of the handle to the top of the head. The width of the racquet head cannot exceed 31.75 cm. The string surface must not be greater than 39.37 cm in length and 29.21 cm in width. Racquet weight varies from 280 to 448 g with 14 g for the strings (Maylack, 1988; Collins & Hollander, 1994). Racquets of 280 g are the modern design. These racquets are powerful and highly manoeuvrable because of the lighter weight. Lightweight racquets can also cause less arm strain compared with heavier racquets.

Racquet type, string tension and location of ball impact on the string surface are some of the determinants of racquet frame vibration. The location on the strings where ball impact causes the least vibration is the node (Brody, 1979; Roetert *et al.*, 1995) (Fig. 37.2). Balls that impact outside the node cause more sting and racquet frame vibration. Vibration may be a factor in causing injury. Several factors influence the transmission of vibration and force to the wrist and forearm: the distance of the impact from the racquet node, the speed of the ball and racquet velocity, the tightness of the strings and the stiff-

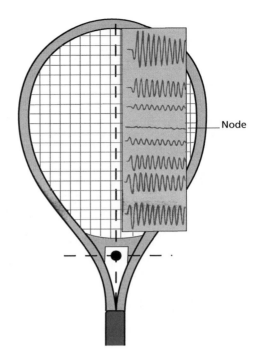

Fig. 37.2 Oscillations of a tennis racquet with different ball impact locations. The location where the ball produces the least vibration is called the node. (From Roetert *et al.*, 1995 with permission.)

ness of the racquet frame. The preferred racquet type for injury protection is a mid-size racquet of graphite composition, which is lightweight and has medium flexibility (Nirschl, 1995). Injuries can often be traced to the use of a new racquet, improper grip size, an increase in racquet string tension or poor stroke technique. It is important to choose the correct racquet grip size for the individual player. The common method to determine size is to measure the ring finger along the radial border from the proximal palmar crease to the tip of the ring finger (Nirschl, 1988) (Fig. 37.3).

The racquet can be strung with a wide variety of string types. Traditionally strings were made of cow gut, but their expense and limited durability have led to a market in synthetic strings. Good-quality synthetic strings, in thinner gauges for more responsive play and thicker gauges for

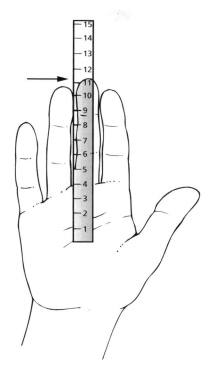

Fig. 37.3 Measurement of hand size to determine proper grip handle size. A good technique is to measure the ring finger along the radial border from the proximal palmar crease to the ring finger tip. (From Nirschl, 1988 with permission.)

practice play, are used by most players. They should be strung at the racquet manufacturer's recommended range of tension. A high string tension gives more control but increases the torque and vibration. When returning to play after a lay-off for an upper extremity injury, the player should have the racquet strung at 1.35–2.25 kg less pressure for the first few weeks.

Balls

Tennis balls have not undergone much modification, except for the change from white to yellow to aid visibility. Balls are made of hollow rubber spheres with felt covering. ITF rules specify the amount of deformation and bound when dropped 254 cm. For play at altitudes above 1219 m, non-pressurized balls can be used (ATP and ITF rules, Collins & Hollander, 1994). Ball speed at impact is 80–225 km·h^{-1} (Maylack, 1988). Worn balls require more stroke energy and bounce lower and may be a factor in injury production. This is the reason the professional players use new balls every seven to nine games.

Courts

The original court surface was grass but there are many other surfaces available now. Each type of court surface predisposes to different types of injuries (Lehman, 1988). Grass is fast and balls have an irregular low bounce, favouring quick players with a serve-and-volley game. Players bend to reach balls, resulting in low back, gluteal and piriformis injuries. Agility training helps a player prepare for grass court play. Clay and indoor carpet courts are the most cushioned and are easier on the joints. Balls bounce higher on clay surfaces, giving the player more time to reach the ball and favouring backcourt players and long rallies. The longer rallies can lead to more thigh and forearm strains from overuse. Stretching routines are helpful. The newest surface, Rebound Ace, is very fast and has a very hard surface with a low amount of cushioning. Low back problems, sprains and ankle injuries are common. Dynamic trunk stabilization, strength training and ankle taping can help players prevent injuries on this surface. Hard courts that heat up result in a tacky surface that causes the foot to stick and results in more foot friction (blisters) and deceleration trauma. Hard surfaces transmit more force to the entire kinetic chain and can be a factor in overload injuries and heel bruises. More protective and well-fitted cushioned shoes, foot powder and socks are important for hard-court players.

Injuries

'Tennis is a complex neurophysiological sport, involving the actions of running, catching, hitting, and throwing in many body segments' (Nirschl, 1995). Since tennis involves the entire body, many different injuries are seen in the sport, particularly those due to overuse or overload.

Types of injuries

Injuries result from a combination of factors, including imbalances in underlying muscle strength, prior injuries, flexibility or inflexibility, age, racquet, technique, surface and conditioning. The biomechanical analysis of tennis is in its infancy, although it is known that for effective movement the body must be linked in the kinetic chain. Motions and forces of all body parts must work together in order best to generate power and force. The kinetic chain in tennis starts with the ground reaction forces of the feet and legs, which are funnelled through the trunk and into the shoulder, elbow and hand, eventually reaching the racquet for ball contact (Fig. 37.4).

Researchers have determined the contribution of each link in the kinetic chain to total energy and force development by using the formulas for kinetic energy ($KE = \frac{1}{2}mv^2$) and force ($F = ma$). Calculations on élite tennis players found that 51% of total kinetic energy and 54% of total force are developed in the leg–hip–trunk link. The

shoulder contributes 13% of total energy and 21% of force (Kibler, 1995). The muscular activity of the shoulder is most effective in stabilizing the shoulder rather than generating a great deal of force. The shoulder therefore acts like a funnel to transfer, direct and concentrate the energy from the legs and trunk into the upper extremity. If the shoulder is well balanced, the transfer of energy is efficient. If there are imbalances in the shoulder, lowered efficiency and performance and clinical symptoms of injury may result.

Anatomical adaptations

There are several adaptations found in tennis players caused by the demands of the sport on the dominant side of the body to generate muscular force at high speed. The characteristic posture of élite and senior tennis players is a drooping or depression of the dominant shoulder, with increased muscular girth of the dominant arm (Priest & Nagel, 1976). The depressed shoulder may be due to stretching of the posterior shoulder capsule and the shoulder-elevating muscles because of either repetitive overhead motions or the increased weight of the dominant arm (Ellenbecker, 1995). Depression of the shoulder may produce or exacerbate rotator cuff impingement, tendinitis or thoracic outlet syndromes. Grip strength is greater in the dominant hand. Other differences in strength between the dominant and non-dominant arms of skilled tennis players are greater isokinetic strength of the dominant arm for internal rotation, extension and flexion of the shoulder as well as for extension and flexion of the wrist and pronation of the forearm (Ellenbecker, 1992). All these strengths are specific for actions relevant to tennis skills.

Of particular interest are the consequences of increased strength of the dominant arm on postural alignment and range of motion. In both male and female tennis players, limitation of internal shoulder rotation by as much as 10° has been found in the dominant shoulder (Chinn et al., 1974; Kibler et al., 1988; Chandler et al., 1990; Ellenbecker, 1992, 1995) (Table 37.1). For standardization, shoulder range of motion is

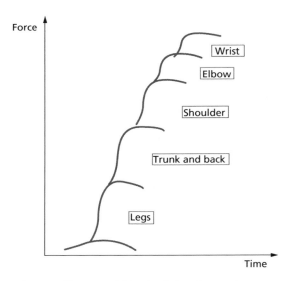

Fig. 37.4 The normal kinetic chain of a tennis serve. (From Kibler, 1995 with permission.)

Table 37.1 Range of motion (in degrees) of internal and external shoulder rotation in 147 élite junior tennis players aged 11–15. (From Ellenbecker, 1995 with permission)

Motion	Dominant arm		Non-dominant arm	
	Mean	SD	Mean	SD
External rotation				
Boys	94.6	26.0	95.9	21.3
Girls	104.9	10.0	103.5	10.1
Internal rotation				
Boys	54.5	23.6	65.4	16.8
Girls	53.6	11.2	62.7	9.8

Data generated with 90° of glenohumeral joint abduction with scapular stabilization.

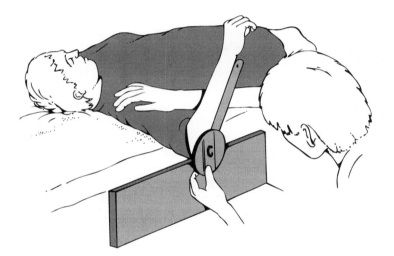

Fig. 37.5 Measurement of the internal rotation of the glenohumeral joint, with stabilization of the scapulothoracic joint being accomplished with anterior support from the examiner's hand; 90° of abduction was used during measurement. (Adapted from Ellenbecker, 1995.)

assessed in the supine patient with the shoulder at 90° of abduction and the scapulothoracic joint stabilized by the examiner placing a hand over the anterior glenohumeral joint (Fig. 37.5). The decrease in internal rotation is attributed to posterior capsular tightness and is associated with increases in external rotation that may indicate anterior and inferior capsular laxity. The changes in shoulder range of motion may be due to the repetitive demands of the tennis serve and the overhead shot. The decrement in internal rotation may predispose to anterior subluxation and

instability of the shoulder and is a contributing factor for shoulder rotator cuff instabilities and tendinitis.

Specific injuries

Young players

Epidemiological studies in young athletes show that injuries are sport specific and occur in different body structures compared with injured adults (Cahill & Pearl, 1993). While bones are still growing during puberty, injuries occur around the growth plate at the end of the long bones. Such injuries are well documented in young players in sports such as baseball, for example Little Leaguer's elbow. Pubertal tennis players are also at risk for these problems (Kibler *et al.*, 1988).

The other types of injury seen in adolescents are due to overload, cumulative injuries that result from overuse plus improper training and underlying anatomical malalignment. In a study of élite junior tennis players, 63% of all injuries were due to overload, 25% were strains and 12% were fractures (Kibler *et al.*, 1988) (Table 37.2). The result of overload injuries is pain and dysfunction, with reduction in strength, flexibility, joint range of motion and function. Chandler *et al.* (1990) showed that junior tennis players had less flexibility in the shoulder, low back and hamstring musculotendinous units compared with other junior athletes. These patterns of inflexibility in young tennis players result in abnormal mechanics during tennis strokes that can lead to further injury, overload and imbalances.

Lateral epicondylitis

This painful, often chronic problem was recognized before tennis was popular. Although it is now called 'tennis elbow', previously it was named 'housemaid's elbow' after one of several occupations with which it was connected. Lateral elbow pain is most common in recreational players over the age of 3 years and accounts for as much as 50% of their chronic injuries (Nirschl, 1995). Medial epicondylitis is less frequent, accounting for 10% of chronic injuries. Lateral epicondylitis is associated with the backhand stroke and medial epicondylitis

Table 37.2 Incidence of injury. (From Kibler *et al.*, 1988 with permission)

	Élite juniors (%)	Recreational (%)
Overload	63	62
Sprains	25	22
Fractures	12	14
Other		2

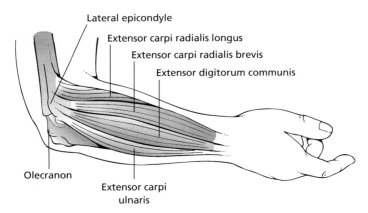

Fig. 37.6 The lateral epicondyle serves as a site of attachment for the forearm and wrist muscles. In patients with lateral epicondylitis (tennis elbow), faulty backhand technique places a strain on the extensor carpi radialis brevis, the extensor digitorum communis, the extensor carpi radialis longus and the extensor carpi ulnaris muscles. Resulting high forces on the extensor supinator origin may cause inflammation and pain. The ulnar nerve travels under the medial epicondyle and is covered by a retinaculum. It can be injured easily. In some patients, the nerve is poorly fixed and actually subluxes or dislocates out of its normal position within the groove. (From Shaffer & O'Mara, 1997 with permission.)

with the forehand, serve or overhead. The cause of lateral epicondylitis is postulated to be microtrauma to the tendon insertions of the wrist extensors at their common origin on the lateral humeral epicondyle (Fig. 37.6).

Repetitive microtrauma may be caused by concentric muscle overload, overuse of forearm muscles and/or transmission of vibrations from the racquet frame to the forearm muscles and tendons (Roetert *et al.*, 1995). Microtrauma at the origins of the extensors can lead to microtears that heal through fibrosis and granulation tissue. The result is a mucinoid degeneration of the tendons at their origin. Under pathological inspection there is non-inflammatory, oedematous, grey tissue with loss of the normal resilient parallel fibres. The normal tendon fibres are disrupted by fibroblastic invasion and vascular overgrowth, referred to as angiofibroblastic hyperplasia (Nirschl, 1995). This condition has been called a tendinosis instead of a tendinitis because it is more of a degenerative process than a true inflammation.

Risk factors for the development of lateral epicondylitis include overuse, poor stroke technique, improper equipment, age over 35, inadequate muscular and cardiovascular conditioning, and postural defects such as thoracic kyphosis and tight shoulder adductors and internal rotators (Field & Alcheck, 1995; Nirschl, 1995; Roetert *et al.*, 1995).

Proper stroke technique, with motion coupling rotation of the trunk with shoulder and arm acceleration during the stroke, is important in order to decrease overload to the forearm muscles. Unskilled players, who do not use the entire body in stroke production, lead with their elbow and use a one-handed backhand stroke, are at most risk. These faults create more forearm torque, muscle overload and strain and, if the ball is hit off-centre, more vibration. A two-handed technique on the backhand reduces these forces. The position of the ball at contact should be in front of the player, giving effective energy transfer to the ball from the racquet speed generated by trunk rotation (Roetert *et al.*, 1995; Sobel *et al.*, 1995) (Fig. 37.7).

The clinical symptoms of lateral epicondylitis are morning stiffness and day-long aching pain at the lateral elbow. Night pain or neck or shoulder pain may reflect referred pain or an underlying pathological process such as infection or tumour (Shaffer & O'Mara, 1997). Symptoms of locking, snapping or catching may be due to loose bodies or articular cartilage tears in the elbow joint. On physical examination, pain is reproduced by palpation distal and anterior to the lateral epicondyle and with resisted wrist

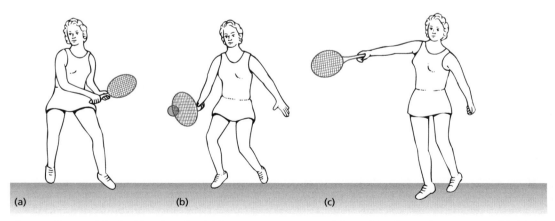

Fig. 37.7 Stages of the backhand stroke. (a) Racquet preparation is followed by the acceleration stage (b); (c) the stroke is completed with follow-through. (From Field & Altchek, 1995 with permission.)

extension. Pain may also be elicited by resisted extension of the middle finger when the elbow is extended. A complete evaluation to determine the specific cause of the injury is needed. Differential diagnosis includes arthritis or osteochondritis dissecans of the radial capitellar joint, loose bodies, bursitis and radial nerve compression (radial tunnel syndrome). X-rays of the elbow, computed tomography for loose bodies and nerve conduction studies are used in the evaluation (Field & Alcheck, 1995; Shaffer & O'Mara, 1997).

Management includes rest, local application of ice for 10–20 min two or three times a day and 1–3 weeks of oral anti-inflammatory medication to decrease the pain and any associated inflammation. The forearm extensor muscles should be protected so that activities of daily living are pain-free. Sufferers can lift bags and briefcases with a palm-up motion. A counterforce brace applied below the elbow will constrain extensor muscles and thereby reduce muscle contractile tension (Nirschl, 1988) (Fig. 37.8). The brace is used daily until symptoms produced by resisted wrist extension are lessened. Steroid injections are used infrequently, as this injury is not felt to be an inflammatory process. If used, there should not be more than three injections in one year (Field & Alcheck, 1995; Shaffer & O'Mara, 1997). Only 1–5% of cases of lateral epicondylitis are resistant to conservative measures and require surgical intervention. Acupuncture has been used for centuries to treat this common overuse syndrome. Specific acupuncture sites are used for pain relief and three or more treatments may be needed. When done by an experienced licenced practitioner using sterilized needles, acupuncture can be well tolerated and considered part of conservative treatment (Baldry, 1993).

Early in the course of management the patient should be referred to a physical therapist for gentle passive, then active, range of motion exercises in symptom-free range of motion. A common deficit is lack of mobility of the radio-ulnar joint, especially in supination. This deficit should be addressed and corrected. Joint mobi-

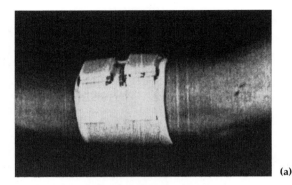

(a)

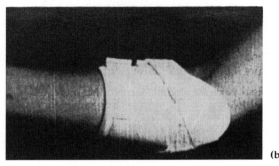

(b)

Fig. 37.8 (a) Lateral counterforce elbow brace. Counterforce bracing is used to decrease pain and control abusive force overloads. Adequate design includes multiple tension straps and wide bracing for full patient control. Curved contours allow accurate fit to key areas in the conically shaped extremities. (b) Medial counterforce elbow brace. Medial protection adds extra support for the common flexor origin. (From Nirschl, 1993 with permission.)

lization by a trained manual physical therapist can be part of therapy. Therapists may use modalities such as ultrasound, iontophoresis and phonophoresis with or without topical anti-inflammatory medications. Some clinicians advocate cross-fibre tissue massage to aid in healing; others feel that this aggressive massage worsens the pain and causes a synovitis (Sobel *et al.*, 1995).

When the athlete is pain-free, therapy is not completed. It is important to include strengthening exercises and a coordinated rehabilitative exercise programme to build strength and endurance of the forearm muscles in all motions. The athlete must also review equipment and, if necessary, learn proper stroke technique with the therapist or a coach (Ellenbecker, 1995). The therapist works to achieve reduction of tissue overload and total arm rehabilitation, not only for the wrist and elbow but also for the shoulder and scapular muscles.

Prevention of tennis elbow injuries

Reducing the known risk factors for elbow injuries can reduce the probability of these injuries. Emphasis on correct stroke technique is essential in reducing risk of this and other overuse injuries. Proper stroke technique requires coordination between trunk rotation and movement of the entire arm and contact with the ball as the angular momentum of the body begins to move forward in a coordinated manner. When these motions are properly coupled, the force of trunk rotation is transferred through the arm to the racquet. If uncoupled, the forces of hitting the ball are not coordinated, resulting in excessive isolated arm motions and overload of the arm and shoulder muscles and soft tissues (Field & Alcheck, 1995) A two-handed backhand technique is protective. A forehand stroke hit late with wrist snap also increases the risk of lateral elbow injury (Roetert et al., 1995; Sobel et al., 1995).

The racquet should have correct grip size. String tension can be lowered by 1.35–2.25 kg and new balls should be used in order to minimize the added stroke energy required for hitting older, deader balls (Field & Alcheck, 1995). Devices on the strings to reduce vibration have not been shown to be of any benefit. Mid-sized racquets with medium flexibility ratings are recommended (Nirschl, 1988; Ellenbecker, 1995). A counterforce brace applied distal to the elbow joint can help decrease elbow angular acceleration and muscle activity (Nirschl, 1988). If the player has postural distortions such as kyphosis, these should be evaluated and addressed as part of the therapy in correcting underlying risk factors.

Age eligibility in women's professional tennis

A new era for tennis began in the late 1970s when it became a sport played not only for enjoyment but also for financial gain. In 1972, Title IX legislation in the USA mandated equal access and facilities for sport for boys and girls in federally funded programmes. With increased opportunities came increased participation by girls and women in all sports, an improved image of athletic girls, and greater access to coaching, facilities and rehabilitation. In the world of tennis, this new era of sport provided more opportunities for not only participation but also the possibility of a college scholarship, turning professional or making a living as a coach. The professional world of sport provided the chance of prize money, endorsements and fees for exhibition play. As the stakes in tennis increased, so did the pressures.

A new era of tennis training began to emerge, with young girls starting early in life because of the unproven notion that the earlier the training, the more likely the chance for success. Girls as young as 8 or 10 years and their families uprooted their lives and moved to tennis academies to train year round, while girls as young as 13 and 14 turned professional. Between the ages of 10 and 18, girls pass through two critical developmental phases, puberty and adolescence. Training for, and competing in, professional tennis can interrupt and add stress to these developmental phases. It is not uncommon for girls to spend up to 6 hours a day training and playing. This can lead to high levels of physical, financial and psychological demands on the girls and their families, and can disrupt normal patterns of schooling, socialization, pubertal psychosocial development, and family life. It is important to remember that for every player who 'makes it' on the tour, there are dozens if not hundreds of others who do not achieve success.

In the late 1980s and early 1990s some of these younger players had visible problems that received widespread publicity. Some young professionals left the game before the age of 20 due to repetitive injuries and burnout. The media reported allegations of parental abuse and drug abuse among some of the youngest players. Individuals in tennis administration, coaching and sports science raised the alarm regarding the adverse effects of intensive early training on the mental and physical health of young athletes (Cahill & Pearl, 1993; Gould *et al.*, 1996; Skolnick, 1996).

The first governing body to respond to these concerns and to change the rules was the Women's Tennis Council. The Council is the governing body of international professional tennis and is composed of player representatives, tournament representatives and leaders from the ITF and the WTA Tour (Women's Tennis Association, the governing body of the professional tour). The WTA Tour sets the regulations for play and age of participation on the professional women's tour. In 1992, girls could begin limited professional play at age 13 and play unrestricted at age 16. Spurred by the requests of the players, in particular Pam Shriver, the president of the Players' Advisory Board, the Women's Tennis Council and the ITF formed an independent voluntary commission of seven experts in sports science and sports medicine to review the age eligibility rule in women's professional tennis. The Age Eligibility Commission was charged with not only reviewing the rule but also identifying factors that would contribute to career longevity and enhance well-being and health on the women's professional tour.

The Commission established a base of evidence and information from diverse sources and held a consensus conference in 1994 to review the evidence and make recommendations. They reviewed the scientific literature and solicited and received written and oral testimony from everyone in the tennis community: agents, sponsors, coaches, parents, spouses, athletes, tournament directors, athletic trainers, media, physicians and manufacturers. They also obtained a detailed statistical analysis of the career longevity of the top 225 players on the WTA Tour from 1981 to 1993 (Otis, 1994; Otis *et al.*, 1999). This review showed that the average

age of players was 22.8 years with a range of 16–37 years. There were only two players in the top 225 under the age of 16 (Otis *et al.*, 1999). The average age of the top 20 international players has been remarkably stable since 1980, ranging from a low of 21.7 years (1990) to 24.45 years (1981). Analysis of the top-ranked American women from 1980 to 1992 found that the average age ranged from 22.2 to 23.3 years (Galenson, 1995). The belief that success comes at an early age is derived from the prominence of a few 'phenoms', players who achieve high rankings while young. Precocious talents have been identified and developed in many fields, from music to science to sport and entertainment. However, these individuals are the rare exception. Contrary to the prevailing notion that to be successful in professional tennis one must achieve success early, statistical analysis showed that success at an early age was rare: only 11 women under the age of 17 have ever been ranked in the top 20 (1981–93). Early success may make a media star, but the price may be high. Analysis showed that the younger a girl started playing professional tennis, the shorter her career. Of girls who turned professional before the age of 15, 19% left the tour before the age of 20 ($n=26$) compared with only 3% of girls who turned professional between the ages of 15 and 17 ($n=262$) (Otis *et al.*, 1999) (Fig. 37.9).

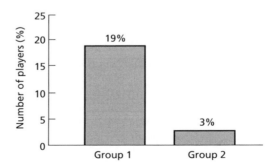

Fig. 37.9 Percentage of players leaving the WTA Tour before the age of 20 years. Group 1, players starting aged 13–14 ($n=26$); Group 2, players starting aged 15–17 years ($n=262$). (From Otis *et al.*, 1999 with permission.)

Direct, coded oral and written testimony from 91 different members of the tennis community was obtained by the Age Eligibility Commission about the appropriateness of the age rule in professional tennis, the proper 'dose' of tennis for young players, and the risks and stressors of professional tennis. Of the respondents, 97% felt that the 1993 age eligibility rules were not appropriate, while 88% felt that a 'phased-in' approach to playing professional tennis was appropriate, with the majority favouring no unrestricted play until 18 years of age. The stressors described included the competitiveness of the tour, injuries, financial issues, pressure from agents, families and media, loneliness and isolation, travel and night matches. The players who gave testimony ranked the pressures from the media and parents and families as their greatest stressors, followed by travel, competition, loneliness and pressures from agents.

Review of the literature and testimony from sports scientists and physicians identified the risks of early participation, including acute and chronic musculoskeletal imbalances and injuries, impaired social and educational development, disruption of normal menstrual cyclicity, and acute and chronic psychological problems such as depression, anxiety, drug abuse, low self-esteem and burnout (Kibler *et al.*, 1988; Otis, 1994; Gould *et al.*, 1996; Skolnick, 1996). These problems are difficult to quantify as there is no literature about professional women players. Moreover, these problems are often hidden, vary greatly among individuals and may not appear until years after a woman finishes her career.

In order to reduce the risks and pressures, the Commission recommended not only changing the age of participation but also trying to ameliorate the known stressors. The Commission also recommended that there should be no unrestricted play on the professional tour until age 18 (Table 37.3). Play is gradually phased in at age 14, with only five tournaments on the satellite ITF circuit and no play on the WTA Tour above the Tier III level until age 16. The Commission also recognized the dangers associated with young players becoming 'revenue producers', participating in unlimited exhibition matches staged by promoters and agents and receiving wild-card entries into tournaments. Therefore, players aged between 14 and 17 are permitted to play in a limited number of exhibition matches (Otis, 1994; Worcester & Otis, 1995). These rules allow the gifted adolescent player to adjust to participation in professional tennis and become exposed gradually to the physical and psychological demands of the professional tennis world.

To lessen the stressors, other rules were recommended and adopted in a multifaceted programme (Women's Tennis Association, 1997). The athlete is required to undergo annual detailed medical and musculoskeletal examinations and to meet the educational requirements of her country of origin. Her coaches and agent are required to register with the tour and to sign a code of conduct. Night matches are forbidden for players under age 18. To monitor these rules, the WTA Tour made some changes in its structure. A Player Development Program was created to track younger players and to monitor their wild-

Table 37.3 New age-eligibility rules 1995

Age	Total events	WTA Tour events	ITF Tour events	Grand Slam events	Non-Tour events	Events under prior rule
13	0	0	0	0	0	3 ITF
14	5	0	4	0	1	12 + championships
15	9	4 (tier III/IV)	8	0	1	17 + championships
16	14	10 + championships		All	3	Unrestricted
17	18	13 + championships		All	4	Unrestricted

ITF, International Tennis Federation; WTA, Women's Tennis Association.

card entries, educational requirements and physical examination. In addition, the WTA Tour adopted the Commission's recommendation for mandatory educational and orientation courses for young players to learn about the tour and about injury prevention, nutrition, periodization of training and coping with the media. A girl's parents or guardian also are required to attend courses. A mentor programme was adopted, where older or retired players are connected to younger players as a source of advice and support. The Commission also recommended increased safeguards for players on the road by recommending the presence of athletic trainers at all levels of tournament play on the ITF satellite circuit and additional trainers for the WTA Tour, with greater access to medical, psychological and career counselling services (Otis, 1994; Howard, 1995; Worcester & Otis, 1995; Otis *et al.*, 1999).

The investigation of the problems and the adoption of these rules in 1994 was a trailblazing move by the Women's Tennis Council and the chief executive officer of the WTA Tour, Anne Person Worcester, and the director of the ITF women's division, Debbie Jevans. The problems identified and their solutions are not unique to tennis. Tennis has led the way and set the standard for sports governing bodies to recognize and implement changes that will improve the health, well-being and long-term success of players. It is hoped that the rest of the world will listen and follow suit.

References

Baldry, P.E. (1993) *Acupuncture, Trigger Points and Musculoskeletal Pain*. Churchill Livingstone, London.

Brody, H. (1979) Physics of the tennis racquet. *American Journal of Physics* 6, 482–487.

Cahill, B.R. & Pearl, A.S. (eds) (1993) *Intensive Participation in Children's Sports*. Human Kinetics Publishers, Champaign, Illinois.

Chandler, T.J. (1995) Exercise training for tennis. *Clinics in Sports Medicine* 14, 33–46.

Chandler, T.J., Kibler, W.B. & Uhl, T.L. (1990) Flexibility comparisons of junior elite tennis players to other athletes. *American Journal of Sports Medicine* 18, 134–136.

Chinn, C.J., Priest, J.D. & Kent, B.E. (1974) Upper extremity range of motion, grip strength, and girth in highly skilled tennis players. *Physical Therapy* 54, 474–482.

Collins, B. & Hollander, Z. (eds) (1994) *Bud Collins' Modern Encyclopedia of Tennis*, 2nd edn. Visible Ink Press, Detroit.

Ellenbecker, T.S. (1992) Shoulder internal and external rotation strength and range of motion of highly skilled junior tennis players. *Isokinetics and Exercise Science* 2, 1–8.

Ellenbecker, T.S. (1995) Rehabilitation of shoulder and elbow injuries in tennis players. *Clinics in Sports Medicine* 14, 87–108.

Field, L.D. & Altcheck, D.W. (1995) Elbow injuries. *Clinics in Sports Medicine* 14, 59–78.

Galenson, D.W. (1995) Does youth rule? Trends in the ages of American women tennis players, 1960–1992. *Journal of Sport History* 22, 46–59.

Gould, D., Tuffey, S., Udry, E. & Loehr, J. (1996) Burnout in competitive junior tennis players. *Sport Psychologist* 10, 322–340.

Groppel, J.L. & Roetert, E.P. (1992) Applied physiology of tennis. *Sports Medicine* 14, 260–268.

Howard, R.R. (1995) Rule changes in women's tennis target medical issues. *Physician and Sportsmedicine* 23, 25–26.

Kibler, W.B. (1995) Biomechanical analysis of the shoulder during tennis activities. *Clinics in Sports Medicine* 14, 79–86.

Kibler, W.B., McQueen, C. & Uhl, T. (1988) Fitness evaluation and fitness findings in competitive junior tennis players. *Clinics in Sports Medicine* 7, 403–417.

Lehman, R.D. (1988) Surface and equipment variables in tennis injuries. *Clinics in Sports Medicine* 7, 229–232.

Maylack, F.H. (1988) Epidemiology of tennis, squash and racquetball injuries. *Clinics in Sports Medicine* 7, 233–243.

Nirschl, R.P. (1988) Prevention and treatment of elbow and shoulder injuries in the tennis player. *Clinics in Sports Medicine* 7, 289–308.

Nirschl, R.P. (1993) Muscle and tendon trauma: tennis elbow. In B.F. Morrey (ed.) *The Elbow and Its Disorders*, 2nd edn, pp. 63–85. W.B. Saunders, Philadelphia.

Nirschl, R.P. (1995) Tennis injuries. In E. Hershman & J. Nicholas (eds) *The Upper Extremity in Sports Medicine*, 2nd edn, pp. 789–803. Mosby, Philadelphia.

Otis, C.L. (1994) A review of the age eligibility commission report. *USTA Sport Science Newsletter* Fall, 1–3.

Otis, C.L., Roetert, E.P., Loehr, J. *et al.* (1999) Age eligibility in women's professional tennis. (Draft in submission.)

Priest, J.D. & Nagel, D.A. (1976) Tennis shoulder. *American Journal of Sports Medicine* 4, 28–42.

Roetert, E.P., Brody, H., Dillman, C.J., Groppel, J.L. &

Schulties, J.M. (1995) The biomechanics of tennis elbow: an integrated approach. *Clinics in Sports Medicine* **14**, 47–57.

Shaffer, B. & O'Mara, J. (1997) Common elbow problems. *Journal of Musculoskeletal Medicine* **14**, 61–75.

Skolnick, A.A. (1996) Health pros want new rules for girl athletes. *Journal of the American Medical Association* **275**, 22–24.

Sobel, J., Pettrone, F.A. & Nirschl, R.P. (1995) Prevention and rehabilitation of racquet sport injuries. In E. Hershma & J. Nicholas (eds) *The Upper Extremity in Sports Medicine*, 2nd edn, pp. 805–822. Mosby, Philadelphia.

Tennis Industry Association (1997) *Participation Report*. Tennis Industry Association, 200 Castlewood Drive, N. Palm Beach, Florida 33408, USA.

Women's Tennis Association (1997) *The Official Corel WTA Tour Rules*. COREL WTA Tour Corporate Headquarters, 1299 East Main Street, Fourth Floor, Stamford, Connecticut 06902-3546, USA.

Worcester, A.P. & Otis, C.L. (1995) Explaining the wisdom of the ages. *Tennis* March, 24.

Yeomans, P.H. (1987) *Southern California Tennis Champions Centennial*. Southern California Committee for the Olympic Games.

Chapter 38

Basketball

SUSAN W. RYAN

Introduction

Women's basketball has enjoyed a tremendous rise in popularity. In the USA, participation in girls' youth basketball has outnumbered all other sports for the first time, while in the last decade the attendance at women's college basketball has tripled. In fact, in the 1996 National Collegiate Athletic Association (NCAA) Basketball Championships, the women's final drew more spectators than the men's final and had the highest television rating in the history of women's basketball. Women also have an opportunity to compete in professional leagues in the USA and Europe (Fig. 38.1).

A great deal of interest has been sparked in the field of sports medicine because of the increased participation in women's basketball. As has often been the case in other sports, the female athlete's psychological and physiological responses to participation in sport has been extrapolated from studies on male athletes. Books such as this serve to identify the particular risks to women in their sports and hopefully will encourage the scholars of science and sports medicine to carry out further research on the impact of female athleticism.

Injury rates

Basketball injuries in men and women are generally similar in their severity and frequency. There are a few exceptions, which are highlighted in this chapter. In general, collegiate and profes-

sional basketball for both men and women involves considerable physical exertion, which puts the athlete at greater risk for injuries.

Injuries are often defined as a traumatic or chronic problem that requires diagnosis and treatment from either the team physician or trainer. The time lost as a result of the injury further distinguishes the severity or complexity of the problem. In 1982, the NCAA Injury Surveillance System was created in order to gather data on collegiate athletic injuries. This has proved to be a current and reliable source of data that involves an enormous sampling pool. Trends can be identified that may prevent future injuries by modification of training regimens or equipment standards.

During the 1991–92 NCAA women's basketball season, acute injuries accounted for 77% of musculoskeletal complaints presenting to the attending medical staff. Nearly 60% of injuries are noted to occur during practice (National Collegiate Athletic Association Injury Surveillance System, 1991–1992). It has often been noted that despite the increased intensity of competition more time is spent in practice, which exposes an athlete to increased probability of injury. According to this same NCAA data, injuries due to contact with another athlete (36%) and those due to non-contact (28%) do not differ greatly. The two most likely areas of the body to be injured are the ankle and the knee, accounting for 45% of all basketball injuries in women. The guard position in basketball is also noted to be at greater risk of injury than either the forward or centre

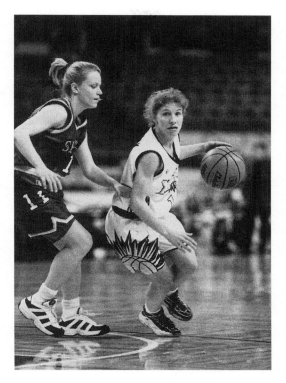

Fig. 38.1 A player for the Colorado Xplosion team brings the ball downcourt in a game with the Seattle Reign team. (Photo courtesy of Brian Lewis.)

position. A guard also is more likely to suffer from lower extremity injuries, while the forward and centre positions receive more upper extremity and facial trauma injuries.

Lower extremity injuries

Ankle

The ankle is the joint most commonly injured in basketball as well as in many other sports. The most common mechanism for ankle sprain is inversion on a plantar flexed foot (Ray *et al.*, 1991). This occurs with cutting manoeuvres, as well as when an athlete lands on another player's foot. Depending upon the severity of the injury, the lateral ligaments are stretched or torn, beginning with the anterior talofibular ligament and

progressing through the calcaneofibular ligament to the posterior talofibular ligament.

An immediate physical examination is valuable in assessing swelling, tenderness and ability to bear weight. Stress testing of the ligaments can provide some information about their integrity. These tests are most valuable if carried out prior to the development of significant swelling and guarding. A positive anterior drawer test, performed with the foot in a neutral position and pulled forward against a secured tibia, reveals disruption of the anterior talofibular ligament. The talar tilt or inversion test assesses the stability of the lateral calcaneofibular ligament. Pain usually prevents active strength testing of the ankle at the time of injury.

Guidelines for determining the need for radiographic testing exist. It is generally agreed that most ankle sprains do not require radiographic examination; however, if the physical examination reveals bony tenderness over the distal 6 cm of the tibia, fibula or the tarsals or metatarsals, radiographs are warranted. Radiographs are also necessary if pain with weight-bearing persists despite an otherwise negative physical examination.

Standard protocols for the treatment of musculoskeletal injuries should be followed. Ice and early range of motion are critical components. Proprioceptive training is another key element in the treatment of ankle sprains and is crucial to prevention. Numerous studies have been carried out on various preventative programmes. Ankle taping is effective in restricting motion initially, although its value decreases rapidly with activity. Many standardized motion-controlled braces are more effective than taping and more economical; they also reduce the rate of ankle injuries by 50% (Ashton-Miller, 1996). High-top shoes and strengthening of the peroneals have also been added to many basketball programmes with good success.

Ankle sprains are so common that many are treated with little regard to some serious complications that may develop or are overlooked initially. The examination should include palpation of the peroneal ligaments as they course behind the lateral malleolus. The peroneal brevis attaches to the base of the fifth metatarsal and occasionally to the cuboid as well. Tenderness over the bony attachments warrants radiographs in order to rule out an avulsion fracture of the proximal end of the fifth metatarsal. Tearing or stretching of the retinaculum can also cause subluxation of the peroneals as a late complication of ankle sprains.

High ankle sprains involve the syndesmosis or interosseous membrane between the tibia and fibula. Initial testing to determine this injury includes direct palpation over the tissue, as well as dorsiflexing and externally rotating the foot to stress this structure. Compression at the proximal ends of the tibia and fibula can also elicit symptoms distally. Treatment with rigid, pneumatic compressive braces can aid significantly in returning the athlete to an active rehabilitation programme. These injuries can be quite problematic in the recovery phase and can delay the return to play by several weeks. Because of the tremendous forces involved with this injury, tenderness along the proximal fibula should be evaluated radiographically to rule out a Maisonneuve's fracture.

Late complications of ankle sprains include capsular scarring, anterior impingement and occult talar dome injuries, including osteochondritis dissecans and chondral defects. Late instability of the ankle can be identified by stress radiographs but is still best treated by non-operative exercises that accentuate muscle strengthening and proprioception.

Foot

Injuries to the foot can present with symptoms similar to those of an ankle sprain. In the acute setting, it is important to consider injuries to the hindfoot and midfoot in the assessment.

Navicular fractures of the foot can be quite a problem for an athlete. Avulsion fractures alone account for more than 50% of injuries to this bone. The mechanism for these injuries is acute eversion of the foot, which places tension on the fibres of both the deltoid ligament and the poste-

rior tibial tendon of the medial ankle. It is often missed initially but fortunately is not a significant cause of chronic dysfunction in the athlete. Large fragments that are symptomatic may need to be surgically excised.

Os trigonum injuries are sustained in basketball when a player steps on the foot of another, causing a forceful plantar flexion of the foot. The os trigonum is an accessory bone of the lateral tubercle of the talus and is found in about 10% of the population. An acute fracture can cause posterior lateral ankle pain as well as pain with ankle motion. The flexor hallucis longus tendon travels through this area. Hyperextension of the great toe can reproduce this pain as the tendon is dragged across the fracture site. Treatment is difficult as protection from weight-bearing for 4–6 weeks is often necessary. Occasionally, surgical attention must be given to this problem.

Calcaneal beak fractures occur through a similar mechanism to os trigonum fractures except that the anterior structures of the foot are under extreme tension. The bifurcate ligament connects the anterior process of the calcaneus to the cuboid and navicular bones. Most commonly, patients present with pain anterior to the lateral malleolus. Despite a good prognosis in the long term, convalescence is tediously slow for the athlete eager to return to play. Most often, a non-weight-bearing cast is required for 4–6 weeks.

Acute rupture of the Achilles tendon is usually seen in the older, recreational athlete unaccustomed to the explosive demands of a sport such as basketball. However, tendinopathies of this area are extremely common. Pain is fairly well localized to the distal tendon and, depending upon the degree of fibrous degeneration and inflammation of the peritendinous structures and the tendon itself, palpation reveals a certain bogginess to the tissue. Recommended treatment includes an aggressive regimen to prevent further deterioration of the condition. This includes heel wedges and curtailing activities, along with the usual approaches to reducing pain and inflammation. Ogilvie-Harris and Gilbart (1995) have found that ultrasound offers little advantage to ice and exercise for this and other tendinous injuries. However, many others still contend that ultrasound serves as a useful adjunct to other therapeutic approaches. Even more controversial is the use of steroids in this area. While many feel comfortable with phonophoresis as the delivery method, injections of corticosteroid remain potentially risky.

Insertional Achilles tendinitis is often seen as a distinct entity. It has been associated with Haglund's disease or 'pump bumps'. This is where the bony prominence of the posterosuperior calcaneus can impinge upon the tendinous insertion, which causes a collection of debris and fibrosis that may occasionally need surgical débridement. Inflammation of the retrocalcaneal bursa, located in this same area, can mimic this problem.

Posterior tibial tendinitis can be caused by an acute injury or repetitive forces, causing pain along the medial aspect of the midfoot and radiating along the length of the muscle more proximally. Patients often present with pain with heel raises and weakness with inversion of the foot. Often seen with this condition is collapse of the longitudinal arch, which then leads to abduction of the forefoot and associated genu varum. Viewing the foot from behind while standing reveals the 'too many toes sign', which indicates progressive perisubluxation of the talus. Complete disruption of this ligament is rare in younger athletes and most respond well to symptomatic treatment and the use of heel cups or orthotics that limit heel valgus and support the longitudinal arch.

Heel pain from plantar fasciitis is another common problem seen in basketball players. Both a flat foot and a cavus foot predispose the athlete to this problem but differ in their mechanisms. The cavus foot is subject to repetitive stretching at its attachment to the calcaneal tuberosity. In the flat foot, however, pronation and valgus changes in the heel cause instability during the gait that strains the plantar fascia. Viscoelastic heel cushions help significantly and night splints have recently become a popular and effective treatment option. During sleep, the foot falls into an equinus position, allowing shorten-ing of the plantar fascia and the Achilles tendon. The first step in the morning can be excruciating as these tissues are abruptly stretched. Splinting in a neutral 90° of dorsiflexion or even an additional 5 or 10° allows the inflamed tissue to heal in a functional position. Stretching and ice continue to play an important role in the recovery.

In the forefoot, sesamoiditis is common. Acute fractures occur but can be difficult to distinguish from bipartite sesamoids. A roughened, irregular margin on plain films can help with this distinction but bone scans are sometimes necessary. Steroid injections, rest and occasionally surgical excisions may be necessary to improve the symptomatology.

Hallux rigidus is a degenerative arthritic response to repetitive trauma at the metatarsal joint of the great toe. It is a progressive problem that begins with extreme positions of dorsiflexion at the joint, as is seen in basketball with sudden starting and jumping. A synovitis occurs that later leads to dorsal lipping across the joint. Pain and limitation of motion bring the athlete in for examination. Initial treatment is to provide a more rigid sole to decrease motion. Surgical treatment is often necessary at some point in the future.

Lower leg

Problems of the lower leg are seen in basketball because of the unforgiving court surface and repetitive running and jumping (Fig. 38.2). Medial tibial stress syndrome is the term that has replaced 'shin splints', which was originally proposed by Drez (Mubarak *et al.*, 1982). It is thought to represent a condition of chronic overload of the posterior tibial tendon but can also include periostitis, fascial shearing of the muscle and stress fractures of the tibia. The pain initially is felt with exertion but progresses to pain at rest. Some describe it as a sharp, lancinating pain, while others perceive it as a dull ache. Diagnosis is often aided by radiological studies. Plain films may show hypertrophy and periosteal thickening of the posterior cortex of the tibia secondary to remodelling due to repetitive stresses (Michael

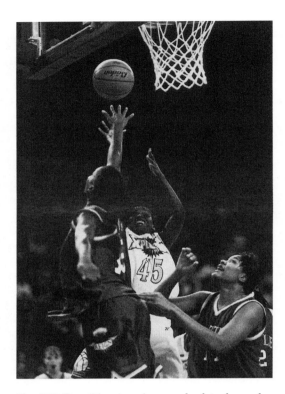

Fig. 38.2 Repetitive jumping can lead to lower leg injuries. (Photo courtesy of Brian Lewis.)

& Holder, 1985). These authors also noted that subperiosteal lucency and scalloping can be seen on the tibia. Numerous studies have documented that the characteristic findings of triple-phase radionuclide bone imaging distinguishes medial tibial stress syndrome from a true stress fracture (Rupani *et al.*, 1985). The syndrome shows increased activity along the posterior border of about one-third of the tibia on delayed images. The radionuclide angiogram and blood pool images, phase 1 and 2, are always normal. A stress fracture, on the other hand, shows a focal, intense reaction with a typical fusiform appearance.

In either injury, evaluation of the biomechanics of the foot, ankle and knee is important. Close examination of the conditioning programme is necessary in order to correct factors that lead to muscle fatigue and failure due to the rhythmic

repetitive actions of basketball. Diagnosis of a stress fracture should alert the physician to the possible presence of the female athlete triad (see Part 6).

Knee

Injuries to the knee are second only to the ankle in frequency but account for more serious problems (Sonzogni & Gross, 1993). Acute injuries commonly include ligamentous tears, meniscal contusions and tears, and patellar dislocations. In basketball, the most common mechanism of acute injury is rapid deceleration with a valgus and external rotatory force (Sonzogni & Gross, 1993).

The diagnosis of anterior cruciate ligament (ACL) tears is relatively straightforward. The athlete often notes an audible pop and may experience an acute effusion. On-site examination offers an invaluable chance to obtain a positive Lachman test, which is the most sensitive test for an ACL tear. There is considerable discussion in the medical community about the higher incidence of ACL disruption in female athletes. This is particularly true in women's basketball, where ACL injuries occur at three times the rate in men's basketball (Arendt & Dick, 1995). Current consensus is that the cause is probably multifactorial and includes some anatomical considerations, such as a smaller femoral condylar notch and a greater Q-angle. Others point to physiological reasons, such as a relative imbalance of the hamstring complex to the quadriceps muscles and a weaker vastus medialis muscle. Proprioception, which develops in early childhood play, is undoubtedly an important factor. Oestrogen receptors and the effect of circulating oestradiol is an area of recent discussion and controversy. Studies are continuing to investigate why women might be more at risk for ACL injuries and hopefully these will provide insight into ways that these injuries can be prevented. Treatment of an ACL tear includes early control of pain, swelling and initiation of range of motion. This is followed by a rehabilitation programme that precedes the surgical repair. After surgery, an aggressive rehabilitation protocol should be designed by the team physicians and training staff.

Meniscal tears can occur with rotatory or compressive forces in a hyperflexed knee. A small tear can be elusive but suggestive findings include joint line tenderness and a positive McMurray's or Apley's grind test. With a large tear, it is common to have an effusion as well as limitation of joint motion. Plain films offer little aid in this diagnosis and although magnetic resonance imaging (MRI) is a valuable tool it is relatively expensive. Treatment is surgical for large tears but small tears are followed symptomatically.

Patellar dislocations are usually obvious to the observer. The patella is found laterally and the athlete resists movement of the knee. Most reduce spontaneously but, like subluxations of the patella, require careful physical examination. There is usually an effusion and tenderness along the medial retinaculum. The patellar facets may be tender and there is usually apprehension with lateral movement of the patella. Protected range of motion while stabilizing the patella allows the tissues to heal in a functional manner. These injuries have a high rate of recurrence so rehabilitation is designed to strengthen the quadriceps. Adjuncts such as McConnell taping and patellofemoral sleeves can help prevent patellar subluxation.

Basketball exposes the joint to tremendous repetitive microtrauma. 'Jumper's knee', a common ailment, is an example of an overuse injury to the knee. It includes a tendinitis anywhere along the quadriceps extensor mechanism, although many consider it limited to the bone–tendon junction at the tibial tuberosity (Molnar & Fox, 1993). It is easy to see that the rapid, eccentric forces of jumping and sprinting associated with basketball are the cause of this condition. Highly specific training schedules using eccentric loads must be incorporated into the preseason as well as the rehabilitation conditioning programme. It is critical to intervene early in order to prevent a chronic inflammatory condition. Aggressive use of modalities along

with rest can help. Counterforce bracing of the patellar tendon may allow the athlete to continue to play. Steroid injections should be avoided in this area because of the tremendous forces acting on this tendon (Kennedy & Willis, 1991). Rarely is surgical débridement necessary except in the most recalcitrant cases.

Patellofemoral pain plagues many female athletes and basketball players appear even more susceptible to this problem. Many factors play a role in the maltracking of the patella, including femoral anteversion, increased genu valgus or varus deformities and excessive Q-angles. In the lower leg, increased tibial torsion and pronation or supination of the foot can contribute to this condition. Physical examination can sometimes reveal crepitation of the patella, facet pain or retinacular tenderness. Observation of patella alta or a lateral tilt is important. Standard radiographs contribute little to the diagnosis (Merchant et al., 1974). Newer techniques such as kinematic MRI offer some insight into this abnormality but come at a prohibitive price (Shellock et al., 1989). Treatment is directed at strengthening the quadriceps within a pain-free arc. This is often carried out with the knee in extension from zero to 30° (Huberti & Hayes, 1984) in order to minimize the contact forces across the patellofemoral surfaces. Functional 'closed-chain' exercises are preferred along with McConnell taping (McConnell, 1986) until proper strength and function are restored. Selective training of the vastus medialis obliquus using biofeedback is another useful tool in the rehabilitation process (Wise et al., 1984).

Back injuries

Serious back injuries are uncommon in basketball players (Jackson & Mannarino, 1984). During the 1991–92 basketball season, back complaints accounted for less than 7% of the musculoskeletal injuries noted that year by the NCAA Injury Surveillance System. Some genetic predisposing factors, such as spondylolysis, spondylolisthesis, spinal stenosis, scoliosis and leg length discrepancies, can contribute to back dysfunction. However, the most common factor is mechanical overload leading to structural fatigue (Jackson & Mannarino, 1984). When there is a breakdown in form and mechanics due to fatigue, injuries can occur. The majority of back problems respond to the usual anti-inflammatory regimens. They can be prevented from recurring by following a well-balanced strength and flexibility programme that includes pelvic and core stabilization.

Defects in the pars interarticularis can cause **spondylolysis** or **spondylolisthesis**. The pain **may be unilateral and accentuated** by hyperextension and twisting. It is uncommon to see any neurological defects on examination (Jackson & Mannarino, 1984). Radiographs usually clinch the diagnosis but bone scans can help distinguish a relatively acute stress fracture from a chronic or congenital defect. Low-grade spondylolisthesis with less than 50% slippage, as well as spondylolysis, usually respond to restriction of activity and physiotherapy within a few months. Formal lumbosacral bracing is selectively indicated and should be considered on an individual basis. Progression of symptoms or slippage warrants a surgical opinion.

Upper extremity injuries

Basketball is a fast-paced sport that requires skilful hands. It predisposes the hand and fingers to acute trauma. Hand injuries that appear inconsequential initially may have devastating long-term consequences. It is imperative that the medical staff have familiarity with the anatomy and subtle nuances of hand injuries.

Fingers

Injuries to the fingers include distal tuft fractures, interphalangeal fractures, shaft fractures and metacarpal–phalangeal fractures. The integrity and congruence of the articular surface must be maintained in order to minimize the potential disabilities of phalangeal fractures. Because of the extensive ligamentous and tendinous attach-

ments, a thorough examination must be carried out to reveal any avulsion that may interfere with future functioning of the extremity. Radiographs should be obtained to complete this examination in cases where there is any suggestion of a fracture.

The proximal interphalangeal joint is the most commonly injured part of the hand (Wilson & McGinty, 1993). Injuries include collateral ligament tears, volar plate disruptions and dorsal capsule injuries involving the central extensor slip. The evaluation of all these injuries includes **active range of motion, localized tenderness and deformity**, along with plain films. Stress testing is carried out last to determine the degree of joint instability. All this information then determines the treatment plan. Most of these injuries allow for splinting and return to play.

Common complications of volar plate injuries include the development of persistent flexion contractures called 'boutonnière' and 'swan-neck' deformities (Wilson & Liechty, 1986). These can be prevented by proper treatment initially but may require correction by surgery later. They should be splinted in 30° of flexion for 2–3 weeks followed by 'buddy-taping' to the adjacent finger.

Mallet finger can result from a blow to the distal tip with a sudden flexion force. It results in a closed avulsion of the terminal extensor tendon from the distal phalanx. Splinting the distal joint alone in full extension for 4–6 weeks may prevent the extension lag that is characteristic of this injury. Similarly, avulsion of the flexor digitorum profundus occurs on the opposing side of the phalanx and is frequently overlooked. Examination reveals a lack of active flexion at this joint. This injury is equally responsive to appropriate splinting in flexion, unless the tendon had retracted significantly.

Hand

Injuries to the hand are usually the result of falls. Localization of pain and deformity guide the examiner to order appropriate radiographs and treatment. Scaphoid fractures are the most notorious of hand injuries to escape detection and have the most serious consequences (Culver & Anderson, 1992). The goal of treatment is to establish anatomical alignment and prevent non-union. The prognosis is dependent upon the degree of disruption to the vascular supply, which enters dorsally (Taleisnik, 1985). All patients with tenderness over this bone should be treated with a thumb spica cast until radiographs are negative at 2 weeks. The supporting ligaments of the scapholunate are also subject to disruption. Clenched fist radiographs along with standard views of the wrist usually demonstrate this altered relationship (Wilson & McGinty, 1993). Pinning is usually required to maintain the stability of these bones.

Facial trauma

Of the sports that do not use protective gear, few pose such a risk of facial trauma as basketball. Injuries to the head and face account for almost 10% of the injuries seen in a typical basketball season (National Collegiate Athletic Association Injury Surveillance System, 1991–1992). There is increasing physical contact at the collegiate and professional level of competition and serious injuries can occur.

Nose

Broken noses are relatively common in sports. An inadvertent elbow can not only fracture but also displace the nasal bones and cartilage. Epistaxis is a common result and initial attention must be given to controlling the bleeding, which is aided by the use of intranasal tampons, direct pressure and ice. Topical vasoconstrictors in the form of a nasal spray can be used with great effectiveness. If initial attempts fail, a more serious posterior bleed is possible that may require instrumentation and nasal packing. Examination must include evaluation of airway obstruction due to displacement of the bones or cartilage as well as of the development of mucosal haematomas. This latter problem can cause necrosis of the surrounding tissue if not evacuated. Protective masks are available, although most players opt to return to play without them. Cosmetic repair can be carried out within a few weeks or at the completion of the season or the player's career.

Eyes

An elbow to the eye poses a serious threat to both the globe of the eye and the surrounding bony orbit. Orbital fractures require a high degree of suspicion because there is rarely crepitance or a palpable depression of the ridge. More commonly, there is significant pain and a complete eye examination rules out entrapment of the muscles to the eye. Frequently, computed tomography is necessary to appreciate these fractures. Involvement of a subspecialist is appropriate.

Direct injuries to the eyeball are common. Most are the result of finger pokes that result in minor corneal abrasions and blepharospasm. Observation of pupil size, reactivity and extraocular movement, along with a fundoscopic examination, are necessary. The use of a topical anaesthetic, such as 0.5% tetracaine hydrochloride solution, can relieve the pain and allow examination. Fluorescein staining demonstrates any corneal abrasions or foreign bodies. These can be cared for with irrigation, removal of the offending irritant, instillation of antibiotic drops, cycloplegics and possibly an eye patch. It has been common automatically to patch the eye but because of the rapid epithelialization of the cornea and the beneficial effects of tears, it may not be necessary in all cases.

An acute hyphaema or haematoma collection within the anterior chamber is a serious but fortunately rare occurrence. With the athlete in a seated position, blood will pool in the inferior aspect of the chamber allowing visualization without specialized equipment. The athlete then needs to be transported in an upright position for more extensive evaluation and observation.

Teeth

Dental trauma is seen on occasion and referral to a dentist is usually necessary. Initial management of the injury can determine the potential success of reparative work. Any loose teeth should be left in place and dislodged teeth should be replaced or at least left in the mouth until seen by the dentist.

Medical issues

Bleeding from any source needs to be taken seriously. Universal precautions mandate the use of protective gloves and eyewear. Prompt removal of the athlete with active bleeding minimizes the risk of exposure to other players. Regulations require the removal of blood-soaked uniforms, although transmission of an infection from this source has never been documented. Control of the bleeding, whether via direct pressure or suture placement, is appropriate and dictated by the injury. Return to play is possible.

Sudden cardiac death

The greatest medical threat in basketball is sudden cardiac death. Although this is relatively rare, it has gained increased attention because of some televised and publicized episodes, including the death of Hank Gathers in March 1990. The cause of sudden death in athletes under the age of 35 is usually hypertrophic cardiomyopathy. This accounts for about half the cases, the remaining being due to congenital anomalies of the coronary artery, ruptured aorta due to cystic medial necrosis associated with Marfan's syndrome, myocarditis and idiopathic left ventricular hypertrophy (Maron *et al.*, 1986).

Identifying athletes at risk is essential. The preparticipation examination is an opportunity to identify some of these athletes. Attention to a family history of sudden death, as well as any history of collapse in the athlete, warrants further investigation. Echocardiography is not practical nor feasible for all athletes so reliance on a diligent history and physical examination is necessary.

The adolescent athlete

In addition to the injuries that plague all basketball players, the adolescent player suffers some unique injuries. As in adults, the rate of injuries is slightly greater for girls than boys (Chandy & Grana, 1985). During adolescence, not only are there changes in emotional and psychological development, there are also rapid changes in body composition, muscular strength and conditioning. Young 'roundball' enthusiasts may play in the driveway for hours. Younger players may not have adequate coaching and conditioning programmes to prevent some injuries.

As in the adult, the ankle is the most vulnerable joint followed by the knee (Micheli, 1986). Upper extremity injuries are quite infrequent. When evaluating adolescents for musculoskeletal injuries, special consideration must be given to the potential for growth plate injuries. Physeal injuries can mimic sprains so suspicion must be maintained in any adolescent with pain over a growth plate. Virtually all adolescent injuries that are serious enough for the child to miss play warrant radiography (Nicholas & Herschman, 1986).

Pain at the heel can include Achilles tendinitis, retrocalcaneal bursitis, calcaneal apophysitis or Sever's disease, and stress fractures of the calcaneus. The symptoms may overlap and when radiographs are obtained may show fragmentation and sclerosis, which is normal. Parental reassurance is usually indicated as these injuries respond nicely to rest, stretching, heel pads and regular ice.

Stress fractures are a particular concern with adolescent athletes. They are vulnerable because of the combination of training errors, improper mechanics, equipment, training surfaces and a rapidly changing body. The diagnosis and treatment are similar to the protocols used in an adult.

ACL tears

ACL tears in the young present a unique management problem. Since the injury is sustained at an early age, there is more time for development of meniscal tears and arthritic damage to the knee (Fetto & Marshall, 1980). These authors have also noted that within 5 years of ACL tears, 70% of these young athletes subsequently develop a meniscal tear. Drilling across the growth plate to reconstruct the ACL poses a challenge to the orthopaedic surgeon. Some consider a rehabilitation programme necessary, while others deem it appropriate to perform the repair. This matter remains controversial and is best managed on an individual basis.

Anterior knee pain

The differential diagnosis of 'jumper's knee' in a younger athlete must include two apophyseal injuries, Osgood–Schlatter disease and Sinding–Larsen syndrome. Both involve traction of the patellar tendon on either the tibial tubercle or the inferior pole of the patella. Rapid growth and relatively inflexible quadriceps contribute to this problem. There is minimal risk of rupture of either the tendon or its bony attachment (Bowers, 1981). This is well managed by ice, relative rest and stretching.

Patellofemoral dysfunction is very problematic in adolescent girls. All the anatomical variants previously noted are beginning to play a greater role. With the increasing demands of sport participation, coupled with these physiological changes, it is common to see anterior knee pain in young girls. Treatment is directed at balancing strength and flexibility of the quadriceps mechanism in an attempt to ameliorate some of the causative factors.

Conclusion

Basketball is increasing in popularity among women in the USA and greater opportunities exist for women to play this sport at both the collegiate and professional levels. This increasing participation has led to an increasing awareness of injuries in women's basketball. Further investigation into injury trends, prevention and treatment is promising.

References

Arendt, E. & Dick, R. (1995) Knee injury patterns among men and women in collegiate basketball and soccer. NCAA data and review of literature. *American Journal of Sports Medicine* **23**, 694–701.

Ashton-Miller, J.A. (1996) What best protects the inverted weight-bearing ankle against further inversion? Evertor muscle strength compares favorably with shoe height, athletic tape and three orthoses. *American Journal of Sports Medicine* **24**, 800–809.

Bowers, K.D. Jr (1981) Patellar tendon avulsion as a complication of Osgood–Schlatter's disease. *American Journal of Sports Medicine* **9**, 356–359.

Chandy, T.A. & Grana, W.A. (1985) Secondary school athletic injuries in boys and girls. A three year comparison. *Physician and Sportsmedicine* **13**, 106–108.

Culver, J.E. & Anderson, T.E. (1992) Fractures of the hand and wrist in the athlete. *Clinics in Sports Medicine* **11**, 101–128.

Fetto, J.F. & Marshall, J.L. (1980) The natural history and diagnosis of anterior cruciate ligament insufficiency. *Clinical Orthopaedics* **147**, 29–38.

Huberti, H. & Hayes, W. (1984) Patellofemoral contact pressures. *Journal of Bone and Joint Surgery* **66A**, 715–721.

Jackson, D.W. & Mannarino, F. (1984) Lumbar spine in athletes. In W.N. Scott, B. Nisonson & J.A. Nicholas (eds) *Principles of Sports Medicine*, pp. 130–147. Williams and Williams, Baltimore.

Kennedy, J.C. & Willis, R.B. (1976) The effects of local steroid injections on tendons: a biochemical and microscopic correlative study. *American Journal of Sports Medicine* **4**, 11–21.

McConnell, J. (1986) The management of chondromalacia patellae: a long term solution. *Australian Journal of Physiotherapy* **33**, 215–222.

Maron, B.J., Epstein, S.E. & Roberts, W.C. (1986) Causes of sudden death in competitive athletes. *Journal of the American College of Cardiology* **7**, 204–214.

Merchant, A.C., Mercer, R.L., Jacobsen, R.H. & Cool, C.R. (1974) Roentgenographic analysis of patellofemoral congruence. *Journal of Bone and Joint Surgery* **56A**, 1391–1396.

Michael, R.H. & Holder, L.E. (1985) The soleus syndrome. A cause of medial tibial stress. *American Journal of Sports Medicine* **13**, 87–94.

Micheli, L.J. (1986) Pediatric and adolescent sports injuries: recent trends. *Exercise and Sport Sciences Reviews* **14**, 359–373.

Molnar, T.J. & Fox, J.M. (1993) Overuse injuries of the knee in basketball. *Clinics in Sports Medicine* **12**, 349–362.

Mooney, V. & Robertson, J. (1976) The facet syndrome. *Clinical Orthopaedics* **115**, 149–156.

Mubarak, S.J., Gould, R.N., Lee, Y.F., Schmidt, D.A. & Hargens, A.R. (1982) The medial tibial stress syndrome. A cause of shin splints. *American Journal of Sports Medicine* **10**, 201–205.

National Collegiate Athletic Association Injury Surveillance System (1991–1992) *Women's Basketball.* NCAA, Overland Park, Kansas.

Nicholas, J.A. & Herschman, E.B. (1986) *The Lower Extremity and Spine in Sports Medicine.* Mosby, St Louis.

Ogilvie-Harris, D.J. & Gilbart, M. (1995) Treatment modalities for soft tissue injuries of the ankle: a critical review. *Clinical Journal of Sport Medicine* **5**, 175–186.

Ray, J.M., McCoomb, W. & Sternes, R.A. (1991) Basketball and volleyball. In B. Reider (ed.) *Sports Medicine: The School-aged Athlete*, pp. 84–126. W.B. Saunders, Philadelphia.

Rupani, H., Holder, L.E., Espinola, D.A. & Engin, S.I. (1985) Three-phase radionuclide bone imaging in sports medicine. *Radiology* **156**, 187–196.

Shellock, F.G., Mink, J.H. & Deutsch, A. (1989) Kinematic magnetic resonance imaging for evaluation of patellar tracking. *Physician and Sportsmedicine* **17**, 99–106.

Sonzogni, J.J. & Gross, M.L. (1993) Assessment and treatment of basketball injuries. *Clinics in Sports Medicine* **12**, 221–237.

Taleisnik, J. (1985) *The Wrist.* Churchill Livingstone, New York.

Wilson, R.L. & Liechty, B.W. (1986) Complications following small joint injuries. *Hand Clinics* **2**, 329–348.

Wilson, R.L. & McGinty, L.D. (1993) Common hand and wrist injuries in basketball players. *Clinics in Sports Medicine* **12**, 265–291.

Wise, H.H., Feibert, I.A. & Kates, J.L. (1984) EMG biofeedback as treatment for patellofemoral pain syndrome. *Journal of Orthopedic Sports Physical Therapy* **6**, 95–114.

Chapter 39

Soccer

MARGOT PUTUKIAN

Introduction

Soccer is the world's game: it is by far the most popular sport worldwide, with an estimated 200 million participants internationally and 42 million in the USA (Barkley, 1997). Most of the world knows it as 'football' but in the USA it has been called 'soccer' to differentiate it from rugby as well as other types of football, including American and Canadian football. The World Cup draws the biggest global television audience for a sporting event. In the USA, although the overall growth of participation in soccer has been remarkable, the increased involvement of girls and women is even more impressive. Women account for 22% of soccer players worldwide and close to 40% of soccer players in the USA (Brewer & Davis, 1994). Soccer is a physically challenging team sport that emphasizes intermittent high-intensity activity as well as endurance performance in combination with sport-specific skills. Soccer is safely enjoyed by all age groups and body types. Understanding the sport-specific medical issues of this tremendous sport is useful in taking care of soccer players and allowing them to enjoy participation safely.

There are many challenges facing the sports medicine team taking care of female soccer athletes and this chapter attempts to present some of these issues as well as the sport itself, which in many ways is poorly understood from a sports medicine perspective. Despite the extensive history of soccer, information about the physiology and biomechanics of the game, nutrition, strengthening and conditioning, injury patterns and injury prevention is sparse. The sport involves many specific activities that are very different from other team sports, such as use of the head, chest, thigh and feet. In fact, it is one of the rare sports where use of the upper extremities is limited. Information that pertains specifically to the female athlete is even more difficult to find. This chapter presents the sport-specific medical problems and, as far as possible, relates them specifically to the female soccer player.

Physiology

Soccer is a sport whose physical demands require a mixture of endurance running as well as discontinuous sprinting. In addition, due to the complex nature of the skills and tactics involved, there is also an emphasis on quick turns, pivots, jumps in the air, and both forward and backward running. All surfaces of the body can be used, with the exception of the arms and hands, although these are used during throw-ins as well as by the goalkeeper. The legs are used most frequently, and many different surfaces of the thigh and foot may be employed to control the ball and maintain possession by passing it to teammates. Most of the sport-specific activities that occur involve balancing on one leg while controlling or kicking the ball with the other. The most effective players make use of both feet equally.

The demands of the women's game are similar to those of the men's game. In a study by B.

Ekblom and P. Aginger (unpublished observations) of élite Swedish players, women covered a similar total distance (8471 m) compared with their male counterparts and sprinted an average of 14.9±5.6 m over 100 times per game. Blood lactate measurements made at half-time and after a game were 5.1±2.1 and 4.6±2.1 mmol·l^{-1} respectively. These measurements are slightly lower than those reported by Ekblom (1986) for male players (range 8.0–12.0 mmol·l^{-1}). Average heart rates during three full-sided women's games were roughly 175±11 beats·min^{-1}, 89–91% of the mean peak heart rate (Ekblom, 1994). $\dot{V}o_{2max}$, or aerobic capacity, has been reported to be between 47.1 and 57.6 ml·kg^{-1}·min^{-1} (Rhodes & Mosher, 1992; Jensen & Larsson, 1993), with the latter value improving from 53.3 ml·kg^{-1}·min^{-1} during a 15-month training programme. Colquhoun and Chad (1992) assessed anaerobic power in élite Australian soccer players and found that peak anaerobic power averaged 47.8±11.2 W. These athletes were able to maintain 62.1% of peak power output at the end of the test.

Flexibility and strength

There are data to suggest that inflexibility of the lower leg musculature is common in soccer players and that a programme of flexibility and prophylactic ankle taping can lead to a decrease in injuries over a season (Ekstrand & Gillquist, 1982). While inflexibility may increase the risk of lumbar spine problems as well as muscle injuries, it may be protective for anterior cruciate ligament (ACL) injuries. In a prospective study of female collegiate athletes, Knapik *et al.* (1991) demonstrated that flexibility and imbalances of >15% in lower extremity strength were associated with a 2.6-fold increase in injury rate. These data emphasize the importance of proper flexibility as well as strengthening as part of the conditioning programme for soccer players.

Biomechanics

Soccer has many specific skills that make it different from most other sports. The reliance on the foot as well as use of the head and potentially all surfaces of the body except the upper extremities is unique. The variety of kicking styles along with the surfaces presented by the foot, thigh and chest to control the ball and pass it to teammates are complex skills that require continuous practice to master. The majority of these techniques require placing one's full weight on one leg while controlling or striking the ball with the other. Understanding the biomechanics of basic soccer techniques can help the healthcare provider understand injury mechanisms as well as individualize treatment programmes.

The inside of the foot is commonly used for short passing and redirecting the ball with accuracy. It provides a large surface that minimizes error but limits the velocity with which the ball can be struck. The foot and hip are externally rotated roughly 90° and the knee is slightly flexed as the ball is struck (Fig. 39.1). The foot is maximally dorsiflexed to 'lock' the ankle, which creates a rigid surface and increases accuracy. This skill can be associated with specific injury. If an athlete has a prominent tarsal navicular bone, ball contact in this area can create pain due to trauma. If the ball makes contact towards the toes, instead of properly at the space between the medial malleolus and the tarsal navicular bone, it can create an external rotation force at the foot and place a stretch on the medial structures, most notably the posterior tibialis tendon. In addition, because of the external rotation that occurs at the hip, there can be overuse of the adductor, sartorius and gracilis musculature.

The inside of the foot is also used for block tackles, when a player attempts to take the ball away from an opponent with the ball on the ground. Often, both players strike the ball at the same time, both using the inside of the foot. Proper technique is essential in order to avoid injury. If performed properly, the player's weight is balanced over the tackling leg and the ball, providing strength and support to the tackling leg. However, if the player extends the leg so that the body is leaning back, the weight of the leg is all that is behind the tackle and often the player not only loses the ball but also sustains an injury. Poor tackling technique puts the medial aspect of

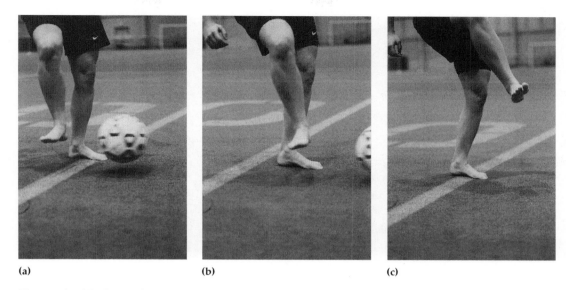

(a)   **(b)**   **(c)**

Fig. 39.1 (a–c) Technique for controlling the ball with the inside of the foot, illustrating the position of the foot and knee. (Courtesy of Steven Manuel.)

the knee at risk for valgus stress, which can result in injuries to the medial collateral ligament and pes anserinus.

The outside of the foot can be used for short passing, a natural motion associated with running, as well as for striking the ball to produce a curve or 'bend' to its flight that can deceive a goalkeeper or defender. The foot is plantar flexed and inverted, with the ball striking the junction between the lateral aspect of the tibiotarsal junction and the cuboid (Fig. 39.2). A varying amount of spin is applied depending on how the foot strikes the ball. When the foot is in this position, it may be at risk for forceful inversion plantar flexion injuries, midfoot and forefoot ligament sprains and peroneal tendon problems. If the foot is 'locked' and ball contact occurs correctly, injuries are less likely to occur. If the ball is struck incorrectly, the anterior tibialis and peroneal muscle groups can be stressed, and injuries to the metatarsal or tarsal bones can result. In the young athlete, these mechanisms can lead to apophysitis or avulsion fractures at the base of the fifth metatarsal.

The instep kick is used for power, although there is less surface area for contact and the degree of error in striking the ball accurately is consequently larger. The foot is maximally plantar flexed and again 'locked', an action that attempts to decrease the motion that occurs at the ankle and provides an increase in the force transmitted. During the approach and ball-strike phases of the instep kick, a varus torque of >200 N·m and an extension torque of 280 N·m is generated on the proximal tibia; during the follow-through phase, an extension torque of 230 N·m is produced on the proximal tibia (Gainor *et al.*, 1978). Although a total of 2000 N·m can be generated during a kick, only 15% of this is transferred to the ball, the remainder being absorbed by eccentric contraction of the hamstring muscles (Gainor *et al.*, 1978). Understanding the tremendous forces generated in kicking explains the predominance of lower extremity injuries in soccer.

If the ball is on the ground, most players often approach it from an angle in order to prevent the toe from striking the ground. If the ball is in the air, it is easier to strike the ball straight on, although it is more difficult to control. Injury mechanisms associated with the instep kick are usually related to the ankle

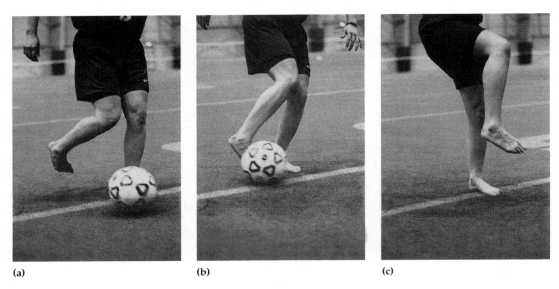

(a)   (b)   (c)

Fig. 39.2 (a–c) Technique for controlling the ball with the outside of the foot, illustrating the position of the foot and knee. (Courtesy of Steven Manuel.)

position of extreme plantar flexion. Injuries to the tarsal navicular bone, other tarsal bones or metatarsals can occur. Muscle overuse injuries generally involve the anterior tibialis musculature, although posterior impingement can also occur. This may be more likely in those athletes with os trigonum or in individuals with posterior tibialis tendonitis.

All these surfaces used to strike the ball can also be used to take the ball out of the air and 'control' it. When the ball is in the air it must be controlled and prepared for whatever the player wants to do next. This often entails complex skill and preparation by the player prior to receiving the ball. A player often decides what to do with the ball before it arrives and then uses the first touch to prepare it for the next move. In controlling the ball, significant velocity may need to be absorbed, and these skills are difficult to perform well. The contact surface must be presented early, and good balance and proprioception are essential. Once initial contact occurs, the surface is generally withdrawn such that the energy on the ball is absorbed and its incoming direction and velocity controlled. The biomechanics of

controlling the ball in soccer are similar to catching a ball. If the surface is held out rigidly, the ball will bounce away as opposed to being controlled. The specific skill of ball control in soccer is one of the most difficult tasks to learn and master.

Any surface of the body except the arms can be used to control the ball and pass it to teammates. This includes the chest, which is a difficult skill to teach the female athlete. Many are uncomfortable when first learning the 'chest trap', and inexperienced coaches may be reluctant to teach this skill to their female players. The ball can be comfortably controlled if it is taken on the sternum, with relaxation of the upper torso as the ball strikes. If the athlete is afraid to use this part of her body, she effectively excludes a large surface area with which she can control the ball. The chest can be used to direct the ball downwards towards the feet, forwards or to the side. Players should be taught this skill early so that they realize it can be performed easily and safely.

Probably the most difficult skill in soccer is heading. This complex activity is unique to the game and one where proper technique is very important. The ball is struck with the middle of the forehead where the skull is thickest. The action of heading has been compared to a catapult, where both the upper and lower parts of the trunk are extended prior to striking the ball. The head is brought back with the low back arched and the chin tucked down by the chest. The eyes are open and the ball is struck with the head brought forward through the ball. Just before contact the trunk flexors, hip flexors and knee extensors contract strongly, creating the major forces in heading. In skilled players, the muscles of the neck become rigid at impact (Burslem & Lees, 1987), which reduces the angular acceleration of the head and decreases the risk of injury to the head and neck (Tysvaer, 1992).

Technique is important, and improper execution may be related to headaches or other neurological symptoms. Players are taught not to strike the ball on the top of the head or over the temple and also to keep their eyes open and strike through the ball. They are also told to strike the ball instead of letting the ball strike them. Proper technique can minimize injury and this is especially important for the young soccer player. For younger players learning proper technique, the use of a smaller, lighter ball is useful in avoiding injury. In addition, some players are afraid to head the ball and using a lighter ball to overcome this apprehension is helpful for the beginner.

Sortland et al. (1982) reported degenerative changes in 40-year-old soccer players equivalent to those seen in 50–60-year-old non-players that were felt to be secondary to repetitive heading. Although there has been concern regarding head injury as a result of chronic repetitive heading, little substantive evidence for this exists. This topic is discussed in greater detail later in the chapter.

Fluid and nutrition

Because soccer is played for 90 min, it is very important to optimize fluid and nutrition so that energy stores and fluid balance can be maintained. This becomes even more important if the athlete is playing numerous games over a short span of time or if the ambient conditions are severe. Nutritional deficiencies, although uncommon in individuals consuming a well-balanced diet, are important to consider in athletes, especially if they complain of fatigue or poor exercise tolerance. Iron deficiency is the most common nutritional deficiency seen in the female athlete and can directly affect performance (see Chapter 21).

Fluid ingestion during exercise serves two major purposes: to provide an energy source to supplement the body's limited stores and to supply water and electrolytes to replace those lost through sweating. Decisions regarding the optimal fluid intake depend on the intensity and duration of exercise, the ambient temperature and humidity, and the individual characteristics of the athlete (see Chapter 4). As there is tremendous individual variability in sweating rates, weight loss can be used to predict the amount of sweat loss (1 kg weight loss is equivalent to 1 litre sweat). It has been reported that during a 90-min match, female soccer players had a fluid intake of 1.4 litres and a drop in body mass of 0.9 kg, suggesting an overall decrease of 2.3 kg. Studies have demonstrated that exercise performance is impaired when as little as 2% of body weight is lost; when dehydration reaches 5%, work capacity can decrease by roughly 30% (Saltin & Costill, 1988).

The most serious side-effect of dehydration resulting from a failure to replace fluids during exercise is impaired dissipation of heat, which can lead to heat exhaustion and heat illness (see Chapter 4). The effects of heat stress on a youth soccer tournament in Minnesota were well illustrated by Elias et al. (1991). Modifications made as the tournament progressed, such as shortened playing periods, more water breaks and more player substitutions, decreased the number of heat-related illnesses. The wet-bulb globe temperature (WBGT) index can be used to measure the relative risk of heat injury. This measurement integrates absolute temperature, humidity and solar radiant energy into a formula. If the WBGT is >27.8°C (82°F), unnecessary activity should be curtailed. General recommendations for fluid replacement and exercise have recently been updated by the American College of Sports Medicine (1996).

The benefits of carbohydrate and fluid ingestion on performance in soccer have been examined by several researchers and have been reviewed recently (Kirkendall, 1993). Leatt and Jacobs (1989) investigated the effect of glucose polymer ingestion before and during a soccer match on muscle glycogen utilization. They performed a biopsy of the vastus lateralis muscle before and after the game and gave 10 players 0.5 litre of 7% glucose polymer solution 10 min before the match and at half-time and compared the results with players given a placebo. They found that the change in muscle glycogen was significantly less in the experimental group compared with the placebo group (111 vs. $181 \pm$ 24 mmol·kg^{-1}, $P < 0.001$). This correlates to a muscle glycogen concentration 31% higher in those subjects given glucose polymer. Ekblom (1986) showed that soccer players with the lowest glycogen reserves at half-time had a slower average speed and covered less ground than other team members during the second half of the game.

Injury statistics

Overall, the incidence of injury in outdoor soccer is favourable, with one-fifth the number of injuries of American football (Pardon, 1977; Pritchett, 1981). The injury data for indoor soccer are less well known.

The injury rate for outdoor soccer is well established, although the results have varied somewhat. In the Norway Cup (an outdoor tournament) in 1975 and 1977, the injury rates for boys and girls were 23.0 and 44.0 per 1000 player hours respectively (Nilsson & Roaas, 1978). In the same tournament in 1984, the injury rates for boys and girls were 8.9 and 17.6 per 1000 player hours respectively (Maehlum et al., 1986). In these studies, the definition of injury used was any medical problem for which attention was sought and thus included mild abrasions and blisters. Schmidt-Olsen et al. (1991) examined injuries in youth players over a 1-year span and

Table 39.1 Soccer injuries per 1000 player hours in boys and girls

Reference	Girls	Boys
Ergstrom et al. (1991)*	12	5
Nilsson & Roaas (1978)	32	14
Maehlum et al. (1986)	17.6	8.9
Schmidt-Olsen et al. (1991)	17.6	7.4
Sullivan et al. (1980)*	1.1	0.5

*Studies using time lost from practice/play as definition of injury.

found an injury incidence of 7.4 and 17.6 per 1000 player years for boys and girls respectively. Their definition included time-loss injuries as well as those requiring 'special bandaging or medical attention' in order for the player to continue to participate. In most of the studies that have assessed both girls and boys, girls have almost twice the injury rate (Table 39.1).

There is good documentation of injuries through the National Collegiate Athletic Association (NCAA) Injury Surveillance System (ISS) in collegiate soccer in the USA. The ISS reports injuries from several NCAA institutions and uses a definition of injury as one that requires medical attention and results in time lost from practice or play. The injury data collected by the ISS are rates expressed as the number of injuries per athlete exposure. In NCAA ISS data from 1986 to 1996, the injury rates in women per 1000 athlete exposures were 17.8 and 6.0 for games and practices respectively. This compares with the rates in men of 20.8 and 4.9 for games and practices respectively during the same time span. During this period, the injuries seen in women's soccer were predominantly mild, with 72.9% resulting in time loss of less than 7 days (vs. 74.9% in men). The ankle, upper leg and knee are the parts injured most frequently. In the 1995–96 season, ISS data reveal that the injury rates during games in men's and women's soccer are 20.2 and 17.3 per 1000 athlete exposures respectively. Similarly, in 1995–96 the injury rates during practice in men's and women's soccer are 4.8 and 5.8 per 1000 athlete exposures respectively. These rates

Table 39.2 Injury rates per 1000 athlete exposures in practice and games. (Adapted from Dick, 1996)

Sport	Practice	Games
American football	4.1	36.1
Wrestling	7.2	30.6
Women's gymnastics	8.1	21.4
Spring football	9.4	20.8
Men's soccer	4.8	20.2
Women's soccer	5.8	17.3
Ice hockey	2.3	16.9
Men's gymnastics	4.7	15.7
Men's lacrosse	3.8	15.7
Men's basketball	4.6	10.1
Women's basketball	4.4	9.4
Field hockey	4.2	9.4
Women's lacrosse	3.5	7.2
Baseball	2.2	6.2
Women's volleyball	4.6	5.2
Women's softball	3.3	4.9

for games and practice compare favourably with football, wrestling and women's gymnastics and are slightly greater than the injury rates of other NCAA sports (Table 39.2).

Two recent studies have evaluated indoor soccer injuries, assessing the rate of injury and including data for women as well as men. Lindenfeld *et al.* (1994) examined the injury rate over 7 weeks of indoor league play and found injury rates of 5.04 and 5.03 per 100 player hours for men and women respectively. They defined injury as any injury in which a player left the game or requested medical attention, as well as any injury that required stoppage of play. In a study assessing injuries during a 3-day indoor tournament, Putukian *et al.* (1996) found that the rates of injury were 5.79 and 4.74 per 100 player hours in men and women respectively. In this study, the definition of injury was time lost from play. The difference between the incidence of injury in men and women was not significant, and there was no difference in the knee injuries seen. In this study, 65.8% of the injuries seen were mild, where time lost from play or practice was less than 1 week. Moderate injuries (15.8%) were defined as those where time lost was between 1

week and 1 month; severe injuries (18.4%) were defined as more than 1 month of time lost. As the injuries increased in severity, they were more likely to have a non-contact mechanism. A majority of the injuries occurred in the lower extremities (71.4%).

The upper leg, ankle and knee account for the three main body parts injured for both men and women in the NCAA ISS data. Between 1986 and 1996, these three body parts comprised 49–58% of the men's total injuries and 50–61% of the women's total injuries. Therefore, it appears that indoor and outdoor soccer result in a similar pattern of injuries in both their location and severity. Because the indoor game is often played on an artificial surface, there may be more abrasions and more injuries that relate specifically to the surface than the game itself.

Specific musculoskeletal injuries

In the following sections, emphasis is placed on those injuries that occur most commonly in soccer. Some of these injuries are discussed in detail in Chapter 15 and therefore in these sections more attention is given to specific rehabilitation or training issues than in discussing how these injuries occur.

Head

In the NCAA data for 1996–97, the injury rates for concussion in men's and women's soccer were 0.44 and 0.46 per 1000 athlete exposures respectively, accounting for 4.7% and 4.4% of the total injuries seen. Soccer is a sport where the head can be used to contact the ball and pass it to teammates, clear it from the defensive area or strike it at goal (Fig. 39.3). Generally, the acute head injuries seen in soccer occur from impact of the head with another player, the ground or the goalposts. These mild injuries are often termed concussions and are generally the head injuries that are reported.

The assessment of head injuries should always include the possibility of cervical spine injury. The most important and often most difficult part

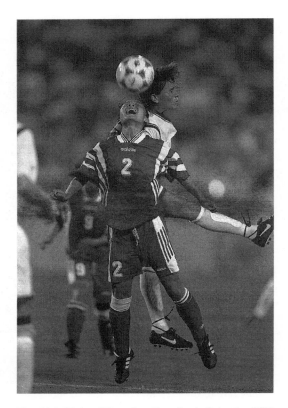

Fig. 39.3 Liping Wang heading the ball in the 1996 Olympics. (© Allsport / David Cannon.)

of assessing a head injury is detection. Many head injuries occur without being obvious. A concussion is defined as an immediate and transient impairment of neurological function that occurs as a result of mechanical forces. The athlete may be disoriented, may or may not lose consciousness and may have impairment in memory both prior to the injury and after the event. They may complain of headache, nausea, visual changes, dizziness or difficulty with concentration.

If an athlete is unconscious it is essential that care is taken to protect the cervical spine and that more significant focal brain injuries such as subdural or epidural haematomas be considered. These athletes should be transported to a hospital for further testing and close observation. If there is loss of consciousness, computerized

tomography (CT) should be obtained to assess for skull fracture or other focal bleeding after radiographs have precluded cervical spine abnormality. Neuropsychological testing may provide more sensitive assessment of cognitive function and may demonstrate deficits in function when other tests, such as magnetic resonance imaging (MRI), CT and electroencephalography, are 'normal' (Putukian *et al.*, 1996). Head-injured athletes should be watched closely for complications such as postconcussive syndrome, seizures or repetitive trauma.

Although there are several systems in the literature that define classification and return to play, the one recommended by Kelly and Rosenburg (1997) is the one most often used (Table 39.3). No matter which classification system is utilized, it is more important that the physician and athletic trainer agree to embrace the same system and be consistent. It may also be more useful to use descriptive terms, e.g. loss of consciousness, retrograde and/or post-traumatic amnesia, in describing these injuries.

There has been concern that cumulative encephalopathy, similar to the 'punch-drunk' syndrome in boxing (Jordan & Zimmerman, 1990), can occur over time due to repetitive minor head impacts with the ball. One study of Norwegian professional soccer players found central cerebral atrophy on CT and that these changes were more likely to be present if a player was a 'typical header' (likely to head the ball) (Sortland & Tysvaer, 1989). In another study, electroencephalographic changes were seen in soccer players with acute or protracted complaints secondary to heading, some of these changes persisting months or years (Tysvaer *et al.*, 1989). These studies have been criticized because of methodological problems, including lack of good control groups and lack of screening for other problems such as alcohol use. A more recent well-controlled study of national players in the USA using MRI assessment found no statistical differences between soccer players and track athletes (Jordan *et al.*, 1996). This is an area where much more work is needed, especially as it relates to the female athlete.

Table 39.3 Guidelines for the management of concussion in sport. (From Kelly & Rosenburg, 1997)

Grade I: Transient confusion, no LOC, concussion symptoms or mental status abnormalities on exam resolve in <15 min
Remove from contest
Examine immediately and at 5-min intervals for development of mental status abnormalities or post-concussive
    symptoms at rest and with exertion
May return if abnormalities/symptoms clear within 15 min
Second grade I concussion in same contest eliminates player from contest, returning only if asymptomatic for
    1 week at rest and exertion

Grade II: Transient confusion, no LOC, concussion symptoms or mental status abnormalities last >15 min
Remove from contest, no return that day
Examine on site frequently for signs of evolving intracranial pathology
Re-examine athlete following day
Neurological exam by doctor 1 week after asymptomatic before return to sports
CT or MRI where headache or other symptoms worsen or persist for >2 weeks
Following second grade II concussion, return to play deferred until at least 2 weeks after athlete is symptom free at
    rest and with exertion
Terminating season mandated by any abnormality on CT or MRI consistent with brain swelling, contusion or other
    intracranial pathology

Grade III: Any LOC, either brief (seconds) or prolonged (minutes)
Transport from field to hospital by ambulance if unconscious or worrisome signs; consider cervical spine
    immobilization
Thorough neurological exam immediately, including appropriate neuroimaging procedures
Admit if any signs of pathology or mental status abnormalities
If normal evaluation, may send athlete home
Neurological status should be assessed daily thereafter until all symptoms have stabilized or resolved
Prolonged LOC, persistent mental status alterations, worsening symptoms or abnormalities on neurological exam
    requires urgent neurosurgical evaluation or transfer to trauma centre
After brief (seconds) grade III concussion, athlete should be withheld from play until asymptomatic for 1 week at
    rest or with exertion
After prolonged (minutes) grade III concussion, athlete should be withheld from play until asymptomatic for
    2 weeks at rest and with exertion
Following second grade III concussion athlete should be withheld from play for a minimum of 1 asymptomatic
    month; doctor may elect to extend that period beyond 1 month, depending on clinical evaluation and other
    circumstances
CT or MRI recommended for athletes whose headache or other associated symptoms worsen or persist for >1 week
Any abnormality on CT or MRI consistent with brain swelling, contusion or other intracranial pathology should
    result in termination of the season for that athlete and return to play in the future should be seriously
    discouraged in discussions with athlete

CT, computerized tomography; LOC, loss of consciousness; MRI, magnetic resonance imaging.

Neuropsychological assessment techniques have been developed to quantify brain functioning reliably by examining brain–behaviour relationships. These techniques and instruments are used to assess the broad range of function, from simple motor speed to complex problem-solving skills. The techniques have been shown to be effective in detecting mild head injuries (Rimel *et al.*, 1981, 1982; Levin *et al.*, 1987; McLatchie *et al.*, 1987; Tysvaer & Lochen, 1991; Porter & Fricker, 1996). They have also been used specifically in soccer players (Abreau & Echemendia, 1996, 1990; Tysvaer & Lochen, 1991). It is possible to use neuropsychological tools to assess the effect of acute and chronic head injury on cognitive function (Alves *et al.*, 1987; Putukian & Echemendia, 1996). Although currently there are no data to support the theory that heading itself is dangerous, more research is needed to investigate both the acute and chronic effects of heading in soccer.

Cervical spine

Cervical spine injuries are not common in soccer. However, given the significant long-term effects of cervical spine injury, it is important to remember that every head injury is a possible neck injury. Any athlete who complains of considerable neck pain or stiffness should have radiographs of the cervical spine. In Scotland, soccer activity accounted for 6% of all paraplegic and quadriplegic injuries. There have been case reports of cervical spine disc herniation (Tysvaer, 1985), cervical spine fracture, and subluxation. Scopetta and Vaccario (1978) reported a case of central cord syndrome felt to be associated with a hand-sewn waterlogged ball and insufficient muscle preparation prior to heading.

Minor cervical spine injuries include strains and occasionally sprains. The mechanisms can be similar to those in more severe injury or can be due to a quick upper extremity motion including the neck. Occasionally, the head strikes another opponent or the ground and results in a cervical sprain or strain. These injuries are best evaluated with radiographs if there is pain centrally, limitation of motion or neurological symptoms. If these symptoms occur acutely, they should be treated as though they represent a fracture by placing the athlete in a cervical collar and removing her from play until X-rays are obtained along with careful neurological assessment. Once routine radiographs are obtained and are normal, flexion and extension views may help in determining if an instability pattern is present. Further treatment will depend on the type and severity of injury sustained.

Maxillofacial/dental injuries

Maxillofacial/dental injuries account for roughly 5% of injuries seen and tend to occur more commonly in goalkeepers. Generally, the injury occurs as a result of contact with an opponent, a goal-post or the ground. Significant dental or ophthalmological injuries should be treated expeditiously by referral to the appropriate specialist. The use of mouth-guards, although not well tolerated by athletes, can significantly diminish the dental injuries that occur and some have advocated their use as an anticoncussive device as well.

Upper extremity

Most of these injuries occur in goalkeepers and other players falling on an outstretched hand or directly on the shoulder. For the most part, they are treated as they would be in other athletes, the exception being that it may be easier to return the athlete to sport-specific activity. Examples of the most common injuries that occur in the upper extremity include fractures of the clavicle, shoulder separations (acromioclavicular joint), shoulder dislocations (glenohumeral joint), ulnar collateral ligament injury (at the metacarpophalangeal joint), fractures of the humerus, radial head and distal radius, and fractures to the scaphoid, metacarpals and phalanges. Wrist and hand injuries are more commonly seen in goalkeepers, although the remainder of the injuries can occur in any field player. These are covered in greater detail in Chapter 15.

Lumbar spine

The two most important entities to discuss are disc disease and spondylolysis. It is important to differentiate these more serious problems from the more common muscular strains that occur commonly in soccer. Annular tears of the intervertebral disc, or degenerative disc disease, are not uncommon and should be considered in the soccer player who complains of back pain that is made worse with flexion, sneezing, coughing or laughing. The athlete should be questioned about previous back pain, the presence of radiating symptoms and whether they experience numbness or tingling, weakness and/or any difficulty with bowel or bladder function. On physical examination, they often have central intervertebral pain, pain with flexion and a positive straight-leg test. Their neurological function should be fully tested. Plain radiographs may be normal but occasionally reveal a narrow disc space or other changes consistent with degenerative disc disease. In addition, radiographs are important for assessing the presence of stress fractures, tumour or infection. MRI is often useful in assessing the presence of disc disease as well as spinal stenosis and provides better demonstration of the soft-tissue structures of the spine.

The other important aetiology of back pain in the soccer player is spondylolysis. This is common in the young athlete, and occurs in soccer players because of the hyperextension that sometimes happens while kicking the ball. Spondylolysis generally occurs in extension-type activities and thus is seen in goalkeepers or players who jump to head the ball. These athletes often have pain in the paralumbar region and increased pain when bending backwards, specifically when performing one-legged extension.

Radiographs are very helpful but only if the symptoms have been present for a long time. Oblique radiographs will demonstrate a 'scotty dog' with a 'collar' or 'broken neck', which represents the defect in the pars interarticularis defining spondylolysis. It appears that the presence of spina bifida increases the risk of spondylolysis. If there is evidence for spondylolysis, flexion and extension views are important in assessing for spondylolisthesis, where one vertebral body slides forward on to the other. This implies bilateral spondylolysis.

Technetium bone scanning is very useful in detecting these stress fractures early; bone scan with single photon emission computerized tomography (SPECT) is the gold standard. In addition, in the athlete who gives a long history of back pain and presence of spondylolysis on radiographs, bone scanning can help determine if the injury is acute or chronic. Early detection is very important because the earlier treatment is initiated, the more likely these injuries are to heal. Treatment includes avoidance of extension activities, a neutral spine strengthening programme and, if detected early on, an antilordosis brace.

Mechanical back pain secondary to muscle overuse is also very common in the soccer player.

It generally appears more with flexion-type activity although it can have a mixed aetiology. It is helpful to look for inflexibility patterns, especially in the hamstrings. Muscular back pain is common in soccer players, especially since many have significant hamstring inflexibility. Treatment generally includes ice, modalities such as electrical stimulation to reduce pain and spasm, flexibility exercises and non-steroidal anti-inflammatory medication. Once the acute pain has subsided, these athletes generally respond to a neutral spine stabilization programme along with abdominal strengthening. Flexibility work is essential in preventing recurrent injury.

Chest/thorax/abdomen

These injuries are uncommon; however, when a player jumps to head the ball or when a goalkeeper makes a save, this region of the body is exposed and can be at risk for injury. Rib fractures can occur and it is important to assess for intra-abdominal organ rupture and specifically for spleen or kidney damage. The spleen can be enlarged due to infectious mononucleosis, in which case it is at risk for rupture. Any evidence of intravascular compromise (athlete is dizzy, light-headed or becomes unresponsive) should prompt emergency transportation to a medical facility.

There is often undue concern with injury to the breasts as a result of ball contact. When the chest trap is performed correctly, contact is made on the upper portion of the sternum. The ball should not directly traumatize the breast tissue even if an individual is large-breasted. Injury can occasionally occur if the ball strikes off-centre or if the player is not expecting it and it is struck at close range by an opponent. In this situation, the pain is generally self-limiting, and these injuries can be treated as other contusions or haematomas. Occasionally, nipple irritation occurs from rubbing against the shirt or bra and is generally alleviated by using Vaseline lubrication. Female players should be taught proper chest control techniques early on so that they realize that this body surface can be used safely and without discomfort.

The kidneys are also at risk when the athlete is struck from behind. It is helpful to perform a dipstick on the urine; if blood is present, the athlete should be sent to the hospital for further evaluation. If negative, close assessment with interval monitoring of the urine for the presence of blood is useful. Intravenous pyelography is helpful for detecting renal abnormalities, and CT is valuable for assessing intra-abdominal trauma to the spleen and other organs.

Groin

Groin pain is common in soccer players, although it tends to be one area where male players have more difficulty than female players for reasons that remain unclear. Common aetiologies of injury include osteitis pubis, hernias, muscle strains (adductor, abdominal, rectus femoris, iliopsoas), stress fractures and fractures, and nerve entrapments. Chronic groin pain, or athletic pubalgia, is also referred to as Gilmore's groin in the soccer player (Gilmore, 1993). In female players it is important to consider stress fractures, especially if any of the features of the female athlete triad are present that would put them at increased risk for femoral stress fractures.

Greater trochanteric bursitis

Greater trochanteric bursitis is common in the female soccer player and can occur as a result of direct trauma to the bursa or as a result of overuse. It is not uncommon for a goalkeeper to experience acute traumatic bursitis from repetitive landing on the lateral aspect of the hip. If the bursal swelling after an acute event is large, aspiration is occasionally warranted. Padding to prevent recurrent injury is indicated, along with ice and anti-inflammatory medication. Greater trochanteric bursitis due to an overuse injury is often seen in combination with tight iliotibial band (ITB) structures. Repetitive running,

kicking and abduction-type activities can create pain. On physical examination, both acute and overuse bursitis present with localized pain and tenderness over the greater trochanteric region and occasionally swelling of the trochanteric bursa. The deep bursa lies underneath the gluteus medius muscle, whereas the superficial bursa generally is more easily palpable just over the greater trochanter. Treatment consists of ice, flexibility exercises, non-steroidal anti-inflammatory medication and corticosteroid injection if these measures fail. Paramount in treatment is an assessment for biomechanical or training errors that may be the cause.

Knee injuries

LIGAMENT INJURIES

Ligament injuries are of particular concern for the female soccer player and represent the most common severe injuries. ACL injuries are often due to a non-contact injury when the player is pivoting or landing and are common in the soccer player. These athletes often report a 'popping' sensation as their knee buckles, are unable to continue play and have swelling within 1–2 hours. As apparent from the NCAA data on female and male soccer players, ACL tears represent the single most important injury in the female player and occur more often in women than in their male counterparts (see Chapter 15).

It is important that those caring for the female soccer player look for certain biomechanical problems that may put the female athlete at particular risk for ACL injuries. Although much research is still being done in this area, it is reasonable to suggest that the soccer player strengthens both the hamstring as well as the quadriceps muscles, maintains good flexibility and preserves cardiovascular fitness to avoid fatigue. It is also important that players practise sport-specific skills such as jumping and landing so that they become agile and can maintain their balance. Balance on one leg is particularly useful, especially when one considers the multitude of soccer skills that require balancing, pivoting and jumping off one foot. It may be helpful for the soccer player to concentrate on landing from a jump with their knees flexed. All these areas need further research in order to elucidate the causative factors involved in ACL injuries in the female athlete.

MENISCAL INJURIES

Meniscal injuries are common in soccer players, especially older players. The mechanism of acute injury is no different from that in other sports, although the rotational forces that occur when the ball is kicked can contribute to the occurrence of this injury. This is particularly true when the ball is crossed into the centre of the field from the sideline so that the planted foot is facing the direction the ball will ultimately travel. Hence, the planted foot may be at an angle of close to 90° from the direction the player may be running. The athlete with a meniscal injury often presents with a knee effusion, joint line tenderness, pain in deep flexion and positive McMurray's as well as Apley's tests. A useful screen is to ask the individual to assume the squat position and then take a few steps. This test may be painful in an acute injury and thus is better used in the preparticipation setting.

These injuries are often very disabling especially if there is an ACL injury. In a retrospective study of 77 soccer players with both anterior cruciate and meniscal injuries, Neyret *et al.* (1993) found that 5 years after a rim-preserving meniscectomy individuals with an intact ACL were more likely still to be playing soccer (75% vs. 52%), more likely to be happy with their knees (97% vs. 74%) and less likely to have radiographic evidence of osteoarthritis (24% vs. 77%). Because of the intense demands on the lower extremities in soccer, it is imperative that aggressive rehabilitation occurs after such injuries. In addition, because players rely on numerous one-legged movements for specific activities, complete rehabilitation is essential.

PATELLOFEMORAL DYSFUNCTION

Patellofemoral dysfunction is extremely common in the female athlete and the most common cause of anterior knee pain. It is common in the soccer player, and presents and is treated as in other athletes (see Chapter 15). An important point to make in terms of rehabilitation is that soccer activity is one of the few examples that demonstrates the sport specificity of open-chain strengthening exercises. In general, therapists have moved away from the use of open-chain exercises because they lack sport specificity. However, in the soccer player open-chain exercises such as leg extension, short arcs and straight leg exercises are sport specific.

PATELLAR TENDONITIS

Patellar tendonitis is very common in the soccer player, generally due to repetitive kicking and jumping activity. These injuries can be frustrating and painful, but usually respond to treatment that includes ice, flexibility and modalities to decrease swelling and inflammation. Occasionally it is helpful to have the athlete work on jumping off their other foot or kick with the other foot; in general, activity should be decreased somewhat.

ILIOTIBIAL BAND FRICTION SYNDROME

ITB friction syndrome is common in soccer players, especially females. ITB friction can occur in association with greater trochanteric bursitis as well as patellofemoral dysfunction. Individuals often have inflexibility, especially of their lateral leg structures, and an increased Q-angle. The increased reliance on one-legged activities in soccer, as well as the direction of forces when the ball is kicked, make this injury a common and often very painful one. The athlete often initially complains of sharp lateral knee pain during running or kicking, which can sometimes be reproduced by repetitive resisted knee extensions. There is pain in the mid-arc region of extension when the ITB courses over the lateral femoral condyle. Eventually, the athlete may complain of aching or radiating lateral thigh pain. Other problems to consider in the differential diagnosis of lateral knee pain include lateral meniscus injuries, defects in the trochlear groove articular surface, osteochondral defects and lateral collateral ligament insufficiency. It is also important to remember that disc disease of the lumbar spine can present with radiating lower leg pain or aching. These other disorders can usually be differentiated by history and physical examination.

ITB friction syndrome appears frequently in association with patellofemoral dysfunction, patellar tendonitis and pronation. It is important to assess the biomechanics of the foot and ankle in addressing these injuries so that they do not recur. It is also important to assess for leg length discrepancies, which can also be a cause of these injuries. Leg length can be assessed clinically by measuring from the medial malleolus to the anterior superior iliac spine on both sides, although often a standing radiograph of the pelvis that includes both femoral heads and iliac crests can be used accurately to assess as well as quantify the leg length discrepancy. Leg length discrepancies should be corrected by instituting a heel lift in the shoe on the shorter leg. Often only a partial correction is necessary (i.e. if the right leg is 1.4 cm short, a 7-mm heel lift should be placed in the right shoe). Orthotics are occasionally necessary to correct for rearfoot and forefoot abnormalities and can also incorporate a heel lift if a concurrent leg length discrepancy exists.

Medial tibial stress syndrome

Medial tibial stress syndrome is common in soccer players, particularly at the beginning of a new season. This is especially true of indoor soccer players as their participation intensifies and also when they move on to artificial turf. Medial tibial stress syndrome represents an overuse injury that can be a precursor to periostitis as well as stress fracture. It is important to identify risk factors for overuse injuries in

the soccer player, especially at the foot and ankle since these structures are integral to participation.

Posterior/anterior tibialis tendonitis

These injuries are commonly due to overuse, although they can result from an acute injury. In general, they are easy to detect and treat if attention is paid to the normal anatomy of the foot and ankle. The anterior tibialis tendon is stretched during the instep kick and the kick with the outside of the foot and flexed during the pass with the inside of the foot. The anterior tibialis muscle can be stressed during all these activities. Similarly, the posterior tibialis tendon can be stressed directly or indirectly during passing and kicking; it can also routinely suffer overuse injury due to running activity. Pain is often elicited over these structures and can occasionally be associated with tenosynovitis as well. Pain is elicited with resisted motion of the affected tendon. Treatment is geared at providing relative rest, ice, flexibility, taping, antiinflammatory medication and, most importantly, identification of risk factors.

Ankle sprains

Ankle sprains account for the majority of injuries in soccer; fortunately, they tend to be mild injuries with little time lost from practice or play. They generally occur secondary to a plantar flexion/inversion mechanism. The kick with the outside of the foot can also be a common preceding activity. These injuries are no different in soccer than in other sports, but may be very debilitating if not addressed aggressively with early treatment and rehabilitation. Because soccer players rely heavily on their mobility and 'touch' on the ball, it may be more difficult to return them to complete functional activity.

The athlete generally presents with localized pain and swelling over the lateral ankle ligaments. The ligaments involved include the anterior talofibular ligament, calcaneofibular ligament and posterior talofibular ligament laterally, and the deltoid ligament medially, along with the distal tibiofibular syndesmosis centrally. Usually, the anterior talofibular ligament is the most commonly involved, followed by the calcaneofibular and posterior talofibular ligaments. Close assessment for associated injuries, such as those of the midfoot or forefoot, or fractures should be performed. In addition, if the injury involves the syndesmosis (tenderness over the distal anterior tibiofibular ligament, positive tibiofibular compression test, pain with passive external rotation of the foot), it can be more difficult to treat. Assessment for injuries to the base of the fifth metatarsal or peroneal tendons should also be carried out and a high index of suspicion for osteochondral lesions or occult fractures maintained if the athlete does not respond appropriately to conservative management.

Radiographs should be obtained if the individual cannot bear weight or there is tenderness along the posterior medial malleolus or posterior lateral malleolus, at the base of the fifth metatarsal or over the navicular tuberosity. Standard radiographs should include anteroposterior, mortise and lateral views of the ankle and anteroposterior view of the foot. Bilateral weight-bearing mortise views can help in detecting significant syndesmotic injuries. It is also important to consider repeating X-rays or other diagnostic tests if swelling and inability to bear weight persist despite initially negative evidence of occult fractures.

Ankle injuries should be treated aggressively with a compression dressing, anti-inflammatory medication, ice and elevation. Crutches should be used if weight-bearing is painful or normal gait is altered. Occasionally with significant injury, immobilization for a short period of time may be helpful. Weight-bearing is allowed as tolerated. Range of motion exercise, isometric strengthening, proprioceptive work and modalities to decrease swelling should be initiated at the first opportunity. Progressive resistance exercise is initiated as tolerated, with return to sport-specific activities as soon as possible. The use of taping or bracing may allow earlier return to play and augment physical therapy measures.

Although ankle sprains occur frequently and are generally minor, it is important to address them early and emphasize rehabilitation. In addition, if significant ankle laxity is detected during the preparticipation physical examination, a strengthening and proprioceptive programme should be initiated and consideration given to prophylactic taping or bracing.

There is a subgroup of ankle sprains that go on to develop ankle impingement syndromes. Impingement syndromes should be considered in the setting of anterolateral pain, the absence of instability and history of prior ankle sprains. Athletes often complain of pain while trying to pivot or push off from one foot, as well as difficulty and pain while kicking the ball with the instep. Impingement syndrome occurs as a result of hypertrophic scar formation, synovium, and fibrocartilage in the anterolateral tibiotalar space extending from the anterior capsule posteriorly into the lateral gutter. In soccer players McCarroll et al. (1987) have described these as 'meniscoid' lesions after inversion ankle sprains. Stress radiographs generally do not reveal significant ligamentous laxity, although anterior spurring of the tibia may be present and increase the soft-tissue impingement.

Knapp and Mandelbaum (1996) have recommended a classification of ankle impingement syndrome that describes four grades: (i) normal radiographs, anterolateral capsular thickening seen on MRI and verified arthroscopically; (ii) extra-articular or intra-articular osteophytes with articular surfaces entirely normal; (iii) bony abnormalities involving articular surface (osteochondritis dissecans); and (iv) previous intra-articular fracture. If aggressive physical therapy and rehabilitation does not provide resolution of impingement problems, these lesions often respond well to arthroscopic débridement.

An impingement syndrome can also occur posteriorly, especially if an os trigonum is present. Other problems to consider in the posterior ankle include Achilles tendonitis, retrocalcaneal bursitis, Haglund's deformity, posterior tibialis tendonitis and tarsal tunnel syndrome. These can usually be detected by careful history and physical examination, occasionally supplemented with additional testing.

Peroneal tendonitis

Peroneal tendonitis is one of many overuse injuries common in the soccer player. Because soccer activities rely on presenting many different foot surfaces, the muscles that control ankle and foot motion are used constantly. When an athlete starts the season, overuse injuries are common because so many of these movements are specific to soccer. Peroneal tendonitis generally presents with pain and occasionally swelling behind the lateral malleolus, with a predictable increase in pain when the player uses the outside of the foot for passing or shooting. Pain with resisted eversion also reproduces the symptoms. Treatment is designed to decrease swelling, increase flexibility and investigate precipitating biomechanical factors. Non-steroidal anti-inflammatory medication, ice, stretching and modalities are all useful. In addition, assessment for orthotics to correct biomechanical problems at the foot and ankle is also important.

Plantar fasciitis

Plantar fasciitis may be difficult to treat in soccer players given the high running and jumping demands the sport entails. The athlete presents with arch pain, initially worse in the morning and better after a gentle warm-up. Generally, these athletes have point tenderness at the calcaneal insertion of the plantar fascia. Athletes usually respond to non-steroidal anti-inflammatory medication, ice, stretching and massage techniques, modalities and arch supports; treatment should also address biomechanical problems. An orthosis that keeps the plantar fascia stretched throughout the night (night splints) are very useful in treating these injuries, although they can be somewhat cumbersome to use. In those individuals unresponsive to this management, phonophoresis, iontophoresis or a localized injection of corticosteroid followed by relative rest is often helpful.

Achilles tendonitis

Achilles tendonitis is another common overuse problem seen in soccer players due to repetitive running, jumping and cutting activities. Overuse injuries appear most frequently before the season starts. The athlete complains of pain in the posterior heel associated with jumping activity and can develop a tenosynovitis with palpable crepitus in the tendon sheath. These injuries should be treated aggressively. A stretching programme, in association with ice, non-steroidal anti-inflammatory medication and activity modification, is generally indicated. In addition, using heel pads bilaterally can help decrease the tension on the Achilles complex and thus decrease pain. The athlete should understand that a stretching programme is essential in treatment. Attention must also be given to potential biomechanical factors that may predispose the athlete to this injury.

Turf toe and reverse turf toe

Turf toe is used to describe a chronic hyperextension of the first metatarsophalangeal joint. This is often due to the repetitive, high-energy forces that occur at this joint in a relatively flexible shoe. Reverse turf toe, commonly called 'soccer toe', is due to chronic hyperflexion of the metatarsophalangeal joint when the ball is struck during an instep kick or when the foot inadvertently strikes the ground. Hallux rigidus is commonly associated with these conditions. These injuries are quite painful and can be debilitating for the soccer player. Treatment includes ice, anti-inflammatory medication, range of motion and taping, as well as shoe modifications.

Fractures

Fractures of the fibula or tibia are uncommon in soccer but can occur, especially if shin-guards are not worn or are used incorrectly. These injuries usually occur as a result of a forceful kick to the leg. The use of shin-guards can decrease the risk of lower leg fractures (Bir *et al.*, 1995). Athletes with tibial fractures are generally unable to tolerate weight-bearing and thus are easy to identify. Fibular fractures may be more difficult to recognize because the fibula is a non-weight-bearing bone and thus players commonly carry on after sustaining this type of injury. A fibular fracture may take longer to heal because of the reduced stress on the bone due to its non-weight-bearing nature. The use of protective shin-guards should be enforced to avoid these injuries. These fractures are treated the same in soccer players as in other athletes, although return to play may be more difficult because of the high demands on the lower leg musculature in soccer.

Metatarsal fractures

Metatarsal fractures are common in soccer due to the high demands placed on the lower extremities. Non-displaced fractures of the metatarsal neck and shaft tend to be quite stable. Symptomatic treatment with strapping and a supportive shoe often suffice. A fair amount of mediolateral angulation can be accepted in metatarsal neck and shaft fractures, with no complications unless cross-union occurs or fragments are displaced.

Displaced fractures of the metatarsal neck and shaft are a different matter and care must be taken with these injuries. The most common complication of metatarsal fractures is late transfer metatarsalgia, where asymmetry of the metatarsal heads in the dorsoplantar plane can lead to a change in the load-bearing forces through the depressed metatarsal heads. Radiographs of the forefoot with the toes extended, similar to a sesamoid view, can help in making decisions about the treatment of these injuries. Referral to an orthopaedic surgeon for consideration of open reduction with internal fixation may be necessary if closed treatment is not successful. In general, the metatarsal injuries seen in soccer tend to be mild, and respond well to conservative management. If there are multiple metatarsal injuries or the athlete has sustained a Lisfranc fracture–dislocation pattern, careful attention to the soft tissue should be maintained for signs of compartment syndrome.

Fractures of the fifth metatarsal deserve special attention. These are generally divided according to their location, with tuberosity or avulsion fractures and shaft and neck fractures treated very differently from fractures that occur at the metaphyseal–diaphyseal junction (so-called Jones fractures). Fractures that involve the styloid process can be either articular or extra-articular and occur at the insertion of the peroneus brevis tendon. The foot is often in the plantigrade position when the injury occurs. It is important to differentiate acute fractures from anomalies and variations in normal growth patterns.

Extra-articular fractures can be treated symptomatically with shoe modifications, relative rest and return to activity as tolerated. Fracture fragments can be excised if they remain or become painful. Treatment for intra-articular fractures is controversial. If they are non-displaced, they tend to respond to casting and rest from weight-bearing (Dameron, 1975; Torg et al., 1984). If the fracture is large or displaced, they can be treated with internal fixation. This may allow athletes to resume activities sooner than with non-operative treatment, although given the good results with non-operative management the treatment should be individualized.

Fractures of the Jones type, which occur at the junction of the metatarsal shaft and base within 1.5 cm of the tuberosity, are unique and merit special attention. These injuries commonly occur in jumping sports when the metatarsophalangeal joints are extended and the heel elevated with loading of the lateral aspect of the foot. These fractures are notoriously difficult to treat conservatively and there is a high incidence of delayed union, non-union and refracture, especially in high-demand athletes (Dameron, 1975; Kavanaugh et al., 1978; Torg et al., 1984).

Jones fractures are subdivided according to whether they are acute fractures or whether they are seen in the setting of chronic stress or previous injury (Torg et al., 1984). The latter can be recognized radiographically or by a history of pain at or near the base of the fifth metatarsal preceding the fracture (DeLee, 1986). Jones fractures that are truly acute can be treated with casting and rest from weight-bearing; however, in the high-demand athlete or others wishing aggressive treatment, percutaneous intramedullary screw fixation is indicated (DeLee *et al.*, 1983; Rettig *et al.*, 1992; Mindrebo *et al.*, 1993). Intramedullary screw fixation is also indicated if there is evidence for stress reaction or previous injury. Delayed unions and symptomatic nonunions are treated by curettage and bone grafting via a dorsolateral incision, supplemented with intramedullary fixation. The use of an external bone growth stimulator can be considered in all these fractures in an attempt to speed healing.

Stress fractures of the base of the fifth metatarsal are treated aggressively as recommended above. Stress fractures of the other metatarsals can usually be treated conservatively with relative rest, activity modification and gradual return to sport-specific activity.

Stress fractures

Stress fractures are due to repetitive submaximal forces that ultimately overwhelm the skeletal system and lead to fracture. The most common stress fractures seen in soccer players are in the lower extremity. In a study of stress fractures in athletes diagnosed by bone scan, Matheson *et al.* (1987) reported the most common sites to be the tibia (49.1%), tarsals (25.3%), metatarsals (8.8%), femur (7.2%), fibula (6.6%), pelvis (1.6%), sesamoids (0.9%) and spine (0.6%). It is important to differentiate stress fractures from insufficiency fractures. In stress fractures, repetitive submaximal forces overwhelm the reparative process but the bone itself is initially normal. In insufficiency fractures, normal stresses on a bone that has decreased resistance to fracture because of an underlying condition such as osteoporosis lead to fracture.

Stress fractures are often difficult to diagnose because they are not associated with a clear traumatic injury. They generally present with a dull pain aggravated by activity and relieved by rest. This progresses to pain at the fracture site associated with localized swelling and erythema and

eventually the athlete can no longer participate because of the pain. The athlete often avoids medical attention until she can no longer participate in activity without pain. The average time to diagnosis in the study by Matheson *et al.* (1987) was 13 weeks.

Predisposing factors to consider include both training and equipment errors as well as biomechanical errors. In the study by Matheson *et al.* (1987), training errors accounted for 22.4% of the stress fractures. Training and equipment errors include an abrupt change in playing surface, an abrupt change in the training schedule including increased distance, intensity or speed, or insufficient recovery time between sessions (Reeder *et al.*, 1996). Inappropriate shoes may be implicated in the development of stress fractures; this may be particularly important in soccer players as many of the soccer cleats worn are often poor at controlling rearfoot and forefoot motion. Biomechanical issues include leg length discrepancies, foot pronation, femoral anteversion or increased knee valgus (Reeder *et al.*, 1996). These problems should be assessed at the time of the athlete's preparticipation physical examination as well as in those who present with an overuse injury or stress fracture.

It is essential to ask female athletes with stress fractures and other overuse injuries about their menstrual history as well as their overall body image. Menstrual dysfunction, as well as eating disorders, are associated with low oestrogen and low bone mineral density and together are known as the female athlete triad (Yeager *et al.*, 1993; Putukian, 1995). Decreased bone mineral density has been associated with an increased incidence of stress fractures.

On physical examination, athletes with stress fractures may have localized tenderness at the fracture site and occasionally swelling, erythema or local warmth. Hopping on the affected limb may elicit pain. Other positive findings include a positive compression test (either tibia–fibula or metatarsal), a positive heel strike (tibia, calcaneus, femur, pelvis), pain with one-legged extension (spondylolysis) or axial loading of the involved bone (metatarsals). In addition, pain is often elicited with a tuning fork or even with ultrasound, which is thought to cause pain because damaged periosteum absorbs ultrasound energy and transforms it to heat. This test is occasionally useful and has been shown to be 93% accurate in detecting acute fractures (Devas, 1983).

Radiographs may show small cortical interruptions followed by periosteal reaction and eventually dense callus formation. The initial radiographic changes may appear at 10–14 days but are often delayed for more than 3 weeks. Technetium bone scanning is useful in athletes with suspected stress fractures who have normal radiographs and in those with old fractures (of 6–12 months' duration). Bone scans generally show areas of increased uptake consistent with stress fracture at 6–72 hours. It is important to remember that bone scans, although sensitive, are not specific and thus a differential diagnosis including osteochondral or acute fractures, Ewing's sarcoma, eosinophilic granuloma or osteogenic sarcoma should be kept in mind. A normal scan usually excludes stress fracture and allows athletes to return to activity sooner. Although technetium bone scanning is the gold standard, other types of diagnostic test have also been used. Multiple grading systems exist and two of these (Zwas et al., 1987; Fredericson et al., 1995) are shown in Table 39.4. Grades 1 and 2 are generally only minimally symptomatic and require 3–4 weeks to heal, whereas grades 3 and 4 are usually symptomatic and require up to 4–6 weeks to heal.

Treatment of stress fractures requires relative rest until the fracture heals followed by gradual resumption of activities. It is important to identify the potential biomechanical problems, such as pronation or other foot biomechanics, that predispose the athlete to recurrent injury. It is often useful to assess the athlete closely while running and initiate shoe modifications or orthotics if necessary. A careful analysis of training patterns and discussion with the staff responsible for coaching or strength and conditioning may also be helpful. Athletes can maintain their cardiovascular conditioning by using a stationary bike, running in a pool or, if possible, running on an unloaded harness system treadmill. This allows athletes to run with a small percentage of their body weight removed and thus allows them to exercise without pain. Pain is the most useful

Table 39.4 Two systems of grading stress fractures based on bone scan and MRI

Grade	Bone scan*	MRI†
1	Small, ill-defined cortical area of mildly increased activity	Periosteal oedema, mild to moderate on T2 images
2	Better-defined cortical area of moderately increased activity	Periosteal oedema, moderate to severe on T2 images; marrow oedema on T2 images
3	Wide to fusiform, cortical–medullary area of highly increased activity	Periosteal oedema, moderate to severe on T2 images; marrow oedema on T1 and T2 images
4	Transcortical area of intensely increased activity	Periosteal oedema, moderate to severe on T2 images; marrow oedema on T1 and T2 images; fracture line clearly visible

*Grading system of Zwas et al. (1987).
†Grading system of Fredericson et al. (1995).

guide in terms of progression of activities. Activities should be as specific to the sport as possible. For the soccer player this means allowing weight-bearing as soon as there is no pain and heading or hitting a ball against a wall gently prior to running.

Prevention of stress fractures, as with all overuse injuries, should be the goal of those taking care of soccer players. It is important to look for and identify risk factors during the preparticipation physical examination. This includes an assessment of not only biomechanical or training errors but also menstrual function, body image abnormalities and nutritional patterns. Encouraging a good strengthening and conditioning programme can help avoid many overuse injuries before they occur.

Contusions/haematomas

These are probably the most common injuries seen in soccer and are usually due to direct trauma with another player or the ball. Most contusions result in acute trauma to, and bleeding of, muscle tissue with localized haematoma formation. Contusions are generally self-limiting and do not result in a time-loss injury; however, if they occur to the head, thorax or abdomen, they can be life-threatening.

Muscle contusions can be intramuscular, where bleeding does not spread outside the epimysium, or intermuscular, where the haemorrhage extends to the muscle fascia and subcutaneous tissue. The latter are generally benign and do not cause problems. Because intramuscular haematomas are contained within the muscle sheath they can create increased intramuscular pressure and pain and ultimately require surgical drainage. Acute compartment syndrome is a complication of a large haematoma and must be detected should it occur. This is a medical emergency as tissue damage may be irreversible if treatment is delayed.

The most common location of muscle contusions in soccer is the quadriceps muscle, usually as a result of direct trauma to the muscle from the knee or foot of an opposing player. Another common area is the anterior compartment of the lower leg; these injuries can be diminished with the use of shin-guards. Treatment should include ice, compression wrap and rest from activity. In large contusions of the quadriceps muscle it is often useful to flex the knee to roughly 120° and apply a compressive wrap in this position for 24 hours (Aronen & Chronister, 1992). It is also reasonable to initiate non-steroidal anti-inflammatory medication in an attempt to prevent fibrosis and heterotopic bone formation.

Large haematomas are occasionally evacuated surgically via aspiration followed by a compressive dressing. This decreases the intramuscular pressure and pain effectively, but should be avoided if possible because there is a high risk of infection. Early rehabilitation efforts should be focused on regaining full range of motion, and cardiovascular fitness maintained by using arm isokinetic machines or swimming while 'dragging' the involved extremity. Isometric exercise can be initiated early in rehabilitation and may help stimulate muscle regeneration. Once the athlete is able to demonstrate full range of motion and has no palpable defect or pain with resisted motion, then a slow return to activity can be allowed.

It is important to follow these injuries closely and observe the range of motion so that complications can be avoided. Heterotopic bone formation and myositis ossificans occur in 9–20% of all quadriceps contusions (Saartok, 1996). Heterotopic bone formation occurs in the muscle, although it can progress to myositis ossificans which extends to the bone. These can require several months of treatment. Other complications of contusions and haematomas are compartment syndromes and nerve palsies. Therefore, close assessment of these seemingly unimportant injuries is essential.

Subungual haematomas and ingrown nails

These injuries are common in the soccer player and are generally a result of trauma to the nail within the soccer shoe. Subungual haematomas are common when a player is stepped on or has kicked the ground. The athlete complains of significant pain, which is a result of blood beneath the nail in an enclosed space. This is easily resolved by creating a hole, either by twisting an 18-gauge needle slowly until the nail is pierced or by heating the end of a paper clip and burning through the nail. Special drills or a jeweller's drill can be used for the same purpose.

Ingrown nails are also common and occur when the nail grows into the lateral skin and becomes embedded. The lateral nail folds then become painful after trauma and occasionally can also become infected. These are often treated with digital anaesthetic block followed by partial nail removal. Infections are treated by antibiotics that provide good skin coverage for *Staphylococcus* and *Streptococcus*. The athlete should be instructed on proper nail-cutting techniques and shoe fitting.

Muscular strains/overuse injuries

Muscular strains/overuse injuries probably represent the most common injury in soccer, although they do not often result in time lost from play. These injuries often occur after an acute load or as a result of chronic overuse. The major muscle groups involved in soccer players include the hamstring, quadriceps and adductor muscles. Another common overuse injury is that to the pes anserinus, where the gracilis, sartorius and semitendinosus tendons converge along the anteromedial aspect of the proximal tibia. This structure is often stressed by the pass with the inside of the foot or by direct trauma and is commonly associated with a bursitis. Other commonly involved areas are the muscles of the lower leg and foot. The athlete describes pain when performing a certain movement and occasionally describes a 'popping' sensation. These athletes may often have point tenderness in the muscle belly itself or pain can be reproduced by resistive testing of the particular muscle group.

On examination of these injuries, the presence of echymosis, swelling, the amount of point tenderness and the presence of a palpable defect should be determined and noted. Occasionally,

recording the circumference of the body part involved is also helpful. The early treatment of these injuries is with ice, compression for 48 hours and rest in the flexed position. It is important to avoid massage or heat initially because these modalities increase bleeding into the area and worsen the injury. Non-steroidal anti-inflammatory medication serves as an adjunct for pain and prevents fibrosis and should be initiated when not contraindicated. Return to play is allowed when the athlete has full range of motion, full strength and can perform sport-specific skills. It will often be difficult to return the athlete to full sprinting activity. During rehabilitation it is important that an attempt is made to match muscle use with speed-specific as well as sport-specific activities. The time to return to full activity is variable and may range from a few days to 6–8 weeks.

It is unclear if some of the acute muscle strain injuries can be avoided, although there are data to demonstrate that a muscle with more length requires more tension prior to tearing. This would imply that increased flexibility is beneficial for decreasing the risk of muscle injury. If an athlete is unconditioned and not accustomed to long practices or high sprinting demands, she may be at increased risk for acute muscle overuse and strain. A comprehensive conditioning and flexibility programme may be beneficial in avoiding these injuries.

Injuries in the adolescent player

Injuries to be concerned about in the adolescent soccer player include apophyseal fractures, apophysitis and Osgood–Schlatter disease. Where major tendons originate or insert into bones, accessory growth plates, or apophyses, occur. These areas are generally weaker than the bone or muscle–tendon junction and as a result of stress can be a site of failure in the young athlete. The apophyses can be avulsed by a strong contraction of the muscle. In soccer players, these tend to occur in the pelvis. It is important to consider avulsion fractures if the athlete gives a history of significant pain or swelling after a forceful contraction, especially if they have difficulty bearing weight. The kicking motion places great tension stress on the anterior inferior iliac spine and the ischial tuberosity due to rectus femoris and hamstring forces respectively. These fractures most commonly occur in girls aged 14–17 years. Avulsion fractures of the tibial tubercle require special mention because these are serious injuries that can occur in the adolescent soccer player. The tibial tubercle has a separate ossification centre that eventually fuses with the tibial epiphysis prior to full closure of the growth plate. A fracture in this location can involve only the tubercle or can extend through the epiphysis; if displaced, this injury often requires early surgical reduction and fixation management. Occasionally, these injuries are not apparent on plain radiographs and MRI or CT can be useful.

Apophysitis is considered an overuse injury of the apophyses and in the soccer player is most often seen at the iliac crest and the calcaneal tuberosity. Iliac crest apophysitis often occurs in females before 14 years of age, when the apophyses usually close. The athlete complains of pain that is often present along the anterior aspect of the iliac crest. Radiographs may show increased widening of the apophyseal line, although this finding may be subtle. Because the muscle structures that attach here are integral to soccer activity, these injuries often take 4–8 weeks to heal fully, and activity modification and play as tolerated by pain are the basic treatment guidelines.

Calcaneal apophysitis, or Sever's disease, is also common in the adolescent athlete, although it can also occur as early as 7–8 years of age. The pain is generally located at the insertion of the Achilles tendon at the posterior aspect of the calcaneus. The pain is generally made worse with jumping activity. Radiographs may be helpful, although it is often difficult to differentiate from normal variants in calcaneal apophyseal ossification centres. Treatment is again conservative, with relative rest, ice and anti-inflammatory medication for pain. Often a heel cord stretching programme, along with bilateral heel lifts to put the Achilles tendon complex at rest, can provide some relief. In addition, shoe modifications may also be useful.

Osgood–Schlatter disease is very common in all young athletes involved in jumping activity and therefore also in the soccer player. It is not a true apophysitis in that it does not occur at the apophyseal growth plate but at the junction between the tuberosity and the tendon when the tuberosity is transforming from cartilage to bone. Osgood–Schlatter disease generally presents in young girls at the age of 9–13. Pain is generally located at the tibial tubercle and is aggravated by jumping, running and kicking activities. On physical examination, localized pain and swelling is present and pain is elicited with resisted leg extension. It is important to ensure that the quadriceps mechanism is intact. Radiographs may be helpful in assessing the presence of fragmentation and ruling out avulsion fracture. Treatment is generally symptomatic, with quadriceps flexibility, ice after activity and activity modification as needed. It is important to reassure the athlete and parents that this condition is self-limiting and will eventually resolve.

Sinding–Larsen–Johansson disease is similar to Osgood–Schlatter disease except that it occurs at the inferior pole of the patella. Physical examination helps differentiate the location of pain and radiographs may be confirmatory. The most important activity modification is to avoid jumping, although depending on the severity of symptoms some players may be unable to tolerate prolonged running. If the athlete cannot run without pain, she can still participate in sport-specific skill work. Increasing flexibility and maintaining cardiovascular fitness with an alternative form of exercise such as cycling or swimming may be useful as an adjunct to rehabilitation.

Conclusion

Soccer is a tremendously exciting sport that is growing exponentially, especially for girls and women. The sport is challenging in that it demands high levels of aerobic as well as anaerobic fitness, requires acquisition and mastery of skills, and does not select for a particular body type. Because of the demands of the sport, flexibility, strengthening and conditioning, and proper nutrition are essential. Soccer enjoys a low injury rate, especially when played by the rules, and the injuries that do occur tend to be mild. In the future, research into the more significant injuries, such as ACL and other ligament injuries and head injuries, should continue to improve the medical care available to soccer athletes and increase safe and enjoyable participation.

References

Abreau, F., Templer, D.I., Schuyler, B.A. & Hutchinson, H.T. (1990) Neuropsychological assessment of soccer players. *Neuropsychology* **4**, 175–181.

Brewer, J. & Davis, J. (1994) The female player. In B. Ekblom (ed.) *Football (Soccer). Handbook of Sports Medicine and Science*, pp. 95–99. Blackwell Scientific Publications, Oxford.

Alves, W.M., Rimel, R.W. & Nelson, W.E. (1987) University of Virginia prospective study of football-induced minor head injury: status report. *Clinics in Sports Medicine* **6**, 211–218.

American College of Sports Medicine (1996) Position stand on exercise and fluid replacement. *Medicine and Science in Sports and Exercise* **28**, i–vii.

Anon. (1994) Injuries associated with soccer goal posts: United States 1979–93. *Morbidity and Mortality Weekly Report* **43**, 153–155.

Aronen, J.G. & Chronister, R.D. (1992) Quadriceps contusions; hastening the return to play. *Physician and Sportsmedicine* **20**, 130–136.

Barkley, K.L. (1997) In Mellion, M. (ed.) *The Team Physician's Handbook*, 2nd edn, pp. 672–684. Hanley & Belfus, Philadelphia.

Bir, C.A., Cassatta, S.J. & Janda, D.H. (1995) An analysis and comparison of soccer shin guards. *Clinical Journal of Sports Medicine* **5**, 95–99.

Burslem, I. & Lees, A. (1987) Quantification of impact accelerations of the head during the heading of a football. In T. Reilly, A. Lees, K. Davids *et al.* (eds) *Science and Football: Proceedings of the First World Congress of Science and Football*, pp. 243–248. E. & F.N. Spon, London.

Colquhoun, D. & Chad, K.E. (1992) Physiological characteristics of Australian female soccer players after a competitive season. *Australian Journal of Science and Medicine in Sport* **18**, 9–12.

Dameron, T.B. (1975) Fractures and anatomical varia-

tions of the proximal portion of the fifth metatarsal. *Journal of Bone and Joint Surgery* **57A**, 788–792.

DeLee, J.C. (1986) Fractures and dislocations of the foot. In R.A. Mann (ed.) *Surgery of the Foot*, pp. 592–808. Mosby, St Louis.

DeLee, J.C., Evans, J.P. & Julian, J. (1983) Stress fracture of the fifth metatarsal. *American Journal of Sports Medicine* **11**, 349–353.

Devas, M. (1983) Ultrasonic assessment of stress fractures. *British Medical Journal* **286**, 1479–1480.

Dick, R. (1996) *NCAA Injury Surveillance System 1995–1996*. National Collegiate Athletic Association, Overland Park, Kansas.

Ekblom, B. (1986) Applied physiology of soccer. *Sports Medicine* **3**, 50–60.

Ekblom, B. (ed.) (1994) *Football (Soccer)*. Handbook of Sports Medicine and Science. Blackwell Scientific Publications, Oxford.

Ekstrand, J. & Gillquist, J. (1982) The frequency of male tightness and injuries in soccer. *American Journal of Sports Medicine* **10**, 75–78.

Elias, S.R., Roberts, W.O. & Thorson, D.C. (1991) Team sports in hot weather: guidelines for modifying youth soccer. *Physician and Sportsmedicine* **19**, 67–78.

Ergstrom, B., Johannsson, C. & Tornkvist, H. (1991) Soccer injuries among elite female players. *American Journal of Sports Medicine* **19**, 372–375.

Fredericson, M., Bergman, A.G., Hoffman, K.L. & Dillingham, M.S. (1995) Tibial stress reaction in runners: correlation of clinical symptoms and scintigraphy with a new MRI grading system. *American Journal of Sports Medicine* **23**, 472–481.

Gainor, B.J., Piotrowski, G., Puhl, J.J. & Allen, W.C. (1978) The kick: biomechanics and collision injury. *American Journal of Sports Medicine* **6**, 185–193.

Gilmore, O.J. (1993) Gilmore's groin. *Sportsmedicine and Soft Tissue Trauma* **3**, 2–4.

Jensen, K. & Larsson, B. (1993) Variations of physical capacity in a period including supplemental training of the Danish soccer team for women. In T. Reilly, J. Clarys & Stibbe (eds) *Science and Football II*, pp. 114–117. E. & F.N. Spon, London.

Jordan, B.D. & Zimmerman, R.D. (1990) Computed tomography and magnetic resonance imaging comparisons in boxers. *Journal of the American Medical Association* **263**, 1670–1674.

Jordan, S.H., Green, G.A., Galanty, H.L., Mandelbaum, B.R. & Jabour, B.A. (1996) Acute and chronic brain injury in United States national team soccer players. *American Journal of Sports Medicine* **24**, 205–210.

Kavanaugh, J.H., Brewer, T.D. & Mann, R.V. (1978) The Jones fracture revisited. *Journal of Bone and Joint Surgery* **60A**, 776–782.

Kelly, J.P. & Rosenburg, J.H. (1997) Diagnosis and management of concussion in sport. *Neurology* **48**, 575–580.

Kirkendall, D.T. (1993) Carbohydrate supplementation and performance in soccer players. *Medicine and Science in Sports and Exercise* **25**, 1370–1374.

Knapik, J.J., Baumn, C.L., Jones, B.H., Harris, J.M. & Vaughan, L. (1991) Pre-season strength and flexibility imbalances associated with athletic injuries in female collegiate athletes. *American Journal of Sports Medicine* **19**, 76–81.

Knapp, T. & Mandelbaum, B.R. (1996) Ankle sprains and impingement syndromes. In W.E. Garrett, D.T. Kirkendall & S.R. Contiguglia (eds) *The US Soccer Sports Medicine Book*, pp. 360–368. Williams & Wilkins, Baltimore.

Leatt, P.B. & Jacobs, I. (1989) Effect of glucose polymer on glycogen depletion during a soccer match. *Canadian Journal of Sports Science* **14**, 112–116.

Levin, H.S., Amparo, E., Eisenberg, J.M. *et al.* (1987) Magnetic resonance imaging and computerized tomography in relation to the neurobehavioral sequelae of mild and moderate head injuries. *Journal of Neurosurgery* **66**, 706–713.

Lindenfeld, T.N., Schmidtt, D.J., Hendy, M.P., Mangine, R.E. & Noyes, F.R. (1994) Incidence of injury in indoor soccer. *American Journal of Sports Medicine* **22**, 364–371.

McCarroll, J.R., Schrader, J.W., Shelbourne, K.D., Rettig, A.C. & Bisesi, M.A. (1987) Meniscoid lesions of the ankle in soccer players. *American Journal of Sports Medicine* **15**, 255–257.

McLatchie, G., Brooks, N., Galbraith, S. *et al.* (1987) Clinical neurological examination, neuropsychology, electroencephalography and computed tomographic head scanning in active amateur boxers. *Journal of Neurology, Neurosurgery and Psychiatry* **50**, 96–99.

Maehlum, S., Dahl, E. & Daljord, O.A. (1986) Frequency of injuries in a youth soccer tournament. *Physician and Sportsmedicine* **14**, 73–79.

Matheson, G.O., Clement, D.B., McKenzie, D.C., Taunton, J.E., Lloyd-Smith, D.R. & MacIntyre, J.G. (1987) Stress fractures in athletes: a study of 320 cases. *American Journal of Sports Medicine* **15**, 46–58.

Mindrebo, N., Shelbourne, D., Van Meter, C.D. & Rettig, A.C. (1993) Outpatient percutaneous screw fixation of the acute Jone's fracture. *American Journal of Sports Medicine* **21**, 720–723.

Neyret, P., Donell, S.T., DeJour, D. & DeJour, H. (1993) Partial meniscectomy and anterior cruciate ligament rupture in soccer players. A study with a minimum 20-year follow-up. *American Journal of Sports Medicine* **21**, 455–460.

Nilsson, S. & Roaas, A. (1978) Soccer injuries in adolescents. *American Journal of Sports Medicine* **6**, 358–361.

Pardon, E.T. (1977) Lower extremities are site of most soccer injuries. *Physician and Sportsmedicine* **5**, 42–48.

Porter, M.D. & Fricker, P.A. (1996) Controlled prospec-

tive neuropsychological assessment of active experienced amateur boxers. *Clinical Journal of Sports Medicine* **6**, 90–96.

Pritchett, J.W. (1981) Cost of high school soccer injuries. *American Journal of Sports Medicine* **9**, 64–66.

Putukian, M. (1995) Female athlete triad. *Sports Medicine and Arthroscopy Review* **3**, 295–307.

Putukian, M. & Echemendia, R.J. (1996) Managing successive minor head injuries. Which tests guide return to play? *Physician and Sportsmedicine* **24**, 25–38.

Putukian, M., Knowles, W.K., Swere, S. & Castle, N.G. (1996) Injuries in indoor soccer. The Lake Placid Dawn to Dark Soccer Tournament. *American Journal of Sports Medicine* **24**, 317–322.

Reeder, M.T., Dick, B.H., Atkins, J.K., Pribis, A.B. & Jartinez, J.M. (1996) Stress fractures: current concepts of diagnosis and treatment. *Sports Medicine* **22**, 198–212.

Rettig, A.C., Shelbourne, K.D. & Wilckens, J. (1992) The surgical treatment of symptomatic nonunions of the proximal (metaphyseal) fifth metatarsal in athletes. *American Journal of Sports Medicine* **20**, 50–54.

Rhodes, E.C. & Mosher, R.E. (1992) Aerobic and anaerobic characteristics of elite female university soccer players. *Journal of Sports Sciences* **10**, 143–144.

Rimel, R.W., Giordani, B., Barth, J.T., Boll, T.J. & Jane, J.A. (1981) Disability caused by minor head injury. *Neurosurgery* **9**, 221–228.

Rimel, R.W., Giordani, B., Barth, J.T. & Jane, J.A. (1982) Moderate head injury: completing the clinical spectrum of brain trauma. *Neurosurgery* **11**, 344–351.

Saartok, T. (1996) Contusions and hematomas. In W.E. Garret, D.T. Kirkendall & S.R. Contiguglia (eds) *The US Soccer Sports Medicine Book*, pp. 318–325. Williams & Wilkins, Baltimore.

Saltin, B. & Costill, D.L. (1988) Fluid and electrolyte balance during prolonged exercise. In E.S. Horton & R.L. Terjung (eds) *Exercise, Nutrition and Metabolism*, pp. 150–158. Macmillan, New York.

Schmidt-Olsen, S., Jorgensen, U., Kaalund, S. & Sorenson, J. (1991) Injuries among young soccer players. *American Journal of Sports Medicine* **19**, 273–275.

Scopetta, C. & Vaccario, M. (1978) Central cervical cord syndrome after heading a football. *Lancet* **i**, 1269.

Sortland, O. & Tysvaer, A.T. (1989) Brain damage in former association football players. *Neuroradiology* **31**, 44–48.

Sortland, O., Tysvaer, A.T. & Storli, O.V. (1982) Changes in the cervical spine in association football players. *British Journal of Sports Medicine* **16**, 80–84.

Sullivan, J.A., Gross, R.H., Grava, W.A. *et al.* (1980) Evaluation of injuries in youth soccer. *American Journal of Sports Medicine* **8**, 325–327.

Torg, J.S., Balduini, F.C., Zelko, R.R., Pavlov, H., Peff, T.C. & Das, M. (1984) Fracture of the base of the fifth metatarsal distal to the tuberosity: classification and guidelines for non-surgical and surgical management. *Journal of Bone and Joint Surgery* **66A**, 209–214.

Tysvaer, A.T. (1985) Cervical disc herniation in a football player. *British Journal of Sports Medicine* **19**, 43–45.

Tysvaer, A.T. (1992) Head and neck injuries in soccer. Impact of minor trauma. *Sports Medicine* **14**, 200–213.

Tysvaer, A.T. & Lochen, E.A. (1991) Soccer injuries to the brain. A neuropsychologic study of former soccer players. *American Journal of Sports Medicine* **19**, 56–60.

Tysvaer, A.T., Storli, O.V. & Bachen, N.I. (1989) Soccer injuries to the brain: a neurologic and electroencephalographic study of former players. *Acta Neurologica Scandinavica* **80**, 151–156.

Yeager, K.K., Agostini, R., Nattiv, A. & Drinkwater, B. (1993). The female athlete triad: disordered eating, amenorrhea, osteoporosis. *Medicine and Science in Sports and Exercise* **25**, 775–777.

Zwas, S.T., Elkanovitch, R. & Frank, G. (1987) Interpretation and classification of bone scintigraphic findings in stress fractures. *Journal of Nuclear Medicine* **28**, 452–457.

Chapter 40

Canoeing and Kayaking

KATHERINE KENAL AND PATRICIA TRELA

Introduction

Canoeing and kayaking are activities that allow participants to enjoy the diversity of the outdoors. The popularity of these paddling sports is evidenced by the fact that several European countries have chosen canoeing as their national sport. Currently, the American Canoe Association estimates that over 24 million Americans are involved in these sports. Originally, canoeing and kayaking provided transportation for hunting, gathering and trade by the Native Americans of North America and the Inuit of the Arctic. By the turn of the century these popular leisure activities had evolved into competitive sports. Consequently, the International Canoe Federation (ICF) was formed in 1924 to provide administrative and technical guidance and to sanction races for participants throughout the world.

The sport of canoeing and kayaking was admitted to Olympic competition in 1936 at the XIII Olympic Games in Berlin. Flatwater racing has been a part of the Summer Olympic Games since that time, with women's kayaking events being added in 1948. However, whitewater slalom racing has only been a part of the official games in 1972, 1992 and 1996. Its entry into the games is left to the discretion of the host country. Australia will host whitewater slalom racing at the Olympic Games in Sydney in 2000.

The technical skills required, combined with the need for strength and endurance, challenge participants in both flatwater and whitewater environments. Several popular forms of paddling sports exist, including canoe sailing, outrigger canoe, sea kayaking and surf skiing. Competitive marathon regattas involve distances from 10 km to several hundred kilometres, while rivers challenge whitewater enthusiasts to the extremes of 'playboating' during rodeo events (Fig. 40.1).

Technological advances in equipment and specific training programmes have allowed an even greater number of women to become involved recreationally and competitively. At the 1997 World Championships for flatwater canoe and kayak in Halifax, Nova Scotia, women competed in kayaking at the 200 and 500 m distances and, for the first time, the 1000 m distance. Women race kayaks over 500 m in three events: K1, K2 and K4 (K4 having been added to the schedule in 1984). The goal is to gain entry to the final race, which may take as many as three races spread out over several days. All competitors start in heats that are not seeded; typically the top three finishers (determined by the number of entries) in each heat go directly to the semi-final. The others get a second chance to progress to the semi-final from the *repêchage*. The semi-finals determine who will progress to the final; the best of the rest compete in a petit-final. In ideal flatwater conditions, without wind or current, women can complete the 500 m race in under 1 min 45 s, a feat that requires power and sustained endurance along with precise placement of each stroke.

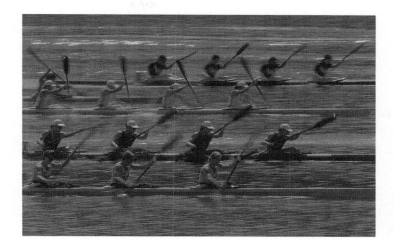

Fig. 40.1 Women's four-person flatwater kayak race, Atlanta 1996. (© Allsport / Pascal Rondeau.)

Whitewater slalom competition at the Olympics takes place in four events. Men compete in C1, C2 and K1, whereas women compete in K1 only. The 1996 Olympic Games in Atlanta were held on a 490-m semi-natural course with strong currents and rapids. There were a total of 25 gates, 19 downstream and 6 upstream, which required the athlete to approach the gate against the current. The athlete's head, shoulder and torso must pass between the gate's poles. Touching a pole results in a 5-s penalty, while missing a gate results in a 50-s penalty added to the elapsed time of the run. Each racer is allowed two runs and the best time, including penalties, is taken. These times typically approximate 2 min. While speed and precision are necessary, there is a much greater skill to conditioning ratio compared with flatwater competitions.

Equipment

Kayaks

The whitewater kayak comes in a multitude of designs, the uniqueness of the design determining its action on the river. In general, the boats are constructed of fibreglass, Kevlar or plastic. Fibreglass is lighter but more susceptible to breakage, whereas plastic is heavier but more durable. Competition boats are typically made of fibreglass or Kevlar. Olympic flatwater kayaks are narrow, enclosed craft that are fast and unstable. They accommodate one, two or four paddlers. They must adhere to the weight, length and width regulations of the ICF (Fig. 40.2). No concave surfaces or surface treatments that improve the hull's wetted surface and therefore speed are allowed. The kayaker sits inside the craft and uses a double-bladed paddle. The person seated in the bow of a team boat or a single kayaker steers the boat with a foot-controlled rudder.

A spray skirt is used to prevent water from entering a kayak; in team boats it is used to prevent the spray of paddlers from entering the boat. In a head wind, a skirt streamlines the boat to prevent wind from entering and slowing it down. The skirt can also trap body heat in the boat and can be used during warm-up and later removed for the race. In 1936, offset paddle blades were introduced. Perhaps the biggest revolution in design since has been the invention of the wing paddle by Stefan Lindeburg, former coach of the Swedish national canoe and kayak team. In the mid-1980s this change in blade configuration, and a change in paddle shaft composition from wood to the harder but lighter

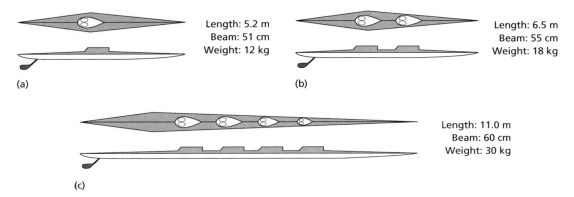

Length: 5.2 m
Beam: 51 cm
Weight: 12 kg

(a)

Length: 6.5 m
Beam: 55 cm
Weight: 18 kg

(b)

Length: 11.0 m
Beam: 60 cm
Weight: 30 kg

(c)

Fig. 40.2 Olympic kayaks: (a) K1, (b) K2 and (c) K4 kayaks.

carbon fibre, altered stroke paddling technique significantly.

Canoes

The canoe, on the other hand, is rudderless and open-topped, making it particularly vulnerable to wind and water. It is built from a wide variety of materials, including fibre-reinforced plastic, wood and aluminium. As with the kayak, the longer the canoe at the waterline, the faster it will go. Traditional canoes are made for one or two people to paddle on flatwater but can also handle small rapids. The paddlers sit freely and comfortably in these canoes. Whitewater canoeists prefer a canoe that is relatively closed, or 'decked', to minimize water entering the boat in rapids. The paddlers kneel with both knees fixed by straps or a padded brace. The paddle is constructed of varying material depending upon its intended use. The longer the race, the lighter the paddle desired. Marathon paddles have a bent shaft, allowing the blade to be angled up to 15°, which increases power. However, only the power side of the blade can be used. Whitewater paddles have a handle grip that is easy to control and a wide blade that is protected at its tip.

Safety equipment

Safety dictates the use of two other important pieces of equipment. The personal flotation device (PFD), commonly called a life-jacket, is self-descriptive. In addition to providing flotation, its insulation properties help prevent hypothermia. It also makes an excellent improvised splint and can be used effectively to aid in relocating a dislocated shoulder. Helmets should be worn by all whitewater canoeists and kayakers. Surveys have shown that head trauma after capsizing comprises >15% of all kayaking accidents (Kizer, 1987). Proper clothing is an important protective factor and is dictated by the environment.

Technique

Participation in kayaking and canoeing has increased significantly in the last couple of decades, both recreationally and competitively. Women are training more often and with greater intensity so that it is important to address the mechanics of paddling. Studies indicate that intense high-volume on-water training, less-than-optimal mechanics of the paddling stroke and dry-land maximum strength training are the precipitating factors in paddling injuries (Pelham *et al.*, 1995).

The mechanics in canoeing and kayaking are mutually exclusive. In kayaking, the athlete has a double-bladed paddle and strokes on both sides of the kayak. Traditionally, it has been taught that the paddler should put her paddle in the water and pull her body and boat past the blade rather than pull the paddle through the water past her body. Proper technique minimizes slip, the backwards movement of the blade in the water. Using good body rotation from the hips to the shoulders is crucial, because it allows effective use of the large muscle groups of the shoulders, back and legs. This rotation ensures that the paddle remains vertical longer and is closely linked to good balance. At the catch, the entire blade should be pushed into the water vertically, as close to the side of the boat as possible. About 25% of the force on the paddle is derived from the top arm (non-control arm) pushing on the shaft, while the other 75% of the force is derived from the bottom arm (control arm) pulling on the shaft. It is important to relax the grip of the non-control hand as the paddle moves forward, allowing the paddle shaft to rotate through this hand. It is best to achieve maximum power as soon as possible in the stroke and to maintain that power evenly throughout the stroke. The power is then transferred to the boat via the legs to the feet, which are placed close together on the footrest just touching the rudder. The knees should be drawn up towards the chest, enough to facilitate hip and torso rotation and alternate extension of the knees during the stroke.

It becomes difficult to adhere to proper technique when paddling on rivers because of the challenges of water hydraulics and obstacles. The low and high brace are useful techniques for maintaining an upright boat. A low brace is used when there is a slight loss of stability. Force is applied to the back side of the paddle with elbows kept close to the trunk. The power side of the blade is used in a high brace to recover from more extreme instability of the boat (Fig. 40.3). Improper technique places the hands above the shoulders with the arms in abduction and external rotation. In this position, too much opposing force results in injuries to the shoulder, such as anterior dislocation and traumatic impingement. It is important to keep the arms close to the trunk and the elbows below shoulder height.

The Duffek stroke (named after Milo Duffek) is an advanced technique ideal for entering and exiting eddies. Key points for proper technique are never to place the blade behind the body, properly rotate the trunk to minimize stress to the shoulders and use the upper hand as a pivot

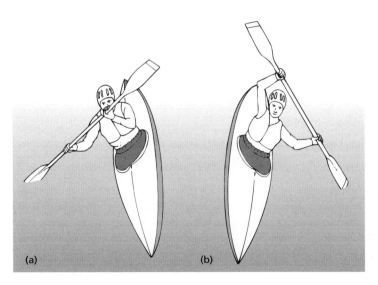

Fig. 40.3 High brace technique: (a) correct and (b) incorrect technique.

(a)   (b)

in front of the forehead. When a boat capsizes it is necessary to return it to its upright position and this is most commonly achieved using the eskimo roll. To increase the paddler's confidence and prevent injury, proper instruction and individual practice of this manoeuvre is necessary until it becomes automatic.

The conoeist has a paddle with one blade that she strokes on her preferred side. Power is generated as the torso rotates and pulls the blade in a vertical position with the arms and shoulders.

Orthopaedic injuries

Traumatic injuries, overuse injuries and various other medical problems result from the physical demands of the paddling sports and the adversity of the environment in which they take place. Improper stroke mechanics and repeated overloading of the musculotendinous unit leads to the common medical problem of overuse. Combined with this is fatigue, which can negatively alter the biomechanics and create an imbalance towards inappropriately applied muscular forces. It must be remembered that nearly half of all injuries occur out of water as a result of dryland training, scouting, and entering or exiting a body of water. Flatwater racers tend to experience proportionately more overuse injuries, whereas whitewater paddlers are exposed to obstacles and technical manoeuvres that place them at risk for traumatic injuries. Orthopaedic injuries are categorized in Table 40.1; diagnosis and complications of orthopaedic injuries are discussed in greater detail in Chapter 15.

Shoulder impingement

The shoulder is considered the most mobile joint in the body and also the most vulnerable to injury and overuse. During shoulder motion, stability of the glenohumeral joint is provided by both dynamic and static components. The rotator cuff muscles, besides allowing for abduction and internal and external rotation, provide the main dynamic stability for positioning the humerus within the glenoid fossa. Capsuloligamentous

Table 40.1 Common musculoskeletal injuries in canoeists and kayakers

Site	Injury
Shoulder	Impingement syndrome, bicipital tendinitis, glenohumeral dislocations/subluxations
Forearm	Tenosynovitis of wrist extensor tendons, flexor tendonitis, carpal tunnel syndrome, forearm compartment syndrome, **medial and lateral epicondylitis of the elbow**
Back	Thoracic and lumbar muscle strains, lumbar disc herniation
Pelvic	Ischial bursitis, hamstring tendonitis, sciatic nerve compression
Miscellaneous	Ankle sprains/fractures, prepatellar bursitis, contusions, finger dislocations

structures afford static stability. Together they prevent anterior migration of the head of the humerus against the acromion process and coracoacromial ligament, which would otherwise cause impingement. Normal functioning of the scapulothoracic stabilizers is essential for the synchrony of scapulohumeral motion.

Optimum strength is essential for the power phase of the flatwater stroke and also during slalom strokes, which demand rapid force production as well as rapid changes in direction of the forces centred in the shoulder joint (Heinrichs, 1991). However, women have relatively weaker shoulder girdle muscles than men and are rarely encouraged to strengthen their upper body musculature (Arendt, 1996). There is also speculation that the cyclical effects of women's hormones on soft tissues may contribute to joint laxity. These factors predispose women to more frequent shoulder injuries than experienced by men.

The most common overuse injury is impingement syndrome, irritation of the rotator cuff muscles and their surrounding soft tissues. The combination of hypovascularity, fatigue, poor stroke mechanics and the progressive instability of a hypermobile joint results in impingement. Chronic inflammation can lead to fibrosis. However, rotator cuff degeneration and tear are rare in this athletic population (Berglund & McKenzie, 1994). Any extremes in internal and external rotation of the arm can lead to frictional irritation of the proximal biceps tendon on the wall of the bicipital groove, resulting in biceps tendonitis.

There are particular positions of the arms during strokes and manoeuvres that place the shoulder in forward flexion, abduction and internal rotation, resulting in repetitive impingement of the soft tissues. The following are a few examples of such strokes: (i) maintaining a high (upper) pivot arm in the canoe paddler (Pelham *et al.*, 1995); (ii) during the recovery phase of the kayak stroke, a high pivot point is also attained; and (iii) during the Duffek stroke, particularly when the body is far from the plant of the blade (Walsh, 1989).

TREATMENT

Modalities, medication and rest can reduce the symptoms. However, specific rehabilitation exercises are most beneficial in returning the athlete to the water. Strengthening and stabilization exercises should be focused on the rotator cuff muscles and parascapular muscles (Kenal & Knapp, 1996). Relative rest with evaluation and elimination of poor biomechanical techniques or modifications to equipment are important in reducing the overload to vulnerable structures. If pain is not recalcitrant, relative rest can be achieved by stroke modification and decreased stroke intensity. The canoe paddler can pull the elbow in slightly to increase relative external shoulder rotation. The kayaker can paddle in base position. Both reduce forward reach. The slalom athlete can train on flatwater gates to reduce force overload. A faulty posture (forward head, slumped shoulders, reduced trunk and hamstring flexibility) that compromises shoulder mechanics must be identified and corrected. Recommendations to canoe paddlers include

angling the T-grip of the paddle and raising the seat.

PREVENTION

Prevention of these injuries needs to address the most common causes. Paddling requires a precise blend of power and endurance and therefore weight-lifting is an integral part of the paddler's overall training programme. However, those programmes that encourage maximal strength training and the use of exercises which place the shoulder in risky positions result in a disproportionate number of shoulder injuries, much to the frustration of athlete, coach and physician. Weight-lifting manoeuvres that produce forced abduction, extension and external rotation, such as military press, flys and behind-the-neck pulldown, should be avoided. Other aggravating manoeuvres are the bench press and dips. In general, paddlers should be instructed to keep their elbows in the plane of their body or anterior to their body during any weight-lifting exercise (Gross *et al.*, 1993). The conditioning programme should also incorporate exercises that allow for the development of adequate muscular and joint flexibility. This is necessary for the athlete's joints to withstand the forces applied by the water on the paddle and boat.

Shoulder dislocations

Anterior shoulder dislocations and subluxations are the most common and disabling shoulder injury in the whitewater slalom athlete. Recurrent episodes can lead to permanent laxity, which may require surgical intervention for further participation. The shoulder is in its most susceptible position when the hand and elbow are above and behind the shoulder. The downward force of the paddle against the upward force of the current pushes the arm beyond the stabilizing limits of the capsule and ligaments surrounding the glenohumeral joint. The increased force ultimately levers the humeral head out of the glenoid fossa. When the arm is abducted to less than shoulder height, the larger, stronger muscles maintain joint stability. However, as the arm is abducted and externally rotated above shoulder height, where only a few weaker muscles are supportive, the shoulder becomes more vulnerable to dislocation. These type of injuries can occur during the following manoeuvres:

• the high brace, used to prevent the boat rolling (not commonly used by the canoe paddler because mechanical advantage is gained as seat height increases);
• the Duffek stroke, used for negotiating holes and gates;
• the roll, used to right a capsized boat;
• accidentally striking a rock with the paddle (often while attempting a roll).

TREATMENT

The on-scene reduction of shoulder dislocation is controversial. However, immediate relief of pain, curtailment of ongoing injury and subsequent ability to function more actively during evacuation are strong reasons favouring it (Weiss, 1995). Several techniques have been advocated for reduction (Reibel & McCabe, 1991). Regardless of technique, the key element is rapid initiation, as delayed reduction may become complicated by

pain and involuntary muscle spasm. Most techniques require a flat and comfortable area upon which to place the injured paddler in the supine or prone position. This can be difficult to find in river and wilderness settings and therefore reduction with the paddler standing should be considered (Weiss, 1995). As soon as the diagnosis is made, the paddler bends forward at the waist while the rescuer grips the wrist and applies steady downward traction and external rotation. While maintaining traction, the rescuer can slowly forward flex the arm until reduction is obtained (Fig. 40.4a). If two rescuers are available, scapular manipulation may be performed simultaneously, augmenting reduction (Fig. 40.4b). Another method uses the injured paddler's PFD to allow one rescuer to apply both controlled traction and countertraction (Dutkly, 1988) (Fig. 40.5). One should always monitor circulation and motor–sensory function to the wrist and hand before and after attempting shoulder reduction. The paddler's arm should then be immobilized across the chest with a sling or swath or by safety-pinning the sleeve of the arm across the chest. If the paddler is in a remote area and further paddling is necessary, the shoulder can be partially stabilized by wrapping an elastic or neoprene covering around the torso and

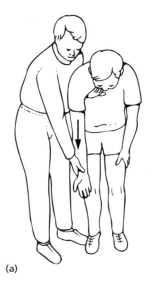

(a)

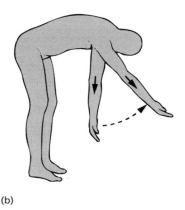

(b)

Fig. 40.4 (a) The rescuer supports the victim's chest with one hand and pulls the externally rotated arm down and forward with the other hand. (b) If two rescuers are available, scapular rotation to assist shoulder relocation can be performed by one rescuer, while the second rescuer pulls the arm down and forward. The inferior tip of the scapula is pushed medially.

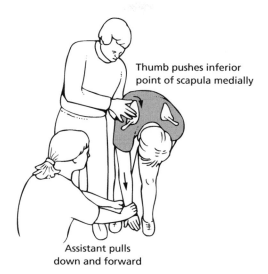

Thumb pushes inferior
point of scapula medially

Assistant pulls
down and forward

Fig. 40.5 Using a life-jacket to assist in countertraction for shoulder relocation with the injured paddler's arm at 90° flexion.

involved arm to limit abduction and external rotation.

Rehabilitation programmes should focus on muscles that reinforce the anterior shoulder (anterior deltoid, subscapularis, pectoralis major), as the most common dislocation is directed anteriorly. The rotator cuff muscles also need to be strong in order to execute effectively the various manoeuvres used in paddling, such as the sudden burst of power needed at the start of a K1 sprint, turning a canoe or kayak to avoid an obstacle, or to enter or exit a racing gate. Rehabilitation exercises are similar to those used for shoulder impingement. Taping methods used by physical therapists may help decrease pain during humeral elevation by facilitating normal scapular positioning and stability while other strengthening and stability problems are addressed (Host, 1995). Those paddlers who have strengthened their shoulder muscles using a vigorous rehabilitation programme are less likely to dislocate again. However, those individuals who conduct recovery exercises with less enthusiasm or return too early tend to experience further problems.

PREVENTION

A conscious effort must be made to alter slalom and whitewater techniques to avoid vulnerability. This is key to prevention. The paddler should stay within their attained level of whitewater experience and only increase the degree of difficulty after the basic manoeuvres have been mastered. Body weight should be centred over the boat by lifting the upstream hip (pulling the boat's upstream edge out of the water) without leaning the torso downstream. The preferred method of bracing is the low brace, in which the arm is held in internal rotation and close to the body. It is an inherently stronger and more versatile manoeuvre. The high brace is an extremely effective stroke, and the risk of dislocation can be reduced by keeping the hands in front of the plane of the shoulders and absorbing the shock of the force of the water with the muscles not the ligaments. If a vulnerably placed brace cannot be avoided, the torso should be quickly rotated to face the shaft of the paddle squarely. During the roll or the high brace the arm should be held close to the trunk or chest wall, thereby diminishing the torque applied to the glenohumeral joint. The forearm should be kept below the level of the forehead when performing the Duffek manoeuvre. Remember particularly that fatigue greatly diminishes concentration and muscle strength.

Wrist and forearm injuries

Power in the stroke is generated most effectively using the stronger muscles of the hip, back and shoulders. This power is transferred to the paddle through the forearm, wrist and hand, which tend to have weaker muscles. Since a key principle of efficient paddling is to keep the blade vertical for as long as possible during the stroke, hip and torso rotation are crucial to proper stroke mechanics.

Paddlers frequently suffer overuse injuries to the wrist and forearm with initiation of on-water training, during high workloads and in conditions of wind and waves. Any deviation of the angle of the wrist during the pull causes inefficient transfer of power to the stroke and puts undue strain on the elbow, forearm muscles and wrist tendons. Aggressive gripping of the paddle to control the boat and maintain proper technique during adverse environmental conditions can also be a source of injury. New technologies in design and materials, such as offset paddles, wing configuration of the blade, carbon-fibre shafts and lighter, less stable flatwater boats, have significantly altered stroke mechanics. With each change, paddlers may experience the onset of new overuse problems that tend to resolve as they become accustomed to the change.

The control hand of the kayak paddler is most commonly affected, as the wrist extensors of this hand are subject to more use. This leads to tenosynovitis of the extensor tendons, the most frequently reported injury. In turn, stresses can be transferred to the lateral elbow, resulting in epicondylitis. Excessive pronation–extension during the crossover phase of the kayak stroke can lead to de Quervain's tenosynovitis, irritation to the extensor tendons proximal to the thumb. Flexor tendonitis is more common in the canoeist who must steer her rudderless boat with her bottom hand. Overuse secondary to aggressive gripping of the paddle is responsible for other forearm injuries. A tight grip of the paddle and repetitive excessive flexion of the wrist can lead to entrapment of the medial nerve of the wrist, causing tingling, numbness, weakness and pain, a condition known as carpal tunnel syndrome. Forearm compartment syndrome can also result from prolonged gripping, the symptoms being very painful, tight, hard flexor compartments, painful resistance of wrist flexion and occasionally numbness in the hand.

TREATMENT

A conservative approach to therapy is useful for most overuse injuries and is directed at decreasing inflammation, stretching, strengthening and relative rest. The wrist can be taped in a neutral position to immobilize excessive flexion and extension. This also serves as a reminder to keep the wrist straight during the pull. Using a looser

grip and a smaller diameter shaft has proved beneficial. On occasion, chronic recurrent injury of the wrist can cause persistent swelling and adhesions of tendons. In such recalcitrant cases a surgical decompression procedure may be necessary.

PREVENTION

Preventive measures are the basis for avoiding these injuries, which can cause an athlete to discontinue training during the period of recovery and treatment. Sound stroke mechanics and appropriately sized equipment are paramount. The seat and footrest in the kayak should be positioned so that the knee bend facilitates torso rotation when reaching forward in the stroke. Too much bend limits hip rotation, a crucial part of body rotation. Proper overall body rotation is important even when the stroke rate is faster, as in team boats and during starts. Generally, the higher the seat, the more leverage and the stronger the catch on the water. However, the lower the seat, the more stable the boat. Beginners should start with a lower seat in order to master technique and gain balance, and then gradually raise the seat over time. A paddle constructed with a 75–80° offset instead of the traditional 90° can reduce wrist stress. Efforts should be directed at holding the wrist in a neutral position and avoiding excessive crossover. Flatwater paddlers should maintain a loose grip during the entire stroke, particularly the pull. Slalom kayakers should relax the grip whenever possible. For stability in the wind and waves, the paddle arc should be lower and wider and air time kept to a minimum.

Back injuries

The power of every stroke is generated by the muscles of the back. In the lower back, they are used as stabilizers in the sitting position. The potential for injury to this area becomes compounded when prolonged sitting with legs extended and minimal back support leads to muscle fatigue and stretched ligaments. A strain of the lumbar myofacial tissue can occur with the repeated flexion and rotation inherent in the mechanics of paddling. It can also occur abruptly with an unexpected torsional force, i.e. performing a brace technique that is countered by the force of the water or an immobile object such as a boulder. Lifting unbalanced water-laden boats and loading boats on to automobiles can also lead to injuries. Lower back pain is most common during heavy training and is a ubiquitous complaint among paddlers older than 25 years of age (Burrell & Burrell, 1982).

Strains to the muscles of the upper back (trapezius and rhomboid muscles) can usually be treated conservatively with stretching to shorten their course of healing. However, low back pain tends to be more chronic in nature. Back pain accompanied by pain radiating to the leg or foot, weakness, numbness or tingling of the leg or foot or, rarely, bowel or bladder dysfunction suggests disc herniation or rupture.

Fractures of the spine have been reported in whitewater kayakers and canoeists (Weiss, 1995). Cervical spine injuries have occurred in kayakers in conjunction with head trauma sustained after flipping upside-down. Compression fractures of the thoracolumbar spine have occurred from axial loading when a kayaker landed flat after paddling over a waterfall. Immediate recognition of these types of injuries and prompt on-site immobilization (minicell blocks from kayaks can be used) until a backboard can be obtained is paramount.

TREATMENT

Initial low back trouble is associated with poor isometric trunk muscle endurance and a hypermobile lumbar spine. Recurrent low back pain is associated with poor hamstring and back flexibility and weak trunk muscles (Biering-Sorensen, 1984). Therefore, stabilization and endurance training are necessary in paddlers when back pain is present. Lumbar spine hypermobilities should be stabilized and the trunk strengthened isometrically to promote strength while promoting stability (Kenal & Knapp, 1996).

Exercises involving isometric cocontraction of lower back muscles (multifidus muscles) and abdominal muscles (particularly transversus abdominis) while maintaining the spine in a static neutral position should help re-educate the stabilizing role of these muscles (Richardson & Jull, 1995). These can be performed in various positions (sitting, standing, quadruped) and monitored with the help of a physical therapist. Ultimately, the athlete should be able to hold a cocontraction of the deep muscles during dynamic functional movements of the trunk.

Abdominal exercises include partial sit-ups and single and double leg-lifts. Hamstring and hip flexor tightness result from prolonged sitting. Hamstring tightness leads to excessive posterior tilt of the pelvis and lengthening of the lumbar muscles, whereas tight hip flexor muscles promote an anterior pelvic tilt and therefore may cause excessive loading on the facet joints of the lumbar spine. Appropriate stretching exercises are warranted.

Surgery is sometimes required for those with a herniated or ruptured disc who do not respond to a long trial of conservative therapy. Experience has shown that athletes may return to full activity following surgery and a prolonged rehabilitation period (Walsh, 1985).

PREVENTION

A consistent programme of stretching specific muscle groups before paddling is key to avoiding these injuries. During extended paddling trips, which lead to fatigue of the paravertebral muscles, periodic breaks to stretch are recommended.

Pelvic injuries

Prolonged sitting and rotational movements in the kayak or canoe can lead to a variety of injuries, such as hamstring tendonitis at the insertion on the ischial tuberosity and ischial bursitis. Both are prevented and managed by proper padding. Sacral furunculosis can be a troublesome lesion. Preventive measures include meticulous attention to hygiene as well as washing and drying all padding before it is used again. Topical, or occasionally oral, antibiotics may be necessary. Compression of the sciatic nerve in the buttock with numbness to the foot is a chronic complaint that can be relieved by moving the position of the seat slightly, using appropriate 'doughnut' padding, or placing a hole in the seat where the compression occurs.

Miscellaneous injuries

The feet and ankles are frequently injured when walking along the banks of a river while attempting to put the boat in, take the boat out or portage around a rapid. Ankle strains can be treated immediately by putting the ankle in cold water, compressing it with an Ace Wrap and elevating it whenever possible. An easy exercise to perform is to write the alphabet (capital letters) in the air using the foot in a pain-free range without moving the leg. Fractured ankles may result from forced dorsiflexion when the bow of the kayak hits an obstruction head-on and the kayaker's heels are pushed under the horizontal toe brace.

Inflammation of the prepatellar bursa occurs very often among paddlers who kneel. Appropriate padding or alternating the side of kneeling can be preventive. Strict hygiene practices must be undertaken to avoid infection of the bursa.

Medical concerns (Table 40.2)

Head

Head and facial trauma is more common in whitewater kayakers and canoeists because of the potential for flipping upside-down while still in the craft. Trauma to these areas can be minimized by wearing a protective helmet and tucking forward instead of leaning backward while rolling.

Frequent exposure of the nasal passages to sudden pressure and temperature changes, including the 'nasal enemas' associated with flipping kayaks, can lead to rhinitis. If an athlete is prone to this, then the best treatment is avoid-

Table 40.2 Common medical problems in canoeists and kayakers

Site	Problem
Head	Concussion, exostosis of the ear canal, rhinitis, ocular trauma
Skin	Hand blisters, finger/heel calluses, sunburn, infections, lacerations
Miscellaneous	Hypothermia, hyperthermia, pregnancy, gastrointestinal infections, entrapments

ance by using nose clips. Decongestant nasal sprays are very effective but must be limited to short-term use of less than 5 days. These can be used prior to an exposure or immediately after exiting the water and then again 15 min later. Rinsing the nose with a saline solution helps to remove contaminants and soothe nasal membranes. Alternatively, steroid nasal sprays can be used.

Chronic recurrent exposure to cold water can lead to reactive changes in the external ear canal producing exostoses. These can impede hearing and hinder clearance of water and foreign particles from the canal. Ear plugs may be the necessary preventive measure.

Skin

Blisters and calluses on the hands are frequently reported in paddlers. Kayakers develop them at the metacarpophalangeal joint of the thumb, whereas canoeists are more likely to have them on the proximal palmar surfaces of the metacarpophalangeal joints. Taping and moleskin application reduce the incidence of this potentially incapacitating problem. Proper padding prevents formation of blisters and calluses on the dorsum of the foot caused by strap friction.

Sunburn is a common problem, overexposure to the sun being the accepted reason for the increasing incidence of skin cancers. Care should be taken to apply an adequate sun protectant factor sun lotion, with repeated applications for prolonged exposures or frequent water exposures.

Miscellaneous

Élite paddlers are now training throughout the year and environmental concerns become problematic when paddlers are exposed to temperature extremes. Immersion in cold water can precipitate two adverse reactions. First, sudden cold water immersion produces profound cardiovascular and respiratory responses. There is a marked increase in blood pressure and heart rate, resulting in lethal dysrhythmias (Keatinge & Hayward, 1981). An immediate and involuntary gasp occurs that results in aspiration of water and laryngospasm, followed by hyperventilation. These responses increase the risk of drowning in rough water.

Second, rapid cooling of the muscles and nerves in the extremities can result in loss of strength and coordination. This preclinical hypothermia impairs the ability to swim, maintain freeboard, avoid obstacles, climb from the river and use appropriate judgement (Keatinge, 1969). Even when the air temperature is warm, paddlers negotiating cold rivers should wear sufficient insulation (splash cover and wet suit) and a PFD and ensure that their boats have enough buoyant support (Berglund & McKenzie, 1994). For flatwater paddlers, a good method of prevention is to teach them that there is just as much good water close to the shore as in the middle of the lake.

Excessive exposure to a hot environment coupled with dehydration can lead to hyperthermic injuries such as heat exhaustion or heat stroke. Adequate hydration and cooling measures should be practised.

The gastrointestinal tract can be exposed to an assortment of aquatic-related infections. In the USA, *Giardia lamblia* has been found to be the most common pathogenic intestinal parasite. Even the most pristine mountain rivers have been contaminated by infected animals that defecate in or near the water. Foreign wilderness travel expands the scope of potential contaminants, and infections of schistosomiasis and pulmonary blastomycosis have been reported. Simple preventive measures, such as drinking only treated water and being aware of local endemic diseases and prophylactic measures, are recommended.

The difficulty of a river generally increases with the volume of flow and the average gradient. An increase in the speed and power of the water make rapids more difficult, although on occasion this can actually make them easier. Serious injuries and drowning can occur with entrapments, such as when kayaks become broached (wrapped sideways around an obstacle such as a boulder) or vertically pinned (when a kayak plunges over a drop and the end of the boat becomes trapped between rocks beneath the surface). In both these situations the plastic kayak can fold over on itself, trapping the occupant upside-down beneath the surface. The potential for entrapment can also occur when swimmers attempt to stand up and walk in swift-moving currents: feet can become wedged between rocks beneath the surface. Swimmers and boaters can also become trapped in strainers, obstacles such as fallen trees or driftwood lodged between rocks or jutting out from the shore. Paddlers should always be accompanied by another boater and be knowledgeable about the appropriate negotiation of obstacles and rescue techniques.

Paddle sports can continue to be a fun and rewarding experience during pregnancy. Women pursuing flatwater training and racing, which has minimal potential for trauma, should follow the guidelines addressed in Chapter 14. However, there are a few specific recommendations for whitewater canoeing and kayaking. The individual should acknowledge her limitations and the level of activity should be well within these in order to avoid trauma. She should also realize that by the third trimester an enlarged abdomen will alter her centre of gravity and therefore her balance. She should always wear a PFD and when the abdomen is larger than the chest a crotch strap should be worn.

Recommendations for future research

Research should be directed at developing the most appropriate dry-land strengthening programme for both preseason and in-season training. This programme should focus on strengthening the female paddler's shoulder muscles as a preventive measure against potential injuries. Development camps organized by the national governing body of each country should be promoted to allow the introduction of more women into the paddling sports. Finally, the ICF needs to develop gender equity within international competition.

Acknowledgements

Appreciation is extended to Buck Tilton, Director of the Wilderness Medical Institute in Pitkin, Colorado and to the United States Canoe and Kayak Team for their valuable information.

References

Arendt, E. (1996) Common musculoskeletal injuries in women. *Physician and Sportsmedicine* 24, 39–48.

Berglund, B. & McKenzie, D. (1994) Injuries in canoeing and kayaking. In P.A.F.H. Renstrom (ed.) *Clinical Practice of Sports Injury, Prevention and Care. Encyclopaedia of Sports Medicine*, Vol. 5, pp. 633–640. Blackwell Scientific Publications, Oxford.

Biering-Sorensen, F. (1984) Physical measurements as risk indicators for low-back trouble over a one-year period. *Spine* 9, 106–119.

Burrell, C.L. & Burrell, R. (1982) Injuries in whitewater paddling. *Physician and Sportsmedicine* 10, 119–124.

Dutkly, P. (1988) A simple method of treating shoulder dislocations for the whitewater enthusiast. *Wilderness Medicine* 5, 9–13.

Gross, M.L., Brenner, S.L., Esformes, I. & Sonzogni, J.J. (1993) Anterior shoulder instability in weight lifters. *American Journal of Sports Medicine* 21, 599–603.

Heinrichs, K.I. (1991) Shoulder anatomy, biomechanics and rehabilitation considerations for the whitewater slalom athlete: Part 1. *National Strength and Conditioning Association Journal* 13, 26–35.

Host, H.H. (1995) Scapular taping in the treatment of anterior shoulder impingement. *Physical Therapy* 75, 803–812.

Keatinge, W.R. (1969) Sudden failure of swimming in cold water. *British Medical Journal* 1, 480–486.

Keatinge, W.R. & Hayward, M.G. (1981) Sudden death in cold water and ventricular arrhythmia. *Journal of Forensic Science* 16, 459–463.

Kenal, K.A.F. & Knapp, L.D. (1996) Rehabilitation of injuries in competitive swimmers. *Sports Medicine* 22, 337–347.

Kizer, K.W. (1987) Medical aspects of white-water kayaking. *Physician and Sportsmedicine* 15, 128–137.

Pelham, T.W., Holt, L.E. & Stalker, R.E. (1995) The etiology of paddler's shoulder. *Australian Journal of Science and Medicine in Sports* 27, 43–47.

Reibel, G.D. & McCabe, J. (1991) Anterior shoulder dislocation: a review of reduction techniques. *American Journal of Emergency Medicine* 9, 180–185.

Richardson, C.A. & Jull, G.A. (1995) Muscle control–pain control. What exercises would you prescribe? *Manual Therapy* 1, 2–10.

Walsh, M. (1985) Preventing injury in competitive canoeists. *Physician and Sportsmedicine* 13, 120–128.

Walsh, M. (1989) Sports medicine for paddlers: the cause, care and treatment of paddler's injuries. *Canoe* 80, 36–38.

Weiss, E.A. (1995) White-water medicine and rescue. In P. Auerbach (ed.) *Wilderness Medicine*, pp. 1234–1250. Mosby, Boston.

Chapter 41

Alpine Skiing

ROSEMARY AGOSTINI

Introduction

Just over 90 years ago, the first organized alpine (downhill) ski competition was held in Kitzbühel, Austria for men. Thirty years later, women made their first appearance in downhill competition at the 1935 World Cup races, followed the next year by the Winter Olympics at Garmisch-Partenkirchen, Bavaria (Wallechinsky, 1993). Today, women's skiing is growing rapidly. In the last 4 years alone, there has been a 104% increase in the number of women competing in ski programmes at National Collegiate Athletic Association (NCAA) Division I colleges in the USA (Anon., 1997). As for recreational skiing, marketing data from sports equipment manufacturers show that 42.1% of the 6–7 million active skiers in the USA are women.

Recognizing a growing demand, the equipment makers have responded. Women's equipment has progressed beyond the 'pretty paint job' it once was. Manufacturers have begun to develop higher-performance, lighter-weight and more versatile skis that fit the specific demands of women. Bindings have been moved slightly forward and the skis have softer, more balanced flexes. Ski boots are being made in smaller sizes, with truer fitting lasts and less-stiff shells.

However, along with the growing participation has come the inevitable injuries. Overall, the incidence of injuries is similar for women and men skiers of comparable skill (Shealy & Ettlinger, 1996), although women appear to have at least twice the rate of knee injuries, especially

of the anterior cruciate ligament (ACL) (Ellman *et al.*, 1989; Shealy & Ettlinger, 1996). The reasons for this increase in knee injuries are not entirely clear, but may relate to a combination of biomechanical and anatomical differences in women as well as contributions from ski equipment (Shealy & Ettlinger, 1996).

Definitions of alpine ski events

An understanding of the risks faced by alpine skiers requires an understanding of the different skiing events. Alpine, or downhill, ski racing consists of four events, which differ in turning radius, speed and length of course (Wallechinsky, 1993; White & Johnson, 1993).

Slalom

Slalom is the shortest of the alpine events and involves weaving between closely set plastic gates on a steep slope. Skiers negotiate these gates by making a series of rapid, short-radius turns in quick succession. The event consists of two runs, each lasting 35–60 s.

Giant slalom

Giant slalom is performed on a longer course but the gates are more widely spaced. Skiers attain moderate speeds and show more fluid progression from gate to gate. The course takes 50–90 s to complete.

Super giant slalom

Super giant slalom is a hybrid of giant slalom and downhill, combining speed and the technical skill of turning. It involves high-speed, short-radius turns on a longer, winding course, with greater distance between the gates. Runs last from 60 to 120 s.

Downhill

Downhill is the longest and fastest of the alpine events. It has a long course that follows the fall line of the mountain, with women skiers achieving speeds of up to 128 km·h^{-1} while negotiating terrain and turns. Runs last approximately 90–140 s.

Freestyle skiing

Freestyle skiing is a recent addition to the Olympics. Not a traditional alpine event, it involves a series of stunts or acrobatics performed on a downhill slope (Wallechinsky, 1993). It consists of several separate events. In mogul skiing, competitors combine 'stunts' and fluidity while skiing on steep, bumpy (mogul) terrain. Aerial skiing involves flips, twists and other acrobatics performed from a ski jump. In ballet skiing, classical ballet moves, such as arabesque, are combined with other dance-like movements on a short, smooth slope. Data on injuries specific to this sport have not yet been published but are likely to be similar to those for other downhill ski events, and potentially include head and neck injuries.

Snowboarding

Snowboarding is another relatively new down-hill sport that is gaining popularity among women. Studies show that the injuries sustained are somewhat different from those in alpine skiing. In snowboarding, impact injuries from falling are seen more commonly than the twisting and bending injuries typical of alpine skiing, with less knee injuries but more arm and wrist

sprains (Shealy, 1993; Bladin & McCrory, 1995; Davidson & Laliotis, 1996). The total injury rate for women is similar to that for downhill skiing (Shealy & Ettlinger, 1996).

Physiology of female skiers

Physiological studies of skiers are being carried out but few focus on gender-specific differences. Studies of body fat composition show that female skiers on the US national alpine team average 13.1% body fat compared with 6.1% in male skiers and 21–29% in non-athletes (White & Johnson, 1993; Gibbs, 1994). In 1980, these body fat values were 20.6% and 10.2% for female and male skiers respectively, showing that lean body mass has increased in these athletes over the past decade.

Skiers tend to have a blend of muscle fibre types, predominantly the slow-twitch type, to meet the high aerobic and anaerobic demands of the sport (Tesch, 1995). Aerobic demands are highest in the longer giant slalom event, although the importance of aerobic power to successful competition in the sport is unclear (White & Johnson, 1993). Anaerobic power appears to contribute about 65% of the energy of alpine skiing and to be a more important determinant of success (White & Johnson, 1993; Bacharach & von Duvillard, 1995).

Alpine skiers demonstrate very high leg strength compared with other athletes, and strength of the leg muscles, particularly the quadriceps and hamstrings, helps predict performance for both men and women (White & Johnson, 1993). In addition, élite female skiers show greater eccentric, but not concentric, knee extensor strength, enabling them to perform the slow, forceful eccentric muscle actions needed during turns in the slalom (Tesch, 1995).

Being a mountain sport, alpine skiing places its participants at altitudes capable of inducing physiological changes. In a recent study by Chapman *et al.* (1998), women were found to respond to hypobaric hypoxia in the same way as men, i.e. increase in red cell mass, haemoglobin level and haematocrit, provided they had sufficient iron available. At altitude, an increase in red cell mass is needed to accommodate the lower amount of oxygen available. If this compensation is inadequate (e.g. as in low iron stores and/or anaemia), it could affect training and performance. Although complete data are not available, preliminary results from European skiers indicate that 20% have low iron stores as reflected by low ferritin levels (mean $11 \pm 5.1\,ng\cdot ml^{-1}$) (N. Meyer, personal communication, 1997). In cross-country skiing, which is more of an endurance sport, 67% of women have been shown to have low iron stores (J. Stray-Gundersen & B.D. Levine, personal communication, 1997).

Incidence of injuries

Estimates for alpine skiing injuries generally lie in the range of two to four serious injuries per 1000 skier-days (Bouter & Knipschild, 1989; Ettlinger et al., 1995). Women have slightly greater rates of injury than men (Ekeland et al., 1993; Shealy, 1993) (Table 41.1). The overall incidence of skiing injuries has declined for both men and women over the past several decades, largely because of improvements in skiing equipment. Most of the decline is in lower extremity injuries, which have decreased from 80% of all injuries in 1960 to 55% in 1980 (Bouter & Knipschild, 1989) and to 40% in 1993 (Ekeland et al., 1993). The pattern of injury in the lower extremity has also changed as there are fewer ankle and foot injuries (45% in 1960 to 10% in 1980) (Bouter & Knipschild, 1989). Fractures of the tibia now account for only 2% of skiing injuries in women,

down from an earlier rate of 25% (Bouter & Knipschild, 1989; Greenwald et al., 1996).

However, while the overall number of lower-leg injuries has declined, the rate of knee injuries has almost tripled since 1972 (Johnson, 1995). Knee injuries now comprise over 40% of all injuries in some studies, with the ACL being most frequently injured (Greenwald et al., 1996). The ACL accounts for 30–50% of all knee injuries (Greenwald et al., 1996) and approximately 15% of all skiing injuries (R.J. Johnson, personal communication, 1997). In fact, skiing ranks as one of the most dangerous activities as regards the ACL, with injury rates near those for American football (Ettlinger et al., 1995) (Table 41.2).

Although men and women have similar rates of injury overall, their rates of knee injury do vary more. Greenwald et al. (1996) surveyed the injuries over a 5-year period at one large Utah ski area and found that the knee accounted for 53% of downhill injuries in women but only 30% in men ($P < 0.0001$) (Table 41.3). In a 2-year nationwide study by Shealy and Ettlinger (1996), knee injuries were twice as common in women skiers as in men (43.5% vs. 22.9%) (Fig. 41.1). On the US skiing team, 85% of the women have torn their ACL compared with 75% of the men (R. Watkins, Medical Coordinator, USA Skiing, personal communication).

The causes of injuries also differ between

Table 41.1 Injury rates for downhill skiing per 1000 skier visits. (Adapted from Shealy, 1993)

	Female	Male
Overall	3.44	2.21
Beginner	9.48	8.38
Intermediate	2.60	2.26
Advanced	0.94	0.88

Table 41.2 Rates of anterior cruciate ligament injury among different activities. (Adapted from Ettlinger et al., 1995)

Activity/study	Rate (per population at risk)
General population	
Miyasaka et al. (1991)	40/100 000 per year
Nielsen & Yde (1991)	30/100 000 per year
American football	
Hewson et al. (1986)	60/100 000 per day
Alpine skiing	
Feagin et al. (1987)	70/100 000 per day
Johnson et al. (1993)	50/100 000 per day
ISSS* (1986)	30/100 000 per day

ISSS (International Society for Skiing Safety) data are unpublished.

males and females. Overall, 70–90% of injuries are due to falls, with 11–20% due to collisions (Bouter & Knipschild, 1989). Impact injuries, resulting from collisions with other skiers or objects or from impact with the snow, are more common in males, as evidenced by their higher percentage of fractures, lacerations and dislocations (Fig. 41.2, Table 41.3). Twisting or bending, resulting in sprains, is a more common mechanism of injury in women (Shealy & Ettlinger, 1996). However, among expert skiers, the rate of impact and trauma injuries is greater regardless of gender (Greenwald *et al.*, 1996).

Fatalities are rare among skiers (0.55 deaths per million skier-days) and even rarer among female skiers (Shealy & Thomas, 1996). Of 329 trauma-related deaths in the USA between 1976 and 1992, only 56 (17.1%) were women. Most deaths resulted from collisions with fixed objects, although a higher proportion of females (particularly preadolescent girls) died from collisions with other skiers, usually being struck by adult males (Shealy & Thomas, 1996).

Risk factors for injury

Risk factors for downhill skiing injury can be divided into several groups, as shown in Table 41.4 (Bouter & Knipschild, 1989). Many of these risk factors are interrelated, making it difficult to isolate the independent contribution of each to an injury, and studies have not defined their relative importance to female compared with male skiers.

Personal characteristics

Children, especially those aged 11–13, and adults over age 40 tend to have a higher rate of injuries. Children have a nine-fold increased risk of leg fractures compared with adult skiers, and a lack

Table 41.3 Type of Alpine ski injuries by gender, 1989–93. (Data from Greenwald *et al.*, 1996)

	Female (%)	Male (%)
Knee	53	30
Upper extremity injury	13	19
Lower extremity fracture	2	3
Upper extremity fracture	5	8
Laceration	3	11
Other	2	6
Miscellaneous trauma	14	18
Miscellaneous medical	6	5

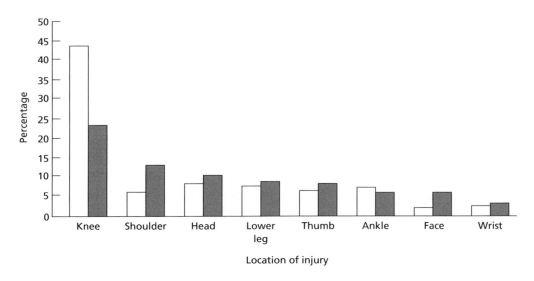

Fig. 41.1 Distribution of ski injuries by gender: women skiers (□) have almost twice the rate of knee injuries as men (■). (Data from Shealy & Ettlinger, 1996.)

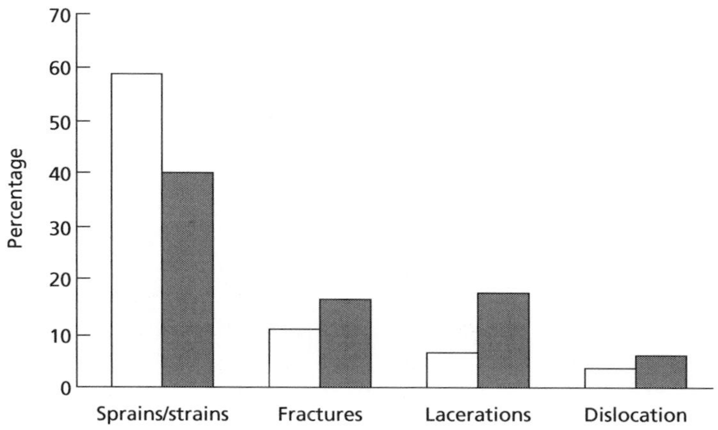

Fig. 41.2 Types of injuries in Alpine skiers by gender: fractures, lacerations and dislocations, often caused by impact injuries, are more common among male skiers (■), whereas strains and sprains (including knee injuries) are 1.5 times more common in women (□). (Data from Shealy & Ettlinger, 1996.)

Table 41.4 Potential risk factors involved in downhill skiing injuries. (Adapted from Bouter & Knipschild, 1989)

Personal characteristics
  Age
  Gender
  Physical conditioning
  Hormonal factors

Skill level
  Ability
  Experience
  Lessons

Equipment
  Bindings/settings
  Boots
  Poles

Behaviour
  Fear
  Risk-taking
  Alcohol
  Nutrition
  Fatigue

Environment
  Snow quality
  Weather conditions
  Difficulty of course
  Time of day
  Altitude

of skill and poorer-quality equipment may be partly responsible (Bouter & Knipschild, 1989; Ekeland *et al.*, 1993).

Good physical conditioning and participation in other sports, despite expectations, do not appear to lower the risk for injury (Bouter & Knipschild, 1989). However, the influence of conditioning may be confounded by increased risk-taking among better-conditioned skiers. Common belief holds that injuries tend to occur more often when skiers are fatigued, usually on their 'last run of the day'. However, epidemiological data are not available to support this view. Nevertheless, the glycogen depletion that occurs in muscle fibres after a day of skiing, plus the additive effects of several days' skiing, may predispose to fatigue and injury. A diet that includes complex carbohydrates may help to maintain glycogen levels and is recommended during skiing trips (Gibbs, 1994; Steadman & Scheinberg, 1995). The higher altitudes of ski slopes may predispose skiers to relative hypoxia before they become acclimatized, compounding the fatigue and risk of injury (Greenwald *et al.*, 1996).

Level of skill and training

Beginners have a considerably greater risk of injury, up to 10-fold higher than that of advanced skiers (see Table 41.1) (Shealy, 1993). Experience or the number of seasons skied appears to relate inversely to the risk of injury, even after skill level (beginner, intermediate, expert) is allowed for in calculations (Fig. 41.3) (Bouter & Knipschild, 1989; Ekeland *et al.*, 1993). Skiing lessons also

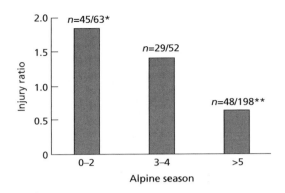

Fig. 41.3 Ratio of lower extremity equipment-related injuries as a function of skiing experience. *n*, number of injured/uninjured skiers; *, $P < 0.01$; **, $P < 0.02$. (From Ekeland *et al.*, 1993 with permission.)

appear to help lower the risk of injury (Ekeland *et al.*, 1993), although some studies dispute this finding (Shealy, 1993).

Equipment

Improvements in equipment, such as release bindings and ski boots, have helped reduce the overall rate of leg injuries by 60% since the 1970s (Johnson *et al.*, 1980). However, despite this reduction, equipment-related injuries still account for approximately 20% of all injuries and 90% of injuries to the lower extremity (R.J. Johnson, personal communication, 1997). These injuries also tend to be severe (Ekeland *et al.*, 1993). In a study of recreational skiers, Ekeland *et al.* (1993) found that 33% of lower extremity, equipment-related injuries required hospitalization, with most of these (60%) involving the knee.

Modern ski equipment, while helping to reduce the number of ankle and tibial injuries, has not reduced risk to the knee. High, stiff ski boots, which rigidly fix the ankle and lower leg, and a new style of ski that carves the snow much more responsively than older models translate forces from the lower leg to the knee. This stress can be compounded by the use of high settings on release bindings (Johnson, 1995).

Failure of bindings to release during falls or stress is a common mechanism of injury (Bouter *et al.*, 1989). Nevertheless, many skiers adjust their release bindings higher than the recommended setting to prevent premature release, especially during racing (Johnson, 1995). Binding adjustments have been shown to average 85% above the recommended settings in individuals who sustain knee injuries and 150% above the recommended settings in individuals who sustain fractures of the tibia (Bouter *et al.*, 1989). For women, the practice of 'cranking down' the binding adjustments may be especially problematic. Some women racers set their release bindings at levels similar to those used by male racers even though the males tend to be 30–45 kg heavier. This setting substantially increases the torsion sustained by the female knee before the ski releases. Release bindings are thus a key focus of injury research.

Types and mechanisms of injury

Knee injuries

Although improvements in ski equipment have resulted in a dramatic decline in lower extremity injuries since the 1950s, knee injuries still account for a significant number of all injuries. Knee injuries result primarily from the twisting and bending of the leg associated with falls (Ekeland *et al.*, 1993), although the stresses associated with competitive ski racing also can induce knee damage without falls (Ellman *et al.*, 1989; Johnson, 1995). Most resulting injuries involve the knee ligaments.

ANTERIOR CRUCIATE LIGAMENT

The ACL is the most common site of knee injury, accounting for 60% of knee injuries in skiers (Steadman & Sterett, 1995). Four common mechanisms of ACL injury are seen in skiers, and these differ from those seen in other sports. The first three mechanisms are common among recreational skiers, whereas the fourth usually occurs in competitive skiers.

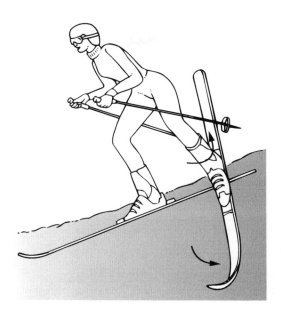

Fig. 41.4 Hyperextension, external rotation and valgus stress on the knee, leading to possible damage to the anterior cruciate ligament and other ligament injury. (Adapted from Steadman & Scheinberg, 1994.)

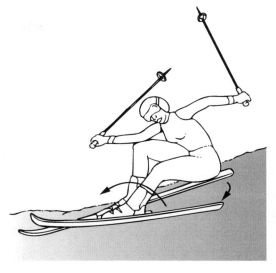

Fig. 41.5 Phantom foot. An internal rotation injury, without hyperextension, occurs when the ski curves inward on its inside edge while a skier falls back or is sliding after a fall. The tail of the ski acts as a lever to twist the foot and lower leg inward, opposite to the natural direction of the foot in this position. (Adapted from Steadman & Scheinberg, 1994.)

1 The first mechanism occurs when the body is moving forward relative to the skis, causing hyperextension of the knee, external rotation of the tibia on the femur and a valgus load to the knee. Such a situation occurs when a skier catches a ski-tip on a gate or in the snow. The torsion across the knee joint leads to possible ACL injury, as well as to injury of the meniscus or medial collateral ligament (Johnson, 1995; Steadman & Sterett, 1995) (Fig. 41.4).

2 The second mechanism involves hyperextension and internal rotation of the knee during a forward fall, such as occurs when a skier crosses the ski-tips or catches the outer edge of the ski in the snow, turning the ski inward.

3 Internal rotation with hyperflexion of the knee may also be seen in association with a backward fall, an injury termed 'phantom foot' (Ettlinger *et al.*, 1995; Steadman & Scheinberg, 1995) (Fig. 41.5). It occurs as the skier falls backward or 'sits down' while the tail of the ski engages the snow with no contact on the front portion. The result is medial rotation of the foot relative to the ski (Ettlinger *et al.*, 1995). This scenario may be the most common mechanism of knee injuries among skiers (R.F. Johnson, personal communication, 1995).

4 The final mechanism of injury, known as boot-induced ACL injury, is seen mostly among competitive skiers. It occurs usually when a skier is landing from a jump, with the skier off balance and leaning backward relative to the skis. The skier instinctively extends the leg and knee in an attempt to recover balance. As the skier lands, the tail of the ski hits first, pushing the top of the boot against the calf, while the skier contracts the quadriceps to hold the leg in rigid extension. When the boot heel hits the snow, the impact drives the boot top forward, pushing the tibia out from under the femur (anterior subluxation) and tearing the ACL (Johnson, 1995; Steadman & Sterett, 1995) (Fig. 41.6).

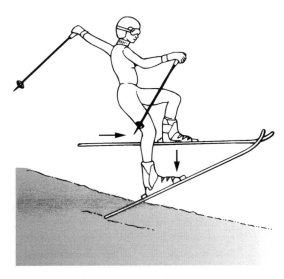

Fig. 41.6 Boot-induced injury to the anterior cruciate ligament. The skier, losing her balance while jumping, attempts to recover balance by extending the leg. On landing, the tail of the ski hits first, pushing the top of the boot against the calf; the skier responds by contracting the quadriceps to hold the leg in extension. As the boot heel strikes, the impact pushes the top of the boot forward and forces the tibia out from under the femur, tearing the anterior cruciate ligament. (Adapted from Steadman & Scheinberg, 1994.)

MEDIAL COLLATERAL LIGAMENT

Injuries to the medial collateral ligament may be the most common knee injury overall but tend to be underreported (Warme et al., 1995). Many minor falls may result in such injuries. These sprains typically result from ski rotation with no binding release or from the boot catching in the snow after binding release. Combined injuries of the anterior and medial collateral ligaments may occur (Duncan et al., 1995; Steadman & Sterett, 1995).

MENISCUS

Isolated tears of the medial or lateral meniscus have been reported in skiers (Steadman & Sterett, 1995).

FACTORS PREDISPOSING TO KNEE INJURIES IN WOMEN

Although the precise reason for the higher rates of knee injury sustained by women remains unknown, several factors have been discussed and are being studied (Arendt, in press; see also Chapter 15). These factors may include:
- imbalance in muscle strength between the quadriceps and hamstring;
- neuromuscular control, including errors in muscle recruitment;
- joint laxity;
- lower extremity alignment;
- pronated foot;
- femoral notch dimension;
- ligament size.

In skiing, it is most likely that an interplay of multiple anatomical and biomechanical factors, combined with extrinsic stresses due to the lever action of the skis and inappropriately set bindings, result in the increased risk of injury.

PROGNOSIS

Despite serious knee injuries, skiers may return to full competitive activity following rehabilitation and, in many cases, fully regain or surpass their world standings before the injury (Ekeland & Vikne, 1995). However, the road to complete rehabilitation can be a long one. An assessment of the psychological reactions to injury shows that social concerns, particularly the loss of fellowship with team members and lack of contact with coaches, are significant sources of stress for injured skiers (D. Gould, unpublished observation). Factors that injured skiers identify as helping to facilitate their recovery include having injured role models for reference, undertaking rehabilitation with others and receiving support from coaches, teammates and friends. Maintaining contact and communication with teammates and coaches helps ease the sense of isolation while waiting for the return to sport. After being cleared to return to skiing, injured skiers often must overcome fear of reinjury, learn technical adjustments to compensate for the previous injury and adapt to initially lower performance expectations (D. Gould, unpublished observation).

PREVENTION

Proposals to reduce the number of knee injuries in skiers have focused on better programmes of muscular conditioning as well as the development of 'smart' ski bindings that sense when dangerous forces are being transmitted to the knee (Johnson, 1995). In one approach, Ettlinger *et al.* (1995) used videotapes to demonstrate the mechanisms of knee injuries and the situations and positions that put the knee at risk, showing these to a population of ski instructors and ski patrol staff. During the 1993–94 winter season, the rate of ACL injuries declined by 62% among trained skiers compared with the rates for the two previous seasons, while there was no decline in a control group. These authors also found that many ACL injuries occurred when skiers 'caught the edge of the ski while sliding' or 'lost control and fought falling'. Among their recommendations to skiers for preventing injury are the following (Ettlinger *et al.*, 1995; Anon., 1996).

• Do not fully straighten the legs when falling; keep the knees flexed.

• Do not try to get up until you have stopped sliding.

• Do not land on your hand; keep the arms up and forward, and do not push off with the hand to recover from a fall.

• Do not jump unless you know where and how to land; land on both skis and keep the knees flexed.

During skiing, 'safe' practice is to keep the arms forward and hands over the skis, keep the skis together with hips above the knees, and maintain balance and control (Anon., 1996). Other safety recommendations include paying attention to weather and snow conditions as well as the boundaries of the ski slope.

Upper extremity injuries

Upper extremity injuries, including sprains and fractures, have increased as lower extremity injuries have declined and now account for about 25% of all injuries (Bouter & Knipschild, 1989; Greenwald *et al.*, 1996).

THUMB

Skier's thumb, a sprain or rupture of the ulnar collateral ligament of the metacarpophalangeal joint of the thumb, may be the most common injury among skiers. It accounts for 7–20% of injuries (Bouter & Knipschild, 1989; Warme *et al.*, 1995). However, because the injury is not immobilizing, it frequently goes unreported. The injury occurs most often during a fall while the hand is grasping the ski pole. As the hand is jammed into the snow, the thumb is forced back into abduction and hyperextension, stressing the ulnar collateral ligament. Alternatively, on the softer snow in the western USA, skier's thumb may occur during a fall when the outstretched hand is jammed into soft snow (Fricker & Hintermann, 1995; Steadman & Scheinberg, 1995).

SHOULDER

Shoulder injuries, including acromioclavicular sprains, dislocations and bruises, are common among skiers but are significantly more frequent and severe among male skiers (Westin *et al.*, 1995; Greenwald *et al.*, 1996). They typically result from impact or collision accidents, which are more common among men (Shealy & Ettlinger, 1996).

Medical issues

Few studies have focused on the medical issues seen specifically in female alpine skiers, although skiers can be assumed to share the problems common to other female athletes. Pertinent data must be extracted from broader studies of mixed populations of athletes.

A study of Canadian athletes preparing for the 1988 Winter Olympics showed that 20% of these female alpine skiers had anaemia and 20% had low serum ferritin levels (Clement *et al.*, 1987). The average rate for anaemia among all female winter athletes was 8%, with the highest rate of 50% being seen among female cross-country skiers. Dietary counselling may be needed for alpine skiers as well as for athletes in general.

Another common problem in female athletes is amenorrhoea, although no studies have identified its incidence specifically among alpine skiers (Ronkainen et al., 1984). Likewise, no published studies have considered eating disorders in female skiers, although these athletes are under the same societal stresses to remain thin as other young women. However, a check of the Swiss alpine ski team has identified several women with amenorrhoea or oligomenorrhoea, including one with an eating disorder (N. Meyer, personal communication, 1997).

Exercise-induced bronchospasm may be aggravated by cold dry air, especially in asthmatics or endurance athletes, i.e. cross-country skiing (Sue-Chu et al., 1996). Metered-dose inhalers for asthma may not work well in the cold and should be kept warm in an inside pocket. A form of motion sickness, termed 'ski sickness', that can be relieved with vestibular suppressants has been described among some women downhill skiers (Hausler, 1995).

Pregnancy

In 1989, Ulrike Maier won the super giant slalom world championship when she was in the early second trimester of pregnancy (tragically, she died in a skiing accident 5 years later). Although few women ski competitively while pregnant, many pregnant women can be assumed to participate in recreational skiing (Farrell, 1986). The risks of skiing for pregnant women remain largely unknown and unstudied. Official guidelines, such as those issued by the American College of Obstetricians and Gynecologists (1994), recommend general exercise during pregnancy but do not address skiing specifically.

The risk of abdominal trauma posed by skiing is minimal. As abdominal or thoracic injuries account for only 5.6% of injuries in female alpine skiers (Shealy & Miller, 1991), skiing should pose little risk during the first trimester provided there are no complications. By the second trimester, the larger uterus becomes more at risk for abdominal injury and skiing should be considered more carefully. As the uterus expands and the woman's centre of gravity shifts, alterations in balance become a theoretical risk (Farrell, 1986). The hormone relaxin, produced during pregnancy, promotes ligamentous relaxation and increases joint laxity, although the effect on injuries is unknown.

Although it is known that fetal birth weight decreases with increasing altitude (Unger et al., 1988), the effect of transient exposure to increased elevations is unknown. A pregnant woman unacclimatized to higher altitudes should avoid intense exercise during the first 3 or 4 days at altitudes above 1980 m; those exposed to altitudes above 3048 m should ascend no more than 305 m a day in order to avoid altitude sickness (Kulpa, 1994). Mild altitude sickness may occur at altitudes above 2438 m and exhibits symptoms of headache, difficulty sleeping, easy fatigue and nausea.

Social issues

In young women and men who regularly travel away from home to compete, social behaviour and coaching relationships should be monitored regularly. Young athletes are psychologically vulnerable. Relationships with coaches may be very positive or problematic, and the potential for abuse, including sexual abuse, must be considered. Recommendations might include a 'buddy' system, so that one athlete cannot be isolated, athlete-advocates, parent-chaperones and a code of ethics for coaches (see Chapter 23).

Conclusion and recommendations for future research

Increasing numbers of women are now participating in alpine skiing at both competitive and recreational levels. The overall rate of injuries is similar for women and men of comparable skill, although women appear to have at least twice the rate of knee injuries, especially those involving the ACL (Shealy & Ettlinger, 1996). Additional research is needed on the mechanisms of

ACL injury in female athletes generally and downhill skiers specifically.

Improvements in the design of ski equipment have already lowered the high rate of ankle and leg injuries, but a new generation of equipment will be needed to address the problem of knee injuries (Johnson, 1995). To prevent injury, an education programme that teaches skiers about the positions and mechanisms that put the knee at risk of injury appears to offer an effective solution (Ettlinger et al., 1995; Anon., 1996), although funding will be needed to develop and implement the programme further. In addition, skiing organizations need to recognize the safety aspects of the release binding (Johnson, 1995) and consider rule changes that do not penalize racers when ski release occurs.

Medical issues among female alpine skiers are largely unstudied, and the menstrual disorders and eating behaviours seen in other female athletes are also possible in this group of athletes. In addition, the influence of hormonal factors on the risk of injury should be investigated further. As in other sports, factors that enhance performance are always a key subject for study; in skiing these include nutrition, equipment, training, iron and mineral supplementation, psychology and coaching. There are still many more unanswered questions than answered ones but we are now beginning to formulate the questions.

Acknowledgements

The author is grateful to the many people with whom she had conversations about this chapter and who generously shared their knowledge and data. They include Karen Briggs, Steadman-Hawkins Foundation, Vale, Colorado; Deanne Eakin, Olin Skis, Seattle, Washington; Dr Dan Gould, University of North Carolina, Greenborough, North Carolina; Dr Robert Johnson MD, University of Vermont, Burlington, Vermont; Nanna Meuer, Trainer, Swiss Alpine Women's Ski Team; Dr Steve Springmeyer MD, Virginia Mason Medical Center, Seattle, Washington; Dawn Straw, Women's Sports Foundation, New York; Dr Jim Stray-Gundersen MD, Dallas; and Dr Richard Watkins MD, USA Skiing, Park City, Utah. In addition, the author is grateful to Ms Anne Robertson, librarian at the Virginia Mason Medical Clinic, for her research assistance; Starr Kaplan of Seattle for her medical illustrations; and Mr Mike Bokulich of Narberth, Pennsylvania for his help in writing the manuscript.

References

Anon. (1996) *ACL Awareness '96*. Videotape, parts 1 and 2. Vermont Safety Research, Underhill Center, Connecticut, USA.

American College of Obstetricians and Gynecologists (1994) *Exercise During Pregnancy and the Postnatal Period*. American College of Obstetricians and Gynecologists, Washington, DC.

Anon. (1997) Title IX: equity in sports: short of the goal (schools close gender gap and women sports show revenue gains). *USA Today*, 4 March, section C, p. 6.

Arendt, E.A. (in press) Anterior cruciate ligament injuries in women.

Bacharach, D.W. & von Duvillard, S.P. (1995) Intermediate and long-term anaerobic performance of elite Alpine skiers. *Medicine and Science in Sports and Exercise* **27**, 305–309.

Bladin, C. & McCrory, P. (1995) Snowboarding injuries: an overview. *Sports Medicine* **19**, 358–364.

Bouter, L.M. & Knipschild, P.G. (1989) Causes and prevention of injury in downhill skiing. *Physician and Sportsmedicine* **17**, 81–94.

Bouter, L.M., Knipschild, P.G. & Volovics, A. (1989) Binding function in relation to injury risk in downhill skiing. *American Journal of Sports Medicine* **17**, 226–233.

Chapman, R.F., Stray-Gundersen, J. & Levine, B.D. (1998) Individual variation in response to altitude training. *Journal of Applied Physiology* **85**(4), 1448–1456.

Clement, D.B., Lloyd-Smith, D.R., Macintyre, J.G., Matheson, G.O., Brock, R. & Dupont, M. (1987) Iron status in Winter Olympic sports. *Journal of Sports Science* **5**, 261–271.

Davidson, T.M. & Laliotis, A.T. (1996) Snowboarding injuries: a four-year study with comparison with alpine ski injuries. *Western Journal of Medicine* **164**, 231–237.

Duncan, J.B., Hunter, R., Purnell, M. & Freeman, J. (1995) Meniscal injuries associated with acute anterior cruciate ligament tears in alpine skiers. *American Journal of Sports Medicine* **23**, 170–172.

Ekeland, A. & Vikne, J. (1995) Treatment of acute combined knee instabilities and subsequent sport performance. *Knee Surgery in Sports: Traumatology and Arthroscopy* **3**, 180–183.

Ekeland, A., Holtmoen, A. & Lystad, H. (1993) Lower extremity equipment-related injuries in alpine recreational skiers. *American Journal of Sports Medicine* **21**, 201–205.

Ellman, B.R., Holmes, E.M., III, Jordan, J. & McCarty, P. (1989) Cruciate ligament injuries in female Alpine ski racers. In R.J. Johnson, C.D. Mote Jr & M.-H. Binet (eds) *Skiing Trauma and Safety: Seventh International Symposium*, pp. 105–111. American Society for Testing and Materials, West Conshohocken, Pennsylvania.

Ettlinger, C.F., Johnson, R.J. & Shealy, J.E. (1995) A method to help reduce the risk of serious knee sprains incurred in alpine skiing. *American Journal of Sports Medicine* **23**, 531–537.

Farrell, M.J.D. (1986) Skiing for two. *Skiing* February, 101–103.

Feagin, J.A., Lambert, K.L., Cunningham, R.R. *et al.* (1987) Consideration of the anterior cruciate ligament injury in skiing. *Clinical Orthopaedics and Related Research* **216**, 13–18.

Fricker, R. & Hintermann, B. (1995) Skier's thumb: treatment, prevention, and recommendations. *Sports Medicine* **19**, 73–79.

Gibbs, P. (1994) Skiing. In R. Agostini (ed.) *Medical and Orthopedic Issues in Active and Athletic Women*, pp. 347–354. Hanley & Belfus, Philadelphia.

Greenwald, R.M., France, E.P., Rosenberg, T.D. & Toelcke, T. (1996) Significant gender-differences in Alpine skiing injuries: a five-year study. In C.D. Mote Jr, R.J. Johnson, W. Hauser & P.S. Schaff (eds) *Skiing Trauma and Safety*, 10th edn, pp. 36–44. American Society for Testing and Materials, West Conshohocken, Pennsylvania.

Hausler, R. (1995) Ski sickness. *Acta Oto-laryngologica* **115**, 1–2.

Hewson, G.F., Mendini, R.A. & Wang, J.B.L. (1986) Prophylactic knee bracing in college football. *American Journal of Sports Medicine* **14**, 262–266.

Johnson, R.J., Ettlinger, C.F., Campbell, R.J. *et al.* (1980) Trends in skiing injuries: analysis of a six-year study (1972–1978). *American Journal of Sports Medicine* **8**, 106–113.

Johnson, R.J., Ettlinger, C.F. & Shealy, J.E. (1993) Skier injury trends 1972–1990. In R.J. Johnson, C.D. Mote Jr & J. Zelcer (eds) *Skiing Trauma and Safety: Ninth International Symposium*, pp. 11–22. American Society for Testing and Materials, West Conshohocken, Pennsylvania.

Johnson, S.C. (1995) Anterior cruciate ligament injury in elite Alpine competitors. *Medicine and Science in Sports and Exercise* **27**, 323–327.

Kulpa, P. (1994) Exercise during pregnancy and post partum. In R. Agostini (ed.) *Medical and Orthopedic Issues in Active and Athletic Women*, pp. 191–199. Hanley & Belfus, Philadelphia.

Miyaska, K.C., Daniel, D.M., Stone, M.L. *et al.* (1991) The incidence of knee ligament injuries in the general population. *American Journal of Knee Surgery* **4**, 3–8.

Nielsen, A.B. & Yde, J. (1991) Epidemiology of acute knee injuries: a prospective hospital investigation. *Journal of Trauma* **31**, 1644–1648.

Ronkainen, H., Pakarinen, A. & Kauppila, A. (1984) Pubertal and menstrual disorders of female runners, skiers, and volleyball players. *Gynecologic and Obstetric Investigation* **18**, 183–189.

Shealy, J.E. (1993) Snowboard vs. downhill skiing injuries. In R.J. Johnson, C.D. Mote Jr & J. Zelcer (eds) *Skiing Trauma and Safety: Ninth International Symposium*, pp. 241–254. American Society for Testing and Materials, West Conshohocken, Pennsylvania.

Shealy, J.E. & Ettlinger, C.F. (1996) Gender-related injury patterns in skiing. In C.D. Mote Jr, R.J. Johnson, W. Hauser & P.S. Schaff (eds) *Skiing Trauma and Safety*, 10th edn, pp. 45–57. American Society for Testing and Materials, West Conshohocken, Pennsylvania.

Shealy, J.E. & Miller, D.A. (1991) A relative analysis of downhill and cross-country ski injuries. In C.D. Mote Jr & R.J. Johnson (eds) *Skiing Trauma and Safety: Eighth International Symposium*, pp. 133–143. American Society for Testing and Materials, Philadelphia.

Shealy, J.E. & Thomas, T. (1996) Death in downhill skiing from 1976 through 1992: a retrospective view. In C.D. Mote Jr, R.J. Johnson, W. Hauser & P.S. Schaff (eds) *Skiing Trauma and Safety*, 10th edn, pp. 66–72. American Society for Testing and Materials, West Conshochocken, Pennsylvania.

Steadman, J.R. & Scheinberg, R.R. (1995) Skiing injuries. In J.A. Nicholas & E.B. Hershman (eds) *The Lower Extremity in Spine and Sports Medicine*, 2nd edn, pp. 1361–1384. C.V. Mosby, St Louis.

Steadman, J.R. & Sterett, W.I. (1995) The surgical treatment of knee injuries in skiers. *Medicine and Science in Sports and Exercise* **27**, 328–333.

Sue-Chu, M., Larsson, L. & Bjermer, L. (1996) Prevalence of asthma in young cross-country skiers in central Scandinavia: difference between Norway and Sweden. *Respiratory Medicine* **90**, 99–105.

Tesch, P.A. (1995) Aspects on muscle properties and use in competitive Alpine skiing. *Medicine and Science in Sports and Exercise* **27**, 310–314.

Unger, C., Weiser, J.K., McCullough, R.E., Keefer, S. & Moore, L.G. (1988) Altitude, low birth weight, and infant mortality in Colorado. *Journal of the American Medical Association* **259**, 3427–3432.

Wallechinsky, D. (1993) *The Complete Book of the Winter Olympics*, pp. 117–152. Little, Brown, Boston.

Warme, W.J., Feagin, J.A. Jr, King, P., Lambert, K.L. &

Cunningham, R.R. (1995) Ski injury statistics, 1982–1993, Jackson Hole Ski Resort. *American Journal of Sports Medicine* **23**, 597–600.

Westin, C.D., Gill, E.A., Noyes, M.E. & Hubbard, M. (1995) Anterior shoulder dislocation: a simple and rapid method for reduction. *American Journal of Sports Medicine* **23**, 369–371.

White, A.T. & Johnson, S.C. (1993) Physiological aspects and injury in elite Alpine skiers. *Sports Medicine* **15**, 170–178.

Chapter 42

Softball

MARGARET M. BAKER

Introduction

A wintry November day in Chicago, 1887, led to the birth of the game we now know as softball. Inclement weather forced some would-be baseballers into the Farragut Boat Club gymnasium. Their efforts to devise a game of indoor baseball resulted in an old boxing glove being laced together to form a soft 'ball'. A smallish 'diamond' was marked off on the gym floor with chalk and the two teams began to play. They discovered, that blustery day, what millions of players around the world now know to be true: this new sport was incredibly fun to play and almost anyone can participate.

In the spring, the young Chicago softballers took their sport outdoors. They named the game 'indoor-outdoors', and its appeal began to spread. By the turn of the century, communities across the USA were playing variations of the game. The city of Minneapolis embraced this new pastime, adapting it for use in the fire department to keep firefighters fit during idle time. One of the local fire companies organized a team called the Kittens. The now popular game became known as Kitten League Ball, then Kitten Ball for short.

The actual name softball did not appear until 1926 when it was suggested by a YMCA official from Denver. Participation in softball boomed, and by the time of the Chicago World's Fair Tournament in 1933 teams were competing in fastpitch, slowpitch and women's divisions. At this time, some confusion existed because of all the local variations in rules and equipment. Once the Amateur Softball Association (ASA) was created, playing rules were formalized. The ASA has also done much to provide guidance on a national level in the USA and to promote widespread participation in the sport.

Over the ensuing decades, thousands of leagues and millions of teams have appeared. Participation by women and girls has rocketed. Less than one generation ago, females rarely played softball. In the early 1970s, fewer than 10000 girls played softball in American high schools; by the 1990s, that number exceeded 220000. Currently, softball is the fourth most popular sport among high-school girls in the USA (Fig. 42.1). Over the last 5 years alone, women's participation in softball has doubled. Women's and girls teams now dominate fastpitch leagues, comprising 75% of all teams in the USA. Over 40 million players enthusiastically participate across the USA, making softball the most popular recreational sport in America. Every culture on earth plays some sport with a stick and a ball, and the International Softball Federation supports growing interest worldwide. Its intense popularity and commitment from countless devoted individuals led to women's fastpitch softball finally becoming an Olympic sport at the Centennial Games in Atlanta in 1996.

From humble beginnings the sport of softball has grown to huge proportions. An estimated 23 million games are played annually in the USA alone. As with other active sports, athletes do

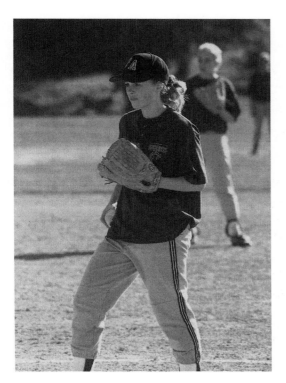

Fig. 42.1 Softball is one of the most popular sports in the USA among high-school girls.

incur injuries from time to time. In the USA, the National Electronic Injury Surveillance System estimates that softball causes more injuries leading to emergency room visits than any other sport (Janda *et al.*, 1992). The rate of softball injury severe enough to require emergency attention is estimated to be 2.26 injuries/1000 players per day, or one injury in every 14.7 games (Shesser *et al.*, 1985). This rate is about half that for recreational ski injuries (Ellison, 1973) and 40% that of recreational soccer (Ekstrand *et al.*, 1983). However, the gross numbers of injury in softball are higher than other sports because of the sheer number of participants. In addition to emergency treatment, countless softball players seek attention for their injuries at outpatient clinics and with private physicians. Because of the difficulty compiling the statistics on non-emergency injury, the true magnitude of the human and economic impact is unknown. In this

day of escalating healthcare costs, what is known is that decreasing the injury and cost burden is critical.

The goal of this chapter is to educate the reader in an effort to minimize the incidence and impact of softball injuries. Injury prevention is the cornerstone, through an understanding of proper biomechanics and by creating a safer environment for play (for clarification of biomechanical terminology, see Chapter 6). Regardless of an athlete's training, education and equipment, some injuries will undoubtedly occur due to the sheer numbers of athletes participating in softball around the world. Sport-specific injuries and appropriate treatment are discussed in this chapter and are related to the mechanism of injury. Treatment of the myriad of upper and lower extremity traumatic musculoskeletal injuries is not the focus of this chapter, as it is covered elsewhere in this volume and extensively in orthopaedic texts (Browner *et al.*, 1992; Green & Swiontkowski, 1992; DeLee & Drez, 1994; Stanitski *et al.*, 1994; Rockwood *et al.*, 1996). Finally, pertinent concerns about equipment safety and areas for future research are also discussed.

Functional anatomy and technique

Windmill pitch

Before one can attempt to diagnose, treat or prevent sports overuse injuries, an understanding of basic biomechanics must be gained. It is critical to understand what normal healthy bones, muscles and joints should be doing during a specific skill. Only then can we really comprehend how things go awry to cause injury. Unfortunately, the vast majority of sports medicine literature in this area deals with baseball. A tiny percentage deals specifically with softball, although most of these articles discuss injuries in slowpitch softball. Very little has been published relating to fastpitch: only one article in the medical literature, to our knowledge, specifically addresses the biomechanics of the windmill pitch (Alexander & Haddow, 1982).

In general, ballistic skills involve transferring momentum from the body to a relatively small projectile. The pitcher's goal is to maximize the horizontal velocity of the projectile and reproducibly to hit a target. Her object is, after all, to strike out the batter. The thrower accelerates body parts in sequence in order to impart maximal momentum to the ball, although in competition not every pitch is intended to be thrown at full speed. Different pitches also have quite different finger positions and grips. To simplify the mechanics, only a 'generic' fastball pitch is detailed here. For the purposes of discussion, the windmill pitch is broken down into six phases (Fig. 42.2): windup, stride, overhead, acceleration, release and follow-through.

Individual pitchers have great variability in the initial phase of the windmill pitch, the windup. This first phase of the pitch includes any motion prior to initiation of the stride. The same pitcher may even wind up differently depending on the defensive situation. The windup, in truth, does little to propel the ball towards the batter. If the shoulder is brought into full extension, tension on the anterior soft tissues may theoretically provide improved muscular contractility during later shoulder flexion. Numerous studies using electromyography (EMG) have been published detailing overhand pitching, but there are none on the windmill pitch to substantiate this theory. The windup begins with the pitcher facing the target, weight balanced evenly between both feet, feet about shoulder width apart and slightly staggered with pivot foot forward. The lead foot (contralateral to the throwing arm) should be pointing towards the target. The trail or pivot foot contacts the front edge of the pitching rubber, pointing at about 45° to the target. During a conventional windup, both hands stay together anteriorly. The trunk flexes as weight is transferred to the trail foot and both shoulders begin to flex. Another common variation is the full-motion windup, where the hands separate and the shoulders swing into extension. Regardless of the style of windup, it should be relaxed and require little or no muscular effort. A pitcher's windup mostly serves to initiate timing of the subsequent sequence of events.

The second phase of the windmill pitch begins as the throwing shoulder begins circumduction and the lead foot leaves the ground in the stride (Fig. 42.3). As the pitcher strides forward, trailing leg drive translates the body's centre of mass towards the catcher. Also, the centre of mass is lowered, releasing stored potential energy. These changes in centre of mass are ultimately transferred into ballistic energy of the ball. The pelvis rotates from perpendicular to the flight path to a more open position. Both shoulders flex, bringing the arms in front of the trunk. The path of the throwing arm begins its oval-shaped arc in a

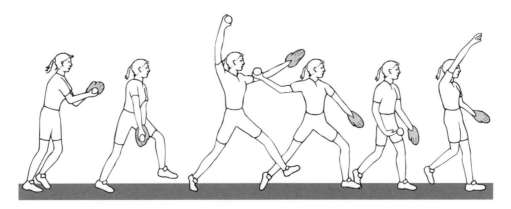

Fig. 42.2 Windmill pitch: windup, stride, overhead, acceleration, release and follow-through.

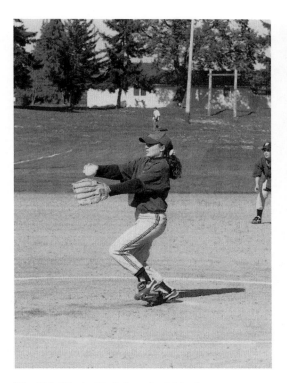

Fig. 42.3 Windmill pitch: early stride phase.

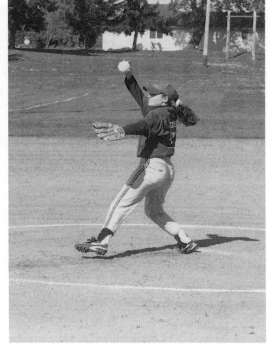

Fig. 42.4 Windmill pitch: early overhead phase.

plane very close to the body. With the arc close to the body, the release point is more reproducible and less stress is placed on the shoulder and elbow.

During the overhead phase, the internally rotated throwing shoulder continues to accelerate to and past the vertical overhead (Fig. 42.4). The elbow is just slightly flexed and the wrist passively volarflexed. At the top of the arc the throwing arm should be fairly straight in order to increase leverage and thus generation of torque. The contralateral upper extremity moves to horizontal, generally pointing at the target to aid in balance. As the lead leg continues to stride forward, the pelvis and trunk rotate completely open (facing third base for a right-handed pitcher). When the arm is overhead it should nearly brush the head (Fig. 42.5). The trail foot now strongly pivots so it is parallel with the pitching rubber. Forcible leg drive is generated

from extension of the trail leg as it pushes off the rubber. This force is transferred to the pelvis and then the trunk as forward rotation towards the target begins. A critical key to force production is often the trunk. If little trunk rotation occurs, leg drive cannot be effectively applied to the upper body and thus increase ball speed.

During the acceleration phase, the lead foot plants and points at the catcher when the throwing arm is at about the 9 o'clock position during the downswing. A common timing problem occurs when the pitcher transfers weight to the stride foot too soon. This tends to neutralize leg drive if the weight shifts forward too early. Proper timing of the weight shift should allow forward leg drive to coincide with downward movement of the throwing arm (Fig. 42.6). As the pitching arm accelerates downward from overhead, the humerus rotates into full external rotation. When the arm is horizontal in the

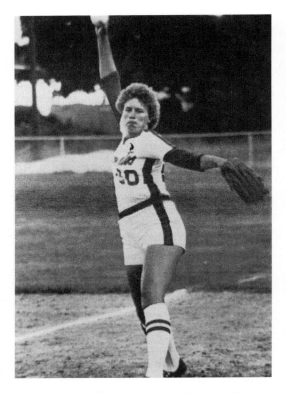

Fig. 42.5 Windmill pitch: arm vertical overhead.

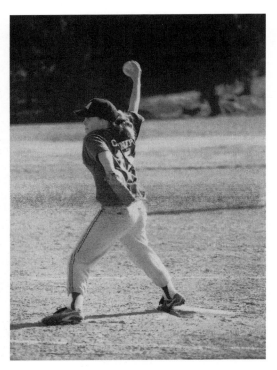

Fig. 42.6 Windmill pitch: early acceleration phase.

downswing, the position of humeral external rotation, extension and abduction is nearly identical to the cocking position of the overhand throw and creates tremendous stress on the shoulder. The elbow flexes to approximately 45° and sustains a valgus force. As the pelvis and trunk initiate turn towards the target, the trailing leg is still driving off the rubber. The power of the legs is transferred to the pelvis, then the trunk and then the arm. The non-throwing arm can also assist in power generation by actively pulling down and backwards to assist in forward rotation of the trunk as the throwing side moves forward. The summation of all the forces from the non-throwing arm, legs and trunk are transferred to the throwing arm in order to gain maximal acceleration. Biomechanical parameters for élite female windmill pitchers were quantified by S. Werner (unpublished data, 1991) at the US Olympic Training Center. Arm speeds of up to $2000°·s^{-1}$ were measured, equivalent to a shoulder circumduction rate of six revolutions per second. Maximal shoulder distraction forces of 100–110% body weight were recorded just prior to ball release. The arm reaches peak angular velocity towards the bottom of the arc, then begins to decelerate and transfer its momentum to the forearm. At release, the elbow now extends to an average of 20° with the forearm in supination. Peak elbow distraction forces of up to 65% body weight have been noted. Momentum is transferred to the ball with a violent flick of the wrist into volarflexion at the instant of release. Ball release should occur from the hip, with the elbow just behind the hip and the arm vertically downwards but close to the trunk (Fig. 42.7). Depending on the desired type of pitch (rise, drop, fastball, curve), the forearm stays supinated or may fully pronate.

Follow-through is the final phase of the wind-

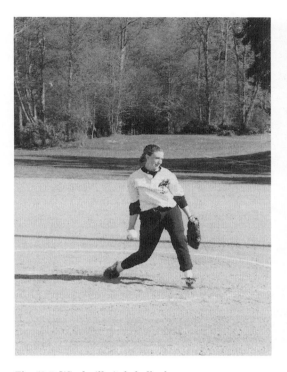

Fig. 42.7 Windmill pitch: ball release.

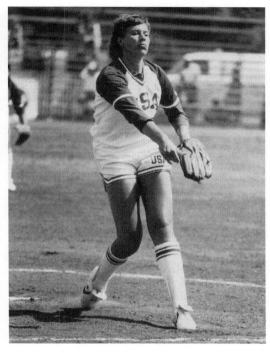

Fig. 42.8 Windmill pitch: follow-through.

mill pitch (Fig. 42.8). This phase serves to decelerate body segments comfortably, dissipating energy into large muscle groups as heat in order to avoid injury. The trail leg has left the rubber, body weight now being borne on the lead leg. A pitcher's rotational momentum causes the pelvis and trunk to close, bringing the trail leg through to plant perpendicular to the target and in a position to field. The throwing shoulder flexes, with eccentric firing of the posterior rotator cuff and periscapular muscles preventing excess tensile loading of the posterior capsule and labrum. The elbow also passively flexes, being slowed by triceps action, and thus decreasing distraction force across it (Fig. 42.9). By flexing the elbow to absorb energy, less distraction stress is applied to the shoulder. Pitchers who maintain a straight elbow in follow-through tend to experience increased shoulder distraction stress that may predispose them to injury. The forearm may experience extreme pronation

in some pitchers that may exceed the tensile strength of bone and put them at increased risk for stress fractures.

In summary, the windmill pitch is a highly skilled performance of complex biomechanics that has been poorly studied. It requires full circumduction of the shoulder, which happens to be the most mobile but intrinsically unstable joint in the body. A coordinated sequence of acceleration–deceleration events occur, controlled and protected by both concentric and eccentric muscle action. Angular and rotational momentum are transferred from each succeeding segment to the projectile. In addition to proper arm motion, pelvic rotation, trail leg drive and follow-through are all key elements in reducing stress on the pitching arm. Skilled performance is dependent on the proper timing of events, and the ability reproducibly to accelerate and decelerate body segments without exceeding the physiological capacity of the tissues.

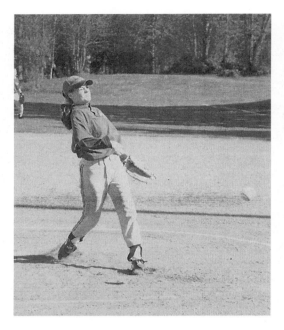

Fig. 42.9 Windmill pitch: elbow flexion in follow-through.

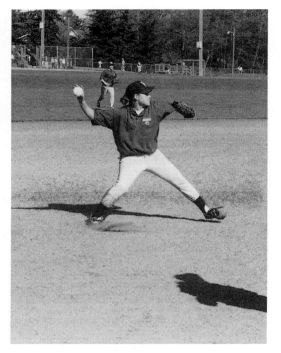

Fig. 42.10 Overhand throw from short-stop.

Overhand throw

Windmill biomechanics are obviously specific only to pitchers; the other eight defensive softball players use the overhand throw (Fig. 42.10). Many sports use an overhead motion to hit or propel an object (volleyball, javelin, tennis) or to propel the athlete (freestyle or butterfly swimming). Although each sport has its specific pattern, these sports have much in common biomechanically. By far the most studied and most extensively described is the baseball pitch. The literature is replete with detailed descriptions of baseball pitching mechanics (Atwater, 1980; Pappas *et al.*, 1985; Feltner & Dapena, 1986; Fleisig *et al.*, 1989, 1995; Dillman *et al.*, 1993; Werner *et al.*, 1993) and EMG analysis (Jobe *et al.*, 1984; Gowan *et al.*, 1987; Sisto *et al.*, 1987; Glousman *et al.*, 1988; Glousman, 1993). The classic baseball pitching windup is not useful for non-pitchers because of the nature of defensive play. Instead, catchers, infielders and outfielders use an abbreviated 'windup' to expedite release of

the ball to where the play is. Otherwise, the biomechanics of overhand baseball and softball throwing are analogous.

The overhand throw is divided into five stages: windup, early cocking, late cocking, acceleration and follow-through (Fig. 42.11). Windup begins when the thrower initiates her first movement and ends when the lead leg lifts and the ball is removed from the glove. Like the windmill windup, it is quite variable depending on the individual and defensive situation. Minimal muscle exertion and tissue stress occur, so the potential for injury during this phase is low.

Early cocking begins when the ball is removed from the glove. The trail leg is planted, extensors contracting to drive the centre of mass towards the target. The body lowers as the lead leg strides, releasing potential energy. The stride should be long enough to generate momentum, but not so long that the athlete cannot rotate her hips and pelvis properly. Maximum stride

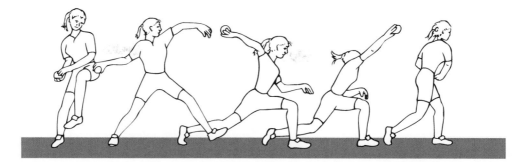

Fig. 42.11 Overhand throw: windup, early cocking, late cocking, acceleration and follow-through.

should be slightly less than the thrower's height. The pelvis and trunk rotate open, parallel to the flight path. The scapula is retracted, elbow flexed, and shoulder abducted, internally rotated and extended. The contralateral upper extremity extends towards the target. Early cocking ends when the lead leg plants.

Late cocking begins as the pelvis and trunk initiate rotation towards the target. Muscular contraction translates into angular velocity as the lower extremity segments accelerate. The legs transfer their momentum to the pelvis, then the trunk and then each more distal segment of the throwing extremity. In late cocking, the throwing shoulder achieves maximal combined external rotation (90–120° between the glenohumeral and scapulothoracic joints). Tremendous tensile stresses are generated at the shoulder anterior capsule, labrum and rotator cuff. A maximum varus torque of up to 120 N·m has been measured at the elbow (Werner *et al.*, 1993).

Acceleration is the fourth phase of the overhand throw. This begins with rapid internal rotation of the humerus and ends with ball release. Acceleration is explosive, lasting only about 50 ms and causing peak angular velocities of 9198°·s⁻¹ (Pappas *et al.*, 1985). As the coiled shoulder is powerfully derotated, the elbow extends and wrist flexes and pronates. During acceleration, considerable muscular activity is seen in the subscapularis, serratus anterior, pectoralis major, latissimus dorsi and triceps.

The goal of follow-through is to decelerate the limb. Muscles, especially the posterior shoulder musculature, fire eccentrically to dissipate kinetic energy as heat to avoid injury. The humerus continues to flex horizontally and rotate internally. The elbow passes from about 20° flexion at ball release to 45° during follow-through. Wrist volarflexion and pronation occur, while the trunk flexes. The trail leg passively lifts off the ground and then swings forward to plant.

In summary, the overhand throw is also a coordinated sequence of events that is a total body activity. Sequential activation of body segments acts as a link system transmitting energy that starts in the legs and ends in the throwing hand. Dramatic shoulder external rotation and elbow valgus stress occur in late cocking and acceleration. During follow-through, muscle and ligamentous forces must counteract forward velocity to decelerate the arm within the physiological tolerance of the tissues. Improper biomechanics will, over time, lead to tissue overload and overuse injury.

Hitting

Compared to the tremendous amount of work that has been done in the development of training and rehabilitation protocols for throwing athletes, there has been little study of hitting. Like throwing, batting is a coordinated sequence of muscle activity beginning with the lower extremities, followed by the trunk and terminating in

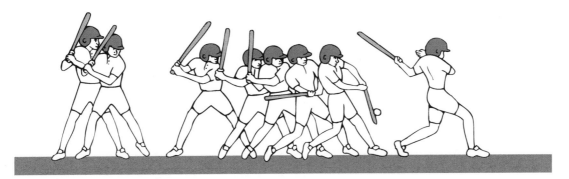

Fig. 42.12 Batting swing: windup, pre-swing, swing and follow-through.

the upper extremities. Understanding the biomechanics of hitting should help physicians, coaches and players design specific training, conditioning and rehabilitation protocols to optimize performance and minimize injuries.

The batting swing is divided into four phases: windup, pre-swing, swing and follow-through (Fig. 42.12). Windup begins with a stride as the lead heel leaves the ground and ends as the lead toe establishes ground contact. Weight first shifts to the trailing leg. The body is rotated in a clockwise direction for a right-handed batter, initiated by the upper extremities and followed by the pelvis. The pelvis rotates to a maximum closed position of 28° 0.35 s before ball contact (Welch *et al.*, 1995). Next the pelvis begins to derotate counterclockwise, while the trunk and shoulders continue to coil clockwise to a maximum of 52° relative to the ball's flight path. Subsequently the shoulders and trunk derotate counterclockwise, following the lead of the pelvis. The arms keep coiling clockwise around the trunk as windup finishes.

Pre-swing begins as the lead foot plants. Mean stride length should be about 380% of hip width and 12° closed (Welch *et al.*, 1995). Weight shifts forward to the lead leg. The gluteus maximus and hamstrings fire maximally in this phase (Shaffer *et al.*, 1993). This creates a counterclockwise acceleration of the pelvis around the axis of the trunk. The arms and shoulders remain maximally coiled, the hands holding the bat near vertical (Fig. 42.13).

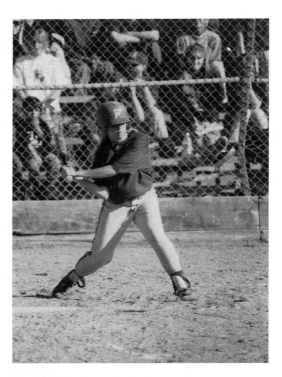

Fig. 42.13 Batting swing: late pre-swing.

The swing phase begins as the posterior deltoid of the lead shoulder fires maximally, which initiates uncoiling of the upper extremities. The hands and bat now begin to move forward. Maximal activity is seen in the erector spinae and abdominal oblique muscles so that power is transmitted from the legs as the body

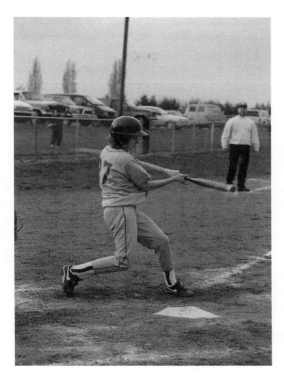

Fig. 42.14 Batting swing: late swing phase with ball contact.

uncoils. The bat accelerates from perpendicular to the ground to parallel during ball contact in late swing (Fig. 42.14). The rotational velocity of the bat has been measured at up to $1588°·s^{-1}$, with linear speeds of $29\,m·s^{-1}$ prior to impact (Welch *et al.*, 1995). Triceps brachii now fire to extend the elbows. The trailing elbow extends near full at the point of impact, transferring the last amount of angular velocity to the uncocking bat. Acting like a block, the lead leg supports about 84% of body weight, with the knee flexed 15°. The trunk is positioned in slight extension, continuous with the lead leg acting as a stable post for continued rotation.

Follow-through begins after ball contact. The body slows itself and the bat via eccentric muscle action, which diffuses energy through large muscle groups. The pelvis, trunk and shoulders finish full counterclockwise rotation, with the lead shoulder ending in maximal abduction and external rotation. Muscular activity of the abdominal obliques and quadriceps femoris, especially the vastus medialis obliquus (VMO), remain high during follow-through.

In summary, little emphasis has been placed on the study of the batting swing in the sports medicine literature. Some limited data from electromyogram (EMG), force plate and cinematographic analysis have been collected. These early results have outlined the basic biomechanics of the hitting swing and reinforced the need for strengthening the erector spinae, abdominal obliques, posterior deltoid, gluteals, hamstrings and VMO. Attention should be given to eccentric as well as concentric muscle strength training.

Injury mechanisms

Injuries due to windmill pitching

Despite the fact that softball is the most popular recreational sport in America, there is a paucity of information on sport-specific injuries. Most of the literature that does exist deals with injuries from slowpitch softball; only a handful of articles pertain to fastpitch. Apparently, the traditional view has been that softball is less physically demanding than baseball and thus more 'suitable' for females. An underhand pitching motion was assumed not to generate much speed and put little stress on the arm compared with the overhand throw. Anyone who has witnessed a competitive women's fastpitch game knows that this is a fallacy. Female fastpitchers can attain ball speeds upwards of $160\,km·h^{-1}$ and have been known repeatedly to strike out male major-league baseball stars.

Perhaps the false belief that windmill pitching is not stressful has led to competitive fastpitchers often being assigned to pitch consecutive double-headers, long batting practices and multiple tournament games. For baseball, even at the Little League level, rules limit pitching time in order to minimize overuse. Such rules are not in effect to protect softball pitchers. One study has verified that fastpitchers have significant injuries related to pitching (Loosli *et al.*, 1992). High-calibre pitchers in National Collegiate Athletic

Association (NCAA) tournament championship teams were surveyed. A total of 26 injuries were identified in 20 of 24 pitchers; 82% of injuries that involved time lost from practice or games were upper extremity injuries. The athletes pitched an average of 139 innings per season (average of 19.9 complete games). The vast majority of injuries (81%) were from overuse, most frequently the shoulder (rotator cuff, tendonitis, biceps, trapezius strain) and elbow (tendonitis, ulnar neuritis, arthralgia). The exact mechanisms of injury and details of the diagnosis were not specified in this study so it is somewhat difficult to determine the aetiology. Extreme shoulder abduction, extension and external rotation during the acceleration phase of the windmill pitch may produce transient anterior glenohumeral subluxation similar to the overhand throw. This can result in secondary impingement and labral tears. Elbow valgus stress just prior to ball release may be responsible for ulnar neuritis and flexor–pronator tendonitis. Improper arm deceleration in follow-through could produce trapezius strain. Further study into windmill biomechanics as related to the aetiology and incidence of injury is definitely warranted.

Radial neuropathy has been reported in competitive windmill pitchers (Sinson et al., 1994). Patients complained of posterior shoulder soreness and progressive weakness without antecedent trauma. Neurological examination and EMG were positive for radial nerve palsy at the level of the triceps. The two pitchers in the report did not improve with non-operative treatment and ultimately underwent surgical exploration and neurolysis. Their radial nerves were found to be scarred and thinned; one had a neuroma. Both patients improved postoperatively. The authors postulated that the nerve may be injured because of the traction forces during the pitch, especially in individuals with tethering of the nerve by an anomalous fibrous arch at the lateral head of the triceps.

One other article specific to fastpitch reported three cases of ulnar stress fractures in pitchers (Tanabe et al., 1991). Patients presented with forearm pain during pitching without any traumatic event. They had tenderness and slight swelling over the mid-ulnar shaft. Radiographs showed a transverse incomplete fracture line in each, with periosteal new bone formation. Cross-sectional computerized tomography of the ulna in six normal volunteers was performed. The diameter of the ulnae were smallest at mid-shaft, exactly where the stress fractures had occurred. The investigators concluded that extreme pronation of the forearm during follow-through resulted in torsional shear on the ulna. Fatigue fracture occurred when bone remodelling and repair could not compensate for repetitive microtrauma.

Unpublished data from team physicians at the 1996 Olympic Games and NCAA Championships also identified an incidence of spine problems in female softball players (J. Henderson, personal communication, 1997). Hyperextension of the spine in pitchers during ball release and exaggerated lordosis in first- and third-base fielders in the crouch position was felt to contribute. Posterior element stress was indicated by specific injuries, including lumbar spondylolysis, facet syndrome, interspinous ligament strain and sacroiliac joint dysfunction. Anterior element stress was indicated by other injuries, including lumbar degenerative disc disease and thoracic endplate apophysitis. Other miscellaneous conditions identified were sacrospinalis spasm, sacral torsion and lumbodorsal fasciitis. Further research in this area would better clarify such sport- and position-specific conditions and allow appropriate training and rehabilitation techniques to be developed.

Injuries due to overhand throwing

Literally hundreds of published articles and texts address injuries specific to overhand throwing. The majority of these studies are centred on baseball pitchers, although non-pitchers also sustain these injuries but with a lesser incidence. Since overhand throwing injuries and their diagnosis, treatment and rehabilitation have been so well delineated in the literature, I briefly outline them here and provide references for more in-depth study.

The shoulder is probably the most frequent site of injury for overhand throwers. The glenohumeral joint is capable of the greatest range of motion of any joint in the body but is also the most unstable. Extreme shear, compressive and tensile stresses during the throwing motion often lead to rotator cuff dysfunction and functional instability (Davidson et al., 1995). Instability may be anterior, inferior, posterior or multidirectional. For the throwing athlete, instability means pain, fatigue and decreased performance. Treatment for recurrent shoulder subluxation begins with functional rehabilitation but may require ligament reconstruction if refractory (Jobe et al., 1991). Glenohumeral instability can result in, or be the cause of, labral tears or detachment. An athlete with a labral tear often complains of recurrent clicking, catching or locking. Several tests on physical examination have been described to aid diagnosis of labral pathology (Kibler, 1995). Arthroscopic treatment of labral injuries has been well described (Snyder et al., 1990; Snyder & Wuh, 1991; Glasgow & Bruce, 1992; Liu et al., 1996). Impingement of the rotator cuff tendons, subacromial bursa and long head of the biceps tendon between the humeral head and inferior acromion can occur primarily or as a result of instability (Jobe & Bradley, 1988; Jobe, 1989). Treatment is directed at addressing the instability if that is the primary problem. If impingement is primary, arthroscopic decompression may be indicated if conservative treatment fails (Savoie, 1993; Roye et al., 1995). Impingement may progress to frank rotator cuff tear; if this occurs in the throwing athlete surgical repair is indicated (Tibone et al., 1986; Snyder & Wuh, 1991; Warner et al., 1991).

Articular and bony lesions can also affect the throwing athlete's shoulder. Ossification at the posterior–inferior glenoid rim (Bennett lesion) has been described as being associated with posterior labral injury and possible partial rotator cuff tear (Ferrari et al., 1994). Physeal fractures, snapping scapulae, glenohumeral loose bodies and humeral head or glenoid chondral injuries are occasionally seen. Spontaneous fractures of the humeral shaft due to throwing a softball (Marymount et al., 1989) or baseball (Branch et al., 1992; DiCicco et al., 1993) have been reported. Humeral stress periostitis, an arm equivalent of shin splints, was shown by Greyson (1995) to correlate with a positive bone scan. Muscular violence has caused avulsion of the triceps, latissimus dorsi, teres major and pectoralis major in overhand throwers.

Other assorted conditions about the shoulder have been reported in association with overhand throwing. Nerve compression can occur at various sites, including thoracic outlet syndrome, quadrilateral space syndrome (Cahill & Palmer, 1983; Redler et al., 1986) and suprascapular neuropathy (Ringel et al., 1990; Glennon, 1992). Axillary artery thrombosis can result from so-called hyperabduction syndrome, with pressure from the pectoralis minor causing vascular occlusion (Rohrer et al., 1990). This potentially limb-threatening condition presents with pain, fatigue and paraesthesias and is diagnosed by arteriogram. Once diagnosed, immediate vascular surgical consultation is recommended.

The elbow is the next most common source of problems for the overhand thrower. Tremendous valgus stress may create medial tensile and lateral compressive overload. Bony injuries include medial epicondyle fracture (so-called Little-Leaguer's elbow), olecranon stress fracture (Nuber & Diment, 1992), olecranon osteophytes, osteochondritis dissecans of the capitellum and intra-articular loose bodies. Flexor–pronator strain or tears, as well as ulnar collateral ligament injuries, occur with tensile overload. The incidence of ulnar collateral injuries is most probably underreported, and may partly be a cause of failure of surgical treatment (Andrews & Timmerman, 1995). Ulnar neuropathy and ulnar nerve subluxation in throwers has been reported to have excellent outcome with surgical transposition (Wojtys et al., 1986; Rettig & Ebben, 1993), although care must be taken not to overlook concomitant occult valgus instability.

Injuries due to collision/impact

The bulk of the literature on softball injuries has been concerned with sliding injuries (Fig. 42.15). Much attention has been given to sliding injuries because of their large public and occupational health impact. Sliding-related injuries have been reported to comprise 42–71% of all softball injuries (Wheeler, 1984; Janda *et al.*, 1992). The average cost of a sliding injury requiring an emergency visit has been estimated to be US$1223 (Janda *et al.*, 1988). Since softball is the most popular recreational sport in the USA and is also responsible for the most visits to the emergency room, the economic impact of sliding injuries is staggering. The armed forces in the USA use softball as a major part of the Morale, Welfare and Recreation Program. Statistics from the US Army reveal that more man-days are lost because of softball injuries each year than any other sport (Wheeler, 1987). The army study also reported that ankle fractures have been the leading cause of sports-related hospital admissions over a 7-year period, and in their prospective studies all ankle fractures were the result of sliding.

Sliding during base running is the act of using the ground and a base to decelerate the body from sprinting to complete stop in the space of a few yards (Fig. 42.16). The injury mechanisms for sliding may include impact, shear and torque. Rapid energy transfer to the small joints and bones of the leading extremity puts the ankle and hand at risk, since the momentum of the entire body must be dissipated as the runner hits a fixed object. Sliding feet first may cause marked axial loading, plantar flexion, version or rotational forces to the ankle. Ankle fractures (Fig. 42.17) and sprains comprise the most frequent major sliding injuries (Nadeau & Brown, 1990). Treatment of ankle and other musculoskeletal injuries related to collision and impact is no different from that outlined in standard orthopaedic and sports medicine texts.

Injuries to the knee also occur during feet-first sliding and collisions between players. Twisting on the flexed knee as it impacts the ground causes meniscal injuries. Valgus, deceleration and external rotation stress in the extended knee as it hits a fixed base can tear the anterior cruciate ligament. Impact on the anterior surface of the flexed tibia may rupture the posterior cruciate ligament. Patellar subluxation, dislocation and osteochondral fractures are not uncommon. The best aid to diagnosis is a thorough examination at the time of injury before the onset of swelling and

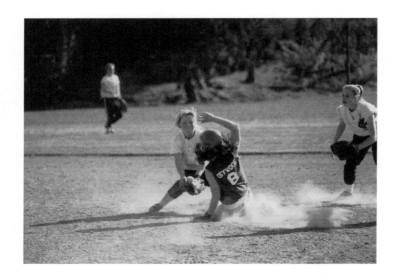

Fig. 42.15 Sliding is a frequent cause of softball injuries.

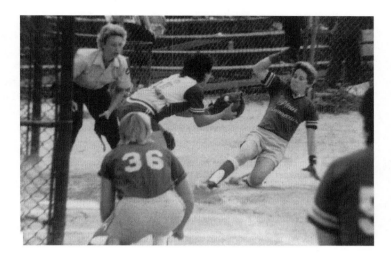

Fig. 42.16 The feet-first slide.

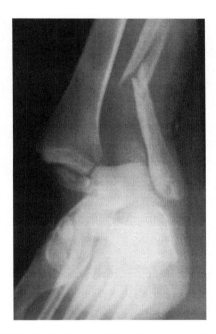

Fig. 42.17 Ankle fracture-dislocation sustained during sliding.

effusion. In head-first sliding, upper extremity, head and face injuries predominate. Contusions, abrasions, digit fractures and sprains, forearm fractures, shoulder dislocations and facial bone fractures are common. Again, treatment is stan-dard and not specific to softball. Anecdotal reports of cervical spine injury have also been attributed to head first-sliding when the head impacts an opponent (American Academy of Pediatrics Committee on Sports Medicine, 1994).

Other collision and impact injuries include those in which a player is hit by a ball, bat, another player or a fixed piece of equipment on the field. The most catastrophic sports injury, death, has been reported for softball. Brunko and Hunt (1988) cited a case of sudden cardiac death in a 30-year-old woman while sliding into second base. Other deaths have been reported during baseball and softball when players have been hit in the head, eye or chest with the ball (Rome, 1995). In the USA between 1986 and 1990, 16 deaths related to softball or baseball occurred in children aged 5–14 (American Academy of Pediatrics Committee on Sports Medicine, 1994). Direct contact with the ball is cited as the most frequent cause of death or serious injury in chil-dren and adolescents, with impact to the head being most common, although impact with the immature, relatively elastic chest can also be lethal.

Facial injuries account for about 5% of all soft-ball injuries (Shesser et al., 1985). Softball ranks second only to skiing as the most frequent cause of maxillofacial fractures sustained in sports

(Tanaka *et al.*, 1996). Mandibular, nasal and dental fractures are caused from impact with balls and bats. Treatment for sports-related facial fractures is no different from that for fractures from other causes. Baseball and softball seem to be the leading cause of sports-related eye injuries in children, with about one-third being caused by impact from a pitched ball. Bat impact has been known to cause both facial and extremity injuries. Aluminium bats break less frequently than wooden bats, although occasionally they do fracture. During one season at a major US university, four aluminium bat fractures were documented that resulted in two lacerations from flying fragments (Strauss & Whitehead, 1982).

Ball impact is responsible for numerous contusions to the extremities and, occasionally, fractures and tendinous injuries. The classic mallet finger is well known to competitive catchers as an injury sustained from impact to a fingertip. The terminal slip of the extensor tendon is avulsed from the base of the distal phalanx, with or without a small piece of bone attached. Baseball catchers have also been reported to sustain digital vessel trauma in the glove hand due to repetitive ball impact (Lowrey *et al.*, 1976). Digital ischaemia typically affects the index finger, and may present as coolness, numbness and paleness especially with cold exposure. The

probability of developing digital ischaemia corresponds to cumulative playing time (Sugawara *et al.*, 1986). I am aware of an identical case of digital ischaemia in the index finger of a collegiate softball catcher (Fig. 42.18). A rare case of a digital artery false aneurysm in the thumb of a softball catcher has been reported by Yasuda and Takeda (1996).

Equipment and safety concerns

Sliding

Since most sliding injuries are probably preventable and because sliding accounts for the brunt of softball injuries, a tremendous reduction in the number of injuries is possible if preventative measures are implemented. Softball and baseball are steeped in tradition, so banning sliding is not an option that would be acceptable to devoted players and fans. However, the American Academy of Pediatrics has recommended a ban on head-first sliding for children less than 10 years of age. Presumably, once players are developmentally mature enough, coaching of proper sliding techniques could be accomplished. For adults, sliding is likely to continue unrestricted. Part of the global appeal of softball is that almost any 'weekend athlete' can

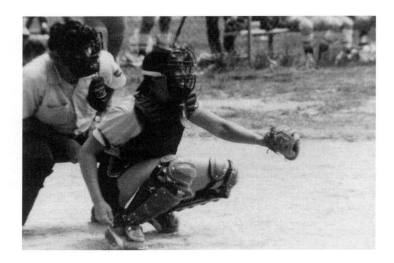

Fig. 42.18 Fastpitch catchers can develop digital ischaemia.

participate. Unfortunately, this also means that skill level and adequacy of proper coaching is quite variable. Analysis of injury data reveals that many injuries happen when the decision to slide is made late and the slide is initiated too close to the base (Wheeler, 1987). Excess momentum is carried to the base and the lead extremity is injured at impact. In addition to poor technique, lack of conditioning and alcohol intake may contribute to the problem. Shesser *et al.* (1985) found that 34% of recreational softball injuries were related to alcohol. Unfortunately, a ban on alcohol would probably be as unpopular among some recreational ball players as a ban on sliding. The fact remains that alcohol impairs both judgement and coordination, so consumption is not recommended during sports participation. Other options to prevent sliding injuries include changes in equipment and improved coaching.

A change in base equipment is a passive preventative measure that would be independent of the athlete, skill level and coaching. The rule books of numerous softball organizations in the USA specify that bases may be up to 12.7 cm in height and must be fixed to the ground. Standard bases are usually bolted to a metal post sunk into concrete. This configuration obviously has little 'give' when a runner collides with it. Recessed bases are one alternative, although this would make it difficult for fielders and umpires to locate them visually from a distance. Break-away bases are now available from various manufacturers in the USA. Models are available for youth, teen, adult and professional levels, each differing in rigidity and the magnitude of force required to break away. Janda *et al.* (1990) showed in a prospective study that use of such break-away bases led to a 98% decrease in the incidence of sliding injuries. If the use of these bases was implemented throughout the USA, 1.7 million injuries could be prevented and US$2.0 billion in medical costs saved annually. A similar study found a comparable rate of injury reduction with a deformable impact-absorbing base (Sendre *et al.*, 1994).

To reduce sliding injuries further, instruction in proper base-sliding technique should be stressed at all levels of play. Coaches should work with inexperienced players to help them gain an understanding that a late slide is dangerous and that it is better not to slide and be called out than to slide late and be out of the game permanently. The decision to slide should be made early, and may be signalled by base coaches and the on-deck batter. The slide should start two to three strides before the base. The body should be relaxed, since tense muscles limit joint flexibility and may predispose to injury. In a feet-first slide, the hands should be raised overhead to protect them from impact. Holding a handful of dirt in each clenched hand reminds the runner not to extend the digits, making them less vulnerable to injury. Impact with the ground should be absorbed by the maximum of body surface area in order to dissipate energy. In the feet-first slide, the buttocks, thighs and lower back should impact the ground first. In a head-first slide, the chest and thighs provide the best large surface for contact. Unfortunately, even in professional players initial ground contact is often made with the hands and knees in the head-first slide (Corzatt *et al.*, 1984). This dangerous technique predisposes vulnerable small body parts to injury. Proper sliding technique can be coached and practised indoors on a gym floor while wearing old sweatpants, using talcum powder and a burlap bag for players to slide on. Once athletes are confident that they can slide safely on a hard gym floor, they tend to be less hesitant on the ball field and have less trouble initiating a slide at the proper time.

Personal equipment

Head injuries are the most frequent serious injury in softball and baseball. Unfortunately, there is no formal requirement for a batting helmet, neither is there a manufacturer's standard for such a helmet. Little research has even been done to quantify the protective capability of batting helmets, unlike the data that has been compiled on testing football and motorcycle helmets. Goldsmith and Kabob (1982) did attempt to quantify and make recommendations

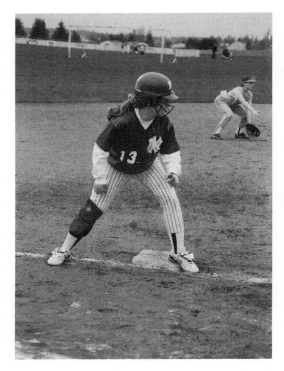

Fig. 42.19 Batting helmets should be worn on the base paths.

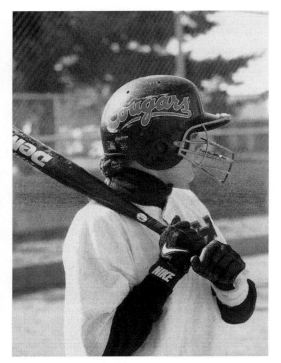

Fig. 42.20 Batting helmet with face mask.

about the performance of batting helmets. Their findings supported the incorporation of shell and suspension modifications to improve the energy absorption of headgear in order to minimize the possibility of head trauma. Batting helmets should be required when batting and base running at all levels of play (Fig. 42.19). For additional eye and face protection, shatter-resistant polycarbonate face shields or wire masks can be added (Fig. 42.20). The American Academy of Pediatrics Committee on Sports Medicine (1994) recommends such face protectors for functionally one-eyed athletes (corrected vision <20/50 in the worst eye) and for athletes with previous eye injury or surgery. They also recommend that the catcher wears a helmet, mask, chest and throat protectors, as well as non-metal spikes.

In the USA, players of American football have been required to use mouth-guards since 1963, resulting in a dramatic decrease in the incidence of dental injury to less than 1% (Wilkins, 1990). Studies have shown that mouth-guards are very effective in preventing orofacial and dental injuries (Thompson, 1982; Garon *et al.*, 1986). Good evidence has also been documented that mouth-guards decrease the potential for brain trauma when a blow to the jaw occurs (Hickey *et al.*, 1967). The modern materials used in fabricating mouth-guards have resulted in improved fit, comfort and compliance rates. New titanium bats entering the market may increase the risk of orofacial injury to infielders, especially third-base fielders. After impact with titanium bats, ball speeds are 4–12% higher (S. Werner & C. Johnson, unpublished data), although fielders' reaction times have not increased. Athletes, especially infielders, should be educated about the advantages of mouth-guards and encouraged to use them by physicians, trainers and coaches.

Facility

Before a practice or a game, part of good warm-up procedure should always be a walk or jog around the field by each player. Athletes should look for soft or wet spots, holes, rocks and debris. If stationary bases are in use, one should make sure they are secure. Each player should check the area of her position thoroughly and get her bearings on distances to poles, fences, dugout and other unyielding objects. Even when playing at home, it is still a good idea to make this check part of the preparticipation routine. Softball players tend to be creatures of habit, and before a game some have specific individualized routines surrounded with superstition. By encouraging the development of good warm-up habits in youngsters, coaches may effect a routine that lasts a lifetime. Proper field maintenance should include regular dragging and raking of the infield and rolling of the outfield. Fences and poles in the playing area should be padded. Dugouts should be fenced to protect occupants from foul balls. For children aged 5–14, the American Academy of Pediatrics recommends elimination of the on-deck circle, use of break-away bases and use of low-impact balls to minimize risk of injury.

Recommendations for future research

Softball has existed as an organized sport for just over 100 years and its worldwide popularity has resulted in it becoming adopted as the newest Olympic sport. Baseball has received far more attention in the literature, presumably because of all the money in professional baseball and the fact that males play baseball and males have done the majority of the research. Very little attention has been given to softball, especially fastpitch softball, so the field is literally wide open for future research. The specific areas that need further investigation include biomechanics of the windmill pitch, EMG analysis of the windmill pitch, epidemiological study of the incidence of fastpitch softball injury, injury mechanisms in fastpitch, windmill pitching injuries, analysis of the effectiveness of hitting technique and visual cues in fastpitch hitting. Some of the past research on male baseball players is applicable to female softball players, although new research on female subjects would be most appropriate. For instance, the only published biomechanical analysis on windmill pitching used male subjects. Do differences in bone, muscle, and joint structure or laxity about the shoulder or elbow make a difference in mechanics or injury risk for women? Should different coaching and training techniques be tailored for women? Should pitching rule limitations be imposed? We will not know the answers to these types of questions until research specific to female fastpitch softball is accomplished.

Much can also be learned in the realm of equipment safety. Universal acceptance of breakaway bases has not occurred despite excellent data showing dramatic reduction of injuries when such bases are used. The protection afforded by batting headgear and face shields needs to be better quantified. Are the current batting helmets effective or should alternative styles be investigated? Before global acceptance of titanium bats, should we further investigate material properties and human reaction times? Should the rules require the wearing of face protectors and mouth-guards and, if so, for what age groups and what levels of play? Certainly, we cannot expect to legislate an end to all sports injuries. Rather, as physicians, trainers, coaches, researchers and administrators the best we can hope to do is learn all we can in an effort to prevent and minimize injuries. Athletes have sustained sports injuries ever since the earliest sports were played, and will undoubtedly continue to hurt themselves from time to time. Today's athletes depend on us to treat their injuries appropriately and, even more importantly, tomorrow's injuries may be prevented by our efforts. Our best defences in the arena of sports medicine are knowledge and commitment to our athletes.

Acknowledgements

I would like to thank Sue Rankin PhD, Sherry Werner PhD, John Henderson DO, Jeannine Gaudreau RN and Kathy Arendsen for technical assistance in the writing of this chapter. My most sincere appreciation goes to Ann Rosecrants for editorial assistance, and to the Port Angeles High School Roughrider Softball team for photographic motion studies. Finally, thanks to my family for all their endless support, ever since my days as a Texas Short-horn on gopher hole field.

References

Alexander, M. & Haddow, J. (1982) A kinematic analysis of an upper extremity ballistic skill: the windmill pitch. *Canadian Journal of Applied Sports Sciences* **7**, 209–217.

American Academy of Pediatrics Committee on Sports Medicine (1994) Risk of injury from baseball and softball in children 5–14 years of age. *Pediatrics* **93**, 690–692.

Andrews, J. & Timmerman, L. (1995) Outcome of elbow surgery in professional baseball players. *American Journal of Sports Medicine* **23**, 407–413.

Atwater, A. (1980) Biomechanics of overarm throwing movements and of throwing injuries. *Exercise and Sport Sciences Reviews* **71**, 43–85.

Branch, T., Partin, C., Chamberland, P., Emeterio, E. & Sabetelle, M. (1992) Spontaneous fracture of the humerus during pitching. *American Journal of Sports Medicine* **20**, 468–470.

Browner, B., Jupiter, J., Levine, A. & Trafton, P. (1992) *Skeletal Trauma*, Vols 1 & 2. W.B. Saunders, Philadelphia.

Brunko, M. & Hunt, M. (1988) Sudden death in a young adult woman. *Journal of Emergency Medicine* **6**, 239–244.

Cahill, B. & Palmer, R. (1983) Quadrilateral space syndrome. *Journal of Hand Surgery* **8**, 65–69.

Corzatt, R., Groppel, J., Pfautsch, E. & Boscardin, J. (1984) The biomechanics of head-first vs. feet-first sliding. *American Journal of Sports Medicine* **12**, 229–232.

Davidson, P., Elattrache, N., Jobe, C. & Jobe, F. (1995) Rotator cuff and posterior–superior glenoid labrum injury associated with increased glenohumeral motion: a new site of impingement. *Journal of Shoulder and Elbow Surgery* **4**, 384–390.

DeLee, J. & Drez, D. (1994) *Orthopaedic Sports Medicine*, Vols 1 & 2. W.B. Saunders, Philadelphia.

DiCicco, J., Mehlman, C. & Urse, J. (1993) Fracture of the shaft of the humerus secondary to muscular violence. *Journal of Orthopaedic Trauma* **7**, 90–93.

Dillman, C., Fleisig, G. & Andrews, J. (1993) Biomechanics of pitching with emphasis upon shoulder kinematics. *Journal of Orthopaedic and Sports Physical Therapy* **18**, 402–408.

Ekstrand, J., Gillquist, J., Moller, M. *et al.* (1983) Incidence of soccer injuries and their relation to training and team success. *American Journal of Sports Medicine* **11**, 63–67.

Ellison, A. (1973) Skiing injuries. *Journal of the American Medical Association* **223**, 917–919.

Feltner, M. & Dapena, J. (1986) Dynamics of the shoulder and elbow joints of the throwing arm during a baseball pitch. *International Journal of Sport Biomechanics* **2**, 235–259.

Ferrari, J., Ferrari, D., Coumas, J. & Pappas, A. (1994) Posterior ossification of the shoulder: the Bennett lesion. *American Journal of Sports Medicine* **22**, 171–176.

Fleisig, G., Andrews, J., Dillman, C. & Escamilla, R. (1995) Kinetics of baseball pitching with implications about injury mechanisms. *American Journal of Sports Medicine* **23**, 233–239.

Fleisig, G., Dillman, C. & Andrews, J. (1989) Proper mechanics for baseball pitching. *Clinical Sports Medicine* **1**, 151–170.

Garon, M., Merkle, A. & Wright, J. (1986) Mouth protectors and oral trauma. *Journal of the American Dental Association* **112**, 663–668.

Glasgow, S. & Bruce, R. (1992) Arthroscopic resection of glenoid labrum tears in the athlete: a report of 29 cases. *Arthroscopy* **8**, 48–54.

Glennon, T. (1992) Isolated injury of the infraspinatus branch of the suprascapular nerve. *Archives of Physical Medicine and Rehabilitation* **73**, 201–202.

Glousman, R. (1993) Electromyographic analysis and its role in the athletic shoulder. *Clinical Orthopaedics and Related Research* **288**, 27–34.

Glousmen, R., Jobe, F. & Tibone, J. (1988) Dynamic electromyographic analysis of the throwing shoulder with glenohumeral instability. *Journal of Bone and Joint Surgery* **70A**, 220–226.

Goldsmith, W. & Kabob, M. (1982) Performance of baseball headgear. *American Journal of Sports Medicine* **10**, 31–37.

Gowan, I., Jobe, F., Tibone, J., Perry, J. & Moynes, D. (1987) A comparative electromyographic analysis of the shoulder during pitching. *American Journal of Sports Medicine* **15**, 586–590.

Green, N. & Swiontkowski, M. (1992) *Skeletal Trauma in Children*. W.B. Saunders, Philadelphia.

Greyson, N. (1995) Humeral stress periostitis. *Clinical Nuclear Medicine* **20**, 286–287.

Hickey, J., Morris, A., Carlson, L. *et al.* (1967) The relation of mouth protectors to cranial pressure and deformation. *Journal of the American Dental Association* **74**, 735–740.

Janda, D., Wojtys, E., Hankin, F. & Benedict, M. (1988) Softball sliding injuries. A prospective study comparing standard and modified bases. *Journal of the American Medical Association* **259**, 1848–1850.

Janda, D., Wojtys, E., Hankin, F., Benedict, M. & Hensinger, R. (1990) A three-phase analysis of the prevention of recreational softball injuries. *American Journal of Sports Medicine* **18**, 632–635.

Janda, D., Wild, D. & Hensinger, R. (1992) Softball injuries. *Sports Medicine* **13**, 285–291.

Jobe, F. & Bradley, J. (1988) Rotator cuff injuries in baseball. *Sports Medicine* **6**, 378–387.

Jobe, F., Giangarra, C., Kvitne, R. & Glousman, R. (1991) Anterior capsulolabral reconstruction of the shoulder in athletes in overhand sports. *American Journal of Sports Medicine* **19**, 428–434.

Jobe, F., Moynes, D., Tibone, J. & Perry, J. (1984) An EMG analysis of the shoulder in pitching. *American Journal of Sports Medicine* **12**, 218–220.

Kibler, W. (1995) Specificity and sensitivity of the anterior slide test in throwing athletes with superior glenoid labrum tears. *Arthroscopy* **11**, 296–300.

Liu, S., Henry, M., Nuccion, S., Shapiro, M. & Dorey, F. (1996) Diagnosis of glenoid labral tears. *American Journal of Sports Medicine* **24**, 149–154.

Loosli, A., Requa, R., Garrick, J. & Hanley, E. (1992) Injuries to pitchers in women's collegiate fast-pitch softball. *American Journal of Sports Medicine* **20**, 35–37.

Lowrey, C., Chadwick, R. & Waltman, E. (1976) Digital vessel trauma from repetitive impact in baseball catchers. *Journal of Hand Surgery* **1**, 236–238.

Marymount, J., Coupe, K. & Clanton, T. (1989) Sports-related spontaneous fractures of the humerus. *Orthopaedic Review* **18**, 957–960.

Nadeau, M. & Brown, T. (1990) The prevention of softball injuries: the experience at Yokota. *Military Medicine* **155**, 3–5.

Nuber, G. & Diment, M. (1992) Olecranon stress fractures in throwers. *Clinical Orthopaedics and Related Research* **278**, 58–61.

Pappas, A., Zawacki, R. & Sullivan, T. (1985) Biomechanics of baseball pitching. *American Journal of Sports Medicine* **13**, 216–222.

Redler, M., Ruland, L. & McCue, F. (1986) Quadrilateral space syndrome in a throwing athlete. *American Journal of Sports Medicine* **14**, 511–513.

Rettig, A. & Ebben, J. (1993) Anterior subcutaneous transfer of the ulnar nerve in the athlete. *American Journal of Sports Medicine* **21**, 836–840.

Ringel, S., Treihaft, M., Carry, M., Fisher, R. & Jacobs, P. (1990) Suprascapular neuropathy in pitchers. *American Journal of Sports Medicine* **18**, 80–86.

Rockwood, C., Green, D., Bucholtz, R. & Heckman, J. (1996) *Fractures in Adults*, 4th edn. Lippincott-Raven, Philadelphia.

Rohrer, M., Cardullo, P., Pappas, A., Phillips, D. & Wheeler, H. (1990) Axillary artery compression and thrombosis in throwing athletes. *Journal of Vascular Surgery* **11**, 761–768.

Rome, E. (1995) Sports-related injuries among adolescents: when do they occur, and how can we prevent them? *Pediatrics in Review* **16**, 184–187.

Roye, R., Grana, W. & Yates, C. (1995) Arthroscopic subacromial decompression: two- to seven-year follow-up. *Arthroscopy* **11**, 301–306.

Savoie, F. (1993) Arthroscopic examination of the throwing shoulder. *Journal of Orthopaedic and Sports Physical Therapy* **18**, 409–412.

Sendre, R., Keating, T., Hornak, J. & Newitt, P. (1994) Use of the Hollywood Impact Base to reduce sliding and base-running injuries in baseball and softball. *American Journal of Sports Medicine* **22**, 450–453.

Shaffer, B., Jobe, F., Pink, M. & Perry, J. (1993) Baseball batting, an electromyographic study. *Clinical Orthopaedics and Related Research* **292**, 285–293.

Shesser, R., Smith, M., Ellis, P., Brett, S. & Ott, J. (1985) Recreational softball injuries. *American Journal of Emergency Medicine* **3**, 199–202.

Sinson, G., Zager, E. & Kline, D. (1994) Windmill pitcher's radial neuropathy. *Neurosurgery* **34**, 1087–1090.

Sisto, D., Jobe, F., Moynes, D. & Antonelli, D. (1987) An electromyographic analysis of the elbow in pitching. *American Journal of Sports Medicine* **15**, 260–263.

Snyder, S. & Wuh, H. (1991) Arthroscopic evaluation and treatment of the rotator cuff and superior labrum anterior posterior lesion. *Operative Techniques in Orthopaedics* **1**, 207–220.

Snyder, S., Karzel, R., DelPizzo, W., Ferkel, R. & Friedman, M. (1990) SLAP lesions of the shoulder. *Arthroscopy* **6**, 274–279.

Stanitski, C., DeLee, J. & Drez, D. (1994) *Pediatric and Adolescent Sports Medicine*. W.B. Saunders, Philadelphia.

Strauss, R. & Whitehead, E. (1982) Hazards of aluminum bats (letter). *New England Journal of Medicine* **307**, 829.

Sugawara, M., Ogino, T., Minami, A. & Seiichi, I. (1986) Digital ischemia in baseball players. *American Journal of Sports Medicine* **14**, 329–334.

Tanabe, S., Nakahira, J., Bando, E., Yamaguchi, H., Miyamoto, H. & Yamamoto, A. (1991) Fatigue fracture of the ulna occurring in pitchers of fast-pitch softball. *American Journal of Sports Medicine* **19**, 317–321.

Tanaka, N., Hayashi, S., Amagasa, T. & Kohama, G. (1996) Maxillofacial fractures sustained during sports. *Journal of Oral and Maxillofacial Surgery* **54**, 715–719.

Thompson, B. (1982) Protection of the head and neck. *Dental Clinics of North America* **26**, 659–663.

Tibone, J., Elrod, B., Kerlan, R. *et al.* (1986) Surgical treatment of tears of the rotator cuff in athletes. *Journal of Bone and Joint Surgery* **68A**, 887–891.

Warner, J., Altchek, D. & Warren, R. (1991) Arthroscopic management of rotator cuff tears with emphasis on the throwing athlete. *Operative Techniques in Orthopaedics* **1**, 236–239.

Welch, C., Banks, S., Cook, F. & Draovitch, P. (1995) Hitting a baseball: a biomechanical description. *Journal of Orthopaedic and Sports Physical Therapy* **22**, 193–201.

Werner, S., Fleisig, G., Dillman, C. & Andrews, J. (1993) **Biomechanics of the elbow during baseball pitching.** *Journal of Orthopaedic and Sports Physical Therapy* **17**, 274–278.

Wheeler, B. (1984) Slow-pitch softball injuries. *American Journal of Sports Medicine* **12**, 237–240.

Wheeler, B. (1987) Ankle fractures in slow-pitch softball: the Army experience. *Military Medicine* **152**, 626–628.

Wilkins, K. (1990) Protective equipment. In J. Sullivan & W. Grana (eds) *The Pediatric Athlete*, pp. 257–261. American Academy of Orthopedic Surgeons Seminar, Park Ridge, Illinois.

Wojtys, E., Smith, P. & Hankin, F. (1986) A cause of ulnar neuropathy in a baseball pitcher. *American Journal of Sports Medicine* **14**, 422–424.

Yasuda, T. & Takeda, R. (1996) False aneurysm of a digital artery in a softball catcher evaluated by sonography: a case report. *Journal of Trauma* **41**, 153–155.

Index

Page numbers in **bold** refer to tables and those it *italic* refer to figures

647